Cardiovascular Disease in Small Animal Medicine

WENDY A WARE

DVM MS Diplomate ACVIM (Cardiology)
Departments of Veterinary Clinical Sciences and
Biomedical Sciences
College of Veterinary Medicine
Iowa State University
Ames, Iowa, USA

MANSON PUBLISHING/THE VETERINARY PRESS

Copyright © 2007 Manson Publishing Ltd

ISBN: 978-1-84076-076-7

A CIP catalogue record for this book is available from the British Library.

For full details of all Manson Publishing Ltd titles please write to:
Manson Publishing Ltd
73 Corringham Road
London NW11 7DL, UK.

Tel: +44(0)20 8905 5150
Fax: +44(0)20 8201 9233

Email: manson@mansonpublishing.com
Website: www.mansonpublishing.com

Commissioning editor: Jill Northcott
Project manager: Julie Bennett
Copy editor: Peter Beynon
Design and layout: DiacriTech, Chennai, India
Colour reproduction: Tenon & Polert Colour Scanning Ltd., Hong Kong
Printed by: Grafos S.A., Barcelona, Spain

Companion animal practice is an ever-changing field. As new research and experience broaden our knowledge, changes in practice, treatment, and drug therapy may become necessary or appropriate. Readers are advised to check the most current product information provided by the manufacturer of each drug to be administered to verify the recommended dose, method and duration of administration, and contraindications. It is the responsibility of the practitioner, relying on his/her own experience and knowledge of the patient, to make diagnoses, to determine best treatment and dosages for each individual patient, and to take all appropriate safety precautions. Neither the publisher nor the author assumes any liability for any injury and/or damage to persons or property related to use of material contained in this book.

Contents

Preface

The extensive use of visual images is a core feature of this book. Over 570 figures and 65 summary tables are used to illustrate various cardiovascular disease conditions and key concepts. The opportunity to write such a richly illustrated book is what drew me to this project. Over twenty years of teaching veterinary students and interacting with veterinary practitioners has convinced me of the importance of visual learning. Most of the images were collected in the course of my practice at the University Veterinary Teaching Hospital. Others are reproduced here with the kind permission of my colleagues and various publishers. I have included multiple graphical examples for a number of important disease conditions in order to reflect some of the variability in clinical appearance that occurs.

My goal was to create a practical clinical reference that would also provide a broad overview of small animal cardiovascular medicine. In writing the text, I have tried to summarize concisely important information about various cardiovascular diseases, the clinical tools used to assess the cardiovascular system, and approaches to disease management. This book was written primarily for veterinary general practitioners and students, although veterinary technicians and others should find it useful as well.

The book is organized into three sections. The initial chapters (1–5) review the normal cardiovascular system and common methods used for cardiac evaluation. Chapters 6–17 contain overviews of common clinical problems, approaches to differentiating these clinical manifestations of disease, and management of heart failure and arrhythmias. Finally, more detailed information about specific cardiovascular diseases is organized anatomically in chapters 18–25. The danger in this organizational structure is the potential for excessive repetition. I have tried to minimize redundancy by cross-referencing among the various chapters. As a consequence, it may be necessary to turn to a different page for the desired information. I hope the reader will forgive such inconvenience in the interest of keeping the book to a more concise length. The chapter reference lists are not exhaustive, but include important and representative resources. Readers who wish for more detailed information, especially related to certain procedures or diseases, are urged to refer directly to individual references.

No one stands alone. What anyone is able to accomplish is intertwined with the work, support, and influence of others. I wish to acknowledge my gratitude to the many colleagues, students, clients, and animals who, over the years and in a multitude of ways, have made it possible for me to write this book. To all my mentors and teachers who helped prepare me for my journey into the world of veterinary clinician/educator, and especially to Drs. John Bonagura and Bob Hamlin, I thank you for sharing your extensive knowledge, dedication, and creativity, and for your high expectations. I am grateful to Mr. Michael Manson and Ms. Jill Northcott of Manson Publishing for asking me to write this book, and for their patience throughout the lengthy process. Thanks are due to Mr. Peter Beynon, Ms. Julie Bennett, and the other members of the Manson Publishing team for all their help and suggestions, as well as to Ms. Kathy Hedges and also Ms. Lori Moran for extensive assistance in preparing the clinical graphics. Most importantly, I wish to express my love and deepest gratitude to my family – thank you for your continued love and support (except for all the times you said "just get the book done…").

Finally, to you the reader, it is my hope that you find this book easy to use and truly helpful in your study and practice.

Wendy A. Ware
Iowa State University

Abbreviations

Ab antibody
ABT aortic body tumor(s)
ACE angiotensin-converting enzyme
Ach acetylcholine
ADH antidiuretic hormone
ADPase adenosine diphosphatase
AF atrial fibrillation
Ag antigen
AHA/ACC American Heart Association and
     American College of Cardiology
ALD aldosterone
ALT alanine aminotransferase
ANP atrial natriuretic peptide
aPTT activated partial thromboplastin time
AR aortic regurgitation
ARVC arrhythmogenic right ventricular
     cardiomyopathy
ASD atrial septal defect
AST aspartate aminotransferase
AT angiotensin
ATP adenosine triphosphate
A-V arterio-venous
AV atrioventricular
AVP arginine vasopressin
BNP brain natriuretic peptide
BP blood pressure
BUN blood urea nitrogen
Ca calcium
cAMP cyclic adenosine monophosphate
CaVC caudal vena cava
CBC complete blood count
CF color flow (mapping)
cGMP cyclic guanylate monophosphate
CHF congestive heart failure
CK creatine kinase
CK-MB (cardiac-specific) isoenzyme of CK
CNS central nervous system
CO cardiac output
CO_2 carbon dioxide
CRI constant rate infusion
CRT capillary refill time
CTD cor triatriatum dexter
CrVC cranial vena cava
CT computed tomography
cTn cardiac troponin
cTnI cardiac troponin protein I

cTnT cardiac troponin protein T
CV cardiovascular
CVP central venous pressure
CW continuous wave (Doppler)
D5W 5% dextrose in water
DADs delayed afterdepolarizations
DC direct current (conversion)
DCM dilated cardiomyopathy
DEC diethylcarbamazine
DHA docosahexaenoic acid
DIC disseminated intravascular coagulation
DLH domestic longhair (cat)
DSH domestic shorthair (cat)
DTI Doppler tissue imaging
DV dorsoventral
EADs early afterdepolarizations
ECG electrocardiogram
EDVI end-diastolic volume index
EF ejection fraction
ELISA enzyme-linked immunosorbent assay
EPA eicosapentaenoic acid
Epi epinephrine
EPSS E point to septal separation
ESVC European Society of Veterinary Cardiology
ESVI end-systolic volume index
ET endothelin
Fab antigen-binding fragments
FDPs fibrinogen/fibrin degradation products
F_IO_2 fraction of inspired oxygen
FS fractional shortening
GFR glomerular filtration rate
GI gastrointestinal
gp glycoprotein
HCM hypertrophic cardiomyopathy
Hct hematocrit
HOCM hypertrophic obstructive cardiomyopathy
HPRF high pulse repetition frequency
HR heart rate
HRV heart rate variability
HSA hemangiosarcoma
HWD heartworm disease
HWs heartworms
ICD implantable cardioverter defibrillator
ICS intercostal space(s)
IL interleukin
IM intramuscular

IMHA immune-mediated hemolytic anemia
ISACHC International Small Animal Cardiac
　　Health Council
IV intravenous
IVRT isovolumic relaxation time
IVS interventricular septum/septal
K potassium
kVp kilovoltage peak
LA left atrium/atrial
LBBB left bundle branch block
L-CHF left-sided congestive heart failure
LMWH low-molecular-weight heparin (products)
LRS lactated Ringer's solution
LV left ventricle/ventricular
LVET left ventricular ejection time
MAP mean arterial pressure
mAs milliamperes x seconds
Mdys mitral valve dysplasia
MEA mean electrical axis
Mg magnesium
MR mitral (valve) regurgitation
mV millivolts
Na sodium
NE norepinephrine
NH neurohormonal
NO nitric oxide
NOS NO synthetase
NT-proANP/BNP N-terminal fragments
　　(ANP and BNP)
NYHA New York Heart Association
O_2 oxygen
PA pulmonary artery/pulmonary arterial
PAI-1 plasminogen activator inhibitor type 1
PaO_2 partial pressure of oxygen in arterial blood
PAO_2 partial pressure of oxygen in the alveolus
PCR polymer chain reaction
PCV packed cell volume
PDA patent ductus arteriosus
PDE phosphodiesterase
PEP pre-ejection period
PEP:ET pre-ejection period:ejection time (ratio)
PH pulmonary hypertension
PISA proximal isovelocity surface area
PMI point of maximal intensity
PNS parasympathetic (cholinergic) nervous
　　system
PPDH peritoneopericardial diaphragmatic hernia
PR pulmonary (valve) regurgitation
PRAA persistent right aortic arch
PRF pulse repetition frequency
PRN *pro re nata* (according to circumstances)

PS pulmonic stenosis
PTE pulmonary thromboembolism
PvO_2 venous partial pressure of oxygen
PVR pulmonary vascular resistance
PVT paroxysm of ventricular tachycardia
PW pulsed wave (Doppler)
RA right atrium/atrial
RAP right atrial pressure
RAAS renin-angiotensin-aldosterone system
RBBB right bundle branch block
RBC red blood cell
R-CHF right-sided congestive heart failure
RCM restrictive cardiomyopathy
RIA radioimmunoassay
RMP resting membrane potential
rt-PA recombinant tissue plasminogen activator
RV right ventricle/ventricular
SA sinoatrial
SAECG signal averaged electrocardiography
SAM systolic anterior motion
SAS subaortic stenosis
SC subcutaneous
SNS sympathetic (adrenergic) nervous system
sPAP systolic pulmonary artery pressure
SR sarcoplasmic reticulum
SSS sick sinus syndrome
STIs systolic time intervals
SV stroke volume
SVT supraventricular tachycardia
TdP torsades de pointes
Tdys triscupid valve dysplasia
TE thromboembolic/thromboembolism
TEE transesophageal echocardiography
TFPI tissue factor pathway inhibitor
TICM tachycardia induced cardiomyopathy
TNF tumor necrosis factor
TNF_α tumor necrosis factor alpha
T of F Tetralogy of Fallot
t-PA tissue plasminogen activator
TR tricuspid (valve) regurgitation
US United States
V/Q pulmonary ventilation/perfusion
VD ventrodorsal
VF ventricular fibrillation
VHS vertebral heart score
VPCs ventricular premature
　　complexes/contractions
VSD ventricular septal defect
VT ventricular tachycardia
WPW Wolff–Parkinson–White (type/syndrome)

Section I
Introduction and Normal Reference Information

1
The Normal Cardiovascular System

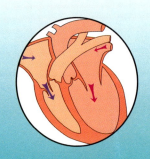

The cardiovascular (CV) system provides nutrient delivery and metabolic waste removal throughout the body. Its two component circulations (pulmonary and systemic) are linked in series. The normal path of blood flow is schematically illustrated (**1**), along with approximate normal pressures. The systemic circulation contains about 75% of the total blood volume, compared with 25% in the pulmonary circulation. Systemic veins act as storage (capacitance) vessels and contain about 67–80% of the systemic blood volume; 11–15% is held within arteries and 5% within the capillaries[1,2]. Blood in the pulmonary

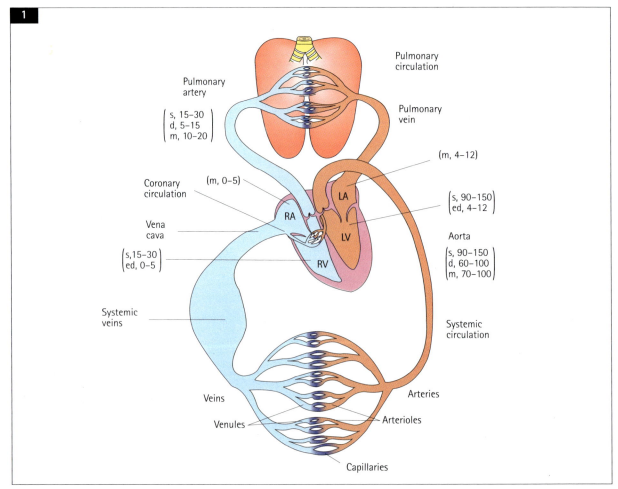

1 Schematic diagram of the cardiovascular system. Examples of normal pressures (mm Hg) in different regions are noted in parentheses: ed = end-diastolic; d = diastolic; m = mean; s = systolic; LA = left atrium; LV = left ventricle; RA = right atrium; RV = right ventricle.

circulation is distributed evenly among arterial, capillary, and venous vessels. Mean blood pressure in the pulmonary circulation is about one seventh of that in the systemic circuit.

THE HEART

EXTERNAL FEATURES

The pericardial sac surrounds the heart. This sac, or pericardium, consists of a thin visceral (epicardial) layer of mesothelial cells that is closely adhered to the heart and reflects back at the heartbase into the serous lining of the fibrous outer parietal layer[3, 4]. The left and right coronary arteries arise from sinuses of Valsalva behind valve leaflets at the aortic root. These arteries course over the external surface of the heart before their branches penetrate into the myocardium (**2**). Smaller coronary veins flow into the great coronary (cardiac) vein, which empties into the coronary sinus in the caudal right atrium (RA). Blood from the body enters the RA through the cranial vena cava, caudal vena cava, and azygous vein (**3**). Inflow to the left heart enters the dorsal left atrium (LA) from several pulmonary veins.

The left ventricle (LV) forms the caudoventral aspect of the heart; its point forms the cardiac apex. The LV is cone-shaped, and is surrounded on the right, cranial, and craniodorsal left sides by the 'U-shaped' right ventricle (RV). The LA is in a dorsocaudal location, above the LV. The aorta exits cranial to the LA, in a central location. The RA occupies the dorsal right aspect, above the RV inflow tract. The pulmonary artery exits the RV on the dorsal left side of the heart.

INTERNAL FEATURES

An endothelial layer covers the internal cardiac surface (endocardium). The valves are thin, flexible fibrous flaps covered with endothelium. Each is attached to a fibrous valve ring (annulus).

Left heart

The LV endocardial surface is fairly smooth. A continuum of myocardial fibers arrayed in varying orientations from epicardium to endocardium and base to apex forms the LV wall. Contraction causes longitudinal shortening as well as reduced circumference of the LV chamber, as blood is pushed toward the outflow region[1]. The mitral (left atrioventricular, AV) valve has two leaflets: septal (anterior; cranioventral) and parietal (posterior; caudodorsal)[4].

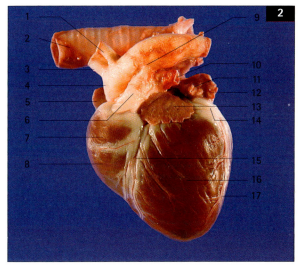

2 Canine heart: external view from the left. a = artery; v = vein; L = left; R = right.
1. L. subclavian a. 2. Trachea 3. Brachiocephalic trunk 4. Aorta 5. R. auricle 6. Pulmonary trunk 7. Conus arteriosus 8. R. ventricle 9. Ligamentum arteriosum 10. L. pulmonary a. 11. Pulmonary v. 12. L. atrium 13. L. auricle 14. Coronary groove (with circumflex branch of L. coronary a.) 15. Cranial (paraconal) interventricular branch of L. coronary a. 16. L. ventricle 17. Caudal (subsinuosal) interventricular branch of L. coronary a.

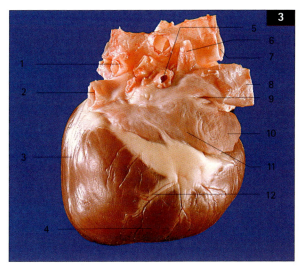

3 Canine heart: external view from the right. a = artery; v = vein; L = left; R = right.
1. Pulmonary v. ostium 2. Caudal vena cava 3. Caudal (subsinuosal) interventricular sulcus 4. R. ventricle 5. R. pulmonary a. 6. Azygous v. 7. Trachea 8. Cranial vena cava 9. Region of sinoatrial node 10. R. auricle 11. R. atrium 12. Branches of R. coronary a.

Stout chordae tendineae attach these leaflets to two large papillary muscles, which arise near the apical region (**4**). The anterior mitral leaflet originates at the caudal aspect of the aortic root. This leaflet functionally separates the LV inflow and outflow tracts (**5**). The 3-cusped (semilunar) aortic valve is located centrally in the heart's fibrous skeleton (**6**). The cranial aspect of the aortic root abuts the interventricular septum (IVS).

Right heart
The RV wall thickness is normally about one third of that of the LV wall, reflecting the much lower systolic pressure here. Muscular ridges (*trabeculae carneae*) characterize the inner RV surface (**7**). A muscular band (septomarginal trabecula, moderator band), which carries conduction system fibers, extends from the IVS to the RV free wall[4].

The tricuspid (right AV) valve has two main leaflets in dogs and cats. The lateral (parietal) leaflet is

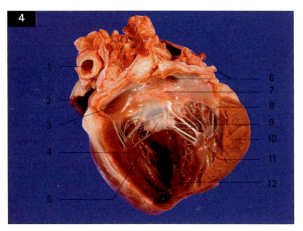

4 Canine heart: left ventricular inflow tract. L = left; R = right; m = muscle; v,=vein.
1. Descending aorta 2. R. ventricular wall (cut) 3. L. auricle
4. Ventral (subauricular) papillary m. 5. Septal (anterior) mitral cusp
6. Pulmonary v. 7. Interatrial septum 8. Parietal (posterior) mitral cusp (cut) 9. Chordae tendineae 10. L. ventricular freewall
11. Dorsal (subatrial) papillary m. 12. Trabeculae carneae

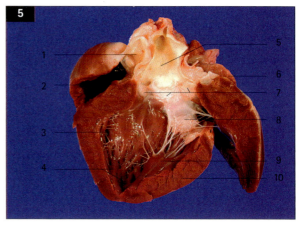

5 Canine heart: left ventricular outflow tract.
L = left; R= right; m = muscle.
1. Pulmonary trunk 2. R. ventricular outflow region (conus)
3. Interventricular septum 4. Trabeculae carneae 5. Ascending aorta
6. L. auricle 7. Aortic valve cusps 8. Septal (anterior) mitral cusp
9. Dorsal (subatrial) papillary m. 10. L. ventricle

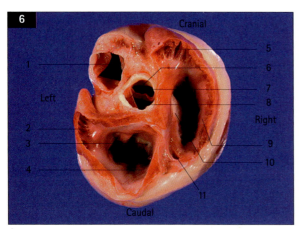

6 Canine heart: dorsal view showing orientation of cardiac valves.
L = left; R = right.
1. Pulmonary valve 2. Pectinate mm in L. auricle 3. Mitral valve: septal (anterior) leaflet 4. Mitral valve: parietal (posterior) leaflet
5. Pectinate mm in R. auricle 6. Aortic valve: left cusp 7. Aortic valve: right cusp 8. Caudal (non coronary) cusp 9. Tricuspid valve: parietal leaflet 10. Tricuspid valve: septal leaflet 11. Coronary sinus

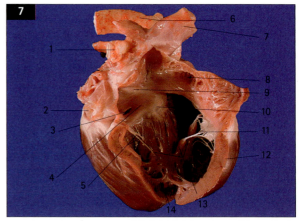

7 Canine heart: right ventricular inflow tract. mm = muscles; R = right.
1. R. pulmonary a. 2. Caudal vena cava 3. Coronary sinus 4. Region of AV node 5. Chordae tendineae 6. Aorta 7. Cranial vena cava
8. R. auricle 9. Interatrial septum 10. Septal tricuspid leaflet
11. Parietal tricuspid leaflet (cut) 12. R. ventricular free wall
13. Papillary mm 14. Trabeculae carneae

larger; the smaller septal (medial) leaflet lies close to the IVS in the area of the membranous septum. Generally, there are three main papillary muscles, but their number and configuration are variable[5]. Inflow and outflow areas of the RV are separated by the muscular supraventricular crest, so that the right AV and semilunar valves are not adjacent as they are in the left heart. The semilunar pulmonary valve is similar in appearance but thinner than the aortic valve (**8**). There are no coronary ostia behind pulmonary valve cusps.

CONDUCTION SYSTEM

The sinoatrial (SA) node is the normal pacemaker of the heart because the specialized muscle cells here have the fastest intrinsic rate of automaticity (spontaneous diastolic depolarization). The SA node is located at the cranial aspect of the RA, near its junction with the cranial vena cava. Electrical impulses originating from SA nodal cells spread into the RA, LA, and via the AV conduction system into the ventricles (**9**). Specialized fibers (internodal pathways) facilitate conduction through the RA and LA to the AV node.

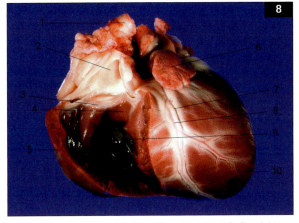

8 Canine heart: right ventricular outflow tract. L = left; R = right; a = artery; v = vein.
1. Aorta 2. Pulmonary trunk (main pulmonary a.) 3. Pulmonary valve 4. Supraventricular crest 5. R. ventricle 6. L. auricle 7. Great coronary v. 8. Cranial interventricular branch of L. coronary a. in cranial (paraconal) interventricular groove 9. Tricuspid valve 10. L. ventricle

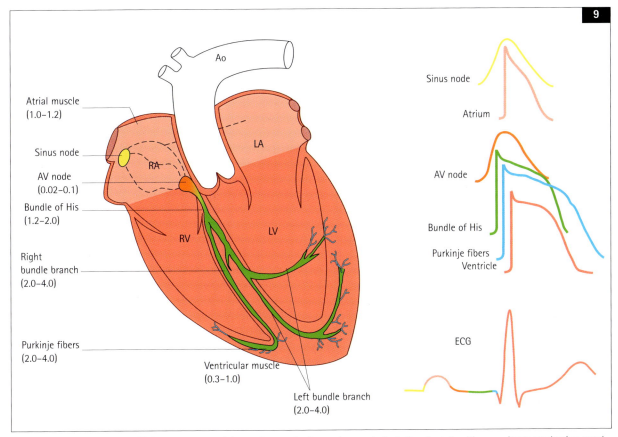

9 Cardiac conduction system. Major components of the cardiac conduction system are indicated on the left, with approximate conduction speed (m/sec) in parentheses. On the right, representative action potentials are color coded to the conduction system components. A composite ECG (below) illustrates the activation sequence of these structures.

The AV node is the electrical 'gatekeeper' to the ventricles. Normally, there is no other pathway for electrical impulses to pass from the atria to the ventricles. The AV node is located in the ventral right side of the interatrial septum, near the septal tricuspid leaflet. AV nodal cells are small and branching. This causes slowed (decremental) conduction of electrical impulses, allowing time for atrial contraction before ventricular activation.

Electrical impulses enter the bundle of His after passing through the AV node. Conduction is rapid through the His bundle and into the left and right bundle branches. The right bundle branch courses down the right side of the IVS and branches distally to activate the RV free wall[6]. The left bundle branch divides into a septal fascicle, a posterior (caudal) fascicle serving the ventrocaudal aspect of the LV wall, and an anterior fascicle serving the craniolateral LV wall. A branching system of Purkinje fibers transmits electrical impulses from the bundle branches into the ventricular myocardium.

CARDIAC ELECTROPHYSIOLOGY

Cardiac action potentials occur in association with changes in cell membrane permeability to sodium (Na^+), potassium (K^+), and calcium (Ca^{++}) ions. Transmembrane movement of these ions depends on the opening and closing of ion-specific channels[7]. The duration of cardiac action potentials is longer than that of noncardiac tissues. Cardiac action potentials also differ among types of heart cells, depending on cellular location and function. There are two main types of cardiac action potentials: 'fast-response' (typical of atrial and ventricular muscle cells, and Purkinje fibers) and 'slow-response' (characteristic of SA and AV nodal cells).

Resting membrane potential

The cardiac cell membrane (sarcolemma) maintains a gradient of certain ions and enzymes between the intra- and extracellular environment. In normal myocardial cells at rest the electrical potential difference across the sarcolemma is about −90 mV; inside the cell is negative compared with the outside[7]. This resting membrane potential (RMP) is largely determined by the equilibrium between chemical and electrostatic forces for K^+ (as described by the Nernst equation[a]). The concentration of K^+ inside the cell is much greater than that outside; conversely, extracellular Na^+ and Ca^{++} concentrations far exceed intracellular concentrations. The resting sarcolemma is relatively permeable to K^+, but not to Na^+ and Ca^{++} as well as negatively charged intracellular proteins. K^+ tends to diffuse outward along its concentration gradient

through K^+-specific channels despite an opposing electrostatic force attracting the positive ions into the cell. A very small inward leak of Na^+ also occurs. Normal RMP is maintained by the membrane's electrogenic Na^+, K^+-ATPase pump, which moves three Na^+ ions out for every two K^+ ions in.

Fast-response action potential

When a stimulus reduces the membrane potential to a less negative 'threshold' level, activation of Na^+-specific membrane channels allows a rapid Na^+ influx, which initiates an action potential (phase 0; 10)[7, 8]. Activation (as well as subsequent inactivation) of these channels depends on the level of membrane potential (i.e. is voltage-dependent), and the inward Na^+ current occurs only briefly. Inactivation (closure) of the Na^+ channels results in an effective refractory period. A return toward RMP, as well as time, is necessary for Na^+ channels to recover from inactivation and become responsive to another stimulus. The steepness of the phase 0 upstroke, as well as its amplitude, influences the velocity of impulse conduction along the myocardial membranes. If the cells are stimulated when membrane potential is less negative than normal RMP, Na^+ channels are partially inactivated and conduction velocity of the resulting action potential is slowed. This predisposes to certain (reentrant) arrhythmias.

The rapid upstroke of the fast-response action potential is followed by a brief partial repolarization in some fibers (phase 1). Voltage-activated membrane Ca^{++} channels (L-type) slowly open during the latter part of phase 0, allowing an inward Ca^{++} current, which is responsible for phase 2 (the plateau). The Ca^{++} that enters the myocardial cells during phase 2 induces electrical–mechanical coupling. As the Ca^{++} channels slowly inactivate, the inward Ca^{++} flux decreases and outward movement of K^+ (through several types of K^+ channels) increases. This leads to repolarization (phase 3).

The effective refractory period (from phase 0 until membrane potential reaches about −50 mV during phase 3) is a time when the cell cannot be reexcited. Immediately following is the relative refractory period, when a stronger than normal stimulus may elicit another action potential, although conduction velocity may be slowed because of partial Na^+ channel inactivation. Normal excitability is achieved only after full repolarization.

Slow-response action potential

Two important properties of the heart are automaticity (the ability to initiate a heartbeat) and rhythmicity (the regularity of this activity). Cells with slow-response action potentials allow the heart to beat spontaneously because, instead of a consistent RMP, they undergo spontaneous diastolic (phase 4) depolarization (**11**). Typically, these cells are in the SA or AV node. They cells have a less negative diastolic membrane potential, and their action potential upstroke (phase 0) depends on slow Ca^{++} channel activation[7, 8]. Conduction velocity in slow-response fibers is much less than in normal fast-response cells, and the refractory period is longer. Consequently, conduction is more easily blocked in these cells.

The SA nodal cells normally have the most rapid intrinsic rate of spontaneous diastolic depolarization. Therefore, they reach threshold first and control the heartbeat. If the sinus rate slows or stops, other slow-response fibers lower in the conduction system (so-called subsidiary pacemakers) can initiate a heartbeat. The rate at which SA cells (or other automatic fibers) activate the heart depends on the slope of their spontaneous phase 4 depolarization, as well as maximal diastolic potential and threshold potential.

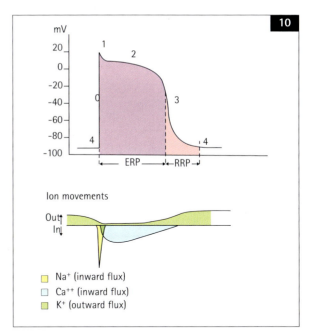

10 Fast-response action potential. Phases of the action potential are indicated (see text for further explanation). Major fluxes of ions into and out of the cell during the action potential are schematically indicated below. ERP = effective refractory period; RRP = relative refractory period; Na^+ = sodium ion; Ca^{++} = calcium ion; K^+ = potassium ion.

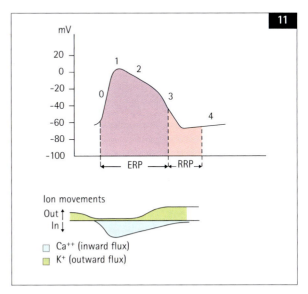

11 Slow-response action potential. Phases of the action potential are indicated (see text for further explanation). Major fluxes of ions into and out of the cell during the action potential are schematically indicated below. ERP = effective refractory period; RRP = relative refractory period; Ca^{++} = calcium ion; K^+ = potassium ion.

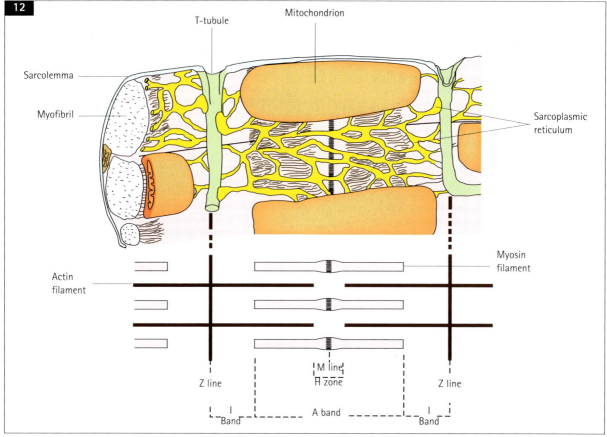

12 Diagram of myocardial cell components involved with excitation and contraction (above) and schematic illustration of the contractile elements (below) (see text for more information).

Electrical–mechanical coupling

The Ca++ influx during phase 2 of cardiac cell activation triggers the intracellular release of more Ca++ from the sarcoplasmic reticulum (SR). The increase in free intracellular Ca++ leads to contraction[1, 2]. This process is known as electrical–mechanical or excitation–contraction coupling. The SR is an intracellular network of tubules surrounding the myofibrils; it sequesters and releases the Ca++ necessary for contraction (12). Invaginations of the cell membrane (T tubule system) facilitate action potential propagation along the cells. Coupling of electrical excitation to mechanical contraction is enhanced by the close proximity of T tubules to parts of the SR.

MYOCARDIAL CONTRACTION

Cardiac myocytes function as a syncytium. Cell to cell conduction and communication are facilitated by gap junctions within the intercalated disks that separate adjacent myocytes[1, 2]. At the subcellular level, sarcomeres (demarcated by Z lines) are the basic

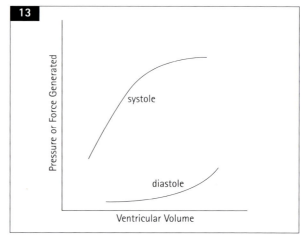

13 Systole: illustration of the effect of increasing ventricular volume (or preload) on the force generated (and stroke output) in systole. This is the Frank–Starling relationship. Diastole: the effect of increasing ventricular volume on filling pressure.

contractile units within myocytes. Thin actin filaments attach to the Z lines and interdigitate with thick myosin filaments. Contraction (sarcomere shortening) occurs as these filaments slide along each other by the cycling of cross-bridges (formed by heavy meromyosin heads interacting with sites on the actin filaments). The actin filaments are composed of two helical chains attached to a twisting tropomyosin support molecule. The troponin complexes consist of proteins (troponins I, C, and T), which regulate contraction; they are attached to the tropomyosin backbone of the actin filaments[9, 10]. Troponin I, in conjunction with the conformation of tropomyosin, inhibits cross-bridge formation during diastole when intracellular free Ca^{++} is low. When Ca^{++} is available (systole), it activates troponin C, which then binds to troponin I. This reduces the inhibitory effect of troponin I and subsequently allows interaction between adjacent actin and myosin filaments[10]. Myocardial injury causes leakage of troponin proteins; clinical assays for circulating troponin I and T can provide a sensitive test for cardiac damage.

Loading conditions

Diastolic stretch of the sarcomeres (to an optimal length) will increase the force of the subsequent contraction by increasing myofilament Ca^{++} affinity. This is the Frank–Starling relationship or Starling's law of the heart (13)[1, 9]. The level of diastolic stretch, or end-diastolic ventricular volume, is known as 'preload'. In the intact heart, as end-diastolic volume (preload) increases, the volume ejected with each contraction increases. But a high preload also raises the (filling) pressure within the chamber (13). Excessive filling pressure leads to venous congestion and edema upstream from that chamber.

'Afterload' refers to the contractile force that must be achieved in order for the sarcomeres to shorten (and for the ventricle to eject blood). It is the force that opposes contraction. In the animal, afterload is largely related to arterial blood pressure, unless there is obstruction to ventricular outflow (e.g. valvular or subvalvular stenosis). The afterload presents opposition to ventricular ejection. Reduced afterload facilitates ejection; increased afterload requires greater force generation for ejection of a given volume of blood.

Contractility

The term 'contractility' refers to the intrinsic strength of contraction at a given preload and afterload. Contractility primarily depends on the amount of free intracellular Ca^{++} available during systole, although adenosine triphosphate (ATP) availability is also important. By increasing intracellular Ca^{++}, positive inotropic agents (e.g. catecholamines, digoxin) increase the peak force of contraction and

reduce ventricular end-systolic volume. Negative inotropic agents (e.g. beta-blockers, calcium channel-blockers) reduce available Ca^{++} and contractility. Indices of myocardial contractility include the maximal rate of pressure generation in the LV during isovolumic contraction (dP/dt_{max}), the slope of the end-systolic pressure-volume relationship (Es, E_{max}, maximal end-systolic elastance), the percent of diastolic volume ejected during systole (ejection fraction, EF), and the percent reduction in LV diameter from diastole to systole (fractional shortening, FS). Other indices are also used sometimes, but all are imperfect. The so-called ejection phase indices (EF, FS) are especially influenced by loading conditions.

MYOCARDIAL RELAXATION

At the end of systole, Ca^{++} influx stops and the SR is not stimulated to release further intracellular Ca^{++}. The SR actively takes up Ca^{++} (via a phospholamban-stimulated Ca^{++} pump in its membrane), which makes it unavailable to the contractile apparatus and leads to inhibition of cross-bridge formation. Although the SR is the major site of Ca^{++} reuptake, some Ca^{++} is transported out of the cell via membrane Na/Ca exchange and Ca^{++} pump mechanisms[10]. Mitochondrial uptake of free Ca^{++} becomes important with pathologically high intracellular Ca^{++} levels. Slowed or incomplete reuptake of Ca^{++} in diastole increases cardiac stiffness and adversely affects filling; impaired myocardial relaxation can contribute to heart failure[10]. Catecholamines accelerate relaxation as well as enhance contractility.

Indices of relaxation include the maximal rate and time constant of LV pressure decline during isovolumic relaxation ($-dP/dt_{max}$ and tau, respectively), and the Doppler echocardiography-derived isovolumic relaxation time (IVRT) and mitral inflow patterns.

THE HEART AS A PUMP

The heart's ability to function as a pump is based on interrelationships between synchronous electrical activation, the level of ventricular contractility, loading conditions (preload and afterload) imposed on the myofibers, and the degree of filling in diastole. Ventricular filling is determined by several factors. Active relaxation of the myocardium is important early in diastole. The amount of venous return to the heart, ventricular compliance, the duration of diastole, and atrial contraction also contribute to ventricular end-diastolic volume (preload). As the heart rate increases, diastole shortens and atrial contraction contributes relatively more to final filling. The loss of atrial contraction (e.g. with atrial fibrillation) may have serious negative effects on cardiac performance.

Ventricular compliance (1/stiffness) affects how much blood flows in during diastole. Filling is impeded when ventricular walls are hypertrophied or infiltrated with fibrous tissue (i.e. causes of increased myocardial stiffness)[11]. External compression of the heart, as with pericardial disease, also impairs ventricular filling and causes diastolic dysfunction. When ventricular compliance is reduced (increased stiffness), higher filling pressure is required for a given diastolic volume. This can result in smaller end-diastolic volumes as well as venous congestion and edema behind the affected ventricle.

Cardiac output

Cardiac output (CO) is the volume of blood pumped from either ventricle over time. It is generally expressed as liters or ml/minute. CO may be indexed to body size (the cardiac index). The normal canine resting cardiac index is about 3.1–4.7 liters/minute/m^2 [9]. Because the right heart and left heart are in series, cardiac output from the RV equals cardiac output from the LV, although minor variation can occur over brief time periods (e.g. during respiration). CO depends on heart rate (HR) and stroke volume (SV); therefore, CO = HR × SV.

SV is the volume ejected with each contraction; this is normally about 65% of the total end-diastolic volume. SV is directly related to the level of myocardial contractility and preload, and inversely related to afterload. Clinical methods used to estimate CO (e.g. thermodilution and others) are based on the Fick principle[b].

Response to excessive pressure or volume loading

Chronic increases in ventricular volume (preload) or systolic pressure generation (afterload) create greater wall tension (stress) according to the LaPlace relationship[c]. Increased wall stress requires greater ATP and O_2 consumption. As a compensatory attempt to normalize wall stress, myocardial hypertrophy occurs by an increase in number of sarcomeres[9, 10]. In general, the pattern of hypertrophy depends on the type of overload. Chronic increases in ventricular volume stimulate the formation of new sarcomeres in series, lengthening the myofibers and creating a larger ventricle of normal wall thickness — so-called 'eccentric' hypertrophy. Diseases causing excessive systolic pressure generation stimulate formation of new sarcomeres in parallel, increasing myofiber diameter and ventricular wall thickness — so-called 'concentric' hypertrophy. With progressive cardiac diseases, normalization of wall stress may not be achieved or sustained.

CARDIAC CYCLE AND GENERATION OF HEART SOUNDS

Understanding the interrelations among electrical, mechanical, and acoustic events during the cardiac cycle is fundamental to understanding both normal and abnormal cardiac function (14). Accurate interpretation of CV examination findings also depends on knowledge of these events. Electrical events (depolarization) always precede mechanical activation (contraction). Atrial contraction (the 'atrial kick') follows the P-wave on ECG and provides final ventricular filling (preload) at end diastole. The QRS complex on ECG, indicating ventricular depolarization, precedes ventricular contraction (systole).

The AV valves close as ventricular pressure exceeds atrial pressure. Vibrations associated with valve closing and tensing are heard as the first heart sound (S_1, 'lub'). The brief time from AV valve closure until ventricular pressure increases enough to open the semilunar valves is known as isovolumic contraction. Ventricular ejection is rapid initially, then decelerates before ventricular relaxation begins. The ventricular walls thicken as ejection progresses. The blood remaining in the ventricles after ejection is known as the residual, or end-systolic, volume.

Ventricular pressure falls quickly as relaxation occurs. As soon as ventricular pressure drops below that in the associated great artery, ejection ceases and the semilunar valve closes. Vibrations associated with closing of these valves create the second heart sound (S_2, 'dub'). This marks the beginning of isovolumic relaxation, where ventricular pressure drops rapidly with no change in volume. When ventricular pressure falls below that in the associated atrium, the AV valves open and rapid (early) ventricular filling occurs. The greatest increase in ventricular volume occurs during this rapid filling phase. A slow filling phase (diastasis) follows. The duration of diastasis depends on heart rate.

During initial ventricular ejection there is a drop in atrial pressure (x descent; 14). A gradual rise in atrial pressure (v wave) follows as blood continues to flow into the atria during ventricular systole. Atrial pressure falls again (y descent) when the AV valves open in early diastole. Continued filling during diastasis produces a gradual rise in atrial (and ventricular) pressure. Atrial contraction causes the final atrial pressure increase (a wave) at the end of diastole.

Normally, only two heart sounds (S_1 and S_2) are heard in dogs and cats. But two other sounds may become audible with certain myocardial abnormalities (14). The S_3 (ventricular gallop sound) results from accentuated low-frequency vibrations associated with the end of early diastolic filling. The S_3 is most likely to be heard in animals with LV dilation and failure (e.g. dilated cardiomyopathy). The S_4 (atrial gallop sound) is associated with blood and tissue oscillations at the time of atrial contraction. The S_4 may be heard with an abnormally stiff or hypertrophied LV (e.g. hypertrophic cardiomyopathy).

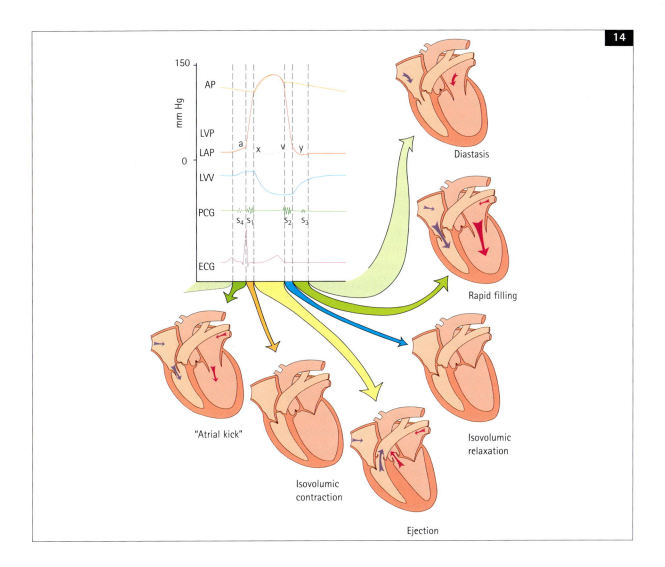

14 Cardiac cycle diagram showing interrelationships among electrical activation; pressures within atrium, ventricle, and associated great vessel; changes in ventricular volume; and heart sounds. Phases of the cardiac cycle are indicated by colored arrows correlating their time of occurrence on the graph with pictoral illustrations of the cardiac events. The timing of the sounds S_3 and S_4 is illustrated, although these sounds are not heard in normal dogs and cats (see text). Similar pressure and volume changes occur in the right heart. (See text for explanation of atrial pressure waves.) AP = aortic pressure; LVP = left ventricular pressure; LAP = left atrial pressure; LVV = left ventricular volume; PCG = phonocardiogram; ECG = electrocardiogram.

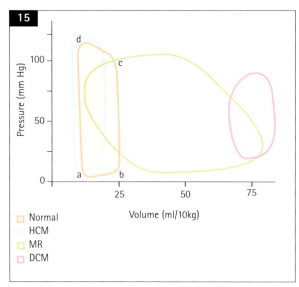

15 The normal left ventricular pressure-volume relationship is illustrated in orange. Ventricular filling occurs from 'a' to 'b'. Mitral valve closure and end-diastolic volume and pressure occur at point 'b'. From 'b' to 'c' is isovolumic contraction and from 'c' to 'd' is ejection. The change in ventricular volume from 'c' to 'd' represents the stroke volume. Isovolumic relaxation occurs from 'd' to 'a', where the mitral valve opens. Changes typical of various chronic heart diseases are also depicted. HCM is associated with increased ventricular stiffness, elevated end-diastolic pressure, and reduced volume. Large end-diastolic and stroke volumes are typical for severe, chronic MR. There is no isovolumic contraction because of the MR. Isovolumic relaxation is also lost because of continued MR after aortic valve closure, followed by rapid inflow from elevated atrial pressure. In DCM, end-diastolic and systolic volumes are both large and stroke volume is small because of the chronically poor contractility and secondary volume retention. Elevated filling pressures develop as ventricular dilation and stiffness increase.

Pressure–volume loops

Depiction of the changes in LV pressure and volume during the cardiac cycle, without regard to timing, can be used to illustrate functional abnormalities. Figure **15** shows a normal pressure–volume loop compared with the changes induced by systolic dysfunction (poor myocardial contractility) and diastolic dysfunction (impaired ventricular filling). Such changes underlie the clinical, radiographic, and echocardiographic findings associated with various heart diseases.

AUTONOMIC CONTROL OF THE HEART
Effects of sympathetic stimulation
Adrenergic receptors are widespread throughout the heart and are mainly of the beta$_1$ subtype. Stimulation of these receptors enhances myocardial contractility and relaxation, as well as HR and conduction velocity. Contractility is increased because more Ca^{++} enters the myocytes and more Ca^{++} is released from the SR. Beta-receptor stimulation also accelerates relaxation via reduced troponin affinity for Ca^{++} as well as accelerated SR reuptake of Ca^{++}. Sympathetic stimulation of the SA node hyperpolarizes the cells and activates an inward flux of Na^+ and K^+ (the so-called I_f); this causes faster spontaneous diastolic (phase 4) depolarization and earlier action potential generation[8]. AV conduction velocity is also accelerated by sympathetic stimulation.

Effects of parasympathetic (vagal) stimulation
Vagal (muscarinic) innervation of the heart is mainly localized to SA and AV nodal tissue; the ventricles have minimal vagal input. Vagal stimulation slows the SA node rate by reducing the slope of diastolic depolarization via an acetylcholine-activated outward K^+ current[8]. AV conduction is also slowed. Thus, the physiologic control of HR, mediated by the autonomic nervous system, is due mainly to changes in the slope of diastolic depolarization in SA nodal cells. Vagal influences predominate normally.

Periodic variation in the sinus rate is called sinus arrhythmia. It is related to reflexly-mediated fluctuations in vagal tone and is usually associated with the respiratory cycle (respiratory sinus arrhythmia). An increase in HR occurs with inspiration and a decrease with expiration. Sinus arrhythmia is often very pronounced in dogs, but it is usually more subtle in cats.

CARDIAC ENERGY SUPPLY
The heart has a high energy requirement in order to support contraction as well as other cellular functions. Coronary arterioles deliver O_2 to the cells via a dense myocardial capillary network. Regulation of coronary arteriolar tone is highly coupled to the energy status of the myocytes, and metabolic vasodilation is the most important control. The myocardium contains a large number of mitochondria, which produce ATP by oxidative phosphorylation; fatty acids are the major source of energy for the heart. Mitochondrial ATP production is impaired when excess intracellular Ca^{++} leads to mitochondrial Ca^{++} overloading.

Coronary blood flow
Overall, coronary blood flow is proportional to the driving pressure across the coronary circulation and is expressed by the relationship:

$$\frac{\text{aortic pressure} - \text{coronary sinus pressure}}{\text{coronary vascular resistance}}$$

Coronary flow varies during the cardiac cycle because of pressure fluctuations within the chambers and ventricular walls. Because the major coronary arteries lie on the external surface of the heart, flow moves in an epicardial to endocardial direction. During systole, when intraventricular pressure rises, coronary flow in subendocardial regions falls or ceases. It may even reverse direction when intraventricular pressure is abnormally high (e.g. with subaortic stenosis). Most coronary flow occurs during diastole. When the active phase of myocardial relaxation is slow, as occurs with ischemia, the early diastolic increase in coronary blood flow is impaired. Furthermore, because the duration of diastole shortens at faster heart rates, coronary flow, as well as ventricular filling, can be further compromised during tachycardia, especially when myocardial stiffness is increased.

Since the direction of coronary flow is epicardial to endocardial, subendocardial regions of the heart are most susceptible to ischemia when coronary flow is inadequate. At the same time, the subendocardial myocardium is also subject to greater mechanical stress and requires greater O_2 uptake. Inadequate coronary blood flow promotes myocardial ischemia and leads to replacement fibrosis. This contributes to the diastolic dysfunction associated with diseases such as hypertrophic cardiomyopathy and severe subaortic stenosis.

THE CIRCULATION

HEMODYNAMIC CONCEPTS

Flow, pressure, resistance relationships

Blood flow (volume/unit time) through any part of the circulation depends directly on the driving pressure and inversely on vascular resistance. These fundamental relationships are summarized by the equation $Q = \Delta P/R$, where Q = blood flow, ΔP = pressure difference across the vessel(s) in question, and R = resistance. When referring to the output from either the left or right heart, Q = cardiac output.

In the systemic circulation, ΔP is the difference between aortic pressure and right atrial pressure, which, averaged over time, is the mean arterial pressure (MAP). Total peripheral (systemic vascular) resistance is R. Therefore, left heart CO = MAP/R. For the pulmonary circulation, ΔP is the difference between pulmonary arterial pressure and left atrial pressure; R is pulmonary vascular resistance. Since the pulmonary and systemic circulations are in series, the output from each ventricle must be balanced over time (left heart CO = right heart CO). Resistance in the pulmonary circulation is normally much less than that in the systemic circulation. This allows perfusion of the lungs at relatively low pressures (see **1**, p. 10).

Resistance

Vascular resistance, or impediment to flow, is an important variable in determining the rate of blood flow. The reciprocal of resistance is conductance, a measure of flow for a given pressure difference. The width of the blood vessel(s) has the greatest impact on resistance and flow. Poiseuille's law summarizes the effects of vessel dimension, flow velocity, pressure, and viscosity on blood flow[d]. According to the relationships described by this law, resistance is inversely proportional to vessel radius to the fourth power (r^4), and directly proportional to blood viscosity[1, 9]. The exponential effect of vessel radius on resistance has important implications in regard to cardiac pathophysiology and therapy.

Viscosity

The apparent viscosity of blood is mainly determined by the hematocrit (or PCV) reading. At higher hematocrit values there is greater friction between successive layers of blood flowing within vessels, and therefore greater viscosity. A normal hematocrit value provides the best balance between ease of flow and ability to deliver oxygen to the tissues.

Blood flow velocity

Blood flow velocity in any area of the circulation is related to cross-sectional area as well as to flow rate. For a given flow (or cardiac output), as total cross-sectional area decreases, velocity increases. For this reason, a narrowed valve orifice abruptly accelerates blood flow velocity. Conversely, blood flow velocity is very slow in the capillary beds because total capillary cross-sectional area is huge.

Laminar and turbulent flow

Blood flowing in smooth vessels tends to form layers (streamlines) that slip over each other; flow is faster toward the center of the vessel, while the outer layers drag along the vessel wall. This laminar flow can easily be disrupted and become turbulent (disorganized). Turbulent flow is characterized by the formation of whorls or 'eddy currents'. Factors that promote turbulence include high flow velocity (e.g. from ventricular outflow obstruction), low blood viscosity (e.g. anemia), wide vessel diameter, sudden change in vessel diameter or direction, and pulsatile flow[1]. A measure of the tendency for turbulence to occur is described by Reynold's number[e]. Reynold's numbers over a 'critical' level (~2,000–2,300) are likely to be associated with an audible murmur. Resistance to blood flow increases when flow is turbulent.

THE VASCULATURE

Arterial system

Arteries provide a high pressure reservoir for the pulsatile cardiac output as well as a conduit for blood to the body's tissues. The strong elastic walls of the large arteries keep systolic pressure from becoming excessively high. Their recoil maintains pressure during diastole, which drives blood toward the peripheral tissues. Smaller arteries are less compliant as the proportion of elastin in their walls is less. Arterioles have more muscular walls, with an increased wall thickness/lumen ratio. The greatest increase in vascular resistance occurs at the arterioles, which act as 'control valves' to the microcirculation[1]. There is rich sympathetic innervation to the smooth muscle within arteriolar walls. The pulsatile pressure in the great arteries is gradually dampened by the elastic recoil of arterial walls and the progressively increasing resistance of the arterial tree. Blood flow in the capillary beds is nonpulsatile.

Arterial blood pressure is expressed as systolic/diastolic, in mm Hg. Systolic pressure is the highest pressure that occurs with each cardiac ejection. Diastolic pressure is the lowest pressure attained just before the next ejection. Pulse pressure is the difference between systolic and diastolic pressures. This is the major determinant of how strong the peripheral arterial pulse feels on palpation. Several factors influence pulse pressure, especially the SV, the compliance of the arterial system, and, to a lesser degree, the character of ventricular ejection. When SV increases, the rise and fall in pressure is greater because a greater volume must be accommodated in the arterial tree with each heartbeat. Pulse pressure is wider at slow HR because SV is greater (CO = HR × SV). When the compliance (distensibility) of the arterial tree is greater, there is less pressure rise with each ejection. So, pulse pressure is directly related to SV and inversely related to arterial compliance. The MAP is estimated as:

MAP = diastolic pressure + 1/3 pulse pressure.

MAP is closer to diastolic pressure because diastole is of longer duration than systole.

Microcirculation and lymphatics

Blood flow to each tissue bed is controlled by the constriction or dilation of the arterioles serving the bed. The level of sympathetic tone and, sometimes, hormonal factors, influence the degree of vasoconstriction; however, precapillary arterioles are strongly influenced by local metabolic (vasodilatory) factors because of their close contact with the tissues they serve. Capillaries, with their single endothelial cell layer, are where nutrient and waste exchange occur.

Fluid movement across the capillary membrane depends on the relationship between hydrostatic and oncotic pressures in both capillary and interstitium (Starling's forces)[f]. Hydrostatic pressure within capillaries tends to push fluid through the membrane pores into the interstitium. Plasma proteins are too large to pass through pores in the capillary membrane (high colloid oncotic pressure within the capillary). Usually, the capillary oncotic pressure tending to hold fluid within the vessel almost balances the outward hydrostatic force (pressure) tending to push fluid into the interstitium, so that there is a small net flow into the interstitium. Most filtered fluid is reabsorbed by the venous side of the capillaries; the rest is removed by lymphatics.

Lymph vessels remove excess fluid from the interstitial space. Some interstitial proteins are also removed, which reduces net fluid flow out of the capillaries. Lymph fluid from most of the body returns to the cranial vena cava via the thoracic duct; return from the right forelimb, neck, and head is by the right lymphatic duct. The rate of lymph flow is increased when interstitial free fluid pressure rises. This can result from increased capillary hydrostatic pressure (e.g. heart failure), decreased plasma colloid oncotic pressure (e.g. severe hypoproteinemia), and increased interstitial proteins (usually from increased capillary permeability). Tissue edema develops when interstitial fluid accumulation exceeds the maximal rate of lymph flow.

Venous system

Veins return blood to the heart; one-way valves help prevent backflow. Because all systemic venous blood eventually reaches the RA, venous return essentially equals cardiac output. Mean systemic venous pressure depends on sympathetic tone (venoconstriction) as well as blood volume. Pressure in the RA and adjoining segments of the vena cavae is also known as central venous pressure (CVP). RA pressure, or CVP, influences pressure in all systemic veins. CVP is usually measured clinically in cm H_2O; in normal dogs and cats it ranges from 0–10 cm H_2O.

Systemic veins can expand to store blood or constrict to return it to the central circulation. The compliance of veins is about 24 times greater than that of arteries, so a large increase in venous volume can occur with little change in pressure. Systemic veins are the major blood reservoir for the body. Venous constriction can maintain arterial flow and pressure when up to 20% of the total blood volume is lost[2]. The spleen also acts as a blood reservoir in the dog and splenic contraction increases venous return.

Normally, venous pulsations are not seen because no pressure pulses are transmitted forward through the capillaries. However, pressure waves can be transmitted backward from the right heart to the large veins, especially when RA pressure is elevated (see Cardiac cycle, p. 19).

CONTROL OF THE CIRCULATION

Regulation of blood flow in the peripheral circulation is under the control of the central (autonomic) nervous system as well as local metabolic conditions. In some situations, humoral factors also contribute. The relative importance of central compared to local control is not uniform across the circulation. For example, neural control predominates in splanchnic tissues, but local metabolic factors are most important in the heart. Constriction and relaxation of arteriolar smooth muscle regulates blood flow distribution throughout the body, total peripheral resistance, and blood pressure. Vascular smooth muscle in most tissues is innervated by only sympathetic fibers. A level of partial contraction (vascular 'tone') exists that appears to be independent of nervous system control. An increase in sympathetic nerve activity stimulates further contraction, while reduced sympathetic nerve traffic allows dilation[12]. Vascular smooth muscle contraction is mediated by increased intracellular Ca^{++}, most often via agonist binding to membrane receptor-operated Ca^{++} channels; intracellular Ca^{++} release from the SR also contributes. Agonists include catecholamines and angiotensin. Voltage-operated Ca^{++} entry can also stimulate contraction.

Local control

Several mechanisms influence blood flow to local tissues. Change in the concentration of vasodilator metabolites produced by the tissues adjusts blood flow according to local metabolic activity (metabolic regulation). Many arterioles have the intrinsic ability to contract (or dilate) in response to increased (or decreased) stretch, so that a steady flow rate is maintained (autoregulation). Endothelial-mediated regulation promotes vasodilation (via nitric oxide release) in response to increased blood flow (shear stress)[9, 12].

Neurohumoral (extrinsic) control

Control of the circulation as a whole is mediated centrally by the autonomic nervous system and also to some extent by humoral controls. The sympathetic (adrenergic) nervous system (SNS) activates the CV system (pressor response) via the neurotransmitter norepinephrine (NE). Sympathetic innervation extends to the veins (capacitance vessels) as well as arteries and arterioles throughout the body. Capillaries are not innervated. Vascular reflexes or humoral stimuli that activate the central pressor region increase the number of efferent sympathetic impulses, which increases NE release at the nerve terminals and, thus, the degree of vasoconstriction. This effect is greater in the small arteries, arterioles, and veins than in larger arteries. Inhibition of the pressor region reduces sympathetic efferent traffic and results in vasodilation.

The parasympathetic (cholinergic) nervous system (PNS) has inhibitory effects on the heart. But parasympathetic activation has minimal effect on total peripheral resistance because the PNS only innervates vasculature in the head and some viscera, not skeletal muscle or skin. Acetylcholine (Ach) is its neurotransmitter.

Vascular receptors

The density and distribution of different receptors in vascular walls varies depending on the organ system and tissue. Postsynaptic alpha$_1$-receptors are most important; stimulation by NE causes vasoconstriction. NE within the synaptic clefts also stimulates presynaptic alpha$_2$-receptors, which inhibit further NE release. Vascular wall alpha$_2$-receptors are extrasynaptic and are usually stimulated by circulating (adrenal-released) catecholamines; they mediate vasoconstriction. Thus, stimulation of vascular alpha$_{(1 \text{ or } 2)}$-receptors increases vascular resistance, reduces compliance, increases venous return to the heart, and ultimately raises systemic arterial pressure[9, 12]. There are vascular beta$_2$-receptors in many tissues (e.g. skeletal muscle); when stimulated by low levels of circulating epinephrine, they mediate vasodilation. They also respond to NE. Epinephrine can also activate alpha-receptors and cause constriction. Some vascular beds (e.g. renal) contain dopaminergic receptors that mediate vasodilation. Overall, however, vasodilation as an autonomic reflex function for blood pressure control is achieved by withdrawal of sympathetic tone and decreased stimulation of alpha-receptors, rather than by stimulation of vascular beta$_2$-receptors.

Vascular reflexes

Central sympathetic and parasympathetic output is influenced by afferent signals from baroreceptors, chemoreceptors, other brain centers, and skin receptors. Widespread activation of sympathetic vasoconstrictor fibers increases peripheral vascular resistance and arterial pressure, stimulates venous constriction (which increases venous return and cardiac output), and increases HR and contractility.

Arterial baroreceptors (pressor receptors), located in the carotid sinuses and in the aortic arch, are stimulated by stretch. They are especially important in the short-term regulation of blood pressure. When stretched by a rise in blood pressure, more afferent impulses are sent to the medulla (solitary tract nucleus) via the vagus nerve (from the aortic arch) or glossopharyngeal nerve (from the carotid sinuses). The solitary tract nucleus acts as a depressor control, which inhibits sympathetic output. Therefore, stimulation of vascular baroreceptors by increased blood pressure inhibits the central sympathetic vasoconstrictor regions, which allows peripheral vasodilation and reduction in blood pressure. Concurrent stimulation of vagal regions also slows HR. Baroreceptors operate over a limited blood pressure range. Maximal receptor firing rates occur at a mean blood pressure of 180–200 mm Hg, while afferent impulses cease at about 50–60 mm Hg. Reduced firing of baroreceptors allows more vasoconstrictor output to the peripheral circulation.

Cardiopulmonary baroreceptors located in the atria, ventricles, and pulmonary vessels are also tonically active and can alter peripheral resistance when stimulated by changes in intracardiac and pulmonary pressures. For example, stretching of atrial receptors mediates reduced sympathetic output to the kidney, increasing renal blood flow and urine output, but enhanced sympathetic output to the sinus node, increasing HR. Cardiopulmonary baroreceptor activation can also alter blood pressure reflexly by inhibiting the vasoconstrictor center in the medulla, as well as inhibiting renin (and thus angiotensin), aldosterone, and antidiuretic hormone release. Changes in urine volume resulting from cardiopulmonary baroreceptor activation are important in the regulation of blood volume. Peripheral chemoreceptors in the area of the aortic arch (aortic bodies) and carotid sinuses (carotid bodies) are sensitive to changes in PO_2, PCO_2, and pH of the blood. They are mainly involved with regulation of respiration but can influence the medullary vasomotor regions to some degree.

Humoral (hormonal) factors

Epinephrine (Epi) and NE can be released into the circulation by the adrenal gland, but this is normally less important in blood pressure control than NE release from sympathetic nerve terminals. Epi in low concentrations dilates resistance vessels (a beta-adrenergic effect) in some tissues (e.g. skeletal muscle); however, in high concentrations, Epi causes vasoconstriction (alpha-adrenergic effect). NE causes vasoconstriction (alpha-adrenergic effect).

Angiotensin (AT) II causes vasoconstriction and increases peripheral resistance and mean circulatory filling pressure. It also reduces sodium and water secretion via direct renal effects and increased aldosterone release from the adrenal cortex. In addition, AT II stimulates thirst, as well as myocardial hypertrophy. AT II production begins with the enzyme renin cleaving the polypeptide angiotensinogen to form AT I. AT I is then cleaved by angiotensin converting enzyme (ACE) to produce the active AT II. Renin is released from the kidney in response to increased sympathetic activation, reduced renal perfusion pressure, and a decreased distal tubular sodium load.

Vasopressin (antidiuretic hormone) is released from the pituitary gland in response to low arterial blood pressure as well as osmotic stimuli. It has a direct vasoconstrictor effect and plays an indirect role in blood pressure regulation via its effect on renal volume retention and thirst stimulation. Endothelins (ET) are a family of potent vasoconstrictors released from endothelial cells.

Atrial natriuretic peptide (ANP) is released from the atrial myocardium in response to stretching. It induces diuresis and vasodilation and, generally, antagonizes AT II effects.

Arterial pressure regulation

Normal blood supply to the body's tissues requires fairly constant arterial blood pressure. The rapidly acting pressure regulatory mechanisms are primarily the neural and hormonal mechanisms, most importantly the arterial baroreceptors. Long-term control of arterial blood pressure also depends on blood volume. This is largely related to renal regulation of sodium and water balance, as well as the neurohumoral mechanisms described above.

ENDNOTES

[a] Nernst equation:
$E_K = -61.5 \log([K^+]_i/[K^+]_o)$
E_K = potassium equilibrium potential;
$[K^+]_i$ = intracellular K^+ concentration;
$[K^+]_o$ = extracellular K^+ concentration.

[b] Fick principle:
The amount of a substance taken up (or released) by an organ per unit time is equal to the arterial-venous concentration difference of that substance × blood flow.

[c] LaPlace relationship:
$\tau = Pr/w$

τ = wall stress; P = transmural pressure; r = chamber radius; w = wall thickness.

[d] Amount of flow in a vessel over a given time:
Q = velocity of flow $([\Delta Pr^2]/8\eta l) \times$ cross-sectional area (πr^2)
r = vessel radius; η = viscosity; l = vessel length.
Rewritten, this is Poiseuille's law:
$Q = (\Delta Pr^4)/8\eta l$
Since Q = flow and ΔP = pressure difference, the rest equals conductance. Because resistance is the reciprocal of conductance: $R = 8\eta l/\pi r^4$.

[e] Reynold's number = $(\sigma/\eta)VD$
σ = fluid density; η = viscosity; V = average velocity; D = vessel diameter.

[f] Starling's forces:
$Q_f = k[(P_c + \pi_i) - (P_i + \pi_p)]$
Q_f = fluid movement; P_c = capillary hydrostatic pressure; P_i = interstitial fluid hydrostatic pressure;
π_i = interstitial fluid oncotic pressure;
π_p = plasma oncotic pressure;
k = filtration constant for capillary membrane.

REFERENCES

1 Berne RM, Levy MN (1997) *Cardiovascular Physiology*, 7th edn. Mosby, St. Louis, pp. 55–81.

2 Stephenson RB (1997) The heart as a pump. In: *Textbook of Veterinary Physiology*, 2nd edn. JG Cunningham (ed). WB Saunders, Philadelphia, pp. 180–197.

3 Dyce KM, Sach WO, Wensing CJG (1996) *Textbook of Veterinary Anatomy*. WB Saunders, Philadelphia, pp. 219–220.

4 Anderson WD, Anderson BG (1994) *Atlas of Canine Anatomy*. Lea & Febiger, Philadelphia, pp. 522–571.

5 Evans HE (1993) *Miller's Anatomy of the Dog*, 3rd edn. WB Saunders, Philadelphia, pp. 586–681.

6 Liu SK (1992) Histopathologic study of the conduction system. In: *Essentials of Canine and Feline Electrocardiography*, 3rd edn. LP Tilley (ed). WB Saunders, Philadelphia, pp. 267–273.

7 Berne RM, Levy MN (1997) *Cardiovascular Physiology*, 7th edn. Mosby, St. Louis, pp. 7–53.

8 Schuessler RB, Boineau JP, Saffitz JE *et al.* (2000) Cellular mechanisms of sinoatrial activity. In: *Cardiac Electrophysiology from Cell to Bedside*, 3rd edn. DP Zipes, J Jalife (eds). WB Saunders, Philadelphia, pp. 187–195.

9 Kittleson MD, Kienle RD (1998) *Small Animal Cardiovascular Medicine*. Mosby, St. Louis, pp. 11–35.

10 Opie LH, Solaro RJ (2004) Myocardial contraction and relaxation. In: *Heart Physiology, from Cell to Circulation*, 4th edn. LH Opie (ed). Lippincott Williams & Wilkins, Philadelphia, pp. 221–246.

11 Hamlin RL (1999) Normal cardiovascular physiology. In: *Textbook of Feline and Canine Cardiology*, 2nd edn. D Sisson, PR Fox, NS Moise (eds). WB Saunders, Philadelphia, pp. 25–37.

12 Berne RM, Levy MN (1997) *Cardiovascular Physiology*, 7th edn. Mosby, St. Louis, pp. 171–194.

2
The Cardiovascular Examination

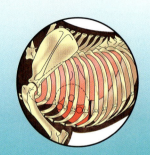

GENERAL CONSIDERATIONS

The CV examination and medical history can reveal evidence of previously unsuspected heart abnormalities as well as provide important information in animals with known CV disease. The patient's signalment should be noted because some congenital and acquired heart abnormalities are more prevalent in certain breeds or age ranges, and some conditions have a gender predisposition (see Chapters 18–25).

SIGNS OF HEART DISEASE AND FAILURE

Cardiac disease can exist without the animal being in 'heart failure'. Signs consistent with heart disease include cardiac murmurs, rhythm disturbances, jugular vein pulsations, and cardiomegaly (see Chapters 6, 7, 10, and 13). Other clinical signs can also suggest cardiac disease or failure, but they may occur with noncardiac disease as well. These include cough, respiratory difficulty, exercise intolerance, weakness, syncope, abdominal distension, tissue edema, excessively weak or strong arterial pulses, and cyanosis (see Chapters 8, 9, 11, 12, 14, and 15).

Most clinical signs of heart failure (*Table 1*) relate to high venous pressure behind the heart (congestive signs) or inadequate blood flow out of the heart (low output signs). Congestive signs related to right-sided heart failure stem from systemic venous hypertension and the elevated systemic capillary hydrostatic pressure that results. Pulmonary venous hypertension and subsequent lung edema result from elevated left heart filling pressure. Chronic elevation of pulmonary venous pressure may increase pulmonary arterial pressure and facilitate the development of right-sided heart failure in patients with chronic left-sided heart failure. Signs of low cardiac output are similar regardless of which ventricle is primarily diseased, because output from the left heart is coupled to that from the right heart.

The medical history and physical findings guide the choice of further tests and initial interventions. Additional diagnostic testing helps identify and more specifically define the severity and progression of the underlying disease.

Table 1 Clinical signs of heart failure.

1) Low cardiac output signs:
   a) Tiring.
   b) Exertional weakness.
   c) Syncope.
   d) Prerenal azotemia.
   e) Cyanosis (from poor peripheral circulation).
   f) Pallor and prolonged capillary refill time.
   g) Cardiac arrhythmias.

2) Congestive signs – left side (high LV filling pressure):
   a) Pulmonary congestion and edema (cough, tachypnea, increased respiratory effort, orthopnea, pulmonary crackles, tiring, hemoptysis, cyanosis).
   b) Secondary right-sided heart failure.
   c) Cardiac arrhythmias.

3) Congestive signs – right side (high RV filling pressure):
   a) Systemic venous congestion (high central venous pressure, jugular vein distension).
   b) Hepatic ± splenic congestion.
   c) Pleural effusion (increased respiratory effort, orthopnea, cyanosis).
   d) Ascites.
   e) Small pericardial effusion.
   f) Subcutaneous edema.
   g) Cardiac arrhythmias.

MEDICAL HISTORY

Historical information of particular interest in patients with CV disease includes that listed in *Table 2*.

OBSERVATION OF THE PATIENT

Prior to the CV examination, the patient's attitude, posture, body condition, level of anxiety, and respiratory pattern should be observed. The animal's appearance depends on the severity of underlying disease and hemodynamic or respiratory compromise, as well as other factors. Chapters 8–15 provide further information about respiratory signs, abnormal body appearance, and other problems the animal may have displayed. The body condition of patients with CV disorders is variable; some animals are thin, some are obese. However, weight loss is common in advanced disease and cardiac cachexia may occur with chronic heart failure (**16**; see also **409**, p. 283)[1].

THE CARDIOVASCULAR EXAMINATION

EVALUATION OF MUCOUS MEMBRANES

Adequacy of peripheral perfusion is estimated by mucous membrane color and capillary refill time (CRT). Oral membranes are usually assessed, but caudal (prepucial or vaginal) membranes also can be used. The ocular conjunctiva can be used if the oral membranes are pigmented. When polycythemia is present, caudal mucous membrane color should be compared with that of the oral membranes, regardless of whether a cardiac murmur is detected.

The CRT is assessed by applying digital pressure to blanch the membrane; color should return within 2 seconds. Dehydration and other causes of decreased cardiac output cause slowed CRT because of high peripheral sympathetic tone and vasoconstriction. Mucous membrane pallor

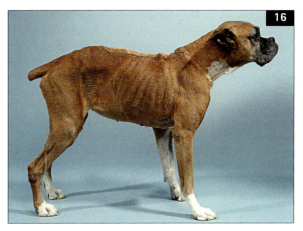

16 Cardiac cachexia is evident in this Boxer with chronic right-sided heart failure. Note the loss of muscle mass dorsally. Ascites caused the abdominal distension.

Table 2 The medical history.
1) Signalment (age, breed, gender).
2) Vaccination status.
3) Diet, as well as any recent changes in food or water consumption.
4) Where animal was obtained and geographical regions where it has been.
5) Housing, whether indoors or out.
6) Any recent change in attitude or activity.
7) Normal level of activity and whether the animal tires easily now.
8) Presence of cough, including timing and description of episodes.
9) Presence of any excessive or unexpected panting or heavy breathing.
10) Any episodes of fainting or weakness, including timing and description of episodes.
11) Whether the tongue/mucous membranes always look pink, especially during exercise.
12) Occurrence of any vomiting or gagging.
13) Any recent change in urinary or bowel habits.
14) Any medications that are being given for the presenting problem. Which? How much? How often? Do they help?
15) Any medications used in the past for this problem. Which? How much? Were they effective?
16) Any other medications or dietary supplements being used.

results from anemia or peripheral vasoconstriction. Anemic animals have a normal CRT unless hypoperfusion is also present, although the CRT can be difficult to assess in severely anemic animals because of the lack of color contrast.

A number of abnormalities can alter the normally pink mucous membrane color (*Table 3* and 17–20)[2]. Cyanotic membranes have a bluish color[3]. This can result from central cyanosis (usually associated with >50 g/l [>5 g/dl] of desaturated hemoglobin) or peripheral cyanosis (associated with extremely poor peripheral perfusion). Differential cyanosis refers to cyanotic caudal membranes with pink cranial membranes; this is associated with 'reversed' patent ductus arteriosus. Petechiae in the mucous membranes suggest a platelet disorder. A yellowish cast (icterus, jaundice) should prompt evaluation for hemolysis and hepatobiliary disease.

EVALUATION OF JUGULAR VEINS
Systemic venous and right heart filling pressures are reflected at the jugular veins. When the animal is standing with its head in a normal position (jaw parallel to the floor), these veins should not be distended. Persistent jugular vein distension occurs when central venous pressure is high, and suggests either high right heart filling pressure or obstruction to cranial vena cava flow (see Chapter 10). Jugular pulsations extending higher than the point of the shoulder in a standing animal are also abnormal.

Sometimes the carotid pulse wave is transmitted through adjacent soft tissues, mimicking a jugular pulse in thin or excited animals. A true jugular pulse can be differentiated from carotid transmission by lightly occluding the jugular vein below the area of the visible pulse. If the pulse disappears, it is a true jugular pulsation; if the pulse continues, it is being transmitted from the carotid artery. Jugular pulse waves are related to pressure changes during atrial contraction and filling (see **14**, p. 19, and Chapter 10).

Testing for hepatojugular reflux can uncover impaired RV filling, reduced pulmonary blood flow, or tricuspid regurgitation, even in the absence of jugular distension or pulsations at rest. To test for this reflux, apply firm pressure to the cranial abdomen while the animal is standing quietly (**21**). This will transiently increase venous return. Jugular distension that persists while abdominal pressure is applied constitutes a positive (abnormal) test. Normal animals have little to no change in jugular vein appearance.

Table 3 Abnormal mucous membrane color.

1) Pale mucous membranes:
   a) Anemia.
   b) Poor cardiac output/high sympathetic tone.
2) Injected, brick-red membranes:
   a) Polycythemia.
   b) Sepsis.
   c) Excitement.
   d) Other causes of peripheral vasodilation.
3) Cyanotic mucous membranes:*
   a) Pulmonary parenchymal disease.
   b) Airway obstruction.
   c) Pleural space disease.
   d) Pulmonary edema.
   e) Right-to-left shunting congenital cardiac defect.
   f) Hypoventilation.
   g) Shock.
   h) Cold exposure.
   i) Methemoglobinemia.
4) Differential cyanosis:
   a) Reversed patent ductus arteriosus (normally oxygenated blood to head and forelimbs, but desaturated blood to caudal part of body via the ductus, which arises from the descending aorta).
5) Icteric mucous membranes:
   a) Hemolysis.
   b) Hepatobiliary disease.
   c) Biliary obstruction.

*Because a blood level of 50 g/dl (5 g/dl) of desaturated hemoglobin is necessary for visible cyanosis, anemic animals may not appear cyanotic even with marked hypoxemia.

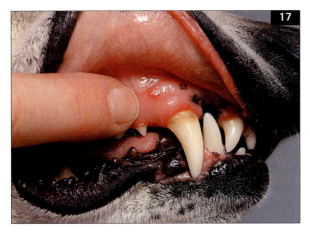

17 Normal pink mucous membrane color. Digital pressure will blanch the membrane and allow determination of CRT.

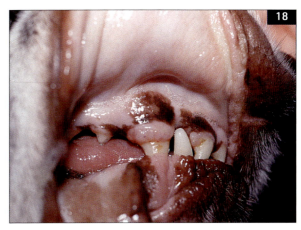

18 Pale mucous membranes can result from high sympathetic tone (slow CRT) or anemia (usually normal CRT).

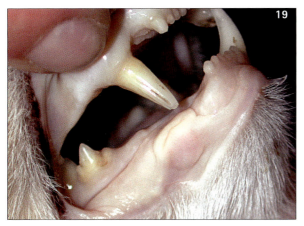

19 Severe anemia, as in this cat, may preclude adequate assessment of CRT.

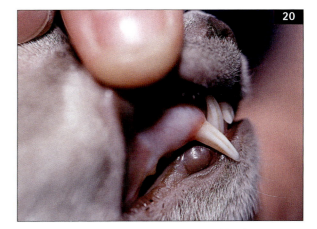

20 Cyanotic membranes are evident in this cat with a right-to-left shunting ventricular septal defect and pulmonary hypertension.

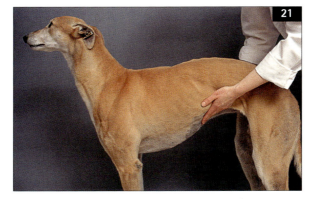

21 Pressure is applied to the cranial abdomen to test for hepatojugular reflux. Jugular vein distension that appears while abdominal pressure is applied constitutes a positive (abnormal) test; normal animals have little to no change in the jugular vein. A normal head and neck position, as shown here, is important when evaluating jugular veins.

EVALUATION OF ARTERIAL PULSES

The strength, regularity, and rate of the peripheral arterial pressure waves are assessed by palpation of the femoral or other peripheral arteries. Subjective evaluation of pulse strength is based on the difference between the systolic and diastolic arterial pressures (see Chapter 1). When the difference is wide, the pulse feels strong on palpation. Hyperkinetic pulses are abnormally strong. When the pulse pressure is small, the pulse feels weak (hypokinetic). The pulse can also feel weak if the rise to maximum systolic arterial pressure is prolonged, as in animals with severe subaortic stenosis. Note that the systolic and diastolic arterial blood pressures cannot be reliably determined by arterial palpation. Both femoral arteries should be palpated and compared; absence of pulse or a weaker pulse on one side may indicate thromboembolism or other vascular abnormality.

Femoral pulses can be difficult to palpate in cats, even when normal. Usually, the pulse can be found by gently working a fingertip toward the cat's proximal femur between the dorsomedial thigh muscles, in the area of the femoral triangle. *Table 4* lists some causes of abnormal arterial pulse strength.

Variations in arterial pulse intensity usually relate to changes in SV[4]. Mild variation normally occurs with the heart rate fluctuations of sinus arrhythmia. Fewer femoral pulses than heartbeats constitutes a pulse deficit. Pulse deficits are detected by simultaneously palpating the femoral arterial pulse rate and counting the direct heart rate, which is obtained by chest wall palpation or auscultation. Various cardiac arrhythmias induce pulse deficits by causing the heart to beat before adequate ventricular filling has occurred; minimal to no blood is ejected for those beats and a palpable pulse is absent (**22**; see also **410**, p. 283). Sometimes, alternately weak then strong arterial pulsations result from a normal heartbeat alternating with a premature beat (bigeminy) or from severe myocardial failure. An exaggerated decrease in systolic arterial pressure during inspiration occurs with cardiac tamponade; weak arterial pulses might be detectable during inspiration in these cases.

PRECORDIAL PALPATION

Normally, the strongest systolic impulse occurs over the area of the left cardiac apex, located at approximately the 5th intercostal space near the costochondral junction. To detect this, the precordium is palpated by placing the palm and fingers of each hand on the corresponding side of the animal's chest wall over the heart. Cardiomegaly or a space-occupying mass within the chest can shift the precordial impulse to an abnormal location. Reduced intensity of the precordial impulse can be caused by obesity, weak cardiac

Table 4 Abnormal arterial pulses.

1) Strong pulses:
   a) Excitement.
   b) Hypertrophic cardiomyopathy.
   c) Hyperthyroidism.
   d) Fever.
2) Very strong, bounding pulses:
   a) Patent ductus arteriosus.
   b) Severe aortic regurgitation.
   c) Fever/sepsis.
3) Weak pulses:
   a) Dilated cardiomyopathy.
   b) (Sub)aortic stenosis.
   c) Pulmonic stenosis.
   d) Shock.
   e) Dehydration.

contractions, pericardial effusion, intrathoracic masses, pleural effusion, or pneumothorax. A stronger precordial impulse on the right chest wall compared with the left can occur with RV hypertrophy or displacement of the heart into the right hemithorax (e.g. by a mass lesion, lung atelectasis, or chest deformity).

The term precordial thrill refers to palpable chest wall vibrations caused by very loud cardiac murmurs. These feel like a focal 'buzzing' sensation on the hand. A precordial thrill is usually localized over the area where the murmur is loudest.

CARDIAC AUSCULTATION

Heart rate and rhythm, heart sounds, and pulmonary sounds are evaluated by thoracic auscultation. Heart sounds are created by turbulent blood flow and associated vibrations in adjacent tissue during the cardiac cycle (see Chapter 1 for a description of heart sounds and their genesis). Many of these sounds are too low in frequency and/or intensity to be heard. Audible heart sounds are classified as transient sounds (those of short duration) and cardiac murmurs (longer sounds occurring during a normally silent part of the cardiac cycle). These sounds can be described by their pitch (frequency), intensity (loudness), duration, and quality (timbre)[5]. The latter is affected by the physical characteristics of the vibrating structures. The turbulence causing audible heart murmurs is generally associated with high velocity flow, abnormal flow disturbance, or reduced blood viscosity (e.g. anemia).

Because many heart sounds are difficult to hear, patient cooperation and a quiet environment are important during auscultation. If possible, the animal should be standing so that the heart is in its normal position. Respiratory sounds can interfere with heart sound assessment and mimic murmurs. Panting in dogs is discouraged by holding the animal's mouth shut. Breath sounds can be decreased further by placing a finger over one or both nostrils for a short time. Purring in cats may be stopped by holding a finger over one or both nostrils (**23**), waving an alcohol-soaked cottonball near the cat's nose, gently compressing the larynx, or turning on a water faucet/tap near the animal. Various other artifacts that can interfere with auscultation include other respiratory noises, shivering or muscle twitching, hair rubbing against the stethoscope (mimics pulmonary crackles), gastrointestinal sounds, and extraneous room noises.

The traditional stethoscope has both a stiff, flat diaphragm and a bell on the chestpiece. The diaphragm is applied firmly to the chest wall; this allows better auscultation of higher frequency heart sounds (and breath sounds) than those of low frequency. The bell, applied lightly to the chest wall, facilitates auscultation of lower frequency sounds such as S_3 and S_4 (see Chapter 1 and Chapter 6). Stethoscopes with a single-sided chestpiece are designed to function as a diaphragm when used with firm pressure, and as a bell when used with light pressure. Ideally the stethoscope should have relatively short, double tubing and comfortable ear tips. The binaural ear tubes should be angled rostrally to align with the examiner's ear canals.

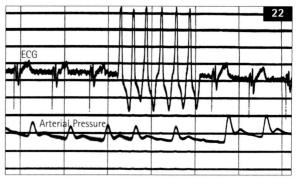

22 Pulse deficits associated with a PVT are shown in this tracing from a Bulldog with atrial fibrillation, 3rd degree heart block, and an endocardial pacemaker. The ECG (top) indicates paced QRS complexes as well as the PVT; arterial pressure waves (bottom) occur following each paced complex, but only sporadically during the tachycardia.

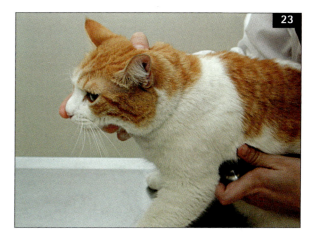

23 Gently occluding one (or briefly both) nostril during auscultation helps slow respiration, minimize lung sounds in dogs, and interrupt purring in cats.

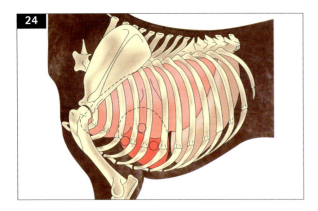

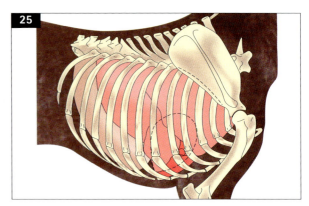

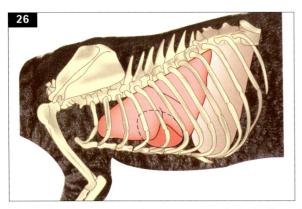

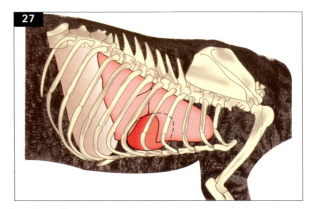

24–27 Approximate locations of cardiac valve areas in the dog (**24, 25**) and cat (**26, 27**).

The orientation of the heart within the thorax varies between cats and dogs and among breeds. The author recommends determining the area of the left apical impulse by precordial palpation, then starting cardiac auscultation at this point. The stethoscope chestpiece is moved gradually to all areas of the precordium from here. Slightly dorsal to this reference point is the mitral valve area. One to two intercostal spaces (ICSs) craniodorsal to this is the aortic valve area; about one ICS cranioventral to the aortic valve is the pulmonary valve. Sounds from the tricuspid valve are best heard over the right hemithorax, slightly cranial to the level of the mitral valve. Because the feline heart lies more horizontally in the chest compared with dogs, it is important to auscultate the areas along the left and right sternal borders in cats. Both sides of the chest should be carefully auscultated in both species, with special focus to the valve areas (**24–27**).

The clinician should concentrate on the individual heart sounds, correlating them to the events of the cardiac cycle, and listen for any abnormal sounds in systole and diastole, successively. The normal heart sounds (S_1 and S_2) are

used as a framework for timing abnormal sounds. It is important to understand the events of the cardiac cycle (see Chapter 1 and **14**, p. 19) and identify the timing of systole (between S_1 and S_2) and diastole (after S_2 until the next S_1) in the animal. The precordial impulse occurs just after S_1 (systole) and the arterial pulse between S_1 and S_2. The point of maximal intensity (PMI) on the chest wall of any abnormal sound(s) should be located. The PMI is generally identified in terms of a particular valve area, ICS, or location at left/right heart base/apex. (See Chapter 6 for information on murmurs and other abnormal heart sounds.) The examiner should focus on cardiac auscultation separately from pulmonary auscultation; full assimilation of sounds from both systems simultaneously is unlikely.

Sometimes, the first (S_1) and/or second (S_2) heart sounds are altered in intensity (*Table 5*) or split. A split or sloppy-sounding S_1 may be normal, especially in large dogs, or it may result from ventricular premature contractions or an intraventricular conduction delay. Normal physiologic splitting of S_2 can be heard in some dogs because of the variation in SV during the respiratory cycle. During inspiration,

Table 5 Altered intensity of heart sounds.

1) Loud S_1:	2) Loud, snapping S_2:	3) Muffled sounds (especially S_1):
a) Thin chest wall.	a) Pulmonary hypertension (e.g. from heartworm disease, a congenital shunt with Eisenmenger's physiology, or cor pulmonale).	a) Pericardial effusion.
b) High sympathetic tone.		b) Obesity.
c) Tachycardia.		c) Diaphragmatic hernia.
d) Systemic arterial hypertension.		d) Dilated cardiomyopathy.
e) Shortened PR intervals.		e) Hypovolemia/poor ventricular filling.
		f) Pleural effusion.

increased venous return to the RV tends to delay closure of the pulmonic valve, while greater pulmonary vascular capacity reduces filling of the LV and accelerates aortic valve closure. Pathologic splitting of S_2 can result from delayed ventricular activation or prolonged RV ejection secondary to ventricular premature beats, right bundle branch block, a ventricular or atrial septal defect, or pulmonary hypertension. Cardiac arrhythmias often cause variation in the intensity, or even absence, of heart sounds.

EVALUATION FOR ABNORMAL FLUID ACCUMULATION

Elevated right heart filling pressure promotes abnormal fluid accumulation within body cavities or, usually less noticeably, in the subcutis of dependent areas (see Chapters 11 and 12). Palpation and ballottement of the abdomen, palpation of dependent areas, and percussion of the chest in the standing animal are used to detect effusions and subcutaneous edema. Fluid accumulation secondary to right-sided heart failure is usually accompanied by abnormal jugular vein distension and/or pulsations, unless the animal's circulating blood volume has been reduced (e.g. by diuretic use). Hepatomegaly and/or splenomegaly may also be palpable in cats and dogs with right-sided heart failure.

REFERENCES

1 Freeman LM, Rush JE, Kehayias JJ *et al.* (1998) Nutritional alterations and the effect of fish oil supplementation in dogs with heart failure. *J Vet Intern Med* **12**(6):440–8.

2 Perloff JK (1983) The physiologic mechanisms of cardiac and vascular physical signs. *J Am Coll Cardiol* 1:184–198.

3 Stepien RL (2000) Cyanosis. In: *Textbook of Veterinary Internal Medicine*, 5th edn. SJ Ettinger, EC Feldman (eds). WB Saunders, Philadelphia, pp. 206–210.

4 Goodwin JK (2000) Pulse alterations. In: *Textbook of Veterinary Internal Medicine*, 5th edn. SJ Ettinger,

EC Feldman (eds). WB Saunders, Philadelphia, pp. 174–179.

5 Braunwald E, Perloff JK (2001) Physical examination of the heart and circulation. In: *Heart Disease: A Textbook of Cardiovascular Medicine*, 6th edn. E Braunwald, DP Zipes, P Libby (eds). WB Saunders, Philadelphia, pp. 45–81.

3
Overview of Cardiac Radiography

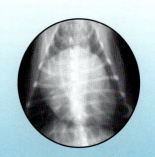

GENERAL PRINCIPLES

Good quality thoracic radiographs can provide vital information about overall cardiac size and shape in dogs and cats with heart disease. Radiographs are the best means of evaluating pulmonary blood vessels, examining the lungs for evidence of edema or other abnormalities, and assessing the pleural space, mediastinum, and diaphragm. However, a major limitation of radiography is that fluid has the same opacity as soft tissue. Because the heart appears as a single fluid/tissue opacity, internal structures cannot be discerned and pericardial effusion cannot be differentiated from cardiomegaly.

RADIOGRAPHIC VIEWS

At least two views should be evaluated: lateral and dorsoventral (DV) or ventrodorsal (VD). Slight changes in cardiac appearance occur with different patient positions[1, 2]; therefore, it is best to be consistent in the views used to evaluate the heart. The right lateral view is generally preferred for cardiac evaluation in dogs and cats[3]. The upper (nondependent) lung fields are accentuated on lateral view. Unilateral pulmonary disease can be better delineated using both right and left lateral views. In general a DV view provides better definition of the hilar area and caudal pulmonary vessels than a VD view. Furthermore, a DV position is better tolerated when respiration is compromised. The heart tends to look more elongated on a VD view compared with a DV view, but a VD view is often better for detecting lung disease and small volume pleural effusion[3].

PATIENT POSITIONING

Proper (not obliquely tilted) patient positioning is important for accurate interpretation of cardiac shape and size, as well as pulmonary parenchyma. For a lateral view the sternum and spine should be equidistant to the cassette so that the ribs are aligned parallel with each other. Chest rotation, with the sternum lower than the spine, increases the apparent size of the LA and heart base[2]. The forelimbs should be pulled forward so the cranial thorax is well visualized. For DV/VD views, the sternum, vertebral bodies, and dorsal spinous processes should be superimposed so that the ribs appear symmetrical and the spine straight. External foreign matter on the body wall (e.g. dirt, water) should be removed.

TECHNIQUE CONSIDERATIONS

High kilovoltage peak (kVp) and low milliamperes × seconds (mAs) radiographic technique is generally recommended for better resolution among soft tissue structures and to minimize respiratory motion (short exposure time)[2]. Exposure is ideally made at the time of peak inspiration to give the best contrast between pulmonary air and soft tissue opacity. On expiration, lung opacity is greater, the heart is relatively larger, the diaphragm may overlap the caudal heart border, and pulmonary vessels are poorly delineated; however, intentional expiratory exposures are useful for identifying dynamic intrathoracic airway collapse.

SYSTEMATIC EVALUATION

The films should be examined systematically. This includes assessing the technique, patient positioning, presence of artifacts, and phase of respiration during exposure. All visible structures should be evaluated. Any observations made must be integrated with the patient's clinical signs and an understanding of anatomy and physiology.

EVALUATION OF THE HEART

NORMAL CANINE CARDIAC SILHOUETTE

Breed differences in chest conformation influence the radiographic appearance of the heart. In dogs with round or barrel-shaped chests, the cardiac silhouette has greater sternal contact and more horizontal orientation on the lateral view (**28, 29**). On DV/VD views, the heart has an oval to rounded shape; this can mimic right heart enlargement, especially if there is increased mediastinal fat[3]. Narrow-chested and deep-chested dogs have an upright and elongated appearance to the heart on a lateral view (**30, 31**). On DV/VD views, the heart looks relatively small and may appear almost circular. Because of the variation in chest conformation, as well as the influences of respiration, cardiac cycle, and positioning on the apparent size of the heart, mild cardiomegaly may be difficult to identify. Occasionally, the cardiac apex is displaced into the right hemithorax on DV/VD views. If there are no other abnormal signs, this may be a normal variation. The cardiac shadow in puppies normally appears slightly large relative to the thoracic size compared with adult dogs. The thymus may obscure the cranial heart border.

Vertebral heart score

Good correlation exists between body length and heart size regardless of chest conformation. Based on this relationship, the vertebral heart score (VHS) can be used to quantify the presence and degree of cardiomegaly in dogs and cats[4]. Measurements for the VHS are obtained using a lateral view (**32**) in dogs. The cardiac long axis (L) is measured from the ventral border of the left mainstem bronchus to the most ventral aspect of the cardiac apex. The short axis (S) is measured in the central third of the heart, perpendicular to L and at the area of maximum cardiac width. Both L and S are compared with the thoracic spine, beginning at the cranial edge of T4; each length is estimated to the nearest 0.1 vertebra. The sum of measurements L and S is the VHS. A VHS between 8.5 and 10.5 vertebrae is considered normal for most breeds, although some variation exists among breeds. For example, in dogs with a short thorax (e.g. Miniature Schnauzers) an upper limit of 11 vertebrae is considered normal, whereas an upper limit of 9.5 vertebrae is normal in dogs with a long thorax (e.g. Dachshunds)[4]. The VHS in normal puppies falls within the reference range for adult dogs[5].

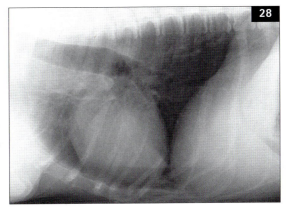
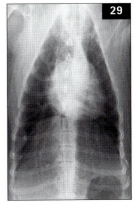

28, 29 Lateral (**28**) and DV (**29**) views from a normal 5-year-old neutered male Basset Hound, showing the wider cardiac silhouette common in breeds with a rounded, barrel-shaped chest.

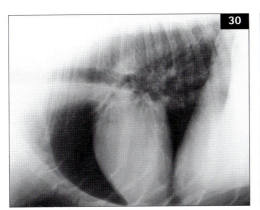
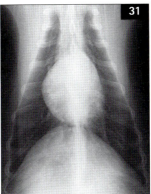
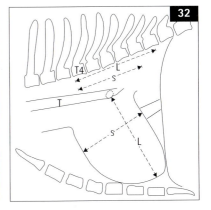

30–32 Lateral (**30**) and DV (**31**) views from a normal 4-year-old neutered male Doberman Pinscher. Note the elongated, upright orientation (**30**) and small DV profile (**31**) common in breeds with a deep, narrow chest. (**32**) This diagram illustrates the method for VHS measurement using the lateral chest radiograph. In this example, L = 5.8 v, S = 4.6 v, therefore VHS = 10.4 v (see text for further information). L = long axis heart dimension; S = short axis heart dimension; T = trachea. (Modified from Buchanan JW, Bücheler J (1995) Vertebral scale system to measure canine heart size in radiographs. *J Am Vet Med Assoc* **206**, 194, with permission.)

NORMAL FELINE CARDIAC SILHOUETTE

In cats the heart on a lateral view is aligned more parallel to the sternum than in dogs (33, 34). This more horizontal orientation is accentuated in older cats[6]. Radiographic positioning as well as patient resistance to restraint can influence the relative size, shape, and position of the heart and trachea. These influences are greater in cats than in dogs because of greater thoracic flexibility[1]. Although there is some variation, the feline heart is usually less than or up to 2 intercostal spaces wide and less than 70% of the height of the thorax on the lateral view. On DV/VD views, the heart is usually no more than one half the width of the thorax[2]. The phase of the cardiac cycle has only a mild influence on heart size and shape, but the effect is greater on a DV view compared with a VD view[7]. In kittens, as in puppies, the relative size of the heart compared with the thorax is larger than in adults because of smaller lung volume[1].

Vertebral heart score

The VHS is also useful in cats. The range of VHSs derived from lateral radiographs in normal cats has been reported as 6.7–8.1 vertebrae, with a mean of 7.5 vertebrae[8]. Cardiac measurement from a DV/VD view is more consistent in cats than in dogs and can be clinically useful. The mean short-axis cardiac dimension taken from a DV/VD view, compared with the thoracic spine beginning at T4 on the lateral view, was 3.4–3.5 vertebrae; an upper limit of normal of 4 vertebrae was identified[8].

GENERALIZED CARDIOMEGALY

Radiographic suggestion of abnormal cardiac size or shape should be considered within the context of the physical examination and other test findings. Also, when a suspected radiographic abnormality is found, one should ask whether other supportive or commonly associated findings are seen.

Generalized enlargement of the heart silhouette on plain radiographs may indicate true cardiomegaly or fluid within the pericardial sac. The contours of different chambers are usually still evident when the heart itself is enlarged, although marked RV and RA dilation can create a round heart appearance (35, 36). Fluid, fat (37), or viscera

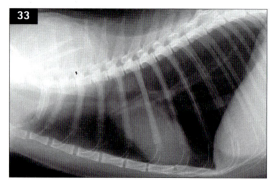
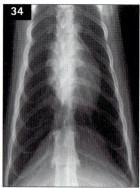

33, 34 Lateral (33) and DV (34) views from a normal, 3-year-old neutered male mixed breed cat.

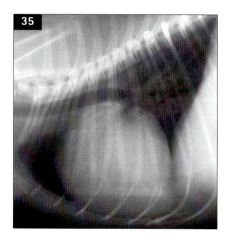
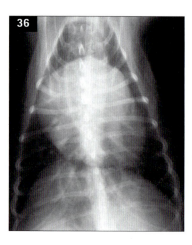

35, 36 Lateral (35) and and DV (36) views in an 8-year-old spayed female mixed breed dog with generalized cardiomegaly that resulted from a large congenital atrial septal defect, tricupid insuffiency, and mitral insufficiency.

within the pericardial sac tends to obliterate specific chamber contours and cause a globoid heart shadow (see Chapter 22). Common differential diagnoses for cardiac enlargement patterns are listed in *Table 6*. Specific chamber enlargement patterns are discussed below.

SMALL CARDIAC SILHOUETTE

An abnormally small heart shadow (microcardia) results from poor venous return (e.g. as with severe hypovolemia). The cardiac apex appears more pointed and may be elevated from the sternum on a lateral view (38). Other findings with hypovolemia include small pulmonary vessels and a thin caudal vena cava.

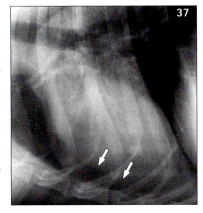 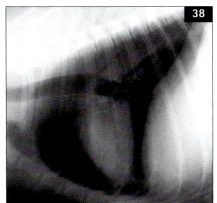

37, 38 (37) Fat accumulation in the pericardium can mimic cardiomegaly. However, in this radiograph from an obese 9-year-old male Vizsla, the demarcation between fat and soft tissue (heart) opacity (arrows) is clearly seen.
(38) Severe dehydration caused an abnormally small cardiac silhouette (microcardia) in this 8-year-old female Collie with pyometra. Note the separation of the cardiac apex from the sternum as well as the small pulmonary vessels.

Table 6 Causes for radiographic cardiomegaly.

1) Generalized enlargement of the cardiac shadow:
   a) Dilated cardiomyopathy (see Chapter 20).
   b) Mitral and tricuspid valve insufficiency (see Chapters 18, 19).
   c) Pericardial effusion (see Chapter 22).
   d) Intrapericardial mass or peritoneopericardial diaphragmatic hernia (see Chapter 22).
   e) Ventricular or atrial septal defect (see Chapter 18).
   f) Tricuspid valve dysplasia (see Chapter 18).
   g) Patent ductus arteriosus (see Chapter 18).
   h) Systemic hypertension (see Chapter 25).
   i) 'Athletic' heart.
   j) Hyperthyroidism.
   k) Acromegaly.
   l) Large arteriovenous fistula.
   m) Chronic anemia.
   n) Intracardiac mass.
   o) (Intrapericardial fat – may mimic cardiomegaly).
2) Left atrial enlargement:
   a) Mild mitral valve insufficiency.
   b) Hypertrophic cardiomyopathy.
   c) Early dilated cardiomyopathy, especially Doberman Pinschers.
   d) (Sub)aortic stenosis.

3) Left atrial and ventricular enlargement:
   a) Mitral valve insufficiency (see Chapters 18, 19).
   b) Dilated cardiomyopathy (see Chapter 20).
   c) Hypertrophic cardiomyopathy (see Chapter 21).
   d) Ventricular septal defect (see Chapter 18).
   e) Patent ductus arteriosus (see Chapter 18).
   f) (Sub)aortic stenosis (see Chapter 18).
   g) Aortic valve insufficiency.
   h) Systemic hypertension (see Chapter 25).
   i) 'Athletic' heart.
   j) Hyperthyroidism.
   k) Mass lesion involving left heart (see Chapter 22).
   l) Acromegaly.
4) Right atrial and ventricular enlargement:
   a) Tricuspid valve insufficiency (see Chapters 18, 19).
   b) Atrial septal defect (see Chapter 18).
   c) Pulmonic stenosis (see Chapter 18).
   d) Heartworm disease (see Chapter 24).
   e) Tetralogy of Fallot (see Chapter 18).
   f) Other reversed-shunting congenital defects (see Chapter 18).
   g) Other causes of pulmonary hypertension (see Chapter 23).
   h) Mass lesion involving right heart (see Chapter 22).

CARDIAC CHAMBER ENLARGEMENT PATTERNS

Most diseases that cause cardiac dilation or hypertrophy affect at least two chambers; rarely is there isolated enlargement of one chamber. For example, mitral insufficiency leads to both LV and LA enlargement; pulmonic stenosis causes RV enlargement, a main pulmonary artery bulge, and, often, RA dilation. Nevertheless, enlargement of specific chambers and great vessels is described individually. The orientation of normal cardiac chambers and major vessels is shown (39–42). Typical enlargement patterns are illustrated (43). Regions of an imaginary clock face superimposed on the cardiac silhouette are often used to describe areas of enlargement, especially on DV/VD views. Specific cardiac chamber enlargement can occur with some diseases even when the overall VHS is normal.

Left atrium

The LA is the most dorsocaudal chamber of the heart, although its auricular appendage extends cranially to the left (39, 40, and 6, p. 12). On a lateral view, the LA bulges dorsally and caudally as it enlarges. The left and possibly right mainstem bronchi are pushed dorsally (44, 45). Left mainstem bronchus compression occurs with severe LA enlargement, especially on expiration. In cats the caudal heart border is normally quite straight on a lateral view; LA enlargement causes subtle to marked convexity of the dorsocaudal heart border, with elevation of the mainstem bronchi (46, 47).

On DV/VD views, the mainstem bronchi are pushed laterally and curve slightly around a markedly enlarged LA; this is sometimes referred to as the 'bowed-legged cowboy sign'. Left auricular enlargement causes a bulge in the 2- to 3-o'clock position of the cardiac silhouette in cats and dogs. LA enlargement increases the opacity of the caudal heartbase. Massive enlargement sometimes appears as a large, rounded soft tissue mass summated over the centro-caudal cardiac silhouette (44, 45).

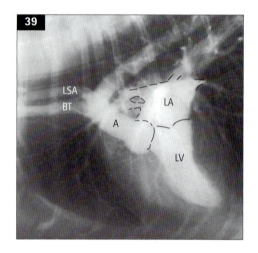

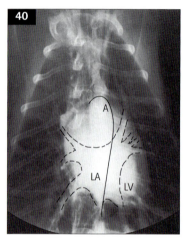

39, 40 Lateral (39) and DV (40) views from a normal nonselective venogram (levo phase) in a 4-year-old dog, showing pulmonary venous inflow, left cardiac chambers, and aorta. A = aorta; BT = brachiocephalic trunk; LA = left atrium; LSA = left subclavian artery; LV = left ventricle.

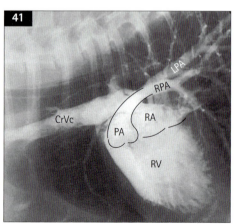

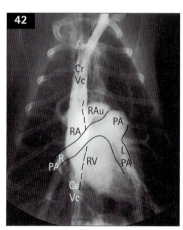

41, 42 Lateral (41) and DV (42) views from a normal nonselective venogram (dextro phase) in a 4-year-old dog, highlighting the cranial vena cava, right cardiac chambers, and pulmonary arterial tree. CaVc = caudal vena cava; CrVc = cranial vena cava; LPA = left pulmonary artery; PA = main pulmonary artery; RA = right atrium; RAu = right auricle; RPA = right pulmonary artery; RV = right ventricle.

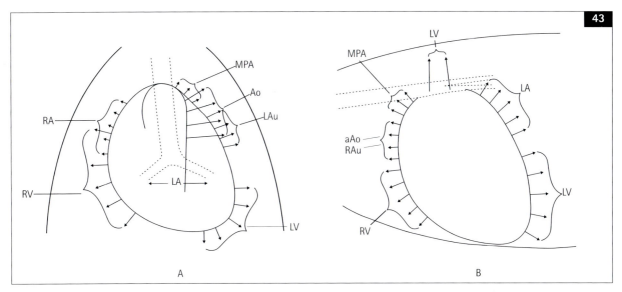

43 Diagrams illustrating common enlargement patterns of heart chambers and great vessels on DV (left) and lateral (right) radiographic views. aAo = ascending aorta; Ao = aorta (descending); LA = left atrium; LAu = left auricle; LV = left ventricle; MPA = main pulmonary artery; RA = right atrium; RAu = right auricle; RV = right ventricle.

44, 45 LV and massive LA enlargement are seen in this 11-year-old neutered male Poodle with chronic mitral insufficiency. Note the tracheal elevation and main bronchus compression on the lateral view (**44**). On the DV view (**45**), the left auricular region is prominently distended and the main bronchi are pushed laterally. The left atrium appears summated over the LV, with its caudal border (small arrows) distinct from the ventricular apex (large arrow).

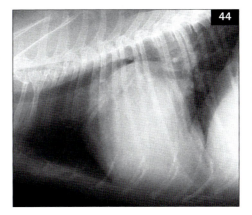

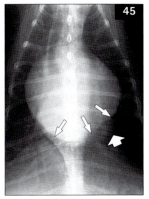

46, 47 Hypertrophic obstructive cardiomyopathy caused marked LA enlargement in this 5-year-old neutered male Burmese cat. Note the mild convexity of the dorsocaudal heart border and tracheal elevation on the lateral view (**46**) and widening of the cranial heart borders on the DV view (**47**). The pointed appearance of the LV apex is maintained, creating a so-called 'Valentine'-shaped heart silhouette. Distended and tortuous pulmonary veins entering the LA (increased opacity just dorsocaudal to the LA on lateral view) result from chronically high left heart filling pressure.

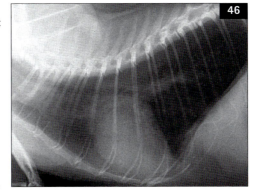

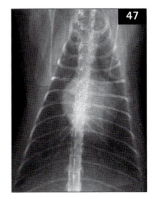

LA size is not only a function of the pressure or volume load imposed, but also the duration of the overload. For example, mitral regurgitation of slowly increasing severity may result in massive LA enlargement without pulmonary edema if there was time for chamber dilation at relatively low pressure. Conversely, rupture of chordae tendineae causes acute valvular regurgitation. When atrial pressure rises quickly, pulmonary edema can develop with little radiographic evidence of LA enlargement.

Left ventricle

LV enlargement is manifested on a lateral view by a taller heart and elevation of the tracheal bifurcation (carina) and caudal vena cava. The caudal trachea appears closer and more parallel to the spine (44, 45). The caudal heart border becomes convex, with the apex still against the sternum.

On DV/VD views, the heart usually looks elongated. There is rounding and enlargement in the 2 o'clock to 5 or 6 o'clock area. Many cats with hypertrophic cardiomyopathy (see Chapter 21) maintain a pointed appearance to the cardiac apex; concurrent atrial enlargement leads to the classic 'valentine'-shaped silhouette (46, 47, p. 39). Other affected cats show apex rounding and more generalized cardiomegaly.

Right atrium

RA enlargement may cause a bulge of the cranial heart border and widening of the cardiac silhouette on a lateral view. Sometimes, the trachea is elevated over the cranial portion of the heart. On DV/VD views, bulging of the cardiac silhouette occurs in the 9- to 11-o'clock position. Because the RA is largely superimposed on the RV, differentiation from RV enlargement is difficult, but concurrent enlargement of both chambers is common.

Right ventricle

RV enlargement (dilation or hypertrophy) usually causes increased widening and convexity of the cranioventral heart border on a lateral view (48, 49). The trachea over the cranial heart border appears elevated. An increased VHS is not always present, especially with RV hypertrophy (pressure overload). With marked RV enlargement and relatively normal left heart size, the apex is elevated from the sternum, especially on the right lateral view. The carina and caudal vena cava are also elevated. Because of breed variation in chest conformation, the degree of sternal contact of the cardiac silhouette is not a reliable sign of RV enlargement.

The heart on DV/VD views tends to take on a reverse-D configuration if left-sided enlargement is absent. The apex may be shifted leftward and the right heart border bulges to the right, with widening and rounding of the 6- to 9- o'clock area.

EVALUATION OF INTRATHORACIC BLOOD VESSELS

AORTA

In cats the aortic arch is often more prominent than in dogs on a lateral view. Older cats especially may have a wavy, undulating appearance to the thoracic aorta (50–52)[2, 6]. On DV/VD views, the aortic arch can become large, with a prominent knob at the junction of the aortic arch and descending aorta[3, 6]. Arterial blood

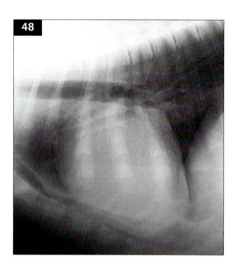
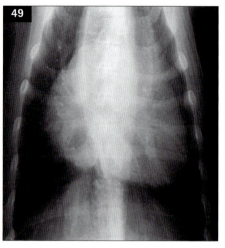

48, 49 RV and RA enlargement resulted from tricuspid valve dysplasia in this 5-month-old male Irish Wolfhound. The heart is widened, with apex elevation on the lateral view (48). On the DV view (49), the right heart border bulges prominently and the apex is shifted leftward.

pressure should be checked, but not all these cats are hypertensive. On DV/VD views in both dogs and cats, it is easier to identify the thoracic aorta near the diaphragm, then follow it cranially to assess its contour.

The aorta and main pulmonary artery tend to dilate in response to chronic arterial hypertension or increased turbulence (e.g. poststenotic dilation). Subaortic stenosis (see Chapter 18) causes the ascending aorta to dilate. Because this region is located within the mediastinum, dilation here may be difficult to see; however, widening and increased opacity of the dorsocranial heart shadow is often observed. Turbulence induced by a patent ductus arteriosus causes localized dilation of the descending aorta just caudal to the aortic arch. This 'ductus bump' is seen on DV/VD views in the 2- to 3-o'clock area (see Chapter 18).

MAIN PULMONARY ARTERY

Dilation of the main pulmonary trunk appears as a bulge superimposed over the trachea at the cranial heartbase on lateral radiograph. On DV/VD views in the dog, main pulmonary trunk enlargement causes a bulge in the 1- to 2-o'clock position; valvular pulmonic stenosis or pulmonary hypertension are the usual causes (see Chapters 18, 23, and 24). In the cat the main pulmonary trunk is slightly more medial and is usually obscured within the mediastinum.

LOBAR PULMONARY ARTERIES AND VEINS

The size and appearance of the pulmonary vasculature should be closely examined. Arteries and veins should be the same size. Four pulmonary vascular patterns are commonly described (see below).

The cranial lobar vessels are easiest to evaluate on a lateral view. Vessels in the nondependent ('up-side') lung are clearest, more ventral, and larger than in the dependent lung[2, 3]. The pulmonary arteries are dorsal to the accompanying veins and bronchi. The right pulmonary artery passes ventral to the carina and appears end-on as a round/oval opacity. The width of the cranial lobar vessels is measured where the vessels cross the 4th rib in dogs, or at the cranial heart border (4th to 5th rib) in cats. These vessels are normally no wider than 0.5–1 times the diameter of the proximal 1/3 of the 4th rib[2, 3].

On DV/VD views, the caudal lobar vessels are easier to see. Caudal lobar arteries originate cranial to the tracheal bifurcation and lie lateral to their accompanying bronchi and veins. Caudal lobar veins enter the heart caudal to the tracheal bifurcation. Caudal lobar vessels are measured where they cross the 9th rib (dogs) or 10th rib (cats). Normal vessels are 0.5–1 times the width of the rib where they cross.

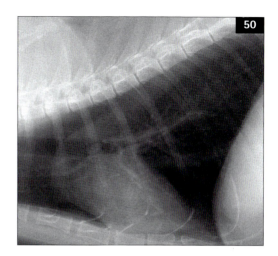

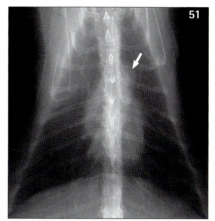

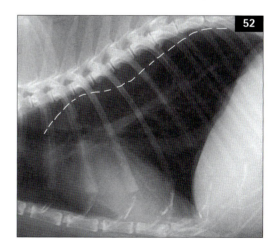

50–52 The heart tends to be more horizontally aligned to the sternum in older cats than in younger cats, as seen in this 15-year-old spayed female Himalayan (50) and this 17-year-old neutered male mixed breed cat (52). A prominent aortic arch and wavy or redundant thoracic aorta may be seen on the lateral views (50 and 52). The large aortic arch creates a knob-like appearance (arrow) on the DV view in the Himalayan (51).

Undercirculation pattern

Pulmonary undercirculation is characterized by narrowed pulmonary arteries and veins, along with an increased lucency of the lung fields (38, p. 37, and 53). Severe dehydration, hypovolemia, obstruction to RV inflow, right-sided congestive heart failure, and tetralogy of Fallot can cause this pattern. Some animals with pulmonic stenosis appear to have pulmonary undercirculation. Pulmonary overinflation and overexposure of radiographs also minimize the appearance of pulmonary vessels.

Overcirculation pattern

An overcirculation pattern occurs when the lungs are hyperperfused (54). Left-to-right cardiac shunts, overhydration, and other hyperdynamic states can

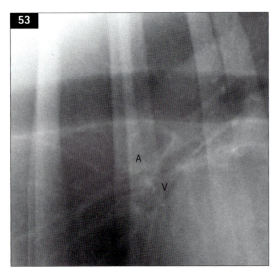

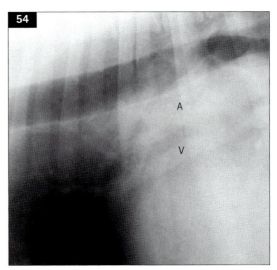

53, 54 Pulmonary vascular patterns. (53) Pulmonary undercirculation pattern (arteries and veins are both small) in a 3-year-old male Rottweiler with untreated hypoadrenocorticism. (54) Pulmonary overcirculation pattern (arteries and veins are both large) in a 2-year-old male Labrador Retriever with left-to-right shunting PDA.

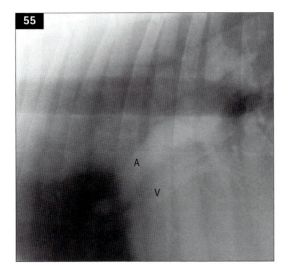

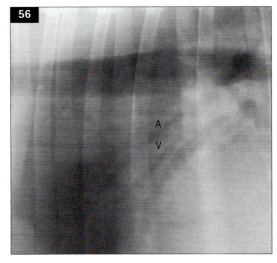

55 Enlarged pulmonary arteries in a 6-year-old neutered male mixed breed dog with pulmonary hypertension from severe heartworm disease. A = artery; V = vein.

56 Distended pulmonary veins caused by left-sided CHF in a 9-year-old spayed female Dalmation with DCM and MR. A = artery; V = vein.

cause this. Pulmonary arteries and veins are both large. The increased pulmonary perfusion also causes a generally increased lung opacity ('haziness').

Pulmonary arteries larger than veins
Pulmonary arteries larger than their accompanying veins indicate pulmonary arterial hypertension (55). The dilated pulmonary arteries can become tortuous and blunted, with poor visualization of the terminal portions. Heartworm disease is a common cause (see Chapter 24); patchy to diffuse interstitial pulmonary infiltrates also are seen often with heartworm disease.

Pulmonary veins larger than arteries
Prominent pulmonary veins are a sign of venous congestion, usually from left-sided congestive heart failure. On a lateral view, the cranial lobar veins are larger and denser than their accompanying arteries and may sag ventrally (56). Dilated and sometimes tortuous pulmonary veins may be seen entering the dorsocaudal aspect of an enlarged LA in dogs and cats with chronic pulmonary venous hypertension. However, dilated pulmonary veins are not always seen in patients with left-sided heart failure, especially after diuretic therapy. Cats with acute cardiogenic pulmonary edema can show enlargement of both pulmonary veins and arteries.

VENA CAVA
The cranial vena cava is not seen as a separate structure, but normally forms the straight ventral border of the cranial mediastinum. The caudal vena cava (CaVC) on a lateral view normally angles cranioventrally toward the heart from its juncture with the diaphragm. Enlargement of either ventricle pushes the CaVC–heart juncture dorsally, causing a more horizontal CaVC orientation.

The diameter of the CaVC is approximately that of the descending thoracic aorta, although its size changes with respiration. Persistent widening of the CaVC suggests increased caval pressure and can be seen with RV failure, cardiac tamponade, pericardial constriction, or other obstruction to right heart inflow (57). Based on a study in dogs with right-sided heart disease, the following ratios between CaVC diameter and other thoracic structures are indicative of abnormal CaVC distension[9]:
- CaVC/aortic diameter (at the same intercostal space as CaVC measurement) >1.5;
- CaVC/length of the thoracic vertebra directly above the tracheal bifurcation >1.3;
- and CaVC/width of right 4th rib (just ventral to the spine) >3.5.

A thin vena cava can be associated with hypovolemia, poor venous return, or pulmonary overinflation.

EVALUATION OF PULMONARY PARENCHYMA

PULMONARY PATTERNS
Increased pulmonary opacity has been categorized into bronchial, vascular, alveolar, and diffuse or nodular interstitial patterns. Prominent bronchial markings can occur from aging changes or bronchial mineralization. Bronchial wall thickening results from accumulation of cellular infiltrates or edema. Thick end-on bronchi have been described as 'donuts'; from the side the thickened parallel walls have been called 'tramlines'. Abnormally dilated bronchi (bronchiectasis) can result from chronic severe airway disease.

Pulmonary overcirculation causes a vascular pattern of increased lung opacity (see above). A diffuse or unstructured increase in interstitial opacity can occur with early or resolving pulmonary edema or some cellular infiltrates (e.g. diffuse lymphoma). However, mild diffuse opacity or 'haziness' is often related to nonpathologic causes such as aging, fat accumulation, expiration, or underexposed film[2]. Obesity tends to reduce maximal lung expansion, which also contributes to increased pulmonary opacity. Nodular interstitial opacities result from end-on vessels, soft tissue masses, granulomas, and external causes (e.g. nipples, ticks).

Alveolar patterns obscure the tissue margins of adjacent structures (such as the heart, vessels, and diaphragm), producing the silhouette sign.

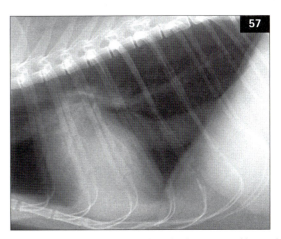

57 Abnormal caudal vena caval distension in a 5-year-old spayed female mixed breed cat with a large ventricular septal defect, moderate pulmonary hypertension, and tricuspid regurgitation.

Air bronchograms become visible as the severity of alveolar infiltration progresses. These are branching lucent lines caused by air-filled bronchi surrounded by fluid opacity. The distribution of an alveolar pattern can be patchy throughout several lung lobes, or localized to certain regions or an individual lobe. Etiologies include edema, infections, contusion, hemorrhage, and some tumors.

Reduced lung opacity can occur with pulmonary hyperinflation (e.g. feline asthma), bronchiectasis, film overexposure, or as a normal variation. Overly lucent lungs can be mistaken for pneumothorax.

PULMONARY EDEMA

Pulmonary edema initially accumulates in the interstitium around vessels and bronchi, causing radiographically ill-defined vessels and thickened bronchial walls[10]. As the edema worsens, areas of fluffy or mottled fluid opacity progressively become more confluent. Alveolar edema produces greater opacity in the lung fields, obscures vessels and outer bronchial walls, and creates air bronchograms.

The distribution of these pulmonary infiltrates often helps characterize their cause. Cardiogenic pulmonary edema in dogs is typically located in dorsal and perihilar areas, and is often bilaterally symmetric

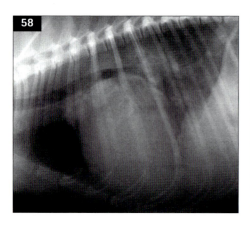

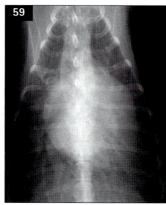

58, 59 The cardiogenic pulmonary edema from chronic MR has a classic dorsohilar, bilaterally symmetric distribution in lateral (**58**) and DV (**59**) radiographic views in this 10-year-old, spayed female Keeshond.

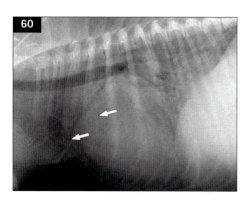

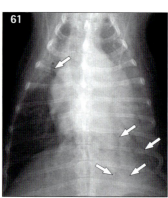

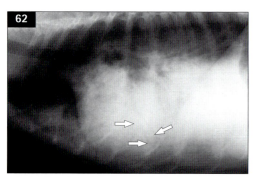

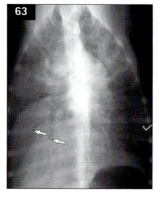

60–63 (**60, 61**) Cardiogenic pulmonary edema from severe, chronic MR is asymmetrically distributed in the right cranial and left lung fields in this 10-year-old male Schnauzer. (**62, 63**) Atypical distribution of cardiogenic edema is also observed in a 10-year-old neutered male Doberman Pinscher with DCM. Arrows indicate air bronchograms.

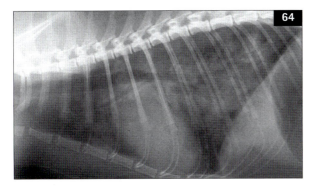

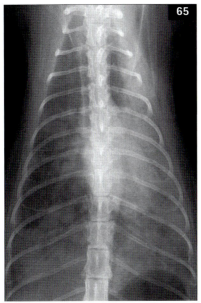

64, 65 Diffuse, patchy interstitial and alveolar infiltrates are common with cardiogenic pulmonary edema in cats. As shown in this two-year-old neutered male cat with HCM. Air in the stomach (aerophagia) is also common with respiratory distress.

(58, 59); however, some dogs with cardiogenic edema have an asymmetric or concurrent ventral distribution of opacities (60–63). Cats with cardiogenic edema usually have an uneven and patchy distribution of opacities, which either extends throughout the lung fields or is concentrated in the middle zones (64, 65).

Other classic patterns of pulmonary infiltrate distribution have been described. Noncardiogenic pulmonary edema tends to be bilateral and dorsocaudal. Infiltrates from bacterial pneumonia usually gravitate to cranioventral regions. Lung lobe atelectasis or torsion tends to be lobar or regional and accompanied by a mediastinal shift[2].

EVALUATION OF THE PLEURAL SPACE

PLEURAL EFFUSION

As free pleural fluid accumulates between lung lobes, wedge-shaped areas of soft tissue/fluid opacity that 'point' toward the center of the chest become visible. On a lateral view, ventral opacity (fluid) separates the lungs from the sternum. On DV/VD views, this opacity separates the lung lobes from each other and the chest wall (66–68). The cardiac silhouette is better visualized on a VD view because the fluid collects at the dorsal aspect of the thorax; however, this position may exacerbate respiratory distress. Large volume pleural effusion causes partial lung collapse, rounding of lobar borders, and silhouetting of the cardiac and mediastinal shadows. Pleural fluid and reduced lung expansion hinder recognition of pulmonary parenchymal infiltrates. Other findings that often accompany cardiogenic pleural effusion include a wide CaVC, cardiomegaly, hepatomegaly, and abdominal effusion.

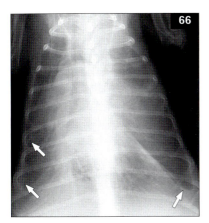

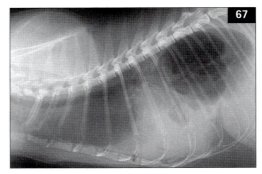

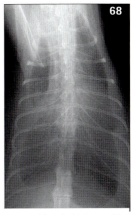

66–68 (66) Mild pleural effusion is seen as narrow, wedge-shaped fluid opacity (arrows) between lung lobes in a 10-year-old male Maltese with chronic heart failure from mitral and tricuspid regurgitation. (67, 68)Large-volume pleural effusion impedes lung expansion, causing retracted and rounded pulmonary borders in a 4-year-old spayed female cat with chronic hypertrophic obstructive cardiomyopathy.

Some conditions can mimic small volume pleural effusion. Pleural fibrosis in old dogs accentuates pleural fissure lines, but the peripheral areas do not look thicker or wedge-shaped, as with effusion. Fat within the caudal mediastinum, between caudally located lung lobes, or lining the chest wall can also mimic pleural effusion.

PNEUMOTHORAX

The lateral view is more sensitive for detecting a small volume of free air in the pleural space[2]. The lung border appears separated from the diaphragm and dorsal thoracic wall; the heart shifts toward the dependent lung and looks 'elevated' off the sternum. On DV/VD views, the lungs retract from the chestwall; a DV view more easily reveals free air, which rises to the widest (dorsal) part of the thorax. With larger amounts of free air, the relatively collapsed lungs appear more opaque.

Pneumothorax is sometimes misdiagnosed on a lateral view when the heart appears to be separated from the sternum, as with hypovolemia (microcardia), very narrow deep-chested conformation, lung hyperinflation, left lateral recumbency, or causes of a mediastimal shift. On DV/VD views, skin folds are sometimes mistaken for pneumothorax. Regions where free air is suspected should be carefully inspected; subtle markings from vessels or bronchi indicate aerated lung is present.

REFERENCES

1 Farrow CS, Green R, Shively M (1994) *Radiology of the Cat*. Mosby, St Louis, pp. 46–130.

2 O'Brien RT (2001) *Thoracic Radiography for the Small Animal Practitioner*. Teton NewMedia, Jackson.

3 Coulson A, Lewis ND (2002) *An Atlas of Interpretive Radiographic Anatomy of the Dog and Cat*. Blackwell Science, Oxford.

4 Buchanan JW, Bücheler J (1995) Vertebral scale system to measure canine heart size in radiographs. *J Am Vet Med Assoc* **206**:194.

5 Sleeper MM, Buchanan JW (2001) Vertebral scale system to measure heart size in growing puppies. *J Am Vet Med Assoc* **219**:57–59.

6 Moon ML, Keene BW, Lessard P *et al.* (1993) Age-related changes in the feline cardiac silhouette. *Vet Radiol Ultrasound* **34**:315–320.

7 Toal RL, Losonsky JM, Coulter DB *et al.* (1985) Influence of cardiac cycle on the radiographic appearance of the feline heart. *Vet Radiol* **26**:63–69.

8 Litster AL, Buchanan JW (2000) Vertebral scale system to measure heart size in radiographs of cats. *J Am Vet Med Assoc* **216**:210–214.

9 Lehmkuhl LB, Bonagura JD, Biller DS *et al.* (1997) Radiographic evaluation of caudal vena cava size in dogs. *Vet Radiol Ultrasound* **38**:94–100.

10 Ware WA, Bonagura JB (1999) Pulmonary edema. In: *Textbook of Canine and Feline Cardiology*, 2nd edn. PR Fox, D Sisson, NS Mose (eds). WB Saunders, Philadelphia, pp. 251–264.

4
Overview of Electrocardiography

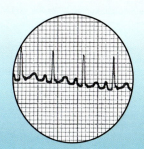

GENERAL PRINCIPLES

The electrocardiogram (ECG) records the electrical activity (depolarization and repolarization) of cardiac muscle from the body surface and provides information on heart rate, rhythm, and intracardiac conduction. ECG findings may also suggest the presence of specific chamber enlargement, myocardial disease, ischemia, pericardial disease, certain electrolyte imbalances, and some drug toxicities. However, the ECG does not record cardiac mechanical activity; therefore, the ECG by itself cannot be used to diagnose congestive heart failure, assess the strength (or even presence) of cardiac contractions, or predict whether the patient will survive anesthetic or surgical procedures.

This chapter reviews basic guidelines for ECG acquisition, interpretation, and ambulatory monitoring. ECG features typical of specific diseases are discussed more fully in the chapters describing those conditions. Approaches to managing abnormal cardiac rhythms are found in Chapter 17. Other means of evaluating cardiac electrical activity, such as intra-cardiac recording[1], high resolution (signal averaged) ECG[2], and heart rate variability (HRV) analysis[3–6] are not discussed here (see references for more information).

The normal cardiac rhythm originates in the sinoatrial (SA) node and follows the cardiac conduction pathway illustrated in figure **9** (p. 13). ECG waveforms, P-QRS-T (**69**), are generated as the heart muscle is depolarized and then repolarized (see Chapter 1). The QRS complex as a whole represents electrical activation of ventricular muscle, regardless of whether individual Q, R, or S components, or variations thereof, are present or absent. The configuration of the QRS complexes depends on the lead recorded as well as the electrical activation pattern of the ventricles; there is some variation from animal to animal. *Table 7* (p. 48) summarizes the events underlying ECG waveforms and time intervals.

ECG LEAD SYSTEMS

Several standard leads are used to evaluate cardiac electrical activity (*Table 8*, p. 48). The orientation of a lead with respect to the heart is called the lead axis. A lead records the depolarization and repolarization waves that are aligned with it. If the direction of myocardial activation parallels the lead axis, a relatively large deflection will be recorded. As the angle between the lead axis and the direction of the activation wave increases (up to 90 degrees), the ECG deflection in that lead becomes smaller. The ECG deflection is isoelectric when the activation wave is perpendicular to the lead axis. Each lead has a positive and a negative pole or direction. A positive ECG deflection will be recorded if the cardiac activation wave moves toward the positive pole (electrode) of the lead. If the wave of

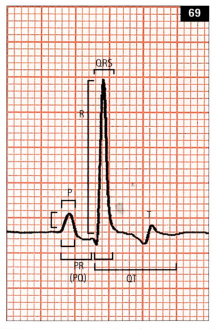

69 P-QRS-T from a dog. Lead II at 50 mm/sec, 1 cm = 1 mV. Waveforms and intervals are indicated. Each small box is 0.02 seconds in duration (X axis) and 0.1 mV in amplitude (Y axis).

Table 7 Normal ECG waveforms.

Waveform	Description
P	Atrial muscle activation wave; normally is positive in leads II and aVF.
PR interval	Also called PQ interval; includes duration of atrial muscle activation, and conduction over the AV node, bundle of His, and Purkinje fibers. Measure from onset of P wave to onset of QRS complex.
QRS comples	Ventricular muscle activation wave; by definition, Q is the first negative deflection (if present), R the first positive deflection, and S is the negative deflection after the R wave.
J point	Junction point between end of QRS complex and ST-T.
ST segment	Represents the period between ventricular depolarization and repolarization (correlates with phase 2 of the action potential).
T wave	Ventricular muscle repolarization wave.
QT interval	Total time of ventricular depolarization and repolarization. Measure from onset of QRS complex through end of T wave.

Table 8 ECG lead systems.

1) Standard bipolar limb leads:

   a) I   RA (−) compared with LA (+).

   b) II   RA (−) compared with LL (+).

   c) III   LA (−) compared with LL (+).

2) Augmented unipolar limb leads:

   a) aVR   RA (+) compared with average of LA and LL (−).

   b) aVL   LA (+) compared with average of RA and LL (−).

   c) aVF   LL (+) compared with average of RA and LA (−).

3) Unipolar chest leads:

   a) V_1, rV_2 (CV_5RL)   5th right ICS near sternum.

   b) V_2 (CV6LL)   6th left ICS near sternum.

   c) V_3 6th left ICS, equidistant between V_2 and V_4.

   d) V_4 (CV6LU)   6th left ICS near costochondral junction.

   e) V_5 and V_6 Spaced as for V_3 to V_4, continuing dorsally in 6th left ICS.

   f) V_{10} Over dorsal spinous process of 7th thoracic vertebra.

4) Orthogonal leads:

   a) X   Lead I (right to left) in the frontal plane.

   b) Y   Lead aVF (cranial to caudal) in the midsagittal plane.

   c) Z   Lead V_{10} (ventral to dorsal) in the transverse plane.

RA = right arm; LA = left arm; LL = left leg; ICS = intercostal space.

depolarization travels away from the positive pole, a negative deflection will be recorded in that ECG lead[7].

Both bipolar and unipolar ECG leads are used clinically. The standard bipolar leads record electrical potential differences between two electrodes on the body surface; the lead axis is oriented between these two points. The augmented unipolar leads employ a recording (positive) electrode on the body surface. The negative pole of the unipolar leads is formed by 'Wilson's central terminal' (V), which is essentially the average of the other electrodes and is analogous to the center of the heart (or zero).

Standard limb leads

The standard limb lead system records cardiac electrical activity in the frontal plane (i.e. that depicted by a DV or VD radiograph). Left-to-right and cranial-to-caudal currents are recorded[8]. The six standard frontal leads (hexaxial lead system), superimposed on the torso, are illustrated (**70, 71**).

Other lead systems

Unipolar chest (precordial) leads 'view' the heart from the transverse plane (**72**). The orthogonal lead system views the heart in three perpendicular planes (*Table 8*).

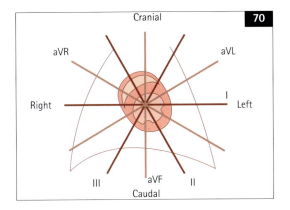

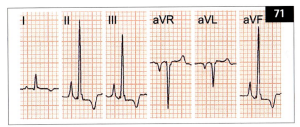

70, 71 (70) Diagram illustrating the orientation of the six standard limb leads with respect to the heart in the frontal plane. The outline of the thorax is drawn around the cardiac ventricles. Note that the leads are labeled at their positive pole. (See text and *Table 8*) (71). ECG complexes from a normal dog. Leads as labeled. Lead II at 25 mm/sec, 1 cm = 1 mV.

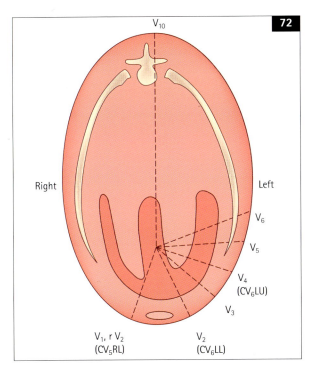

72 Diagram illustrating the orientation of selected chest leads with respect to the heart in the transverse plane. The cardiac ventricles, rib, and thoracic vertebra are indicated within the outline of the thorax. (See text and *Table 8*.)

RECORDING THE ECG

For standard ECG recording, the animal is placed in right lateral recumbency on a nonconducting surface. The forelimbs are held parallel to each other and perpendicular to the torso. Other body positions can alter the recorded waveform amplitudes and affect the calculated mean electrical axis (MEA)[9-11]; however, if the only information needed is heart rate and rhythm, almost any recording position is adequate. The animal is gently held in position to minimize movement artifacts. A better quality tracing is obtained when the animal is relaxed and quiet. Holding the patient's mouth shut to discourage panting or placing a hand on the chest of a trembling animal may be helpful.

Forelimb electrodes are placed at or slightly below the elbows, not touching the chest wall or each other. Hindlimb electrodes are placed at the stifles or hocks. ECG contact paste or, less ideally, alcohol is used to ensure good skin contact when using alligator clip or plate electrodes. Communication between two electrodes via a bridge of paste or alcohol, or by physical contact, should be avoided.

A good ECG recording has a clean baseline, with minimal artifact from patient movement and no electrical interference. The ECG complexes should be centered and totally contained within the printed grid so that neither the top nor bottom of the QRS complex is clipped off. If the complexes are too large to fit entirely within the grid, the calibration should be changed from standard (1 cm = 1 mV) to 1/2 standard (0.5 cm = 1 mV). To measure waveform amplitude, the calibration used for recording each lead must be known. A calibration square wave (1 mV amplitude) should be inscribed during the recording. The paper speed and lead(s) recorded must also be identified.

APPROACH TO ECG INTERPRETATION

A consistent approach to ECG interpretation is recommended. If the tracing is of adequate quality (i.e. all complexes within the grid, minimal artifact), the paper speed, lead(s) used, and calibration are identified. Then the heart rate, heart rhythm, and MEA are determined. Finally, individual waveforms are measured.

The heart rate is the number of complexes (or beats) per minute. This can be calculated by counting the QRS complexes within a 3 or 6 second period and then multiplying by 20 or 10, respectively. Some ECG machines inscribe one-second marks on the paper during recording. Some one-channel recorders use paper with small vertical hash marks at the top margin that can be used to calculate time elapsed (e.g. at 25 mm/sec there are 3 seconds between two marks, at 50 mm/sec there are 1.5 seconds). If the heart rhythm is regular, 3,000 divided by the number of small boxes (at paper speed 50 mm/sec) between the onset (or R wave peak) of successive QRS complexes equals the approximate heart rate. However, because variation in heart rate is common, especially in dogs, estimating the average heart rate over several seconds is usually more accurate and practical than calculating an instantaneous heart rate. *Table 9* lists normal heart rate ranges for sinus rhythms in dogs and cats.

The heart rhythm is evaluated by scanning the ECG for irregularities and identifying individual waveforms. Common rhythm abnormalities are described below. The presence and pattern of P waves and QRS-T complexes are determined first. The relationship between P waves and QRS-T complexes is then evaluated. Calipers are useful for assessing the regularity and interrelationships of the waveforms. Estimation of MEA is described below (p. 60).

Although heart rate and rhythm can be assessed using any lead, waveforms and intervals are usually measured using lead II (**69**). Waveform amplitudes are recorded in millivolts (mV) and durations in seconds. Only one thickness of the inscribed pen line should be included for each measurement. At a paper speed of 25 mm/sec, each small (1 mm) box on the ECG grid is 0.04 seconds in duration from left to right. At a paper speed of 50 mm/sec, each small box equals 0.02 seconds. At standard calibration, a deflection of the pen up or down 10 small boxes (1 cm) equals 1 mV. *Table 9* contains normal ECG reference ranges for cats and dogs. While measurements for most normal animals fall within these ranges, measurements for some subpopulations can fall

Table 9 ECG reference ranges for dogs and cats.

	Dog	Cat
Heart rate	70–160 beats/minute (adults)* to 220 beats/minute (puppies)	120–240 beats/minute
Mean electrical axis (frontal plane)	+40 to +100 degrees	0–+160 degrees
Measurements (lead II)		
P-wave duration (maximum)	0.04 sec (0.05 sec, giant breeds)	0.035–0.04 sec
P-wave height (maximum)	0.4 mV	0.2 mV
PR interval	0.06–0.13 sec	0.05–0.09 sec
QRS complex duration (maximum)	0.05 sec (small breeds) 0.06 sec (large breeds)	0.04 sec
R-wave height (maximum)	2.5 mV (small breeds) 3 mV (large breeds)†	0.9 mV, any lead; <1.2 mV QRS total, any lead
ST segment deviation	<0.2 mV depression <0.15 mV elevation	< 0.1 mV deviation
T wave	Normally <25% of R wave height; can be positive, negative, or biphasic	Maximum 0.3 mV; can be positive (most common), negative, or biphasic
QT interval duration	0.15–0.25 (to 0.27) sec; varies inversely with heart rate	0.12–0.18 (range 0.07–0.2) sec; varies inversely with heart rate
Chest leads		
V₁, rV₂	Positive T wave	R wave 1.0 mV maximum in chest leads
V₂₋₃	S wave 0.8 mV maximum; R wave 2.5 mV maximum†	
V₄₋₆	S wave 0.7 mV maximum; R wave 3 mV maximum†	
V₁₀	Negative QRS; negative T wave (except Chihuahua)	R/Q <1.0; negative T wave

Each small box on the ECG paper grid is 0.02 sec wide at 50 mm/sec paper speed, 0.04 sec wide at 25 mm/sec, and 0.1 mV high at a calibration of 1 cm = 1 mV.

* Range may extend lower for large breeds and higher for toy breeds.
† May be greater in young (under 2 years old), thin, deep-chested dogs.

outside[12, 13]. Manual frequency filters are available on many ECG machines. Activating the frequency filter can markedly attenuate some waveform voltages, although baseline artifact is reduced. The effects of filtering on QRS amplitude may complicate the assessment for ECG chamber enlargement criteria.

CARDIAC RHYTHM ASSESSMENT

SINUS RHYTHM AND VARIATIONS

Sinus rhythm is the normal cardiac rhythm, manifested by the P-QRS-T waveforms described previously (73, 74). The P waves are positive in the caudal leads (II and aVF), the PR (PQ) intervals are consistent, and the QRS to QRS intervals occur regularly, with less than 10% variation in timing. Sinus arrhythmia (described below) is a normal variation. Normal sinus-origin QRS complexes are narrow and upright in leads II and aVF, but, intraventricular conduction disturbance or ventricular enlargement can change this (see below).

The general term 'bradycardia' describes a heart rhythm that is slow, without identifying its site of origin. Conversely, a 'tachycardia' is a heart rhythm with a faster rate than normal. Sinus bradycardia and sinus tachycardia are rhythms that originate in the sinus node, but have a rate that is slower or faster, respectively, than normal for the species. Some causes of sinus bradycardia and tachycardia are listed in *Table 10* (p. 52).

Sinus arrhythmia

This normal rhythm variation is characterized by a cyclic slowing and speeding of the sinus rate. It is usually, but not always, associated with respiration (75). With respiratory sinus arrhythmia, the sinus rate increases on inspiration and decreases with expiration as a result of fluctuations in vagal tone through the respiratory cycle. The term 'wandering pacemaker' refers to a cyclic change in P wave configuration, related to a shift in pacemaker location, that may accompany sinus arrhythmia[14]. The P waves become taller and spiked during inspiration and flatter in expiration. This is considered a normal variation in dogs. Sinus arrhythmia occurs commonly in dogs, especially brachycephalic breeds. It also occurs often in resting cats[15], although it is not usually seen clinically in this species. Exaggerated sinus arrhythmia occurs in some dogs with chronic pulmonary disease.

Sinus arrest

A pause in sinus activity lasting at least twice the duration of the patient's usual QRS to QRS interval is known as sinus arrest (76). Either an escape beat (see below) or resumption of sinus activity can follow. Long pauses cause weakness or syncope. Sinus arrest cannot be differentiated with certainty from SA block by the surface ECG. Sinus arrest is a major feature of the sick sinus syndrome (see Chapter 13, p. 133 and Chapter 17).

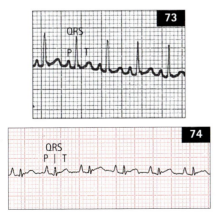

73, 74 Examples of normal sinus rhythm from two cats. Lead II at 25 mm/sec, 1 cm = 1 mV. The QRS complexes can be quite small in normal cats (74).

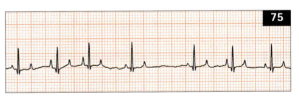

75 Normal sinus arrhythmia with wandering pacemaker in a male English Cocker Spaniel with pneumonia and chronic bronchial disease. The QRS complexes are abnormally small in this case. Lead II at 25 mm/sec, 1 cm = 1 mV.

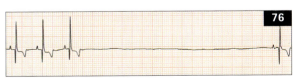

76 Episode of sinus arrest (~4 seconds duration) with resumption of sinus rhythm in an old American Cocker Spaniel with pulmonary carcinoma and hypertension. Lead II at 25 mm/sec, 0.5 cm = 1 mV.

ABNORMAL (ECTOPIC) CARDIAC RHYTHMS

Concepts of origin and timing

Depolarizations originating from outside the sinus node (ectopic complexes) are abnormal and cause an arrhythmia (or 'dysrhythmia'). Ectopic complexes are described by their general site of origin and their timing (77, 78). The configuration of the ECG waveforms is used to surmise whether the ectopic complexes are likely of supraventricular (atrial, AV junctional) or ventricular origin. Impulses of supraventricular origin are usually conducted through the ventricles via the normal conduction pathway, so their QRS is like that of sinus complexes. The configuration of ventricular origin complexes reflects their abnormal (and usually slower) pattern of conduction through the ventricular muscle. Timing refers to whether the ectopic complex occurs earlier than the next expected sinus impulse ('premature') or after a longer pause ('late' or 'escape'). Escape complexes represent activation of a subsidiary pacemaker (see Chapter 1).

Premature ectopic complexes occur singly or in multiples; groups of three or more comprise an

---

Table 10 Causes of sinus bradycardia and tachycardia.

1) Sinus bradycardia:	2) Sinus tachycardia:
a) Hypothermia.	a) Hyperthermia/fever.
b) Hypothyroidism.	b) Hyperthyroidism.
c) Cardiac arrest (before or after).	c) Anemia/hypoxia.
d) Drugs (e.g. certain tranquilizers and anesthetics, beta-blockers, calcium channel-blockers, digoxin).	d) Heart failure.
e) Increased intracranial pressure.	e) Shock.
f) Brainstem lesions.	f) Hypotension.
g) Severe metabolic disease (e.g. uremia, hyperkalemia).	g) Sepsis.
h) Ocular pressure.	h) Anxiety/fear.
i) Carotid sinus pressure.	i) Excitement.
j) Other causes of high vagal tone (e.g. lower airway, pharyngeal or GI obstruction).	j) Exercise.
k) Sinus node disease.	k) Pain.
l) Normal variation (athletic dog).	l) Drugs (anticholinergics, sympathomimetics).
	m) Toxicities (e.g. chocolate, hexachlorophene).
	n) Electric shock.
	o) Other causes of high sympathetic tone.

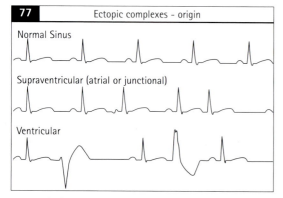

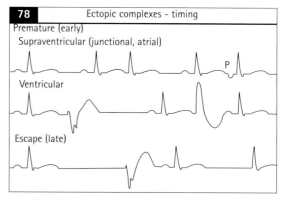

77, 78 (77) Diagram illustrating the concept of supraventricular versus ventricular origin of ectopic complexes. Impulses arising from atrial tissue or the AV junctional region have a QRS configuration similar to the patient's sinus-origin complexes. (78) Concept of premature versus late (escape) timing of ectopic impulses. (Both figures from Ware WA (2003) Diagnostic tests for the cardiovascular system. In *Small Animal Internal Medicine* (3rd edn). (eds RW Nelson, CG Couto) Mosby, St Louis, p.19, with permisssion.)

episode of tachycardia. Episodes of tachycardia can be brief ('paroxysmal') or prolonged ('sustained'). When a premature complex follows each normal QRS, a bigeminal pattern exists; the origin of the premature complexes determines whether the rhythm is described as atrial or ventricular bigeminy.

Supraventricular premature complexes

These originate above the AV node, either in the atria or the AV junctional area. Because their conduction into and through the ventricles occurs via the normal conduction pathway, their QRS configuration is normal (unless an intraventricular conduction disturbance or enlargement is also present). Premature complexes that arise within the atria (i.e. outside the SA node) are usually preceded by an abnormal P wave (positive, negative, or biphasic configuration) called a P' wave (**79–82**). Sometimes, the premature impulse is conducted slowly (prolonged P'Q interval) or with a bundle branch block pattern. If an ectopic P' wave occurs before the AV node has completely repolarized, the impulse may not be conducted into the ventricles (an example of physiologic AV block). Junctional complexes are usually not preceded by a P' wave;

however, conduction backward ('retrograde') into the atria can cause a negative P' wave after, superimposed on, or even preceding the resulting QRS complex.

The more general term 'supraventricular' is used if it is unclear whether the origin of ectopic complex(es) is atrial or junctional. Clinically, distinguishing whether the arrhythmia originates from above the AV node (supraventricular) or below it (ventricular) is most important. Supraventricular premature activity usually depolarizes the sinus node as well. This resets the sinus rhythm and creates a 'noncompensatory pause' (i.e. the interval between the sinus complexes preceding and following the premature complex is less than that of three consecutive sinus complexes).

Atrial tachycardia

Atrial tachycardia originates from an abnormal atrial focus or atrial reentry (repetitive activation from electrical conduction around an abnormal circuit within the atria). P' waves are often hidden within the QRS-T complexes. Atrial tachycardia is usually a regular rhythm unless the rate exceeds the AV node's ability to conduct every impulse, in which case

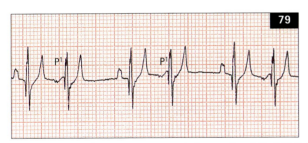

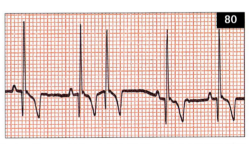

79, 80 Examples of premature supraventricular ectopic activity. (79) Atrial bigeminy in a 6-year-old female Irish Wolfhound several days after surgery for gastric dilatation-volvulus. Note the notched negative P' waves. (80) Junctional premature complex in an older male Doberman Pinscher.

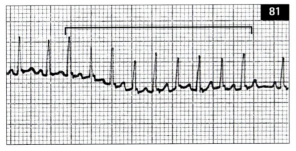

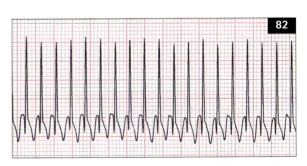

81, 82 (81) Paroxysm of supraventricular tachycardia (bracket) in an old Siamese cat. (82) Sustained supraventricular tachycardia at a rate of 360 beats/minute in a Labrador Retriever puppy with mitral and tricuspid valve dysplasia. All examples are lead II at 25 mm/sec, 1 cm = 1 mV.

physiologic AV block and irregular QRS intervals result (83). A consistent ratio of atrial to ventricular activation (e.g. 2:1 or 3:1 AV conduction) preserves the regularity of this arrhythmia. If atrial tachycardia occurs with delayed intraventricular conduction, causing a bundle branch block pattern on ECG, differentiation from ventricular tachycardia can be difficult (84, 85). Atrial tachycardia in dogs may have a rate of 260–380 beats/minute.

Reentrant supraventricular tachycardia

Supraventricular tachycardia may involve a reentrant pathway incorporating the AV node. This can occur with functional dissociation of slow- and fast-conducting fibers within the AV node, or by means of an abnormal accessory pathway[16, 17]. A premature supraventricular or ventricular impulse can initiate such a tachycardia, which is maintained by impulses looping around the functionally divided AV node or the AV node and accessory pathway. In animals with ventricular preexcitation (see p. 59), episodes of reentrant supraventricular tachycardia often normalize or prolong the PR interval, cause retrograde P' waves, and normalize the QRS complexes (unless a simultaneous intraventricular conduction disturbance is present)[18]. Persistent tachycardia eventually leads to myocardial failure[1, 19].

Atrial flutter

Atrial flutter results from a single (macro-) reentrant wave of electrical activation regularly cycling through the atria[16], usually at >300–400 cycles/minute. The ventricular response rate depends on AV conduction and may be irregular or regular. 'Sawtooth' flutter waves, representing recurrent atrial activation, are seen between QRS complexes on the ECG (86). Atrial flutter is not a stable rhythm; it often degenerates into atrial fibrillation (AF) but may convert to sinus rhythm. Atrial enlargement is a common underlying factor.

Atrial fibrillation

Atrial electrical activation is rapid and chaotic because of multiple small reentrant circuits in AF[16]. The AV node is bombarded by these chaotic electrical impulses; therefore, AV conduction velocity and recovery time determine the (ventricular) heart rate. No P waves are seen on ECG because no uniform atrial depolarization wave occurs. The ECG baseline usually shows irregular undulations known as fibrillation (f) waves (87, 88). Because organized electrical activity is absent, effective atrial contraction is lacking. AF causes an irregular heart rhythm, usually with a rapid rate. Heart rate in patients with AF should be monitored using the ECG because heart rate estimation by auscultation can be highly inaccurate[20]. Most often the QRS complexes are

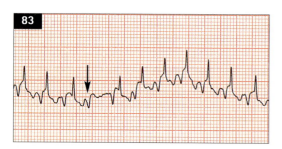
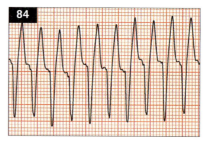
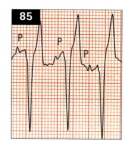

83–85 (83) Atrial tachycardia at a rate of 200 beats/minute in an 11-year-old Yorkshire Terrier. Note the negative P' waves, one of which is not conducted (arrow). Lead II at 25 mm/sec, 1 cm = 1 mV. (84) Wide-complex supraventricular tachycardia in a male Irish Wolfhound with preexisting right bundle branch block is easily mistaken for ventricular-origin tachycardia. (85) Sinus rhythm in the dog in 84. Examples 84 and 85 are lead II at 25 mm/sec, 0.5 cm = 1 mV.

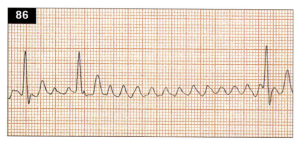

86 Atrial flutter recorded in an older German Shorthaired Pointer with heart failure. Note the sawtooth flutter waves at a rate of about 330/minute. Lead II at 50 mm/sec, 1 cm = 1 mV.

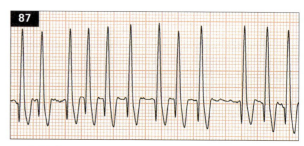

87 Atrial fibrillation with an uncontrolled ventricular rate of 220/minute in a 4-year-old male Labrador Retriever with DCM. Note the irregular R to R intervals and small 'f' waves in the baseline. Lead II at 25 mm/sec, 0.5 cm = 1 mV.

normal in configuration because intraventricular conduction is normal, although minor variation in the height of the QRS complexes is common; however, intermittent or sustained bundle branch blocks can occur. AF tends to be a consequence of severe atrial disease and enlargement in dogs and cats; it is usually preceded by intermittent atrial tachyarrhythmias and, perhaps, atrial flutter. Sometimes, AF occurs spontaneously in giant breed dogs without evidence of underlying heart disease; the heart rate is generally normal in these dogs[21].

Ventricular premature complexes

Ventricular premature complexes (VPCs, or PVCs) originating below the AV node have a different and usually wider QRS configuration compared with the patient's sinus complexes (89–92). VPCs generally are not conducted backward through the AV node

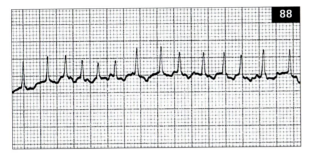

88 AF in a cat with cardiomyopathy and marked LA enlargement. Besides the irregular QRS timing there is some variation in QRS size as well. Lead II at 25 mm/sec, 1 cm = 1 mV.

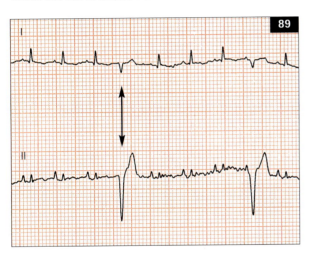

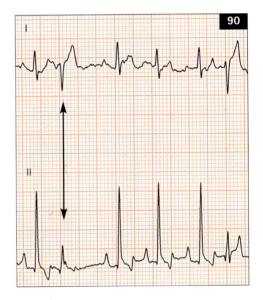

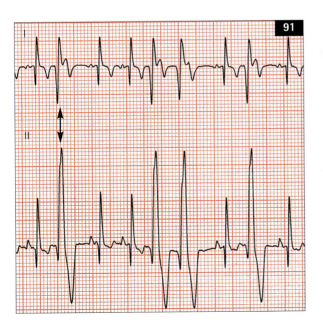

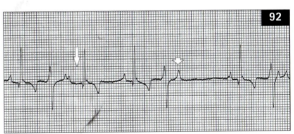

89–92 Examples of VPCs. Various VPC configurations (arrows) are illustrated in leads I and II from a 15-year-old male cat with HCM (89), a young female Great Dane with exercise intolerance (90), and a 4-year-old female Boxer with type III Boxer cardiomyopathy (91), all at 25 mm/sec, 1 cm = 1 mV. (92) VPCs in an old, asymptomatic dog caused concealed retrograde AV nodal conduction as evidenced by PR prolongation after the 1st VPC (arrow) and block of the P wave coinciding with the T wave of the 2nd VPC (arrowhead). Lead II at 50 mm/sec, 1 cm = 1 mV.

into the atria, so the sinus rate continues undisturbed and the VPC is followed by a 'compensatory pause' in the sinus rhythm; however, partial (concealed) retrograde conduction into the AV node may affect conduction of a subsequent sinus impulse (92). When VPC configuration is consistent, the complexes are described as uniform, unifocal, or monomorphic. When the VPCs in an individual have differing ECG configurations, they are said to be multiform or polymorphic. Multiform VPCs (or ventricular tachycardia) may indicate greater electrical instability.

Ventricular tachycardia

Three or more sequential VPCs, generally at a rate >100/minute, constitutes ventricular tachycardia (93–96). Although some variation can occur, ventricular tachycardia usually has regular QRS intervals. Nonconducted sinus P waves may be seen superimposed on or between the ventricular complexes. Successful conduction of a sinus P wave into the ventricles, uninterrupted by another VPC, is known as a 'capture beat'. If the normal ventricular activation sequence is interrupted by another VPC, a 'fusion' complex can result. The configuration of a fusion complex represents a melding of the normal QRS and that of the VPC. Fusion complexes are preceded by a P wave and shortened PR interval; they are often observed at the onset or end of a paroxysm of ventricular tachycardia. Identification of P waves, whether conducted or not, or fusion complexes (95) helps in differentiating ventricular tachycardia from supraventricular tachycardia with abnormal intraventricular conduction.

Polymorphic ventricular tachycardia has QRS complexes that vary in size, polarity, and often rate. Sometimes, the QRS configuration appears to rotate around the isoelectric baseline (96). Torsades de pointes is a specific form of such polymorphic ventricular tachycardia associated with Q-T interval prolongation[16, 22].

Accelerated idioventricular rhythm

Also called idioventricular tachycardia, this rhythm occurs at a rate of about 60–100 beats/minute in the dog (perhaps somewhat faster in the cat). Because the rate is slower than true ventricular tachycardia, it is considered a less serious rhythm disturbance. An accelerated idioventricular rhythm may appear during the slower phases of sinus arrhythmia and be suppressed as the sinus rate increases (97). This is commonly observed in dogs recovering from motor vehicle trauma[23]. Clinically, the arrhythmia may cause no deleterious effects, although deterioration to ventricular tachycardia is possible.

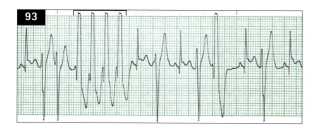

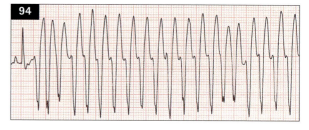

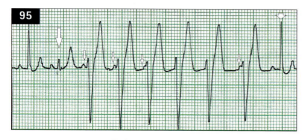

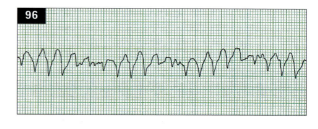

93–96 Examples of VT. (93) Brief paroxysm of upright VT (bracket) as well as multiform VPCs in a young Golden Retriever with syncope from intracardiac rhabdomyosarcoma. (94) Slightly irregular VT at a rate of about 280/minute in a 9-year-old female Dalmation with DCM and episodic weakness. (95) A fusion complex (large arrow) is seen at the onset of paroxysmal VT (~140 beats/minute) in a dog. The sinus complex following the VT is known as a capture beat (arrowhead). Nonconducted sinus P waves can be seen between some of the ectopic ventricular complexes (small arrows). (96) Polymorphic VT (Torsades de pointes) in an 11-year-old Siamese cat with DCM and a prolonged sinus QT interval. All examples are lead II, 25 mm/sec, 1 cm = 1 mV.

Ventricular fibrillation

This lethal rhythm is characterized by multiple reentrant circuits causing chaotic electrical activity in the ventricles (**98**). Consequently, like the atria during AF, the ventricles have no coordinated mechanical activity and cannot function as a pump. Ventricular fibrillation (VF) may be 'coarse', with larger ECG baseline oscillations, or 'fine'. Ventricular flutter, appearing as rapid sine-wave activity on the ECG (**99**), may precede fibrillation. Ventricular asystole is the absence of ventricular electrical (and mechanical) activity.

Escape complexes and rhythms

Escape complexes occur after a pause in the dominant (usually sinus) rhythm. If the sinus rhythm does not resume, the escape focus continues to fire at its own intrinsic rate. Escape rhythms are usually regular. Escape activity can originate from automatic cells in the atria, the AV junction, or the ventricles (**100, 101**). Ventricular escape rhythms (idioventricular rhythms) usually occur at a rate <40–50 beats/minute in the dog and <100 beats/minute in the cat. Junctional escape rhythms usually range from 40–60 beats/minute in the dog. Because escape activity is a cardioprotective mechanism, escape complexes and escape rhythms should not be suppressed with antiarrhythmic drugs.

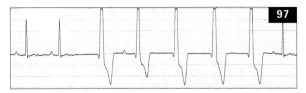

97 An accelerated idioventricular rhythm was manifest when the sinus rate slowed in a dog that had been hit by a car the previous day. This uniform ventricular rhythm, at about 80 beats/minute, caused no hemodynamic instability and resolved spontaneously. Lead II at 25 mm/sec, 0.5 cm = 1 mV.

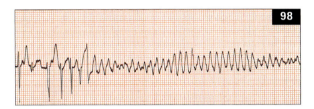

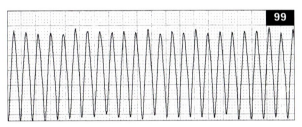

98, 99 (98) Irregular ventricular ectopic activity degenerated into coarse VF at the right side of this strip in a dog under anesthesia. (99) Ventricular flutter in a 7-year-old Great Pyrenees with severe DCM; shortly after this strip was recorded the dog developed VF and could not be resuscitated. Both examples are lead II at 25 mm/sec, 1 cm = 1 mV.

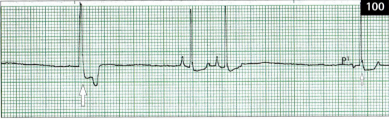

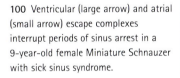

100 Ventricular (large arrow) and atrial (small arrow) escape complexes interrupt periods of sinus arrest in a 9-year-old female Miniature Schnauzer with sick sinus syndrome.

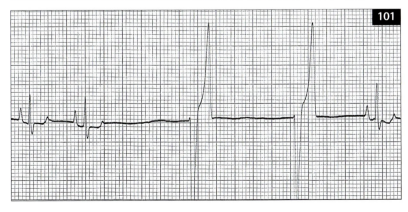

101 A ventricular escape rhythm began after sinus arrest occurred in a 12-year-old, male Scottish Terrier with heart failure and syncope. Both examples are lead II at 25 mm/sec, 1 cm = 1 mV.

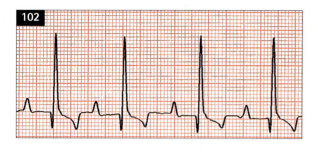

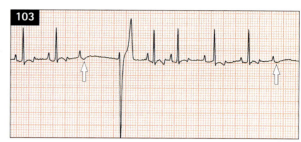

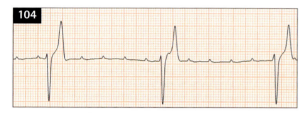

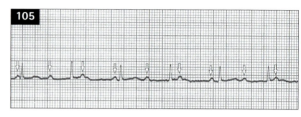

102–105 Examples showing AV block of varying severity. (**102**) Sinus rhythm with 1st degree AV block in a 13-year-old female American Cocker Spaniel receiving digoxin for chronic compensated heart failure from mitral valve disease. PR interval is 0.16 sec; lead II at 50 mm/sec, 1 cm = 1 mV. (**103**) Sinus arrhythmia with 2nd degree AV block in a 12-year-old female West Highland White Terrier with chronic pulmonary disease. Note that the Ta wave (arrows; see text, p. 61) is easily seen after the blocked P waves. A ventricular escape complex also occurred after the first blocked P wave. Lead II at 25 mm/sec, 1 cm = 1 mV. (**104**) 3rd degree (complete) AV block with a ventricular escape rhythm in a 12-year-old male Weimeraner. Note the consistent sinus P waves unrelated to the ventricular-origin escape complexes. Lead II at 25 mm/sec, 0.5 cm = 1 mV. (**105**) 3rd degree (complete) AV block with a ventricular escape rhythm in a cat with cardiomyopathy. The regular sinus P waves are indicated by arrows. Lead II at 50 mm/sec, 1 cm = 1 mV. (**105** courtesy Dr J Tyler.)

ABNORMAL CARDIAC CONDUCTION

Atrioventricular (AV) conduction disturbances
Abnormalities of AV conduction can result from excessive vagal tone, drugs (e.g. digoxin, xylazine, verapamil, and anesthetic agents), and organic disease of the AV node and/or intraventricular conduction system. Three degrees of AV conduction block severity are commonly described (**102–105**):
- First-degree AV block is abnormally prolonged conduction from atria to ventricles, although all impulses are conducted.
- Second-degree AV block is characterized by intermittent AV conduction; some P waves are not followed by a QRS complex. Many nonconducted P waves constitute high-grade 2nd degree heart block. Second-degree AV block has been subclassified. Mobitz type I (Wenckebach) is characterized by progressive prolongation of the PR interval before a nonconducted P wave occurs; it is frequently associated with disorders within the AV node itself and/or high vagal tone. Mobitz type II is characterized by uniform PR intervals preceding the blocked impulses and is more often associated with disease lower in the AV conduction system (bundle of His or major bundle branches). An alternate classification of 2nd degree AV block based on QRS configuration has also been described. Patients with type A 2nd degree block have a normal, narrow QRS configuration; those with type B 2nd degree block have a wide or abnormal QRS configuration, which suggests diffuse disease lower in the ventricular conduction system. Mobitz type I AV block is usually type A, whereas Mobitz type II is frequently type B. Supraventricular or ventricular escape complexes are common during long pauses in ventricular activation.
- Third-degree or complete AV block is present when no sinus (or supraventricular) impulses are conducted into the ventricles. P waves often indicate a regular sinus rhythm or sinus arrhythmia; however, the P waves are not temporally related to QRS complexes, which result from a (usually) regular ventricular escape rhythm.

Intraatrial conduction disturbances
Several abnormalities of intraatrial conduction can occur. SA block is conduction failure between the SA node and the surrounding atrial muscle. This cannot reliably be differentiated from sinus arrest on the ECG, although the interval between P waves is a multiple of the normal P to P interval in SA block. Prolonged sinus arrest or block can be followed by an atrial, junctional, or ventricular escape rhythm.

In atrial standstill, diseased atrial muscle prevents normal electrical and mechanical function,

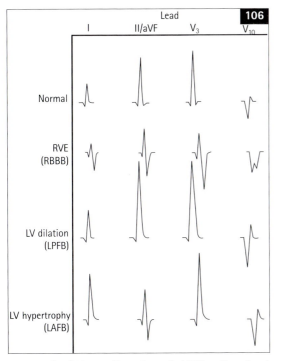

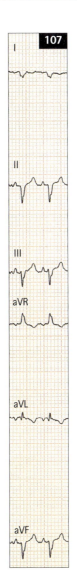

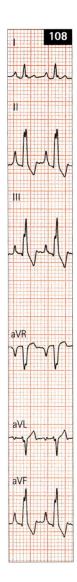

106–108 (106) Diagram illustrating typical QRS configurations in selected leads resulting from ventricular enlargement or conduction delay. (Modified from Ware WA (2003) Diagnostic tests for the cardiovascular system. In *Small Animal Internal Medicine* (3rd edn). (eds RW Nelson, CG Couto) Mosby, St Louis, p.16, with permission.) (107) Sinus rhythm with a RBBB pattern in a Manx cat with restrictive cardiomyopathy but no evidence for RVE. Leads as marked; 25 mm/sec, 1 cm = 1 mV. (108) Sinus rhythm with a left bundle branch block in a 9-year-old female Dalmation with dilated cardiomyopathy; QRS complexes were unusually small in this dog. Leads as marked; 25 mm/sec, 1 cm = 1 mV. LAFB = left anterior fascicular block; LPFB = left posterior fascicular block; LV = left ventricular; RBBB = right bundle branch block; RVE = right ventricular enlargement.

regardless of sinus node activity. P waves are absent and a junctional or ventricular escape rhythm develops. Hyperkalemia interferes with normal atrial function and can mimic atrial standstill (see p. 64).

Intraventricular conduction disturbances

Slowed or blocked impulse transmission within any of the major bundle branches causes an intraventricular conduction disturbance (aberrant conduction). The region of ventricular muscle served by a diseased bundle branch is activated late and slowly, which causes QRS widening and orientation of the terminal QRS forces toward the area of delayed activation (*Table 11* and 106–108). The right bundle branch or the left anterior or posterior fascicles of the left bundle branch can be affected singly or in combination. A block in all three major branches results in 3rd degree (complete) heart block. Right bundle branch block (RBBB) is sometimes identified in otherwise normal

dogs and cats, although it can result from disease or distension of the RV. Left bundle branch block (LBBB) is usually related to clinically relevant underlying disease of the LV (see below and 108). The left anterior fascicular block (LAFB) pattern is common with LV hypertrophy, such as in cats with hypertrophic cardiomyopathy.

Ventricular preexcitation

Early activation (preexcitation) of part of the ventricular myocardium can occur when an accessory conduction pathway bypasses the normal slow-conducting AV nodal pathway[1, 17]. Several types of preexcitation and accessory pathways have been described. Most cause a shortened PR interval. When the accessory pathway lies outside the AV node (extranodal), there is early depolarization of the ventricle distant to where ventricular activation normally begins. This causes early widening and slurring of the QRS by a so-called delta wave (**109**) and is characteristic of Wolff–Parkinson–White (WPW) type preexcitation. Other accessory pathways can connect the atria or dorsal areas of the AV node directly to the bundle of His. These cause a short PR interval, but not early QRS widening. Preexcitation can be intermittent or concealed (not evident on ECG). The danger with preexcitation is that reentrant supraventricular tachycardia can occur using the accessory pathway and AV node (also called AV reciprocating tachycardia). Usually, the tachycardia impulses travel into the ventricles via the AV node (antegrade or orthodromic conduction) and then back to the atria via the accessory pathway; however, sometimes the direction is reversed. Rapid AV reciprocating tachycardia can cause weakness, syncope, congestive heart failure, and death. The presence of the WPW pattern on ECG in conjunction with reentrant supraventricular tachycardia that causes clinical signs characterizes the WPW syndrome.

MEAN ELECTRICAL AXIS

The MEA describes the average direction of the ventricular depolarization process in the frontal plane. It represents the summation of the various instantaneous vectors that occur from the beginning until the end of ventricular muscle activation.

Estimation of the MEA helps the clinician identify major intraventricular conduction disturbances and/or ventricular enlargement patterns that shift the average direction of ventricular activation. Since the MEA is determined in the frontal plane, only the six frontal leads are used. By convention, the reference position of the leads is defined by degrees (from 0° to ±180°) around a circle (**110**). The positive pole (electrode) of most leads lies on the 'positive' side of the circle; however, it is important to note that the positive pole of leads aVR and aVL lie on the 'negative' side of the circle. The MEA can be

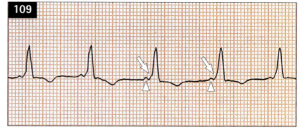

109 Sinus rhythm with ventricular preexcitation in a 4-month-old kitten with occasional syncope (AV reciprocating tachycardia suspected but not documented). Small P waves (arrowheads) are followed by delta waves (arrows), indicating early ventricular activation from an extranodal accessory pathway. Lead V6 at 50 mm/sec, 1 cm = 1 mV.

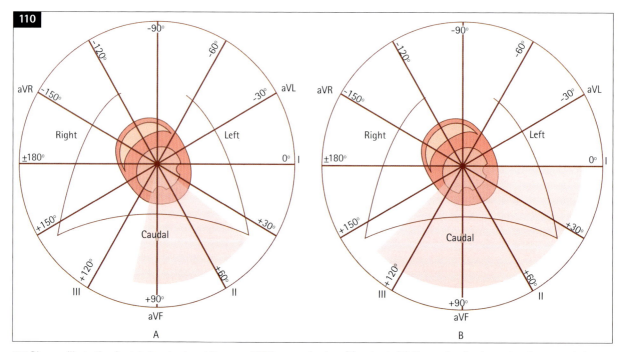

110 Diagram illustrating frontal plane leads and the normal MEA ranges for dogs (A) and cats (B). Conventional ± degree locations around the circle are indicated for all leads (see text). Each lead is labeled at its positive pole. (Modified from Ware WA (2003) Diagnostic tests for the cardiovascular system. In *Small Animal Internal Medicine* (3rd edn). (eds RW Nelson, CG Couto) Mosby, St Louis, p.14, with permission.)

Table 11 Ventricular chamber enlargement and conduction abnormality patterns.

1) Normal:
   a) Normal mean electrical axis.
   b) No S wave in lead I.
   c) R wave taller in lead II than in lead I.
   d) Lead CV6LL R wave larger than S wave.

2) Right ventricular enlargement:
   a) Right axis deviation.
   b) S wave present in lead I.
   c) S wave in V3 (CV6LL) larger than R wave or greater than 0.8 mV.
   d) Q-S (W-shaped QRS) in V10.
   e) Positive T wave in lead V10 (except Chihuahuas).
   f) Deep S wave in leads II, III, and aVF.

3) Right bundle branch block (RBBB):
   a) As for right ventricular enlargement with the end of the QRS prolonged (wide, sloppy S wave).

4) Left ventricular (concentric) hypertrophy:
   a) Left axis deviation.
   b) R wave in lead I taller than R wave in leads II or aVF.
   c) No S wave in lead I.

5) Left anterior fascicular block (LAFB):
   a) As for left ventricular hypertrophy, possibly with wider QRS.

6) Left ventricular dilation:
   a) Normal frontal axis.
   b) R wave taller than normal in leads II, aVF, and CV6LL.
   c) Widened QRS; slurring and displacement of ST segment and T-wave enlargement may also occur.

7) Left bundle branch block (LBBB):
   a) Normal frontal axis.
   b) Very wide and sloppy QRS.
   c) Small Q wave may be present in leads II, III, and aVF (incomplete LBBB, or left posterior fascicular block).

estimated by either of the following methods:
- Find the lead (I, II, III, aVR, aVL, or aVF) with the largest R wave (note: the R wave is a positive deflection). The positive electrode of this lead is the approximate MEA orientation.
- Find the lead (I, II, III, aVR, aVL, or aVF) with the most isoelectric QRS (positive and negative deflections are about equal). Then identify the lead perpendicular to this lead on the hexaxial lead diagram (**70, 71** [p. 49] and **110**). If the QRS in this perpendicular lead is mostly positive, the MEA is toward the positive pole of this lead. If the QRS in the perpendicular lead is mostly negative, the MEA is oriented toward the negative pole. If all leads appear isoelectric, the frontal axis is indeterminate. The normal MEA range for dogs and cats is shown (**110**).

CARDIAC CHAMBER ENLARGEMENT

Certain changes in ECG waveform patterns can suggest enlargement or conduction disturbance related to a particular cardiac chamber; however, cardiac enlargement sometimes occurs without these ECG changes.

ATRIAL ENLARGEMENT PATTERNS
LA enlargement commonly prolongs the P wave duration (also known as 'p mitrale'). Sometimes, the P wave is notched as well as wide. Slowed intraatrial conduction can also cause wide and notched P waves. RA enlargement may be manifest by tall, spiked P waves ('p pulmonale'). Atrial enlargement also often magnifies the usually obscured atrial repolarization (T_a) wave. The T_a wave appears as a brief baseline shift in the opposite direction of the P wave (see **103**, p. 58).

Table 12 Clinical associations of ECG enlargement patterns.

1) Left atrial enlargement:
   a) Mitral insufficiency (acquired or congenital).
   b) Cardiomyopathies.
   c) Patent ductus arteriosus.
   d) Subaortic stenosis.
   e) Ventricular septal defect.

2) Right atrial enlargement:
   a) Tricuspid insufficiency (acquired or congenital).
   b) Chronic respiratory disease.
   c) Interatrial septal defect.
   d) Pulmonic stenosis.

3) Left ventricular enlargement (dilation):
   a) Mitral insufficiency.
   b) Dilated cardiomyopathy.
   c) Aortic insufficiency.
   d) Patent ductus arteriosus.
   e) Ventricular septal defect.
   f) Subaortic stenosis.

4) Left ventricular enlargement (hypertrophy):
   a) Hypertrophic cardiomyopathy.
   b) Subaortic stenosis.

5) Right ventricular enlargement:
   a) Pulmonic stenosis.
   b) Tetralogy of Fallot.
   c) Tricuspid insufficiency (acquired or congenital).
   d) Severe pulmonary hypertension (including heartworm disease).

VENTRICULAR ENLARGEMENT PATTERNS
Right ventricle
Right axis deviation and an S wave in lead I are strong criteria for RV enlargement (or right bundle branch block). Other ECG changes can usually be found as well. Three or more of the criteria listed in *Table 11* are generally present when marked RV enlargement exists. Mild RV enlargement is often not evident on

ECG because LV activation forces are normally so dominant. A right bundle branch pattern can mimic or accompany RV enlargement.

Left ventricle
LV dilation and eccentric hypertrophy (see Chapter 1) often increase R-wave voltage in the caudal leads (II and aVF) and may widen the QRS. A complete LBBB or left posterior fascicular block pattern can mimic or accompany LV dilation. LV concentric hypertrophy is inconsistently associated with left axis deviation (left anterior fascicular block pattern). *Table 11* and **106–108** (p. 59) summarize ECG patterns seen in association with ventricular enlargement or conduction delay. Common clinical associations are noted in *Table 12*.

OTHER ECG ABNORMALITIES AND CONSIDERATIONS

SMALL VOLTAGE QRS COMPLEXES
In dogs, small voltage QRS complexes have been associated with pleural or pericardial effusions, obesity, intrathoracic mass lesions, hypovolemia, and hypothyroidism. They are occasionally seen in dogs without identifiable abnormalities. Small voltage QRS complexes are normal in cats.

ELECTRICAL ALTERNANS
Every other beat alteration in QRS complex size is known as electrical alternans. This is most often associated with large volume pericardial effusions,

which allow the heart to swing back and forth within the pericardium (see Chapter 22 and **485, 486**, p. 324).

ST-T ABNORMALITIES
The ST segment extends from the end of the QRS complex (also called the J-point) to the onset of the T wave, and represents the time between ventricular depolarization and the onset of repolarization. However, in dogs and cats the ST segment slopes into the T-wave without a clear demarcation because repolarization begins immediately after depolarization[24]. ST segment abnormalities can be primary (caused by abnormalities of the repolarization process) or secondary to abnormalities of ventricular depolarization. Deviation of the ST segment from the isoelectric baseline (**111, 112**) as well as changes in duration can occur. Elevation (>0.15 mV in dogs or >0.1 mV in cats) or depression (>0.2 mV in dogs or >0.1 mV in cats) of the J point and ST segment in leads I, II, or aVF can be caused by ischemia or other myocardial injury.

Secondary ST segment deviation occurs with ventricular hypertrophy, aberrant conduction, and some drugs (e.g. digoxin). Prominent T_a waves associated with atrial enlargement or tachycardia can mimic depression (pseudodepression) of the ST segment.

The T wave, representing ventricular muscle repolarization, may be positive, negative, or biphasic in normal cats and dogs. Differences in size, shape, or polarity from previous recordings in an individual animal are probably clinically important. Primary abnormalities of the T wave are related to factors affecting repolarization (**113**). Secondary changes are

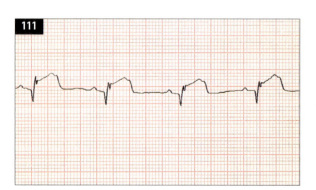

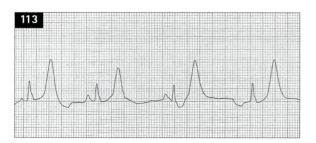

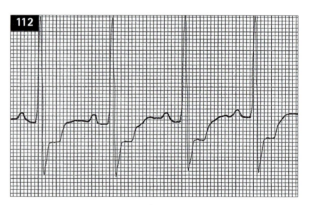

111–113 (111) Sinus rhythm with ST segment elevation in a 2-year-old Pomeranian with severe stenosis of the pulmonary valve. Ischemia of the markedly hypertrophied RV wall was suspected. **(112)** Sinus rhythm with ST segment depression in a 5-month-old Newfoundland with severe SAS and presumed LV ischemia. **(113)** Sinus rhythm with very large T waves in a 12-year-old Yorkshire Terrier without a cardiac murmur. Hypoxia from airway disease was suspected based on the history of cough and dyspnea. All examples are lead II at 50 mm/sec, 1 cm = 1 mV.

Table 13 Causes of ST segment, T Wave, and QT abnormalities.

1) Depressed J point/ST segment:
   a) Myocardial ischemia.
   b) Myocardial infarction/injury (subendocardial).
   c) Hyperkalemia or hypokalemia.
   d) Cardiac trauma.
   e) Secondary change (ventricular hypertrophy, conduction disturbance, VPCs).
   f) Digitalis ('sagging' appearance).
   g) Pseudodepression (prominent Ta).

2) Elevated J point/ST segment:
   a) Pericarditis.
   b) Left ventricular epicardial injury.
   c) Myocardial infarction (transmural).
   d) Myocardial hypoxia.
   e) Secondary change (ventricular hypertrophy, conduction disturbance, VPCs).
   f) Digoxin toxicity.

3) Prolonged QT interval:
   a) Hypocalcemia.
   b) Hypokalemia.

VPC = ventricular premature complex

   c) Quinidine toxicity.
   d) Ethylene glycol poisoning.
   e) Secondary to prolonged QRS.
   f) Hypothermia.
   g) Central nervous system abnormalities.

4) Shortened QT interval:
   a) Hypercalcemia.
   b) Hyperkalemia.
   c) Digitalis toxicity.

5) Large T waves:
   a) Myocardial hypoxia.
   b) Ventricular enlargement.
   c) Intraventricular conduction abnormalities.
   d) Hyperkalemia.
   e) Metabolic or respiratory diseases.
   f) Normal variation.

6) Tented T waves:
   a) Hyperkalemia.

Table 14 Effects of electrolyte abnormalities and selected drugs* on the ECG.

1) Hyperkalemia (see also p. 64 and 114–116):
   a) Peaked (tented) ± large T waves.
   b) QT interval abbreviation.
   c) Flat or absent P waves.
   d) Widened QRS.
   e) ST segment depression.

2) Hypokalemia:
   a) ST segment depression.
   b) Small, biphasic T waves.
   c) QT interval prolongation.
   d) Tachyarrhythmias.

3) Hypercalcemia:
   a) Few effects.
   b) Abbreviated QT interval.
   c) Prolonged conduction.
   d) Tachyarrhythmias.

4) Hypocalcemia:
   a) Prolonged QT interval.
   b) Tachyarrhythmias.

5) Digoxin:
   a) PR prolongation.
   b) Sinus bradycardia or arrest.
   c) 2nd- (or 3rd) degree AV block.
   d) Accelerated junctional rhythm.
   e) Ventricular premature complexes.
   f) Ventricular tachycardia.
   g) Paroxysmal atrial tachycardia with block.
   h) Atrial fibrillation with slow ventricular rate.

6) Quinidine/procainamide:
   a) Atropine-like effects.
   b) QT prolongation.
   c) AV block.
   d) Ventricular tachyarrhythmias.
   e) QRS widening.
   f) Sinus arrest.

7) Lidocaine:
   a) AV block.
   b) Ventricular tachycardia.
   c) Sinus arrest.

8) Beta blockers:
   a) Sinus bradycardia.
   b) PR prolongation.
   c) AV block.

9) Barbiturates/thiobarbiturates:
   a) Ventricular bigeminy.

10) Halothane/methoxyflurane:
   a) Sinus bradycardia.
   b) Ventricular arrhythmias (increased sensitivity to catecholamines, especially halothane).

11) Xylazine:
   a) Sinus bradycardia.
   b) Sinus arrest/sinoatrial block.
   c) AV block.
   d) Ventricular tachyarrhythmias, especially with halothane, epinephrine.

* Adverse or toxic effects

related to abnormalities of ventricular depolarization. Secondary ST-T changes tend to be in of opposite polarity to the main QRS deflection. *Table 13* lists some causes of ST-T abnormalities.

THE QT INTERVAL

The QT interval represents the total time of ventricular activation and repolarization. This interval varies inversely with average heart rate; faster rates have a shorter QT interval. Autonomic nervous tone, various drugs, and electrolyte disorders influence the duration of the QT interval (*Table 13*). Equations to predict expected QT duration have been derived for normal dogs[25] and cats[26] in an attempt to define more clearly the QT interval–heart rate relationship. Inappropriate prolongation of the QT interval can facilitate development of serious reentrant arrhythmias when the ventricular repolarization process is not uniform[27].

EFFECTS OF DRUGS AND ELECTROLYTE ABNORMALITIES ON THE ECG

Digoxin, antiarrhythmic agents, and anesthetic drugs often alter heart rhythm and/or conduction either by their direct electrophysiologic effects or by affecting autonomic tone. *Table 14* summarizes common ECG manifestations of these drug effects.

Abnormalities of potassium homeostasis have marked and complex influences on cardiac electrophysiology and, consequently, on the ECG. Noticeable ECG changes caused by other electrolyte disturbances occur infrequently (*Table 14*).

Hypomagnesemia has no reported effects on the ECG, but it can predispose to digoxin toxicity and arrhythmias and exaggerate the effects of hypocalcemia.

Hyperkalemia

Moderate hyperkalemia actually has an antiarrhythmic effect by reducing automaticity and enhancing repolarization speed and uniformity. However, rapid or severe increases in serum potassium concentration can cause arrhythmias, mainly because they slow conduction velocity and shorten the refractory period. Rising serum potassium concentration causes a progression of ECG changes (**114–117**). The earliest is usually a more narrow and peaked (tented) T wave. T wave changes begin as serum K^+ rises to near 6 mmol/l (6 mEq/l). The characteristic 'tented' T-wave appearance may be more apparent in some leads than in others.

SA nodal cells are relatively resistant to the effects of hyperkalemia and continue to function, although the sinus rate decreases. P waves appear flattened as serum K^+ approaches 7 mmol/l (7 mEq/l) and disappear above about 8 mmol/l (8 mEq/l). Despite progressive unresponsiveness of atrial muscle, specialized fibers can transmit sinus impulses to the AV node, resulting in a so-called sinoventricular rhythm.

Progressive QRS widening from slowing of intraventricular conduction also occurs as serum K^+ rises above 6 mmol/l (6 mEq/l). With severe hyperkalemia (>10 mmol/l [>10 mEq/l]) there may be activation of ectopic pacemakers, but eventually asystole occurs[7]. Hypocalcemia, hyponatremia, and acidosis accentuate

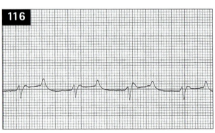

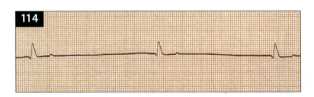

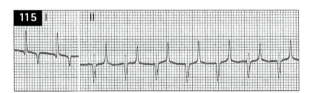

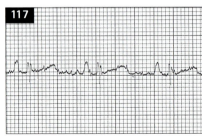

114, 115 Examples of the effects of marked hyperkalemia on the ECG. Note the peaked (tented) T waves, loss of P waves (sinoventricular rhythm), and widened QRS complexes. (114) Lead II at 50 mm/sec, 1 cm = 1 mV from a dog with hypoadrenocorticism; serum K^+ was 10.5 mmol/l (10.5 mEq/l). (115) Leads I and II at 25 mm/sec at 2 cm = 1 mV from a male cat with urethral obstruction; serum K^+ was 10.2 mmol/l (10.2 mEq/l).

116, 117 (116) Lead II at 50 mm/sec, 1 cm = 1 mV from a male cat with urethral obstruction; serum K^+ was not available. (117) Sinus rhythm with normal P waves is now evident 8 hours post-treatment in the cat in 116. The QRS complexes and T waves also appear normal. Some muscle tremor artifact is evident in this strip.

the ECG changes caused by hyperkalemia, whereas hypercalcemia and hypernatremia tend to counteract them.

Therapy for life-threatening hyperkalemia is aimed at promoting intracellular translocation of potassium, as well as removing the underlying cause. Sodium bicarbonate (1–2 mEq/kg, slow IV bolus) is generally effective, but can provoke hypocalcemia in some cats with urethral obstruction and hyperphosphatemia[28]. For severe hyperkalemia from feline urethral obstruction, regular insulin (0.25–0.5 U/kg IV) given with glucose (2 g/U insulin, diluted to a 10% solution) is recommended; subsequent fluid therapy should include 2.5–5 % dextrose. A third therapeutic option for severe hyperkalemia is 10% calcium gluconate (50–100 mg/kg; or 0.5–1.5 ml/kg, slow IV bolus)[28].

Hypokalemia

Hypokalemia may increase spontaneous automaticity of cardiac cells, as well as nonuniformly slow repolarization and conduction. These effects predispose to both supraventricular and ventricular arrhythmias. Hypokalemia can cause progressive ST segment depression, reduced T-wave amplitude, and QT interval prolongation. Severe hypokalemia can also increase QRS and P-wave amplitudes and durations. In addition, hypokalemia exacerbates digoxin toxicity and reduces the effectiveness of class I antiarrhythmic agents (see Chapter 17). Hypernatremia and alkalosis worsen the effects of hypokalemia on the heart. Concurrent magnesium deficiency may exacerbate the effects of and interfere with correction of hypokalemia.

COMMON ECG ARTIFACTS

Artifacts complicate ECG interpretation and can mimic arrhythmias. Some common ECG artifacts are illustrated (118–122). Electrical interference can be minimized or eliminated by properly grounding the ECG machine. Turning off other electrical equipment or lights on the same circuit, placing the animal on an

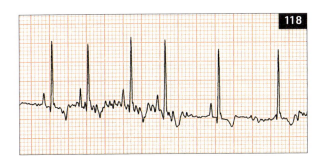

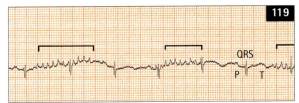

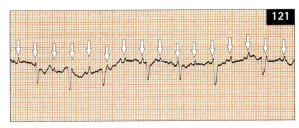

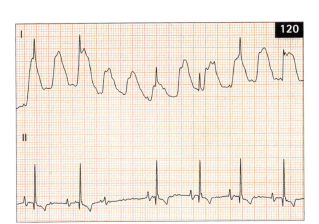

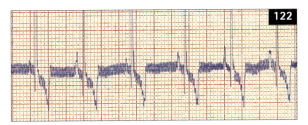

118–122 Examples of common ECG artifacts. (118) Intermittent shiver/muscle tremor artifact in a dog with sinus arrhythmia and wandering pacemaker. Lead II at 25 mm/sec, 1 cm = 1 mV. (119) Sinus rhythm with purr artifact (brackets) as well as mild 60 Hz interference (seen best superimposed on P and T waves and baseline segments in between) from a cat with cardiomyopathy. Lead II at 50 mm/sec, 1 cm = 1 mV. (120) Simultaneous lead I and II recording at 25 mm/sec, 1 cm = 1 mV, from a dog. Left limb movement caused by the dog's panting obscures the rhythm in lead I, but lead II clearly shows sinus arrhythmia with one blocked P wave (Mobitz I [Wenckebach] 2° AV block). (121) Lead III recording at 25 m/sec, 1 cm = 1 mV, from a 9-year-old cat with HCM, moderate pericardial effusion, and multiple myeloma. The large negative deflections could be mistaken for ventricular ectopic complexes; however, closer inspection reveals no accompanying 'T waves' and no disruption of the underlying sinus rhythm. The negative deflections occurred when the cat moved its leg. Arrows indicate sinus QRS complexes. (122) 60 Hz (electrical) interference is evident in the baseline of this lead aVF strip from a dog with sinus rhythm. 25 mm/sec, 1 cm = 1 mV.

electrically insulated pad, or having a different person restrain the animal may also help. ECG artifacts are sometimes confused with arrhythmias, but artifacts do not disturb the underlying cardiac rhythm. In contrast, ectopic complexes often disrupt the underlying rhythm and are followed by a T wave. Determining whether the ECG deflection in question changes the underlying rhythm and is also followed by a T wave usually allows the clinician to differentiate between intermittent artifacts and arrhythmias. Recording more than one lead simultaneously is also helpful.

AMBULATORY ECG

HOLTER MONITORING

Holter monitoring allows the continuous recording of cardiac electrical activity during normal daily activities, exercise, and sleep. Intermittent cardiac arrhythmias can be detected and quantified, and cardiac causes of syncope or episodic weakness can be identified (see Chapter 14). Holter monitoring is also used to assess antiarrhythmic drug therapy efficacy, and to screen for arrhythmias associated with cardiomyopathy or other diseases. The Holter monitor is a small battery-powered tape or digital recorder worn by the patient, typically for 24 hours. Two or three ECG channels are recorded from modified chest leads. During the recording period, the animal's activities are noted in a patient diary for later correlation with simultaneous ECG events. An event button on the Holter recorder can be pressed if syncope or other episode is witnessed.

The digititized Holter recording is analyzed using computer algorithms that classify the recorded complexes. Since fully automated computer analysis can result in significant misclassification of QRS complexes and artifacts from dog and cat recordings, interaction and editing by a trained Holter technician experienced with veterinary recordings is important for accurate analysis. A summary report and selected portions of the recording are enlarged and printed for examination by the clinician. In addition, a full disclosure print-out of the entire recording should be visually scanned and compared with the selected ECG strips as well as with the times of clinical signs and/or activities noted in the patient diary (see references for more information)[15, 29, 30]. Holter monitoring equipment and tape analysis are available through some commercial human Holter scanning services, many university veterinary teaching hospitals, and cardiology referral practices.

Normal animals can experience wide variation in heart rate throughout the day. Maximum sinus rates up to 300 beats/minute have been recorded with excitement or activity in dogs. Episodes of bradycardia (<50 beats/minute) are common, especially during quiet periods and sleep; heart rates as low as 17 beats/minute have been recorded[31]. Sinus arrhythmia, sinus pauses (sometimes for over 5 seconds), and occasional 2nd degree AV block also occur in normal dogs, especially at times when the mean heart rate is lower. In normal cats, heart rates also vary widely over 24 hours (from 68–294 beats/minute in one study)[15]. While regular sinus rhythm predominates in normal cats, sinus arrhythmia is evident at slower heart rates. VPCs occur only sporadically in normal dogs and cats; their prevalence likely increases only slightly with age.

CARDIAC EVENT RECORDING

Cardiac event recorders are smaller than typical Holter units and contain a microprocessor with a memory loop that can store a brief period of a single modified chest lead ECG. The event recorder can be worn for longer time periods, but it cannot store prolonged, continuous ECG activity[32]. Event recorders are used most often to discern whether episodic weakness or syncope is caused by a cardiac arrhythmia (see Chapter 14). When an episode is observed, the owner activates the recorder, which then stores the ECG from a predetermined time frame (e.g. from 45 seconds before activation to 15 seconds after). The stored recordings are sent via telephone to a receiving station for printing and analysis.

REFERENCES

1 Wright KN, Mehdirad AA, Giacobbe P et al. (1999) Radiofrequency catheter ablation of atrioventricular accessory pathways in 3 dogs with subsequent resolution of tachycardia-induced cardiomyopathy. *J Vet Intern Med* **13**:361–371.

2 Calvert CA (1998) High-resolution electrocardiography. *Vet Clin North Am: Small Anim Pract* **28**: 1429–1445.

3 Calvert CA (1998) Heart rate variability. *Vet Clin North Am: Small Anim Pract* **28**:1409–1425.

4 Matsunaga T, Harada T, Mitsui T et al. (2001) Spectral analysis of circadian rhythms in heart rate variability of dogs. *Am J Vet Res* **62**:37–42.

5 Malliani A, Pagani M, Lombardi F (1994) Physiology and clinical implications of variability of cardiovascular parameters with focus on heart rate and blood pressure. *Am J Cardiol* **73**:3C–9C.

6 Häggstrom J, Hamlin RL, Hansson K et al. (1996) Heart rate variability in relation to severity of mitral regurgitation in Cavalier King Charles Spaniels. *J Small Anim Pract* **37**: 69–75.

7 Mirvis DM, Goldberger AL (2001) Electrocardiography. In: *Heart Disease: A Textbook of Cardiovascular Medicine*, 6th edn. E Braunwald, DP Zipes, P Libby (eds). WB Saunders, Philadelphia, pp. 82–126.

8 Detweiler DK, Patterson DF (1965) The prevalence and types of cardiovascular disease in dogs. *Ann N Y Acad Sci* **127**:481–516.

9 Rishniw M, Porciello F, Erb HN et al. (2002) Effect of body position on the 6-lead ECG of dogs. *J Vet Intern Med* **16**:69–73.

10 Coleman MG, Robson MC (2005) Evaluation of six-lead electrocardiograms ontained from dogs in a sitting position or sternal recumbency. *Am J Vet Res* **66**:233–237.

11 Harvey AM, Faena M, Darke PGG et al. (2005) Effect of body position on feline electrocardiographic recordings. *J Vet Intern Med* **19**:533–536.

12 Hinchcliff KW, Constable PD, Farris JW et al. (1997) Electrocardiographic characteristics of endurance-trained Alaskan sled dogs. *J Am Vet Med Assoc* **211**:1138–1141.

13 Constable PD, Hinchcliff KW, Olson JL et al. (2000) Effects of endurance training on standard and signal-averaged electrocardiograms of sled dogs. *Am J Vet Res* **61**:582–588.

14 Miller MS, Tilley LP, Smith FWK. (1999) Electrocardiography. In: *Textbook of Feline and Canine Cardiology*. PR Fox, D Sisson, NS Moise (eds). WB Saunders, Philadelphia, pp. 67–106.

15 Ware WA (1999) Twenty-four hour ambulatory electrocardiography in normal cats. *J Vet Intern Med* **13**:175–180.

16 Olgin JE, Zipes DP (2001) Specific arrhythmias: diagnosis and treatment. In: *Heart Disease: A Textbook of Cardiovascular Medicine*, 6th edn. E Braunwald, DP Zipes, P Libby (eds). WB Saunders, Philadelphia, pp. 815–889.

17 Atkins CE, Wright KN (1995) Supraventricular tachycardia associated with accessory pathways in dogs. In: *Current Veterinary Therapy XII*. JD Bonagura, RW Kirk (eds). WB Saunders, Philadelphia, pp. 807–813.

18 Wright KN, Atkins CE, Kanter R (1996) Supraventricular tachycardia in four young dogs. *J Am Vet Med Assoc* **208**:75–80.

19 Atkins CE, Kanter R, Wright K et al. (1995) Orthodromic reciprocating tachycardia and heart failure in a dog with a concealed posteroseptal accessory pathway. *J Vet Intern Med* **9**:43–49.

20 Glaus TM, Hässig M, Keene BW (2003) Accuracy of heart rate obtained by auscultation in atrial fibrillation. *J Am Anim Hosp Assoc* **39**:237–239.

21 Brownlie SE (2000) Follow-up study of Irish Wolfhounds with three electrocardiographic abnormalities. Abstract. *J Small Anim Pract* **41**:392.

22 Baty CJ, Sweet DC, Keene BW (1994) Torsades de pointes-like polymorphic ventricular tachycardia in a dog. *J Vet Intern Med* **8**(6):439–42.

23 Snyder PS, Cooke KL, Murphy ST et al. (2001) Electrocardiographic findings in dogs with motor vehicle-related trauma. *J Am Anim Hosp Assoc* **37**:55–63.

24 Hamlin RL (2001) The ST segment of the electrocardiogram. In: *Proceedings of the 19th ACVIM Forum*, Denver, p. 88.

25 Oguchi Y, Hamlin RL (1993) Duration of QT interval in clinically normal dogs. *Am J Vet Res* **54**:2145–2149.

26 Ware WA, Christensen WF (1999) Duration of the QT interval in healthy cats. *Am J Vet Res* **60**:1426–1429.

27 Finley MR, Lillich JD, Gilmour RF et al. (2003) Structural and functional basis for the long QT syndrome: relevance to veterinary patients. *J Vet Intern Med* **17**:473–488.

28 Macintire DK (1997) Disorders of potassium, phosphorus, and magnesium in critical illness. *Compend Cont Educ Pract Vet* **19**:41–48.

29 Goodwin JK (1998) Holter monitoring and cardiac event recording. *Vet Clin North Am: Small Anim Pract* **28**:1391–1407.

30 Meurs KM, Spier AW, Wright NA et al. (2001) Use of ambulatory electrocardiography for detection of ventricular premature complexes in healthy dogs. *J Am Vet Med Assoc* **218**:1291–1292.

31 Hall LW, Dunn JK, Delaney M et al. (1991) Ambulatory electrocardiography in dogs. *Vet Rec* **129**:213–216.

32 Cote E, Richter K, Charuvastra E (1999) Event-based cardiac monitoring in small animal practice. *Compend Contin Educ Pract Vet* **21**:1025–1033.

5
Overview of Echocardiography

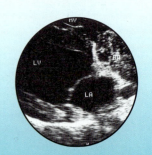

GENERAL PRINCIPLES

Echocardiography is an important, noninvasive tool for evaluating cardiac anatomy and function, as well as surrounding structures. Pericardial fluid, pleural fluid, and mass lesions in or near the heart can also be detected. Three modes of echocardiography are commonly used: M-mode, two-dimensional (2-D, real-time), and Doppler. Each has important and complementary applications, as described below. As with many other diagnostic tests, the echocardiogram should be interpreted within the context of the patient's history, CV examination findings, and any other appropriate tests. The importance of the echocardiographer's technical skill in performing the study and understanding of cardiovascular anatomy and physiology cannot be overemphasized.

This chapter is an introduction to transthoracic echocardiography. Additional echo images related to specific diseases are found in later chapters. The interested reader is referred to other sources for more detailed information on underlying physics, additional technical issues, and other applications[1–4].

BASIC PHYSICS AND TERMINOLOGY

Diagnostic ultrasonography uses pulsed, high-frequency sound waves, which are reflected from body tissue interfaces back to the transducer. When the ultrasound beam meets an interface between differing biologic tissues, it is reflected, refracted, and absorbed, similar to visible light energy. Only the reflected energy can be received and processed by the transducer, which acts as a receiver most of the time. Because the velocity of sound through tissue is known (~1,540 m/sec), the distance from the transducer to the various reflective interfaces can be calculated and the resulting images displayed.

Echo intensity

The strength of received echos depends on several factors. More reflective tissue boundaries (greater mismatch in acoustic impedance, which is related to tissue density) produce stronger echos. Orienting the ultrasound beam perpendicular to the structure of interest produces a stronger echo signal with 2-D and M-mode. Ultrasound beam energy decreases as distance from the transducer increases because of beam divergence, and absorption, scatter, and reflection of wave energy at tissue interfaces. These factors reduce the intensity of echos returning from deeper structures. Very reflective interfaces such as bone/tissue or air/tissue prevent visualization of deeper, soft tissue interfaces. Transducer frequency as well as ultrasound power output and processing controls also influence echo signal intensity.

Transducer frequency

Higher frequency ultrasound waves produce better resolution of small structures; however, higher frequencies have less penetrating ability because more energy is absorbed and scattered by the tissues. Conversely, a transducer producing lower frequency ultrasound will provide greater depth of penetration but less well-defined images; therefore, the highest frequency that allows adequate penetration is used for 2-D and M-mode imaging. Frequencies generally used in small animals range from 3.5 MHz for large dogs to >7.5 MHz for cats and small dogs. A megahertz (MHz) represents 1,000,000 cycles/second.

Descriptive terms

Certain terms are used to describe ultrasound images. Tissues that strongly reflect ultrasound are called hyperechoic or of greater echogenicity. Poorly reflecting tissues are hypoechoic, whereas fluid, which does not reflect sound, is anechoic or sonolucent. Tissue behind an area of sonolucency appears hyperechoic because more ultrasound energy reaches it; this is known as acoustic enhancement. On the other hand, through-transmission of the ultrasound beam is blocked by a strongly hyperechoic object, such as a rib, which casts an acoustic shadow, where no image appears, behind the object.

THE ECHOCARDIOGRAPHIC EXAMINATION

PATIENT PREPARATION

The animal is gently restrained in lateral recumbency (**123**); better quality images are usually obtained when the heart is imaged from the recumbent side. A table or platform with an edge cut out, which allows the echocardiographer to position and manipulate the transducer from the animal's dependent side, is useful. Some animals can be imaged adequately while standing. For most echo examinations, the hair over the transducer placement site is shaved to improve skin contact and image clarity. However, some animals are not shaved for cosmetic reasons. Coupling gel is applied to produce air-free contact between skin and transducer.

Sedation

Most animals do not require chemical restraint; however, if the patient will not lie quietly with gentle restraint, light sedation is usually effective. Buprenorphine (0.005–0.01 mg/kg IV) with acepromazine (0.025–0.03 mg/kg IV) usually works well for dogs and has minimal effect on echo measurements[5]. Butorphanol (0.2 mg/kg IM) with acepromazine (0.1 mg/kg IM) is adequate for many cats, although some require more intense sedation. Acepromazine (0.1 mg/kg IM) followed in 15 minutes by ketamine (2 mg/kg IV) can be used in cats, but this regimen can increase heart rate undesirably. Ketamine administration has been shown to increase IVS and LV wall thicknesses as well as decrease LV diastolic dimension[6]. Xylazine and sodium pentobarbital have negative effects on heart function, so are not recommended for echo sedation[7].

IMAGING

The right and left parasternal transducer positions are used most often. The transducer is placed over the precordial impulse area, or other appropriate site, and its position adjusted to find a good 'acoustic window' that allows clear visualization of the heart (**124**). Minor adjustment of the animal's forelimb or torso position may be required. The transducer is angled or rotated and the echocardiograph's controls, for factors such as gain, focus, and power, are adjusted as necessary to optimize the image. For 2-D and M-mode examinations, optimal visualization is achieved when the ultrasound beam is perpendicular to the structures being imaged.

Artifacts

Image artifacts are common and can mimic cardiac abnormalities. If a suspected 'mass' or 'septal defect' can be visualized in more than one imaging plane, it is more likely to be real. Artifacts can result from misplacement of displayed echos returning from secondary vibrations, not along the primary ultrasound beam path (**125**), reverberation artifact from deeper structures, or from poor lateral resolution, when the structure is aligned parallel, not perpendicular, to the beam[8, 9].

Poor quality images also result from inadequate skin–transducer contact, improper adjustment of the various ultrasound machine controls, a low frequency transducer, and other equipment limitations. Individual patient characteristics also affect the quality of images obtained. Images are often poor in animals with barrel-shaped chest conformation or obesity. Lung artifact and rib interference can prevent good visualization of the entire heart (**126**).

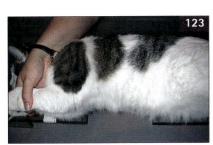

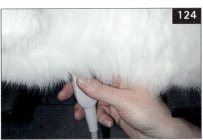

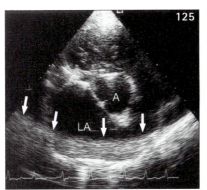

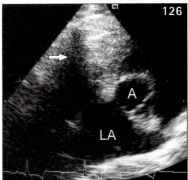

125 A band of 'false' echos caused by side lobe artifact (arrows) can be seen within the enlarged LA (see text). LA= left atrium; A= aorta.

126 Acoustic shadow (arrow) cast by an overlying rib and lung artifact prevent visualization of deeper structures. LA = left atrium; A = aorta.

123, 124 Most small animals are best imaged in lateral recumbency (**123**). An elevated table with an edge cut out allows the probe to be positioned underneath (**124**).

EXAMINATION COMPONENTS

The basic echo examination includes all standard 2-D imaging planes, with cardiac measurements obtained either using M-mode or carefully timed 2-D frames. Off-angle views may also be needed to further evaluate specific lesions. Doppler evaluation of transvalvular flows and any area of suspected flow disturbance provides important additional information. The complete examination can be quite time consuming in some animals.

A systematic approach for evaluating each cardiac chamber, valve, and great vessel is useful. Questions to be answered include:

- Are the anatomic relationships among chambers, valves, and great vessels normal?
- Are the chamber sizes normally proportioned when compared with each other?
- Are ventricular wall and septal thicknesses normal and symmetrical?
- Are the structure and motion of all the valves normal?
- Is pericardial or pleural fluid present?
- Are any masses or other abnormal structures seen?
- Are abnormal blood flow patterns present on Doppler examination?
- Are there abnormalities of ventricular systolic or diastolic function?
- Does any observed chamber enlargement logically fit with the structural or functional abnormalities thought to be present?
- How severe does any hemodynamic (pressure or volume) overload appear to be?

Measurements are usually made; however, the assessment of cardiomegaly remains somewhat subjective, especially regarding right heart chambers. Diastolic RV wall thickness should be <50% (and usually ~33%) of LV wall thickness. Measurements in cats (*Table 15*) are relatively consistent. Because of breed and body size-related variation, standardized values for normal dogs are more problematic (*Table 16*, pp. 72–73).

2-D ECHOCARDIOGRAPHY

A plane of tissue, both depth and width, is evaluated with 2-D echocardiography. Anatomic changes caused by various diseases or congenital defects can be seen. Any suspected abnormality should be scanned in multiple planes to further verify and delineate it. Actual blood flow is not (usually) visualized with 2-D or M-mode imaging alone. Comparisons of wall thickness to lumen size and right heart to left heart structures can be made. LV internal dimensions and wall thickness are usually obtained using M-mode; however, appropriately timed short-axis 2-D frames can also be used and are preferred when the M-mode beam cannot be placed accurately through the area of interest (e.g. to measure an area of localized hypertrophy). There are also several methods that can be used to estimate LV volume and wall mass[2, 4, 7]. Area or volume-based calculations of LV systolic function are best derived from 2-D images. The entire length of the LV can usually be imaged from the right parasternal long-axis view, except in large dogs[10]. 2-D frames selected at maximal systole and end-diastole can be used for measurements, but timing within the cardiac cycle and the plane of interrogation need to be precise.

Table 15 Echocardiographic measurements in normal cats*.

	Sedation	N	Body weight (kg)	HR (beats/min)	LVIDd (mm)	LVIDs (mm)	IVSd (mm)	IVSs (mm)	LVFWd (mm)	LVFWs (mm)	LA (mm)	Ao (mm)	LA/Ao	RVd (mm)	FS (%)
Pipers et al[69]	None	25	4.7 ± 1.2	167 ± 29	14.8 (9.6–20)	8.8 (4–13.6)	4.5 (2.7–6.3)	–	3.7 (2.1–5.3)	–	7.4 (4–10.8)	7.5 (3.9–11.1)	0.99	–	41 (26.4–55.6)
Jacobs and Knight[67]	None	30	4.1 ± 1.1	194 ± 23	15.9 (12.1–19.7)	8 (5.2–10.8)	3.1 (2.3–3.9)	5.8 (4.6–7)	3.3 (2.1–4.5)	6.8 (5.4–8.2)	12.3 (9.5–15.1)	9.5 (7.3–11.7)	1.3 (0.96–1.64)	6 (3–9)	49.8 (39.3–60.3)
Fox et al[66]	Ketamine	30	3.9 ± 1.2	245 ± 36	14 (11.4–16.6)	8.1 (4.9–11.3)	3.6 (2–5.2)	–	3.5 (2.5–4.5)	–	10.3 (7.5–13.1)	9.4 (7.2–11.6)	1.1 (0.74–1.46)	5 (0.8–9.2)	42.7 (26.5–58.9)
Moise et al[68]	None	11	4.3 ± 0.5	182 ± 22	15.1 (11–19)	6.9 (2.5–11)	5 (3.6–5.6)	7.6 (5.2–10)	4.6 (3.6–5.6)	7.8 (5.8–9.8)	12.2 (6.5–16)	9.5 (6.5–13)	1.29 (0.83–1.75)	5.4 (3.4–7.4)	55 (35–75)
Sisson et al[70]	None	79	4.7 ± 1.2	–	15 (11–19)	7.2 (4.2–10.2)	4.2 (2.8–5.60)	6.7 (4.3–9.1)	4.1 (2.7–5.5)	6.8 (4.6–9)	11.7 (8.3–15.1)	9.5 (6.7–12.3)	1.25 (0.89–1.61)	4.6 (1.2–8)	52.1 (37.9–66.3)
DeMadron et al[65] (2D data)	**	13	3.6 ± 1.05	196 ± 30	13.5 (10.7–16.3)	8.4 (5.5–11.3)	3.9 (2.2–5.6)	5.9 (4.3–7.5)	3.5 (2.1–4.9)	5.5 (3.8–7.2)	12.1 (10.3–13.9)	9.6 (7.1–12.1)	–	–	38 (20–56)
DeMadron et al[65] (M-mode data)	**	13	3.6 ± 1.05	196 ± 30	13.4 (11.3–15.5)	8.5 (6.9–10.1)	4.2 (2.8–5.6)	7.0 (5.4–8.6)	4.0 (2.6–5.4)	6.1 (4.5–7.7)	10.9 (8.9–12.9)	8.2 (6.8–9.6)	–	–	36 (26–46)

* Values expressed as mean ± 2 standard deviations (or as a range).

** 6/13 cats were sedated with acepromazine/ketamine; data pooled from both awake and sedated cats.

Comment: LVFWd and/or IVSd measurements >5.5 mm (sensitive) to >6 mm (specific) indicate LV hypertrophy.[3] HR = heart rate; LVIDd = left ventricular diameter in diastole; LVIDs = left ventricular diameter in systole; LVFWd = left ventricular free wall thickness in diastole; LVFWs = left ventricular free wall thickness in systole; IVSd = interventricular septal thickness in diastole; IVSs = interventricular septal thickness in systole; LA = left atrial diameter in systole; Ao = aortic diameter in diastole; LA/Ao = left atrial/aortic ratio; RVd = right ventricular diastolic diameter, FS = left ventricular fractional shortening.

Table 16 Echocardiographic measurements in normal dogs*.

Breed	N	Body weight (kg)	LVIDd (mm)	LVIDdI (mm/m²)	LVIDs (mm)	LVIDsI (mm/m²)	LVFWd (mm)	LVFWdI (mm/m²)	LVFWs (mm)
Miniature Poodle[22]	20	3 (1.4–9)	20 (16–28)	100	10 (8–16)	50	5 (4–6)	25	8 (6–10)
Beagle[18]	20	8.9±1.5	26.3 (19.5–33.1)	61.2	15.7 (8.9–22.5)	36.5	8.2 (4.4–12)	19.1	11.4 (7.6–15.2)
West Highland White Terrier[71]	34	9.4±2.4	27.2 (21.6–32.8)	61.8	16.8 (12.8–20.8)	38.2	6.7 (4.7–8.7)	15.2	9.8 (6.8–12.8)
English Cocker Spaniel[19]	12	12.2 ± 2.25	33.8 (27.2–40.4)	63.8	22.2 (16.6–27.8)	41.9	7.9 (5.7–10.1)	14.9	–
Welsh Corgie[22]	20	15 (8–19)	32 (28–40)	53.3	19 (12–23)	31.7	8 (6–10)	13.3	12 (8–13)
Pointer[24]	16	19.2 ±2.8	39.2 (34.4–44)	54.4	25.3 (20.5–30.1)	35.1	7.1 (5.7–8.5)	9.9	11.5 (8.9–14.1)
Afghan[22]	20	23 (17–36)	42 (33–52)	51.9	28 (20–37)	34.6	9 (7–11)	11.1	12 (9–18)
Greyhound[23]	16	26.6± 3.5	44.1 (28.1–50.1)	49.6	32.5 (25.5–39.5)	36.5	12.1 (8.7–15.5)	13.6	15.3 (10.9–19.7)
Boxer[20]	30	28+7.1	40 (30–50)	43.5	26.8	29.1	10 (6–14)	10.9	15 (11–19)
Greyhound[25]	11	29.1± 3.7	46.9 (40.7–53.1)	49.9	33.3 (28.1–38.5)	35.4	11.6 (8.2–15)	12.3	–
Golden Retriever[22]	20	32 (23–41)	45 (37–51)	44.6	27 (18–35)	26.7	10 (8–12)	9.9	15 (10–19)
Dobermann[29]	23	–	40.1 (34.7–45.5)	–	31.4 (25.9–36.9)	–	8 (5.6–10.4)	–	11.2 (8.3–14.1)
Dobermann[72]	21	36 (31–42)	46.8 (38.5–55.1)	42.9	30.8 (24.2–37.4)	28.3	9.6 (8.4–10.8)	8.8	14.1 (12.4–15.8)
Spanish Mastiff[30]	12	52.4 ± 3.3	47.7 (44.9–50.5)	33.8	29 (26.8–31.2)	20.6	9.7 (8.9–10.5)	6.9	15.2 (14.4–16)
Newfound-land[73]	27	61 (47–69.5)	50 (44–60)	32.1	35.5 (29–44)	22.8	10 (8–13)	6.4	15 (11–16)
Great Dane[73]	15	62 (52–75)	53 (44–59)	32.3	39.5 (34–45)	24.1	12.5 (10–16)	7.6	16 (11–19)
Irish Wolfhound[27]	262	65 (43–93)	53.2 (45.2–61.2)	32.6	35.4 (29.8–41)	21.7	9.8 (6.6–13)	6.0	14.9 (10.6–19.2)
Irish Wolfhound[73]	20	68.5 (50–80)	50 (46–59)	28.6	36 (33–45)	20.6	10 (9–13)	5.7	14 (11–17)

LVIDd = left ventricular diameter in diastole; LVIDdI = left ventricular diastolic diameter index; LVIDs = left ventricular diameter in systole; LVIDsI = left ventricular systolic diameter index; LVFWd = left ventricular free wall thickness in diastole; LVFWs = left ventricular free wall thickness in systole; IVSd = interventricular septal thickness in diastole; IVSs = interventricular septal thickness in systole; FS = left ventricular fractional shortening.

Table 16 Echocardiographic measurements in normal dogs* (continued).

IVSd (mm)	IVSs (mm)	FS (%)	M-Mode LA (mm)	M-Mode Ao (mm)	M-Mode LA/Ao
–	–	47 (35–57)	12 (8–18)	10 (8–13)	1.2
6.7 (4.5–8.9)	9.6 (6.6–12.6)	40 (22–58)			
7.2 (4.6–9.8)	9.7 (7.1–12.3)	36 (26–46)			
–	–	34.3 (25.3–43.3)			
–	–	44 (33–57)	21 (12–24)	18 (15–22)	1.17
6.9 (4.7–9.1)	10.6 (8.6–12.6)	35.5 (27.5–43.5)	22.6 (18.6–22.6)	24.1 (20.7–27.5)	0.94 (0.8–1.08)
–	–	33 (24–48)	26 (18–35)	26 (20–34)	1.0
10.6 (7.2–14)	13.4 (8.2–18.6)	25.3 (12.7–37.9)			
9 (5–13)	13 (9–17)	33 (17–49)	23 (19–27)	22 (18–26)	1.06 (1.04–1.08)
13.4 (10–16.8)	–	28.8 (20.4–37.2)			
–	–	39 (27–55)	27 (16–32)	24 (14–27)	1.13
–	–	21.7 (14.4–29)			
9.6 (8.4–10.8)	14.3 (13–15.6)	34.2 (30.6–37.8)	26.6 (23.6–29.6)	29.9 (25.3–34.5)	0.89
9.8 (9–10.6)	15.6 (14.6–16.6)	39.2	28.5 (26.7–30.3)	27.6 (26–29.2)	1.03
11.5 (7–15)	15 (11–20)	30 (22–37)	30 (24–33)	29 (26–33)	1.0 (0.8–1.25)
14.5 (12–16)	16.5 (14–19)	25 (18–36)	33 (28–46)	29.5 (28–34)	1.1 (0.9–1.5)
9.3 (5.7–12.9)	13.7 (8.9–18.5)	34 (25–43)	32.9 (26.1–39.7)	33.1 (27.7–38.7)	.99
12 (9–14.5)	15 (11–17)	28 (20–34)	31 (22–35)	30 (29–31)	1.0 (0.9–1.5)

* Values expressed as mean, ± 2 standard deviations or (range). Values indexed to body surface area are of group mean divided by mean group body surface area.

Comment: In general, normal FS is considered from 25% to 40% or 45%, although some healthy athletic dogs have FS between 20% and 25%. Most normal dogs have an EPSS ≤6 mm; may be slightly larger in giant breeds.

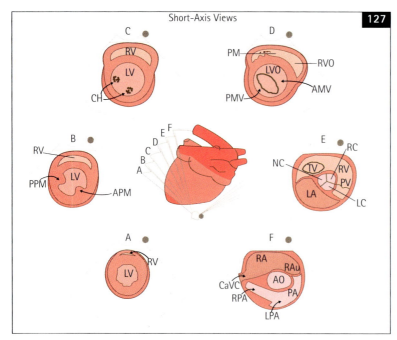

Short-Axis Views

127 Short-axis views from the right parasternal transducer position. Progressive angulation of the transducer yields image planes from cardiac apex to base. (A) apex; (B) papillary muscle; (C) chorda tendineae; (D) mitral valve; (E) aortic root/left atrium; (F) pulmonary artery. (From Thomas WP *et al.* (1993) Recommendations for standards in transthoracic two-dimensional echocardiography in the dog and cat. *J Vet Intern Med* 7, 247-252, with permission.)

Abbreviations for **127–132**. RA = right atrium; RAu = right auricle; RV = right ventricle; RVO = right ventricular outflow tract; TV = tricuspid valve; PV = pulmonary valve; LPA = left pulmonary artery; RPA = right pulmonary artery; CaVC = caudal vena cava; VS = ventricular septum; LA = left atrium; LAu = left auricle; LV = left ventricle; LVO = left ventricular outflow tract; LVW = left ventricular free wall; PM = papillary muscle; CH = chorda tendineae; MV = mitral valve; AMV = anterior (septal, cranioventral) mitral valve cusp; PMV = posterior (parietal, caudodorsal) mitral valve cusp; AO = aorta; LC = left coronary cusp; RC = right coronary cusp; NC = noncoronary cusp; (brown dot = transducer index mark.)

STANDARD 2-D ECHOCARDIOGRAPHIC VIEWS

A variety of planes should be imaged from several chest wall locations to evaluate the heart adequately. Most standard views are obtained from either the right (**127, 128**) or left (**129–132**) parasternal positions (directly over the heart and close to the sternum)[11]. Images are occasionally obtained from subxiphoid (subcostal) or thoracic inlet (suprasternal) positions.

Long-axis (sagittal) views are obtained with the imaging plane parallel to the long axis of the heart, whereas short-axis (transverse, horizontal) views are perpendicular to this plane. Images are described by the location of the transducer and the imaging plane used (e.g. right parasternal short-axis view, left cranial parasternal long-axis view). On the right parasternal short-axis view (**127**), the LV appears round. When the transducer is angled dorsally, the pulmonary artery is positioned on the right side of the image. From the short-axis view, the transducer is rotated 90° counterclockwise to obtain the long-axis views (**128**). The heart base is positioned to the right of the screen and the apex to the left. The left apical 4-chamber view provides good visualization of the ventricular inflow tracts and chamber proportions.

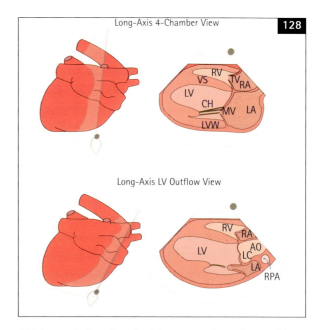

Long-Axis 4-Chamber View

Long-Axis LV Outflow View

128 Long-axis views from the right parasternal transducer position. The transducer is rotated 90 degrees from the position used for the short-axis views. Slight cranial angulation from the 4-chamber view yields the LV outflow view. (Abbreviations list in **127**.) (From Thomas WP *et al.* (1993) Recommendations for standards in transthoracic two-dimensional echocardiography in the dog and cat. *J Vet Intern Med* 7, 247-252, with permission.)

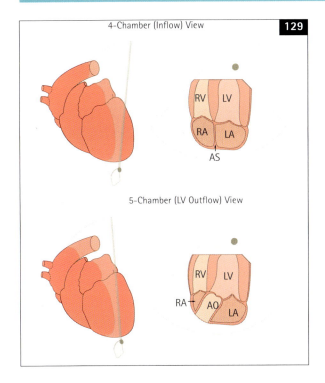

4-Chamber (Inflow) View **129**

5-Chamber (LV Outflow) View

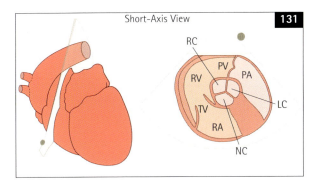

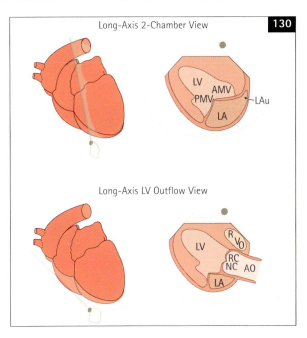

Long-Axis 2-Chamber View **130**

Long-Axis LV Outflow View

Short-Axis View **131**

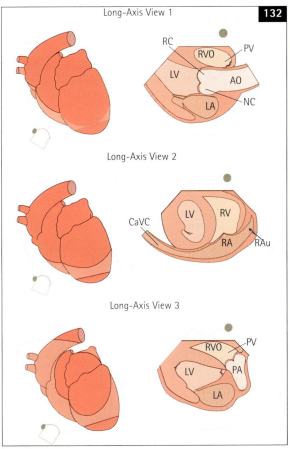

Long-Axis View 1 **132**

Long-Axis View 2

Long-Axis View 3

129 Left caudal (apical) transducer position. The 4-chamber view is obtained by orienting the transducer index mark toward the animal's left and slightly caudal.

130 Left caudal (apical) transducer position. The 2-chamber view is obtained by orienting the ultrasound beam plane parallel to the long axis of the heart, almost perpendicular with the long axis of the body. Rotation of the beam more craniodorsally-to-caudoventrally yields the LV outflow view. (Abbreviations list in **127**.) (From Thomas WP *et al.* (1993) Recommendations for standards in transthoracic two-dimensional echocardiography in the dog and cat. *J Vet Intern Med* **7**, 247-252, with permission.)

131, 132 (131) The left cranial short-axis view is obtained by moving the transducer slightly more cranial on the chest wall (from the left apical position) and rotating the beam so it is almost perpendicular to the long axis of the body and heart. This view usually provides optimal orientation to the right ventricular inflow and outflow tracts. (132) Left cranial parasternal position, long-axis views. The beam plane is rotated almost parallel to the long axis of the heart to align with the ascending aorta (view 1). More medial transducer angulation allows the RV inflow

tract, RA and RAu to be seen (view 2). Lateral angulation of the beam reveals the RV outflow tract and main PA (view 3). (Abbreviations list in **127**.) (From Thomas WP *et al.* (1993) Recommendations for standards in transthoracic two-dimensional echocardiography in the dog and cat. *J Vet Intern Med* **7**, 247-252, with permission.)

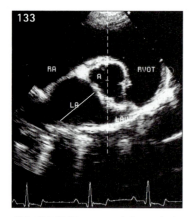
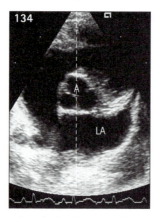
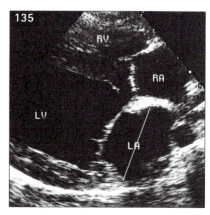

133, 134 Right parasternal short-axis view at the heart base. In dogs the standard M-mode cursor position (dashed line) for measuring aortic root diameter usually transects the LA near its auricle (**133**), therefore underestimating true LA size. In many (not all) cats (**134**), the full extent of the LA can be appreciated in this view. Alternate methods of LA measurement have been used, including LA diameter in diastole (**133**) as indicated by the solid line (see references 12 and 13). A = aorta; RA = right atrium; RVOT = right ventricular outflow tract; LA = left atrium; Lau = left auricle.

Left atrial size

LA size is better assessed using 2-D rather than M-mode, especially in dogs (**133, 134**)[2, 3, 7]. Several methods for LA measurement have been described using either the right parasternal short-axis view at the heart base or the long-axis 4-chamber view. Often, LA size is compared with aortic root dimension[10, 12, 13, 14]. One method is to measure the cranial-caudal diameter (top to bottom on screen) at end-systole (just before mitral valve opening) using a right parasternal long-axis 4-chamber view (**135**). For cats, the LA dimension normally is <16 mm; a diameter >19 mm may pose a greater risk for thromboembolism[2, 15]. Because of the greater variation related to body size in dogs, the LA dimension can be compared with the 2-D aortic root diameter measured across the sinuses of Valsalva in diastole. The LA diameter:aortic root ratio has been reported as between 1.6–1.9 [2, 15] or about 1.6 (with a 95% confidence interval of 1.1–2.0)[12].

CONTRAST ECHOCARDIOGRAPHY

Contrast echocardiography or 'bubble study' is a technique used in 2-D modalitiy (and, occasionally, in M-mode modality) in which a substance containing 'microbubbles' is rapidly injected either into a peripheral vein or selectively into the heart. The passage of these microbubbles into the ultrasound beam generates many tiny echos that temporarily opacify the blood pool being imaged. The microbubbles look like bright sparkles moving with the blood flow. Agitated saline solution, a mixture of saline and the patient's blood, and other substances can be used as echo contrast material. Injection into a peripheral vein will opacify the right heart chambers; bubbles seen in the left heart or aorta indicate a right-to-left shunt (**136, 137**). Saline microbubbles do not pass through the pulmonary capillaries, although some commercially available echo contrast agents do. Echo contrast injection via selective

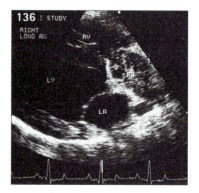

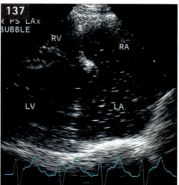

135 The right parasternal long-axis 4-chamber view is good for assessing LA diameter (solid line). (See text for more information.) LA = left atrium; LV = left ventricle; RA = right atrium; RV = right ventricle.
136, 137 Boluses of agitated saline injected intravenously create bright 'bubbles' in these echo contrast (bubble) studies. Both images are right parasternal long-axis 4-chamber views. (**136**) Blood in the RA is opacified with bubbles in this normal dog. A few bubbles are seen in the RV; however, none appear in the LA or LV. Figure **134** shows a similar view in this dog without echo contrast. (**137**) A large right-to-left shunting atrial septal defect is evident in this 18-month-old Akita with pulmonary hypertension. Bubbles have moved from the RA into the LA and are also seen in the LV. LA = left atrium; LV = left ventricle, RA = right atrium; RV = right ventricle.

left heart catheterization can be used to visualize intracardiac left-to-right shunts or mitral regurgitation. Although Doppler echocardiography generally has replaced the use of echo contrast injection, this technique is still helpful for identifying a right-to-left shunting atrial septal defect or patent ductus arteriosus, imaging the abdominal aorta to see the bubbles[2, 16].

M-MODE ECHOCARDIOGRAPHY

The M-mode echocardiogram provides a one-dimensional view (depth) into the heart. M-mode images represent echos from various tissue interfaces that the beam traverses (displayed on the vertical axis) as their relative positions move through time (displayed on the horizontal axis) during the cardiac cycle (**138**)[1–4]. The 2-D imaging mode should be used to guide accurate placement of the M-mode cursor. The M-mode image usually provides cleaner resolution of cardiac borders and more accurate timing of events within the cardiac cycle than 2-D alone because of its high sampling rate. Therefore, measurement of cardiac dimensions and motion throughout the cardiac cycle are often more accurately assessed from M-mode tracings, especially when coupled with a simultaneously recorded ECG; however, difficulty in consistently achieving proper beam placement, as well as translational motion of the beating heart, can be limitations. In animals with localized or asymmetrical ventricular hypertrophy, wall thickness measurements from 2-D images are preferable when the M-mode cursor cannot be optimally aligned.

STANDARD M-MODE VIEWS

Standard M-mode views (**138–141**) are obtained from the right parasternal transducer position. The M-mode cursor is positioned with 2-D guidance using

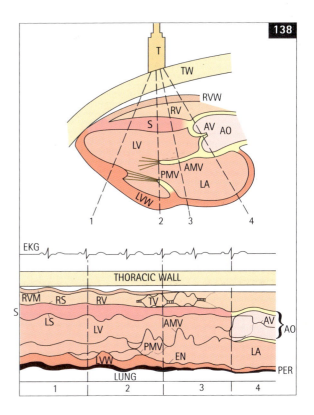

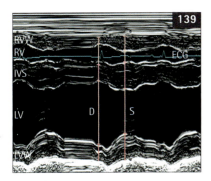

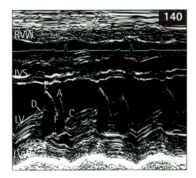

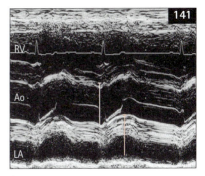

138-141 (138) Schematic diagram illustrating how various tissue interfaces crossed by a one-dimensional ultrasound beam (upper panel) are displayed over time in M-mode echocardiography (lower panel). Although the long-axis view is shown here to depict different levels from apex to base, short-axis views are generally used in practice to guide M-mode cursor placement. (Diagram derived from Feigenbaum H (1972) Clinical applications of echocardiography. *Prog Cardiovasc Dis* 14, 531, with permission.) (139) M-mode image from a normal dog at the ventricular level (corresponding to left side of panel 2 in 138). Diastolic ('D') measurements are made at the onset of the QRS complex of the ECG; systolic ('S') measurements are taken at the time of smallest LV diameter. (140) M-mode image from a normal dog at the mitral valve level. Letters are used to identify anterior leaflet motion: point D = initial valve opening in early diastole; point E = maximal opening of the leaflet during rapid ventricular filling; point F = end of rapid ventricular filling; point A = atrial contraction; point C = valve closure at onset of ventricular contraction. (141) M-mode image from a normal dog at the aortic root/LA level (see 133 for 2-D orientation). During systole in this image, only one aortic leaflet is seen moving downward toward the caudal aortic wall. (See text for more information.) AMV = anterior leaflet of mitral valve; Ao = aorta; AV = aortic valve; EN = endocardium; IVS = interventricular septum; LA = left atrium; LS = left edge of septum; LV = left ventricle; LVW = left ventricular wall; PER = pericardium; PMV = posterior leaflet of mitral valve; RS = right edge of septum; RV = right ventricle; RVW = right ventricular wall; S = interventricular septum; T = transducer; TV = tricuspid valve; TW = thoracic wall.

the right parasternal short-axis view. Precise positioning of the ultrasound beam within the heart and clear endocardial edge resolution are essential for accurate M-mode measurements and calculations. For example, papillary muscles within the LV must be avoided when measuring free wall thickness (**142, 143**).

COMMON MEASUREMENTS AND NORMAL VALUES

The standard dimensions measured with M-mode and their timing within the cardiac cycle are also indicated in figures **138–141** (p. 77). Measurements are generally made using the leading edge technique (i.e. from the edge closest to the transducer [leading edge] of one side of the dimension to the leading edge of the other). In this way, only one endocardial interface is included in the measurement. Uniformly accepted guidelines for cardiac size measurement are lacking; the guidelines for common echo measurements in the Tables should be regarded as approximate. Somatotype, breed, and body size are important in dogs (*Table 16*, p. 72)[2, 3, 7, 10, 17–31]. Endurance training also affects measured parameters, reflecting the increased cardiac mass and volume associated with frequent and sustained strenous exercise[26].

The ventricles

The systolic and diastolic thicknesses of the LV wall and IVS, as well as LV chamber dimensions, should be determined at the level of the chordae tendineae. If the M-mode cursor cannot be aligned properly within the LV or perpendicular to an area of focal hypertrophy,

measurements can be taken from appropriately timed 2-D images. It may be difficult to measure the RV in some animals because of poor near field resolution. Diastolic measurements are made at the onset of the QRS complex of a simultaneously recorded ECG. Systolic measurements of the LV are made from the point of peak downward motion of the septum to the leading edge of the LV free wall endocardium at the same instant.

The septum and LV wall normally move toward each other in systole, although their peak movement may not coincide if electrical activation is not simultaneous. Paradoxic septal motion, in which the septum seems to move away from the LV wall and toward the transducer in systole, occurs in some cases of RV volume and/or pressure overload (**144–146**). This abnormal septal motion can also be visualized on 2-D images; it precludes accurate assessment of LV function using fractional shortening.

Left ventricular function

The fractional shortening (FS; % delta D) is the index often used to estimate LV function, although it has important limitations. FS is the percentage change in LV dimension from diastole to systole (**147, 148**). This index of contractility assumes the ventricle contracts uniformly and, like others taken during cardiac ejection, has the limitation of being dependent on ventricular loading conditions (see Chapter 1). For example, reduced LV afterload, as with mitral insufficiency, ventricular septal defect, or peripheral vasodilation, facilitates ejection of blood from the LV

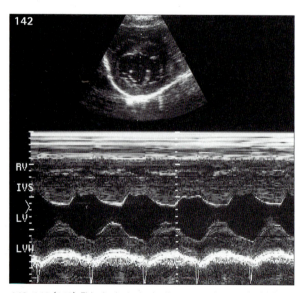

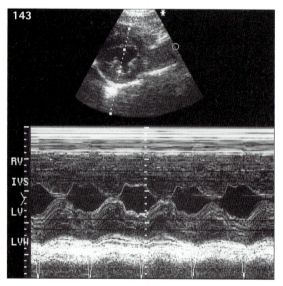

142, 143 (142) This duplex echocardiogram at the ventricular level from a normal cat shows a 2-D image (top) with correct cursor placement, from which the M-mode image (below) is derived. **(143)** Duplex image from the same cat illustrating inaccurate cursor placement and its effect on the M-mode image. The 2-D image plane is slightly more ventral than that in **142** and the cursor transects a papillary muscle; consequently the LVW spuriously appears abnormally thick. RV = right ventricle; IVS = interventricular septum; LV = left ventricle; LVW = left ventricular free wall.

and results in greater FS, although intrinsic myocardial contractility is not increased (**147**). Hence the apparent hypercontractility (exaggerated FS) in patients with severe mitral regurgitation and normal myocardial function. Heart rate and rhythm as well as regional wall motion abnormalities can also affect this index. Normal FS in dogs is between 25–40 or 45%[2, 7]. Some healthy athletic dogs have a FS of about 20–25%, perhaps because of greater apical-basilar shortening[2, 32]. Normal FS in cats is reported as >35% or 30–55%[2, 7]. Other indices of LV performance, such as mean velocity of circumferential fiber shortening (V_{cf}) and percentage change in IVS or LV wall thickness are also used sometimes (*Table 17*, p. 80). Normal V_{cf} is about 1.6–2.8 circumferences/second in dogs and 1.3–4.5 circumferences/second in cats[7].

The use of the calculated end-systolic volume index (ESVI) has been suggested as a more accurate way to assess myocardial contractility in the presence of mitral regurgitation[33]. This index compares LV size after ejection with body size rather than with the volume-overloaded end-diastolic ventricular size. Based on extrapolations from human studies, ESVI <30 ml/m[2] is normal, 30–60 ml/m[2] suggests mild LV systolic dysfunction, 60–90 ml/m[2] suggests moderate LV dysfunction, and >90 ml/m[2] is consistent with severe LV dysfunction[33]. However, volume calculations based on one dimension measurement are potentially fraught with error because of the geometric assumptions that must be made. Estimation of LV volumes and ejection fraction are best done using 2-D imaging and the modified Simpson's rule or area-length methods[34]. The right parasternal long-axis view optimized for maximally visualized LV size is recommended.

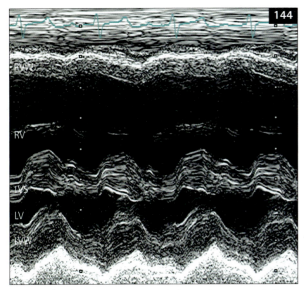

144–146 (**144**) RV dilation with paradoxic septal motion is seen in this M-mode echocardiogram from a 1-year-old Chow Chow with moderately severe pulmonary hypertension and tricuspid valve regurgitation. In diastole, (**145**) higher RV diastolic pressure pushes the IVS toward the LV (septal flattening), but in systole (**146**) LV pressure exceeds RV systolic pressure and the septum is pushed upward toward the RV. RV = right ventricle; RVW = right ventricular wall; IVS = interventricular septum; LV = left ventricle; LVW = left ventricular wall.

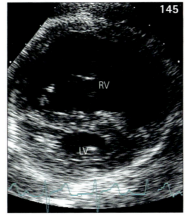
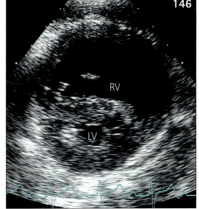

147, 148 M-mode echocardiograms at the ventricular level. (**147**) Reduced LV afterload from MR causes vigorous LVW and IVS motion and a high FS (57%) in this older mixed breed dog with normal LV function. (**148**) LV dilation with reduced FS (11%) is seen in this 4-year-old Labrador Retriever with dilated cardiomyopathy. RV = right ventricle; IVS = interventricular septum; LV = left ventricle; LVW = left ventricular wall.

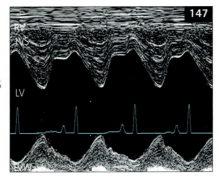
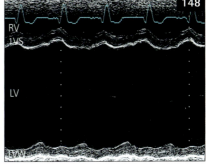

Table 17 Selected echocardiographic measures of LV systolic function.

Fractional shortening (FS) = $\dfrac{\text{LVIDd} - \text{LVIDs}}{\text{LVIDd}} \times 100$

(LV internal dimension measurements taken at chordal level)

End-systolic volume index (ESVI) = $\dfrac{\text{ESV}}{\text{BSA}}$

ESV derived from 2-D:

Short-axis area/long-axis length = $\dfrac{5\text{AL}}{6}$

Long-axis area length = $\dfrac{8\text{A}^2}{3\pi\text{L}}$

Modified Simpson's Rule (Method of Disks) =

$$\sum_{i=1}^{n} \pi r^2 \times \frac{L}{n}$$

(based on dividing the LV along its long axis into a series of disks of equal thickness)

Mitral valve E-point to septal separation (EPSS) = distance between maximal mitral opening in early diastole (E point on M-mode) and endocardial surface of interventricular septum

Mean velocity of circumferential fiber shortening (V_{cf})

$$= \frac{\text{LVIDd} - \text{LVIDs}}{\text{LVIDd} \times \text{LVET}}$$

(LVET is derived from the time between aortic valve opening and closing on M-mode, or the duration of aortic flow signal on Doppler examination)

V_{cf} normalized for heart rate = $\dfrac{(\text{LVIDd} - \text{LVIDs}) \times 100}{(\text{LVIDd} \geq \text{LVET} \times \text{HR})}$

LV free wall thickening (%FWth) = $\dfrac{\text{LVFWs} - \text{LVFWd}}{\text{LVFWd}} \times 100$

A = left ventricular area; BSA = body surface area (m²); ESV = end-systolic volume; HR = heart rate; L = left ventricular length; LVET = left ventricular ejection time; LVIDd = left ventricular internal dimension at end-diastole; LVIDs = left ventricular internal dimension in systole; LVFWd = left ventricular free wall thickness in diastole; LVFWs = left ventricular free wall thickness in systole; n = number of disks; r = disk radius.

Systolic time intervals (see p. 82) and mitral annular motion[32] are other methods of assessing LV function.

Mitral valve

Mitral valve motion is also evaluated using M-mode. The anterior (septal) leaflet is most prominent and has an 'M' configuration. The motion of the smaller posterior (parietal) leaflet appears as a 'W', and is more easily seen in the dilated ventricle. Tricuspid valve leaflet motion is similar. The leaflet motion pattern is identified by letters (**140**, p. 77). Point E is the maximal opening of the valve during rapid ventricular filling. In normal animals the mitral E point lies close to the IVS. Poor myocardial contractility is the most common cause of an increased E point to septal separation (EPSS; **149**). Normal EPSS is generally considered ≤6 mm in dogs, although it may be greater in giant breed dogs[27], and 4 or 5 mm in cats[7]. Atrial contraction opens the valve to point A. Normally, leaflet excursion is greater at point E. With tachycardia, the A point merges with the E point; this is common in cats (**150, 151**).

Dynamic LV outflow obstruction causes the anterior mitral leaflet to be sucked toward the septum during ejection. This is called systolic anterior motion (SAM). SAM causes the normally straight anterior leaflet

echos (between points C and D) to bend toward the septum during systole (**152, 153**). Diastolic flutter of the anterior mitral leaflet is seen sometimes when an aortic insufficiency jet causes the leaflet to vibrate (**154–156**).

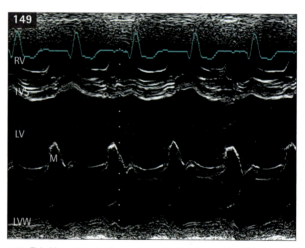

149 This M-mode echo from a Labrador Retriever with dilated cardiomyopathy shows marked LV dilation, poor IVS and LVW motion, and wide E point to septal separation (29 mm). RV = right ventricle; IVS = interventricular septum; LV = left ventricle; LVW = left ventricular free wall; M = mitral valve.

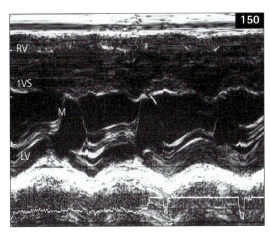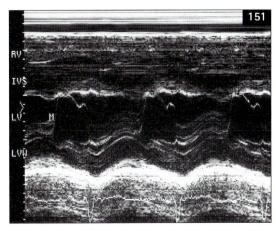

150, 151 (150) M-mode echo at the mitral valve level from a normal cat showing merging of atrial contraction or A point with the initial opening motion of the anterior leaflet (E point). The ECG was malfunctioning during this recording. (151) As the cat's heart rate slows, separate E and A points become evident. The ECG is visible at the bottom of the image. RV = right ventricle; IVS = interventricular septum; LV = left ventricle; LVW = left ventricular free wall; M = mitral valve.

152, 153 Systolic anterior motion of the anterior mitral leaflet is demonstrated (arrows) on M-mode (152) and 2-D images (153) in this 3-year-old Maine Coon cat with dynamic LV outflow tract obstruction associated with hypertrophic cardiomyopathy. RV = right ventricle; IVS = interventricular septum; LV = left ventricle; LVW = left ventricular free wall; M = mitral valve; Ao = aorta.

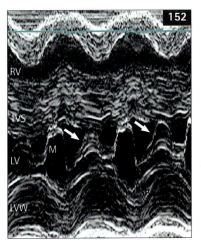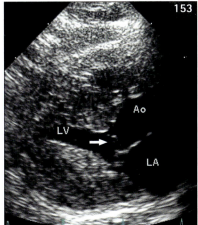

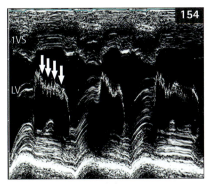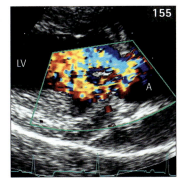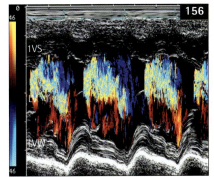

154–156 (154) Diastolic flutter (arrows) of the anterior mitral valve leaflet caused by aortic valve regurgitation in a 6-year-old Pomeranian with endocarditis. The flow disturbance from the regurgitant jet that causes the mitral vibrations can be seen in the right parasternal long-axis 2-D color flow image (155) as well as the color M-mode image (156) at the mitral level, as in 154. IVS = interventricular septum; LV = left ventricle; LVW = left ventricular free wall; A = aorta.

Aortic root

The aortic root diameter and LA are also commonly measured with M-mode (**141**, p. 77). The walls of the aortic root appear as two parallel lines shifting upward in systole. During diastole, one or two aortic valve cusps are seen as a line centered between the aortic wall echoes. At the onset of ejection, the cusps quickly separate to opposite sides of the aortic root and then come together again at the end of ejection; their appearance has been described as a train of boxes attached together by a string. Aortic diameter is measured at end-diastole. The amplitude of posterior to anterior motion of the aortic root is decreased when cardiac output is poor.

Left atrium

The M-mode LA dimension is taken at maximal systolic excursion (**141**, p. 77). In normal cats and dogs the ratio of LA to aortic root diameter is usually about 1:1[3]. Ratios >1.3 suggest LA enlargement[7]. However, this M-mode dimension is an imprecise measure of LA size because, especially in dogs, the portion of the LA imaged is usually the area between the body of the LA and the left auricular appendage (**133, 134**); therefore, this measurement does not usually represent maximal LA size (see p. 75)[2, 3, 12]. In cats the M-mode beam is more likely to cross the body of the LA, but its orientation can be inconsistent. Echo beam placement may be difficult in some animals, and the pulmonary artery can be inadvertently imaged instead.

Systolic time intervals

Systolic time intervals (STIs) can also be used to estimate LV function, although they too are influenced by cardiac filling and afterload[35]. These intervals can be calculated if the opening and closing of the aortic valve are clearly seen on M-mode and a simultaneous ECG is recorded for timing. They also can be derived using Doppler echocardiography. The STIs are LV ejection time (LVET), the duration of time the aortic valve is open); preejection period (PEP) the time from the onset of the QRS to aortic valve opening; and total electromechanical systole (LVET plus PEP). Reduced LV function leads to PEP prolongation and LVET shortening as stroke volume decreases. The PEP/LVET ratio is more sensitive to changes in LV performance.

DOPPLER ECHOCARDIOGRAPHY

Doppler echocardiography detects blood flow velocity and direction in relation to the ultrasound transducer. The most important clinical applications relate to finding abnormal flow direction or turbulence and increased flow velocity. The Doppler modality is based on the detection of a frequency shift between the frequency of the emitted ultrasound energy and the echos reflected back from moving blood cells (the Doppler shift):

$$V = C(\pm \Delta f/2f_0 \cos\theta)$$

where V is the calculated blood flow velocity (meters/sec); C is the speed of sound in soft tissue (1,540 meters/sec); $\pm \Delta f$ is the Doppler frequency shift; f_0 is the transmitted frequency; and θ is the intercept angle (between ultrasound beam and blood flow direction)[1, 3, 36, 37].

Echos from cells moving away from the transducer are of lower frequency, and those from cells moving toward the transducer are of higher frequency than the originally transmitted frequency. The higher the velocity of the blood cells, the greater the frequency shift. In contrast to 2-D and M-mode, lower frequency transducers produce better Doppler signals.

Because blood flow patterns and velocity can be evaluated with Doppler interrogation, valvular insufficiency, obstructive lesions, and cardiac shunts can be detected and quantified. Cardiac output and other indicators of systolic as well as diastolic function can also be assessed. Adequate Doppler examinations are technically demanding and require a good understanding of cardiac anatomy and hemodynamic principles.

DOPPLER BEAM ALIGNMENT

Optimal blood flow profiles and calculation of maximal flow velocity are possible when the ultrasound beam is aligned parallel to the path of blood flow. This is in contrast to the perpendicular beam orientation needed for optimal M-mode and 2-D imaging. With Doppler, calculated blood flow velocity diminishes as the ultrasound beam's angle of incidence and the direction of blood flow diverge from 0 degrees (**157**). This is because calculated flow velocity is inversely related to the cosine of this angle (cosine 0 degrees = 1). As long as the angle between the ultrasound beam and path of blood flow is less than 20 degrees, maximal flow velocity can be estimated with reasonable accuracy. As this angle of incidence increases, calculated velocity decreases. At an angle of 90 degrees, the calculated velocity is 0 (cosine 90 degrees = 0); therefore, no flow signal is recorded when the ultrasound beam is perpendicular to blood flow. The use of angle correction settings for cardiac studies is discouraged because the inability to correct for the elevational (azimuthal) plane can cause additional error[1, 36].

Flow signals are usually displayed with time on the horizontal axis and velocity (scaled in m/sec) on the vertical axis. A zero baseline demarcates flow away from (below baseline) or toward (above baseline) the transducer. Higher velocities are displayed farther from the baseline. Other flow characteristics (e.g. turbulence) also affect the Doppler spectral display.

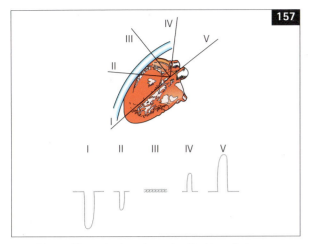

157 Diagram illustrating how the angle of incidence between Doppler beam and blood flow direction affects the maximal recorded flow velocity (see text for more information). Top: solid lines I–V represent different Doppler beam alignments to left ventricular outflow. Bottom: corresponding flow velocity profiles. Maximal peak velocity is recorded when alignment is 0 degrees or 180 degrees. No flow is detected when alignment is 90 degrees. (From Goldberg SJ, Allen HD, Marx GR, Donnerstein RL (1988) *Doppler Echocardiography* (2nd edn). Lea & Febiger, Philadelphia, p. 28, with permission.)

DOPPLER MODES

Several types of Doppler echocardiography are used clinically: pulsed wave (PW), continuous wave (CW), and color flow (CF) mapping. PW and CW are also known as spectral Doppler.

Pulsed wave Doppler

PW Doppler uses short bursts of ultrasound to interrogate a specified area, designated the sample volume, distant to the transducer. This is known as range gating. Its advantage is that blood flow velocity, direction, and spectral characteristics can be calculated from a specific location in the heart or blood vessel (**158–161**). The main disadvantage is that the maximum measurable velocity is limited by the transmitted frequency, the sample volume's distance from the transducer, and by the pulse repetition frequency (PRF). The PRF relates to the time required to send, receive, and process echos returning from the selected location as discreet pulses. Twice the PRF (or the Nyquist limit) defines the maximum measurable velocity, which is influenced by the transmitted frequency and the distance of the sample volume from the transducer.

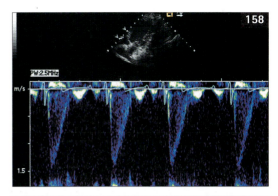

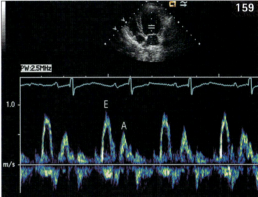

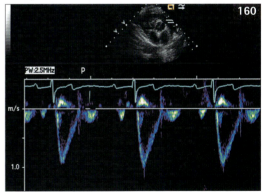

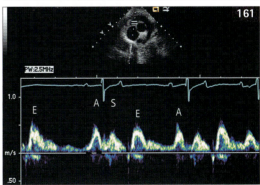

158–161 Pulsed wave Doppler velocity profiles from a normal dog. Normal transvalvular flow patterns are shown: (**158**) aorta; (**159**) mitral; (**160**) pulmonary; and (**161**) tricuspid (systolic wave is also commonly seen here). E = early rapid ventricular filling wave; A = late filling from atrial contraction; S = systolic flow acceleration.

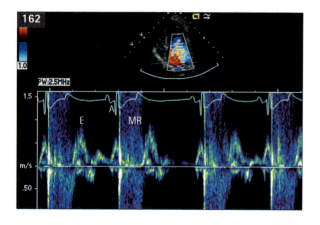

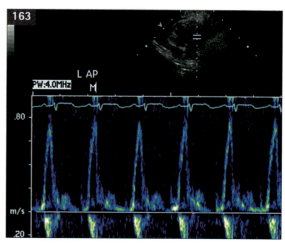

162, 163 (162) Systolic regurgitant flow across the mitral valve is of higher velocity than can be quantified here and aliasing occurs as shown in this dog with mitral regurgitation (see text). (163) Summation of mitral E and A peaks often occurs at the higher heart rates seen in cats. E = early rapid ventricular filling wave; A = late filling from atrial contraction; MR = aliased signal from mitral regurgitant flow.

Lower frequency transducers and closer sample volume placement increase the Nyquist limit. Blood flow velocity higher than the Nyquist limit cannot be measured because of signal 'aliasing' (162, 163). This so-called velocity or range ambiguity is displayed as a broad spectal band extending above and below ('wrapped around') the baseline, so neither velocity nor direction is measurable (162)[1, 2, 3, 7, 36]. High pulse repetition frequency (HPRF) PW Doppler is a hybrid of PW and CW that allows sampling from several depths along the line of interrogation.

When blood cells are traveling in the same direction at a similar velocity within the sample volume, the velocity spectrum displayed across time (time–velocity curve) is relatively thin or tight. Spectral broadening (widening) occurs with disparities in blood cell velocity and direction.

Continuous wave Doppler

CW Doppler uses dual crystals so that ultrasound can be continuously and simultaneously transmitted and received along the line of interrogation. Because the PRF is very high, there is theoretically no maximum velocity limit with CW Doppler and high velocity flows can be measured (164). The disadvantage of CW Doppler is that sampling of blood flow velocity and direction occurs all along the line of interrogation, not in one specified area. This is called range ambiguity.

Color flow mapping (color flow Doppler)

CF mapping can show normal flow patterns and identify areas of abnormal flow. CF mapping is a form of PW Doppler that combines 2-D or M-mode with blood flow imaging. However, instead of one sample volume along one scan line, many are analyzed along multiple scan lines within the region of interest. The mean frequency shifts obtained from these multiple sample volumes are color coded for direction (in relation to the transducer) and velocity. Most systems code blood flow moving away from the transducer as blue and flow toward as red (Blue Away Red Toward or 'BART') (165, 166). Zero velocity is indicated by black; this indicates either no flow or that flow direction is perpendicular to the angle of incidence (according to the Doppler equation)[1, 37]. Differences in relative velocity of flow can be accentuated, and the presence of multiple velocities and directions of flow (turbulence) can be indicated by different display maps that use variations in brightness and color to enhance the visibility of abnormal flow. Aliasing occurs often, even with normal blood flow velocity because the Nyquist limits are usually quite low. Signal aliasing is displayed as a reversal or 'wrap around' of color (e.g. red shifting to blue; 167, 168). Multiple velocities and directions of flow in an area are indicated using a variance map, which adds shades of yellow or green to the red/blue display (169).

During the CF mapping examination all valve areas, the interventricular and interatrial septa, and the proximal great vessels are scanned in several planes to detect abnormal flow patterns. Many normal dogs have trivial to mild physiologic regurgitation of the pulmonary and/or other valves (less often)[38, 39]. Physiologic tricuspid regurgitation appears to be common in cats; however, physiologic regurgitation of the mitral or pulmonic valves is uncommon, and not reported from the aortic valve[40]. Artifacts can be common. Timing within the cardiac cycle is important: valve position and ECG can guide this, but at high heart rates the 2-D color frame may not correlate well

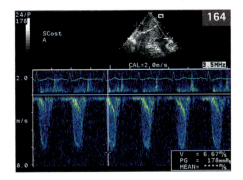
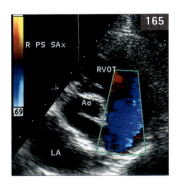
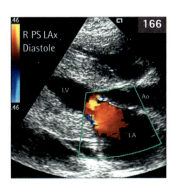

164–166 (164) Continuous wave Doppler allows quantification of higher peak velocities, although velocity is sampled all along the cursor line, not at a specified location (see text). A peak velocity of 6.67 m/sec is recorded here from a 3-month-old female Newfoundland with severe subaortic stenosis (instantaneous pressure gradient estimated at 178 mm Hg according to the modified Bernoulli equation).
(165, 166) In color flow Doppler echocardiography, blood flowing away from the transducer is generally coded blue (165; normal pulmonary outflow in a dog) and flow toward is coded red (166; mitral inflow in a cat with hypertrophic cardiomyopathy).
As blood accelerates from zero (black), the shade of color lightens. Color aliasing occurs at relatively low velocities (note the velocity scale at upper left in the images). Color aliasing is manifest as a 'wrapping around' to the opposite side of the color scale.

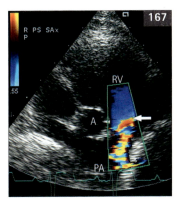
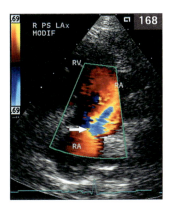
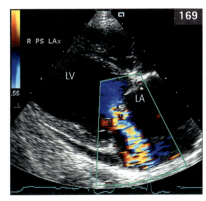

167–169 (167) Aliasing of the color flow signal (arrow) occurs as blood accelerates toward the pulmonary valve in this 3-year-old West Highland White Terrier with valvular pulmonic stenosis. (168) An aliased signal (arrow) is seen as blood accelerates across the opening of an abnormal membrane within the RA of this 4-month-old Staffordshire Terrier with cor triatriatum dexter. Ao/A = aorta, LA = left atrium; LV = left ventricle; RVOT = right ventricular outflow tract; RA = right atrium; RV = right ventricle; PA = pulmonary artery. (169) Turbulent blood flow, here resulting from mitral regurgitation in a 13-year-old mixed breed dog, causes a mixed color pattern of varied flow velocity and direction. LA = left atrium; LV = left ventricle.

with the ECG frame indicator. Color flow-guided spectral Doppler should be used to quantify flow velocity and verify timing whenever turbulent flow is suspected. CF M-mode also can be used for more precise timing. There are several important technical issues to consider when performing CF examinations. The interested reader is referred to additional sources for more specific information[1–3, 7, 37, 41].

Color flow M-mode

The use of CF mapping with M-mode imaging permits more precise timing of flow events within the cardiac cycle. This is done by placing the color sector over the area of interest in 2-D mode, then aligning the M-mode cursor over this and switching to M-mode (156).

NORMAL TRANSVALVULAR FLOW

Characteristic blood flow patterns are obtained from the different valve areas[2, 3, 7, 36, 42–45]. Breed, age, and body weight appear to have little influence on normal Doppler measurements[45]. Flow across both AV valves has a similar pattern; likewise, flow configuration across the semilunar valve areas is similar. Mitral and tricuspid inflow velocities are measured with the sample volume placed at the tips of the opened leaflets. Normal diastolic flow across the mitral and tricuspid valves (158–163, pp. 83, 84) consists of an initial higher velocity signal during the rapid ventricular filling phase (E wave), which is followed by a smaller velocity signal associated with atrial contraction (A wave). Peak velocities are normally higher across the mitral valve (peak E usually about 0.75 m/sec; peak A usually about 0.55 m/sec)[2, 3] compared with the tricuspid valve. A prominent systolic wave is often seen with the tricuspid flow spectrum. Higher velocities occur with greater transvalvular flow, including from severe valve insufficiency, shunts, anemia, and also with tachycardia. As heart rate increases, the time between E and A waves diminishes until they fuse into a single, summated signal. This pattern is typical for cats (163).

The 4-chamber left apical view (129, p. 75) provides optimal alignment for imaging mitral inflow[44]. Usually, the left cranial short-axis ('left middle') view allows good alignment with tricuspid inflow, although sometimes the left apical 4-chamber view, right parasternal short-axis view at the heart base, or the left cranial long-axis position with medial beam angulation can be used.

Flow across the ventricular outflow tracts (158, 160) accelerates quickly during ejection, with more gradual deceleration. The aortic velocity signal is normally more rapid and sharply peaked than the pulmonary flow signal. Peak velocities are recorded at or just distal to the valves[1, 2, 36]. Peak aortic velocity is usually between 0.9 m/sec and 1.6–1.7 m/sec or less. Peak recorded velocity varies with cycle length, ventilation, and translational motion of the heart. Some normal dogs have higher peak aortic velocities related to increased stroke volume, high sympathetic tone, or possibly breed-related LV outflow tract characteristics. Ventricular outflow obstruction causes more rapid flow acceleration, increased peak velocities, and turbulence. In general, aortic velocities over 2.1 or 2.2 m/sec are suggestive of outflow obstruction. However, between 1.7 and around 2.2 m/sec lies a 'grey zone' where very mild LV outflow obstruction (e.g. some cases of subaortic stenosis) cannot be differentiated with certainty from normal but vigorous LV ejection. Maximal aortic/LV outflow velocity readings are obtained in most dogs from the subcostal (subxiphoid) position, although some dogs may have higher aortic velocities recorded from the left apical position (130, p. 75). This region should be interrogated from both positions and the highest velocity recording used.

Peak systolic pulmonary velocity is 1.4–1.5 m/sec or less in most normal dogs. Pulmonary outflow is usually better assessed from left-sided transducer positions rather than right parasternal short-axis view.

ABNORMAL FLOW AND VELOCITY ASSESSMENT

The increased flow velocity, abnormal flow direction, and turbulence that signal abnormal valve function or a cardiac shunt can be detected with Doppler echocardiography. The timing, within the cardiac cycle, of any abnormal flow signals should be determined using spectral or CF M-mode Doppler. The instantaneous pressure gradient across a stenotic or regurgitant valve area, or across a shunt, is estimated using the maximal measured velocity of the flow jet (164, p. 85). Probe angulation into unconventional view planes may be needed to find optimal alignment. CW Doppler is used if aliasing occurs with PW Doppler. 2-D and M-mode evaluation of chamber sizes and wall thicknesses provides more information on the hemodynamic significance of abnormal flow disturbances.

Modified Bernoulli equation

A modification of the Bernoulli equation is used to estimate the instantaneous gradient:

$$\text{pressure gradient} = 4(\text{maximum velocity})^2$$

Other factors involved in this relationship are usually of little clinical consequence and are generally ignored, although they could be influential in some types of flow obstruction[2, 3, 7]. It is important to note that this method of estimating stenosis severity is flow dependent. Doppler estimation of pressure gradients is used in combination with M-mode and 2-D imaging, sometimes with calculation of effective orifice area, to assess the severity of congenital or acquired outflow obstructions.

The maximum velocity of a regurgitant jet can be used also to estimate the peak pressure gradient across the regurgitant valve. For example, the peak velocity of a tricuspid regurgitation jet can be used to estimate pulmonary artery pressure in the absence of pulmonic stenosis. The calculated systolic pressure gradient plus the central venous pressure equals the peak RV systolic pressure, which approximates pulmonary artery pressure.

Semiquantification of valve regurgitation by determining the size and shape of the regurgitant jet is sometimes done with CF Doppler. Although technical and hemodynamic factors confound the accuracy of such assessment, wide and long regurgitant jets are generally associated with more severe regurgitation than narrow jets. Other methods have been used to quantitate mitral regurgitation as well, including the proximal isovelocity surface area (PISA)[37, 46]. Measurement of maximum regurgitant jet velocity is not an indicator of the severity of regurgitation, especially mitral regurgitation. Changes in chamber size provide a better indication of severity with chronic regurgitation. Trivial, brief regurgitation of the tricuspid and pulmonary valves is commonly seen in normal dogs[2, 3, 47].

Left ventricular function

Various Doppler-derived indices of systolic and diastolic LV function have been described[1–4, 7, 34, 48–53]. Cardiac output can be estimated from heart rate and the area under the ventricular outflow signal (velocity–time integral), which is proportional to stroke volume. Doppler spectra with simultaneous ECG can be used to measure preejection period and ejection time (STIs). Aortic signal acceleration time correlates with LV systolic function but is load dependent. LV dP/dt$_{max}$ can be estimated in patients with mitral regurgitation by the acceleration rate of the regurgitant jet velocity signal[36, 54]. Although the quantification of abnormal blood flow and estimation of cardiac output and LV function are subject to numerous sources of error, they are sometimes clinically useful.

There is increasing interest in Doppler-derived indices of diastolic function to evaluate patients with cardiac disease. These include isovolumic relaxation time (IVRT), characteristics of the mitral inflow pattern (see also **447–449**, p. 305), pulmonary venous flow pattern, Doppler tissue imaging (DTI), and others[1–4, 48–50, 52, 55]. Abnormalities of early (active) LV relaxation, LV compliance, and increased LA pressure affect the amplitude and timing of these patterns in characteristic ways (see references for further information).

Doppler tissue imaging

DTI targets the motion of tissue rather than blood cells by altering the signal processing and filtering of returning echos. CF mapping (M-mode and 2-D) and PW spectral DTI techniques are used to evaluate myocardial velocity patterns. Their use is increasing in veterinary medicine. Spectral DTI displays the velocity and direction of motion of a specific location defined by the sample volume (**170**). It allows greater temporal resolution than color DTI, along with the ability to quantitate peak velocities, but it has spatial limitations[4, 56]. The lateral and septal aspects of the mitral valve annulus are commonly used sites that provide information on LV function in both systole and diastole[4, 56–58]. Color DTI methods provide spatial orientation of mean myocardial velocities from different ventricular regions; color M-mode DTI offers greater temporal resolution than 2-D color DTI. Several other analyses used to assess regional myocardial function and synchrony are derived from DTI techniques, including myocardial velocity gradients, strain, strain rate, and velocity vector imaging[4, 59–62].

TRANSESOPHAGEAL ECHOCARDIOGRAPHY

Cardiac structures can be imaged through the esophageal wall with specialized transducers mounted on a flexible, steerable endoscope tip. Transesophageal echocardiography (TEE) can provide clearer images of some cardiac structures (especially those at or above the AV junction) compared with transthoracic echocardiography because interference from the chest wall and lung is avoided[1, 63, 64]. TEE can be especially helpful for defining some congenital malformations, identifying atrial thrombi or tumors, evaluating valves for endocarditis lesions, and guiding cardiac interventional procedures. The need for general anesthesia, or heavy sedation, and the expense of the endoscopic transducers, are the main disadvantages of TEE.

3-D ECHOCARDIOGRAPHY

The ability to acquire and manipulate 3-D images of the heart and other structures is becoming more widespread. With this modality, anatomic and blood flow abnormalities can be viewed from any angle by rotating or bisecting the image. Current technology requires several cardiac cycles in order to acquire sufficient data for 3-D reconstruction of the entire heart, although true 'real time' 3-D echocardiography is on the horizon.

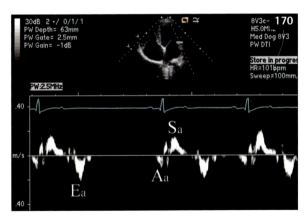

170 Example of pulsed wave Doppler tissue imaging from the left apical 4-chamber view with the sample volume placed at the lateral mitral annulus (small image on top). The two diastolic annular motions occur with early filling (Ea) and atrial contraction (Aa). In this normal dog, the velocity of Ea is greater than that of Aa, similar to the normal transmitral flow velocity pattern; with diastolic dysfunction, Ea diminishes and the Ea/Aa ratio reverses. Comparison of annular motion with transmitral flow velocities is helpful in defining the presence and severity of abnormal diastolic function. The annulus moves toward the ventricular apex in systole (Sa); the systolic velocity has been correlated with ejection fraction.

REFERENCES

1 Armstrong WF, Feigenbaum H (2001) Echocardiography. In: *Heart Disease: A Textbook of Cardiovascular Medicine*, 6th edn. E Braunwald, DP Zipes, P Libby (eds). WB Saunders, Philadelphia, pp. 160–228.

2 Bonagura JD, Luis Fuentes V (2000) Echocardiography. In: *Textbook of Veterinary Internal Medicine*, 5th edn. SJ Ettinger, EC Feldman (eds). WB Saunders, Philadelphia, pp. 834–873.

3 Moise NS, Fox PR (1999) Echocardiography and Doppler imaging. In: *Textbook of Canine and Feline Cardiology*, 2nd edn. PR Fox, DD Sisson, NS Moise (eds). WB Saunders, Philadelphia, pp. 130–171.

4 Feigenbaum H, Armstrong WF, Ryan T (2005) *Feigenbaum's Echocardiography*, 6th edn. Lippincott Williams & Wilkins, Philadelphia.

5 Stepien RL, Bonagura JD, Bednarski RM *et al.* (1995) Cardiorespiratory effects of acepromazine maleate and buprenorphine hydrochloride in clinically normal dogs. *Am J Vet Res* 56:78–84.

6 Jacobs GJ, Knight DH (1985) Changes in M-mode echocardiographic values in cats given ketamine. *Am J Vet Res* 46:1712–1713.

7 Kienle RD (1997) Echocardiography. In: *Small Animal Cardiovascular Medicine*. MD Kittleson, RD Kienle (eds). Mosby, St. Louis, pp. 95–117.

8 Barthez PY, Leveille R, Scrivani PV (1997) Side lobes and grating lobes artifacts in ultrasound imaging. *Vet Radiol Ultrasound* 38:387–393.

9 Kirberger RM (1995) Imaging artifacts in diagnostic ultrasound – a review. *Vet Radiol Ultrasound* 36:297–306.

10 O'Grady MR, Bonagura JD, Powers JD *et al.* (1986) Quantitative cross-sectional echocardiography in the normal dog. *Vet Radiol* 27:34–49.

11 Thomas WP, Gaber CE, Jacobs GJ *et al.* (1993) Recommendations for standards in transthoracic two-dimensional echocardiography in the dog and cat. *J Vet Intern Med* 7:247–252.

12 Rishniw M, Erb HN (2000) Evaluation of four 2-dimensional echocardiographic methods of assessing left atrial size in dogs. *J Vet Intern Med* 14:429–435.

13 Haggstrom J, Hansson K, Kalberg BE *et al.* (1994) Plasma concentrations of atrial natriuretic peptide in relation to severity of mitral regurgitation in Cavalier King Charles Spaniels. *Am J Vet Res* 55:698–703.

14 Abbott JA, MacLean HN (2006) Two-dimensional echocardiographic assessment of the feline left atrium. *J Vet Intern Med* 20:111–119.

15 Bonagura JD (2001) Echocardiography case studies. In *Proceedings of the 19th ACVIM Forum*, Denver, pp. 133–135.

16 Goodwin JK, Holland M (1995) Contrast echoaortography as an aid in the diagnosis of right-to-left shunting patent ductus arteriosus. *Vet Radiol Ultrasound* 36:157–159.

17 Concalves AC, Orton EC, Boon JA *et al.* (2002) Linear, logarithmic, and polynomial models of M-mode echocardiographic measurements in dogs. *Am J Vet Res* 63:994–999.

18 Crippa L, Ferro E, Melloni E *et al.* (1992) Echocardiographic parameters and indices in the normal Beagle dog. *Lab Anim* 26:190–195.

19 Gooding JP, Robinson WF, Mews GC (1986) Echocardiographic assessment of left ventricular dimensions in clinically normal English Cocker Spaniels. *Am J Vet Res* 47:296–300.

20 Herrtage ME (1994) Echocardiographic measurements in the normal Boxer. Abstr. In: *Proceedings of the 4th European Society of Veterinary Internal Medicine Congress*, p. 172.

21 Lonsdale RA, Labuc RH, Robertson ID (1998) Echocardiographic parameters in training compared with non-training Greyhounds. *Vet Radiol Ultrasound* 39:325–330.

22 Morrison SA, Moise NS, Scarlett J *et al.* (1992) Effect of breed and body weight on echocardiographic values in four breeds of dogs of differing somatotype. *J Vet Intern Med* 6:220–224.

23 Page A, Edmunds G, Atwell RB (1993) Echocardiographic values in the Greyhound. *Aust Vet J* 70:361–34.

24 Sisson DD, Schaeffer D (1991) Changes in linear dimensions of the heart, relative body weight as measured by M-mode echocardiography in growing dogs. *Am J Vet Res* 52:1591–1596.

25 Snyder PS, Sato T, Atkins CE (1995) A comparison of echocardiographic indices of the nonracing, heathy greyhound to reference values from other breeds. *Vet Radiol Ultrasound* 36:387–392.

26 Stepien RL, Hinchcliff KW, Constable PD *et al.* (1998) Effect of endurance training on cardiac morphology in Alaskan sled dogs. *J Appl Physiol* 85:1368–1375.

27 Vollmar AC (1999) Echocardiographic measurements in the Irish Wolfhound: reference values for the breed. *J Am Anim Hosp Assoc* 35:271–277.

28 Vollmar AC, Fox PR (2001) Clinical echocardiographic and ECG findings in 232 sequentially examined Irish Wolfhounds. Abstract. *J Vet Intern Med* 15:279.

29 Minors SL, O'Grady MR (1998) Resting and dobutamine stress echocardiographic factors associated with the development of occult dilated cardiomyopathy in healthy Doberman Pinscher dogs. *J Vet Intern Med* 12:369–380.

30 Bayon A, DelpalacioMJF, Montes AM *et al.* (1994) M-mode echocardiography studying growing Spanish mastiffs. *J Small Anim Pract* 35:473–479.

31 Brown DJ (2003) M-mode echocardiographic ratio indices. In *Proceedings of the 21st Annual ACVIM Forum*, Charlotte, pp. 78–79.

32 Schober KE, Luis Fuentes V, McEwan JD *et al.* (1997) Atrioventricular annular displacement in healthy dogs and

dogs with heart disease: relation to left ventricular systolic function. In *Proceedings of the BSAVA Congress*, Birmingham, p. 312.

33 Kittleson MD, Eyster GE, Knowlen GG *et al.* (1984) Myocardial function in small dogs with chronic mitral regurgitation and severe congestive heart failure. *J Am Vet Med Assoc* **184**:455–459.

34 Schiller NB, Shah PM, Crawford M *et al.* (1989) Recommendations for quantitation of the left ventricle by two-dimensional echocardiography. *J Am Soc Echocardiog* **2**:358–367.

35 Atkins CE, Snyder PS (1992) Systolic time intervals and their derivatives for evaluation of cardiac function. *J Vet Intern Med* **6**:55–63.

36 Bonagura JD, Miller MW (1998) Doppler echocardiography I: pulsed and continuous wave studies. *Vet Clin North Am: Small Anim Pract* **28**:1325–1359.

37 Bonagura JD, Miller MW (1998) Doppler echocardiography II: color Doppler imaging. *Vet Clin North Am: Small Anim Pract* **28**:1361–1389.

38 Nakayama T, Wakao Y, Takiguchi S *et al.* (1994) Prevalence of valvular regurgitation in normal Beagle dogs detected by color Doppler echocardiography. *J Vet Med Sci* **56**:973–975.

39 Rishniw M, Erb HN (2000) Prevalence and characterization of pulmonary regurgitation in normal adult dogs. *J Vet Cardiol* **2**:17–20.

40 Adin DB, McCloy K (2005) Physiologic valve regurgitation in normal cats. *J Vet Cardiol* **7**:9–13.

41 Kisslo JA, Adams DB, Belkin RN (1998) *Doppler Color Flow Imaging*. Churchill Livingstone, New York.

42 Kirberger RM, Bland-Van den Berg P, Darazs B (1992). Doppler echocardiography in the normal dog: parts I & II. *Vet Radiol Ultrasound* **33**:370–386.

43 Brown DJ, Knight DH, King RR (1991) Use of pulsed-wave Doppler echocardiography to determine aortic and pulmonary velocity and flow variables in clinically normal dogs. *Am J Vet Res* **52**:543–550.

44 Darke PGG, Bonagura JD, Miller MW (1993) Transducer

orientation for Doppler echocardiography in dogs. *J Small Anim Pract* **34**:2–8.

45 Yuill CD, O'Grady MR (1991) Doppler–derived velocity of blood flow across cardiac valves in the normal dog. *Can J Vet Res* **55**:185–192.

46 Kittleson MD, Brown WA (2003) Regurgitant fraction measured by using the proximal isovelocity surface area method in dogs with chronic myxomatous mitral valve disease. *J Vet Intern Med* **17**:84–8.

47 Nakayama T, Wakao Y, Takiguchi S *et al.* (1994) Prevalence of valvular regurgitation in normal Beagle dogs detected by color Doppler echocardiography. *J Vet Med Sci* **56**:973–975.

48 Schober KE, Luis Fuentes V, McEwan JD *et al.* (1998) Pulmonary venous flow characteristics as assessed by transthoracic pulsed Doppler echocardiography in normal dogs. *Vet Radiol Ultrasound* **39**:33–41.

49 Schober KE, Luis Fuentes V, Bonagura JD (2003) Comparison between invasive hemodynamic measurements and noninvasive assessment of left ventricular diastolic function by use of Doppler echocardiography in healthy anesthetized cats. *Am J Vet Res* **64**:93–103.

50 Luis Fuentes V, Schober KE (2001) Diastology: theory and practice II. In *Proceedings of the 19th ACVIM Forum*, Denver, pp. 142–144.

51 McEntee K, Clercs C, Amory H *et al.* (1999) Doppler echocardiographic study of left and right ventricular function during dobutamine stress testing in conscious healthy dogs. *Am J Vet Res* **60**:865–871.

52 Schober KE, Fuentes VL (2001) Diastology: theory and practice I. In: *Proceedings of the 19th ACVIM Forum*, Denver, pp. 139–141.

53 Koffas H, Dukes-McEwan J, Corcoran BM *et al.* (2003) Peak mean myocardial velocities and velocity gradients measured by color M-mode tissue Doppler imaging in healthy cats. *J Vet Intern Med* **17**:510–524.

54 Chen C, Rodriguez L, Guerroro JL *et al.* (1991) Noninvasive estimation of the instantaneous first derivative of left ventricular pressure using continuous-wave Doppler echocardiography. *Circulation* **83**:2101–2110.

55 Schober KE, Fuentes VL (2001) Effects of age, body weight, and heart rate on transmitral and pulmonary venous flow in clinically normal dogs. *Am J Vet Res* **62**:1447–1454.

56 Waggoner AD, Bierig SM (2001) Tissue Doppler imaging: a useful echocardiographic method for the cardiac sonographer to assess systolic and diastolic ventricular function. *J Am Soc Echocardiog* **14**:1143–1152.

57 Gavaghan BJ, Kittleson MD, Fisher KJ *et al.* (1999) Quantification of left ventricular diastolic wall motion by Doppler tissue imaging in healthy cats and cats with cardiomyopathy. *Am J Vet Res* **60**:1478–1486.

58 Koffas H, Dukes-McEwan J, Corcoran BM *et al.* (2006) Pulsed tissue Doppler imaging in normal cats and cats with hypertrophic cardiomyopathy. *J Vet Intern Med* **20**:65–77.

59 Chetboul V (2002) Tissue Doppler imaging: a promising technique for quantifying regional myocardial function. *J Vet Cardiol* **4**:7–12.

60 Koffas H, Dukes-McEwan J, Corcoran BM *et al.* (2003) Peak mean myocardial velocities and velocity gradients measured by color M-mode tissue Doppler imaging in healthy cats. *J Vet Intern Med* **17**:510–524.

61 Chetboul V, Sampedrano CC, Concordet D *et al.* (2005) Use of quantitative two-dimensional color tissue Doppler imaging for assessment of left ventricular radial and longitudinal myocardial velocities in dogs. *Am J Vet Res* **66**:953–961.

62 Chetboul V, Sampedrano CC, Tissier R *et al.* (2006) Quantitative assessment of velocities of the annulus of the left atrioventricular valve and left ventricular free wall in healthy cats by use of two-dimensional color tissue Doppler

imaging. *J Vet Intern Med* 67:250–258.

63 Loyer C, Thomas WP (1995) Biplane transesophageal echocardiography in the dog: technique, anatomy, and imaging planes. *Vet Radiol Ultrasound* 36:212–226.

64 Kienle RD, Thomas WP, Rishniw M (1997) Biplane transesophageal echocardiography in the normal cat. *Vet Radiol Ultrasound* 38:288–298.

65 DeMadron E, Bonagura JD, Herring DS (1985) Two-dimensional echocardiography in the normal cat. *Vet Radiol Ultrasound* 26:149–158.

66 Fox PR, Bond BR, Peterson ME (1985) Echocardiographic reference values in healthy cats sedated with ketamine HCl. *Am J Vet Res* 46:1479.

67 Jacobs G, Knight DV (1985) M-mode echocardiographic measurements in nonanesthetized healthy cats: effects of body weight, heart rate, and other variables. *Am J Vet Res* 46:1705.

68 Moise NS, Dietze AE, Mezza LE *et al.* (1986) Echocardiography, electrocardiography, and radiography of cats with dilatation cardiomyopathy, hypertrophic cardiomyopathy, and hyperthyroidism. *Am J Vet Res* 47:1476.

69 Pipers FS, Reef V, Hamlin RL (1979) Echocardiography in the domestic cat. *Am J Vet Res* 40:882–886.

70 Sisson DD, Knight DH, Helinski C *et al.* (1991) Plasma taurine concentrations and M-mode echocardiographic measures in healthy cats and in cats with dilated cardiomyopathy *J Vet Intern Med* 5:232–238.

71 Baade H, Schober K, Oechtering G (2002) Echokardiographische referenzwerte beim West Highland White Terrier unter besonderer Bercksichtigung der Rechtsherzfunktion. *Tierärztl Prax* 30:172–179.

72 Calvert CA, Brown J (1986) Use of M-mode echocardiography in the diagnosis of congestive cardiomyopathy in Doberman Pinschers. *J Am Vet Med Assoc* 189:293–297.

73 Koch J, Pedersen HD, Jensen AL *et al.* (1996) M-mode echocardiographic diagnosis of dilated cardiomyopathy in giant breed dogs. *Zentralbl Veterinarmed A* 43(5):297–304.

Section 2

Clinical Manifestations and Management of Cardiovascular Problems

6
Murmurs and Abnormal Heart Sounds

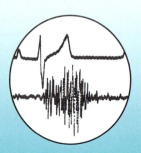

OVERVIEW

Normal heart sounds in dogs and cats are the S_1 sound, associated with closure and tensing of the AV valves and associated structures at the onset of systole, and the S_2 sound, associated with closure of the aortic and pulmonic valves following ejection (see Chapter 1 and **14**, p. 19). Proficiency in recognizing abnormal heart sounds and their origin is not easily achieved[1-4], but this is a skill that can provide important clinical insight. In animals with a murmur or other abnormal heart sounds, it is especially important to understand the cardiac cycle events associated with these sounds and to identify the timing of systole (between S_1 and S_2) and diastole (after S_2 until the next S_1) in the patient.

Identifying abnormal heart sounds as 'systolic' or 'diastolic' is critical to understanding their origin. Besides the paired 'lub-dub' sound of S_1 and S_2 during sinus rhythm, palpation can help the clinician differentiate these sounds (and, thus, the timing of systole). The precordial impulse occurs just after S_1, and the arterial pulse between S_1 and S_2. In addition, subtle changes in the relative intensity of the two sounds occur as the stethoscope chestpiece is moved toward or away from the source of each sound.

Murmurs are defined as audible vibrations of prolonged duration[5]. Although cardiac murmurs often indicate heart disease, some murmurs occur when the heart is structurally normal (innocent or functional murmurs). Audible turbulence is associated with high velocity blood flow, reduced blood viscosity (anemia), and, sometimes, also with flow into a dilated or large vessel. Sympathetic nervous system activation (e.g. with fever, exercise, hyperthyroidism) can increase ejection velocity and worsen any dynamic ventricular outflow obstruction. An increased flow volume, as with a cardiac shunt, also increases transvalvular velocity. Pathologic causes of murmurs usually relate to insufficiency or stenosis of valves or surrounding regions, as well as to shunts.

Transient sounds are vibrations of brief duration[5]. They occur with abrupt changes in blood flow and pressure. Normal transient sounds in dogs and cats are the S_1 and S_2. Changes in the intensity or splitting of the S_1 and/or S_2 sounds sometimes indicate underlying pathology (see Chapter 2 and *Table 5*, p. 33). Split sounds result from asynchronous closure of the left and right heart valves. Diastolic transient sounds are not normally heard.

Many sounds generated by the heart are of too low a frequency and/or intensity to be heard, even with the stethoscope. Any hearing impairment adds further limitation[6]. Low frequency sounds, such as gallop sounds, must be of greater intensity (loudness) than higher pitched sounds to be heard as well. When relatively loud sounds are also present (e.g. a loud murmur or environmental noise), the examiner may not consciously hear any softer sounds because of the phenomenon of 'masking'[6]; therefore, efforts to optimize conditions for auscultation are important. These include using a good quality stethoscope with proper technique; a quiet listening environment; and a calm patient who is breathing quietly and standing in a normal position (see Chapter 2).

CARDIAC MURMURS

MURMUR CHARACTERISTICS
Timing
Cardiac murmurs are described by their timing within the cardiac cycle (systolic or diastolic, or portions thereof; **171**), intensity, PMI on the precordium, pattern of radiation over the chest wall, quality, and pitch. Systolic murmurs may occur in early (protosystolic), middle (mesosystolic), or late (telesystolic) systole, or throughout systole (holosystolic). Diastolic murmurs generally occur in early diastole (protodiastolic) or throughout diastole (holodiastolic). Occasionally, a murmur is heard at the very end of diastole (just before the next S_1); this timing is termed presystolic. Continuous murmurs begin in systole and extend without interruption through S_2 into all or part of diastole[5].

Intensity and radiation

The intensity of a murmur is generally graded on a I to VI scale (*Table 18*). Often, louder murmurs are associated with more severe disease, but this is not always the case, as several factors influence murmur

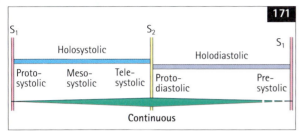

171 The timing of murmurs in relation to the normal heart sounds.

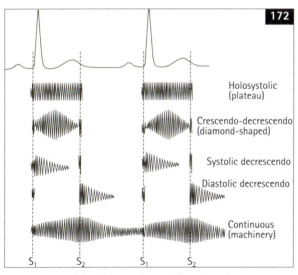

172 Depiction of the (phonocardiographic) configuration and timing of various cardiac murmurs. (From Ware WA (2003) The cardiovascular examination. In *Small Animal Internal Medicine* (3rd edn). (eds RW Nelson, CG Couto) Mosby, St Louis, p. 10, with permission.)

intensity. The PMI is usually indicated by the hemithorax (right or left) and intercostal space or valve area where it is located, or by the terms apex or base. Loud murmurs radiate to other areas over the chest wall. The areas to which a murmur radiates are often characteristic of the source and relate to the direction of abnormal blood flow. The entire thorax, thoracic inlet, and carotid artery areas should be auscultated.

'Shape' and quality

A murmur is also described by its phonocardiographic shape. Figure **172** depicts the configuration of various murmurs. The holosystolic or plateau-shaped murmur begins at the time of S_1 and is of fairly uniform intensity throughout systole. Loud murmurs of this type may prevent distinction of S_1 and S_2 from the murmur. AV valve insufficiency and IVS defects commonly cause this murmur because the turbulent abnormal flow occurs throughout ventricular systole. A crescendo-decrescendo or diamond-shaped murmur starts softly, builds intensity in midsystole, and then diminishes; S_1 and S_2 usually can be heard clearly before and after the murmur. This type is often called an ejection murmur because it usually occurs during blood ejection, most commonly because of ventricular outflow obstruction. A decrescendo murmur tapers from its initial intensity over time; it may occur in systole or diastole.

The pitch and quality of a murmur relate to its various frequency components. Murmurs are usually of higher frequency than transient sounds[6]. 'Noisy' or 'harsh' murmurs contain mixed frequencies; most murmurs can be described as such. 'Musical' murmurs are of essentially one frequency with its overtones.

Grade	Murmur
I	Very soft murmur; heard only in quiet surroundings after listening intently.
II	Soft murmur, but easily heard.
III	Moderate intensity murmur.
IV	Loud murmur, but without a precordial thrill.
V	Loud murmur with a palpable precordial thrill.
VI	Very loud murmur that can also be heard with the stethoscope lifted away from the chest; accompanied by a precordial thrill.

Table 18 Murmur intensity grading.

SYSTOLIC MURMURS

Systolic murmurs commonly are holosystolic (plateau-shaped) or mid-systolic (crescendo-decrescendo or ejection) in configuration. It can be difficult to differentiate these murmurs, especially for the inexperienced listener. However, establishing that a murmur occurs in systole (rather than diastole), determining its PMI, and grading its intensity are the most important steps toward diagnosis. The typical location of various murmurs over different areas of the chest wall are shown (173, 174).

Functional murmurs

Functional murmurs occur with no structural heart abnormality. They tend to be heard best at the left heart base, over the aortic and pulmonic valves and great vessels. They are usually of soft to moderate intensity and have a crescendo-decrescendo configuration. Functional murmurs may have no apparent cardiovascular cause (e.g. 'innocent' puppy murmurs) or can result from an altered physiologic state (physiologic murmurs). Innocent puppy murmurs generally disappear by about 4 (to 6) months of age. Physiologic murmurs have been associated with anemia, fever, high sympathetic tone, hyperthyroidism, peripheral arteriovenous fistulae, hypoproteinemia, an athletic heart, and extreme bradycardia. Some cats with aortic dilation (e.g. with hypertension) have an audible murmur. Dynamic RV outflow obstruction also has been described as a cause of an ejection murmur in cats[7].

Pathologic murmurs

The murmur of mitral regurgitation (insufficiency; MR) is heard best in the area of the mitral valve and at the left apex. Its causes include degenerative mitral valve disease (endocardiosis), infectious endocarditis, congenital malformation of the valve or its supporting structures (chordae, papillary muscles), and diseases causing LV dilation or hypertrophy. MR murmurs radiate well dorsally and often to the left base and right chest wall. Characteristically, MR causes a holosystolic murmur; however, the murmur may be heard in early systole (protosystolic) and taper into a decrescendo configuration, either with mild MR, where the leakage ceases in late systole, or with sudden and severe valve insufficiency, if atrial and ventricular pressures equalize. Occasionally, MR murmurs have a musical or 'whoop-like' quality. The intensity of a MR murmur caused by degenerative valve disease is related to severity[8], but this is not necessarily so with other etiologies. Increased arterial pressure can increase MR murmur intensity, while hypotension can diminish it. MR associated with mitral systolic anterior motion (SAM) from dynamic outflow obstruction varies with the degree of obstruction.

Murmurs caused by ventricular outflow obstruction are crescendo-decrescendo in shape and are most often heard at the left base. A fixed narrowing (e.g. subaortic or pulmonic valve stenosis) or dynamic muscular obstruction (hypertrophic cardiomyopathy or, occasionally, mitral dysplasia) can be the cause. These murmurs become louder as cardiac output or contractile strength increases. The murmur of subaortic stenosis is heard well at the low left base and radiates prominently up the aortic arch (which curves toward the right) to the right base. This murmur also radiates up the carotid arteries and occasionally can be heard on top of the skull (calvarium). The murmur of pulmonic stenosis is best heard high at the left base over the pulmonary valve and main pulmonary artery. Relative pulmonic stenosis occurs when flow through the valve is greatly increased, even though the valve itself may be structurally normal (e.g. with a large left-to-right shunting atrial or ventricular septal defect).

Most murmurs heard on the right chest wall are holosystolic, plateau-shaped murmurs, with the exception of the subaortic stenosis murmur described above. The murmur of tricuspid regurgitation

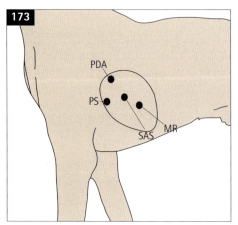 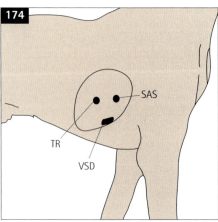

173, 174 The typical PMI for various congenital and acquired murmurs is illustrated on the left (173) and right (174) chest walls. MR = mitral valve regurgitation; PDA = patent ductus arteriosus; PS = pulmonic stenosis; SAS = subaortic stenosis; TR = tricuspid valve regurgitation; VSD = ventricular septal defect.

(insufficiency; TR) is loudest at the right apex over the tricuspid valve and tends to radiate dorsally. A noticeably different pitch or quality from a concurrent MR murmur, a right precordial thrill, jugular pulsations, or signs of right-sided heart failure help differentiate TR from radiation of a MR murmur to the right chest wall. Causes of TR include degenerative disease (endocardiosis), infection, and congenital malformation, as well as diseases that cause RV hypertrophy and/or dilation.

Ventricular septal defects also cause holosystolic murmurs. The PMI is usually at the right sternal border (perimembranous defects), reflecting the direction of the intracardiac shunt. A large ventricular septal defect may also cause the murmur of relative pulmonic stenosis. Prolapse of part of the aortic valve into the defect may cause an audible aortic regurgitation murmur.

DIASTOLIC MURMURS

Diastolic murmurs are relatively uncommon in dogs and cats. Aortic regurgitation (insufficiency; AR) from bacterial endocarditis is the most common cause, although congenital malformation, prolapse associated with ventricular septal defect, or degenerative aortic valve disease occasionally occurs. This diastolic murmur begins at the time of S_2 and is heard best at the left base over the aortic valve; it sometimes radiates to the right base. It is decrescendo in configuration and extends a variable time into diastole, depending on the pressure difference between the aorta and the LV. Some aortic insufficiency murmurs have a musical quality. Clinically relevant pulmonic insufficiency is rare, but an audible murmur would be more likely in the face of pulmonary hypertension. A soft, low diastolic rumble is described in humans with mitral or tricuspid stenosis[5], but this is almost never heard in dogs and cats.

MURMUR IN BOTH SYSTOLE AND DIASTOLE
Continuous murmurs

Continuous (machinery) murmurs begin in systole and continue through S_2 into diastole, indicating that a significant pressure gradient exists continuously between two connecting locations (vessels). At slow heart rates, this murmur may become inaudible toward the end of diastole. Patent ductus arteriosus (PDA) is by far the most common cause of a continuous murmur. The PDA murmur is loudest high at the left base above the pulmonic valve area (main pulmonary artery area). This murmur tends to radiate cranially, ventrally, and to the right. The systolic component is usually louder and heard well all over the chest, whereas the diastolic component is more localized to the left base in many cases. If only the cardiac apical area is auscultated, the diastolic component (and the correct diagnosis) may be missed. Concurrent MR associated with LV dilation is

common. A continuous murmur also occurs with aorticopulmonic window, ruptured sinus of Valsalva aneurysm, and other central arterio-venous (A-V) shunts. Peripheral A-V fistulae may also be associated with an audible continuous murmur (bruit).

Sometimes, both holosystolic and diastolic decrescendo murmurs can occur (e.g. with a ventricular septal defect and aortic insufficiency from loss of aortic root support), but this is not considered a true 'continuous' murmur.

'To and fro' murmurs

Continuous murmurs can be confused with concurrent mid-systolic (ejection) and diastolic decrescendo murmurs. But in these so-called 'to and fro' murmurs, the ejection murmur component tapers in late systole, allowing the S_2 to be heard as a distinct sound. The most common cause of 'to and fro' murmurs is the combination of subaortic stenosis and aortic insufficiency.

ABNORMAL TRANSIENT SOUNDS

GALLOP SOUNDS

The third (S_3) and fourth (S_4) heart sounds occur during diastole (see **14**, p. 19) and are not normally audible in dogs and cats. These transient sounds are lower in frequency and are usually softer than the S_1 and S_2, so they are harder to hear. Because they are of lower frequency than S_1 and S_2, gallop sounds are usually heard best with the bell of the stethoscope (or by light pressure applied to a single-sided chestpiece). When an S_3 or S_4 sound is heard, the heart may sound like a galloping horse, hence the term gallop rhythm. But the presence or absence of an audible S_3 or S_4 has nothing to do with the heart's electrical rhythm. At very fast heart rates, differentiation of S_3 from S_4 is difficult. If both sounds are present, they may be superimposed (called a summation gallop). Gallop sounds indicate ventricular diastolic dysfunction in dogs and cats. Congestive heart failure and increased LA pressure intensify gallop sounds.

S_3 gallop

The S_3, also known as an S_3 gallop or ventricular gallop, is associated with low frequency vibrations during the rapid ventricular filling phase. An audible S_3 in a dog or cat usually indicates ventricular dilation with myocardial failure and poor compliance. The extra sound can be fairly loud or very subtle, and is heard best over the cardiac apex. This may be the only auscultable abnormality in an animal with dilated cardiomyopathy. An S_3 gallop may also be audible in dogs with advanced valvular heart disease and congestive failure.

S$_4$ gallop

The S$_4$ gallop, also called an atrial or presystolic gallop, is associated with low frequency vibrations induced by blood flow into the ventricles during atrial contraction. An audible S$_4$ in dogs and cats often occurs with abnormal ventricular relaxation and increased ventricular stiffness. LV hypertrophy, as with hypertrophic cardiomyopathy or hyperthyroidism, and myocardial ischemia are typical underlying causes. A transient S$_4$ gallop of unknown significance is sometimes heard in older stressed or anemic cats.

OTHER TRANSIENT SOUNDS

Systolic clicks and ejection sounds

Other brief abnormal sounds are sometimes audible. Systolic clicks are mid- to late-systolic sounds that are usually heard best over the mitral valve area. These sounds have been associated with degenerative valvular disease (endocardiosis), mitral or tricuspid valve prolapse, and congenital mitral dysplasia. They are thought to occur with abrupt tension or checking of a redundant valve or abnormal chordae tendineae[5]. A concurrent murmur of valvular insufficiency may be present. In dogs with degenerative valvular disease, a mitral click may be noted before the typical MR murmur develops.

An early systolic, high-pitched ejection sound at the left base is sometimes heard in animals with valvular pulmonic stenosis or other diseases that cause dilation of a great artery. The sound is thought to arise from either the sudden checking of a fused pulmonic valve or the rapid filling of a dilated vessel during ejection[5].

Pericardial knock

Rarely, restrictive pericardial disease causes an audible pericardial knock. This early diastolic sound is caused by sudden checking of ventricular filling by the restrictive pericardium. Pericardial friction rubs are rarely heard in dogs with pericarditis; they can occur as triple sounds heard in mid-systole and mid- and late-diastole.

APPROACH TO THE PATIENT WITH A MURMUR OR ABNORMAL HEART SOUNDS

When assessing an animal with a murmur or another abnormal heart sound, the clinician should consider several questions (*Table 19*, **175**). Information from the medical history, other findings on the physical examination (Chapter 2), and tests such as thoracic radiographs (Chapter 3), ECG (Chapter 4), and echocardiography (Chapter 5) help in answering these questions and guiding appropriate patient management.

Table 19 Approach to the patient with abnormal heart sounds.

1) What is the anatomic origin of the abnormal sound? (See **175**).

2) What is the underlying etiology?

    a) Structural abnormality (e.g. congenital, degenerative, infective)?

    b) Physiologic change (e.g. fever, anemia, hyperthyroidism, etc.)?

3) Are there any adverse hemodynamic or clinical consequences?

    a) What are they (e.g. specific cardiac chamber dilation or hypertrophy, evidence of edema or effusions, myocardial dysfunction, arrhythmias, etc.)?

    b) How severe are they? Base assessment on examination and test results.

4) Is therapy warranted? Determine based on specific disease process involved and answers to the questions above.

5) If therapy is indicated, what specific treatments and dosages should be used?

    a) Refer to other appropriate chapters and sources.

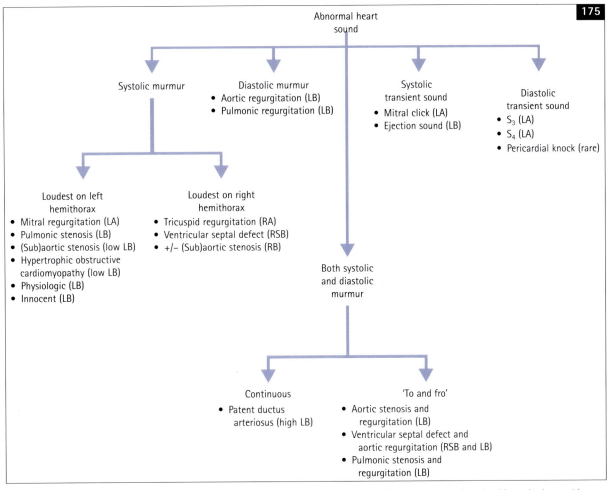

175 Approach to differentiating the origin of various murmurs and abnormal heart sounds. The usual point of maximal intensity is noted in parentheses. LA = left apex; LB = left base; RA = right apex; RB = right base; RSB = right sternal border.

REFERENCES

1 Pedersen HD, Haggstrom J, Falk T *et al.* (1999) Auscultation in mild mitral regurgitation in dogs: observer variation, effects of physical maneuvers, and agreement with color Doppler echocardiography and phonocardiography. *J Vet Intern Med* **13**:56–64.

2 Mangione S Nieman LZ (1997) Cardiac auscultatory skills of internal medicine and family practice trainees. A comparison of diagnostic proficiency. *J Am Med Assoc* **278**:717–722.

3 Mangione S (2001) Cardiac auscultatory skills of physicians in training: a comparison of three English speaking countries. *Am J Med* **110**:210–216.

4 Naylor NJ, Yadernuk LM, Pharr JW, Ashburner JS (2001) An assessment of the ability of diplomates, practitioners, and students to describe and interpret recordings of heart murmurs and arrhythmia. *J Vet Intern Med* **15**:507–515.

5 Braunwald E, Perloff JK (2001) Physical examination of the heart and circulation. In: *Heart Disease: A Textbook of Cardiovascular Medicine*, 6th edn. E Braunwald, DP Zipes, P Libby (eds). WB Saunders, Philadelphia, pp. 45–81.

6 Selig MB (1993) Stethoscopic and phonoaudio devices: historical and future perspectives. *Am Heart J* **126**:262–268.

7 Rishniw M, Thomas WP (2002) Dynamic right ventricular outflow obstruction: a new cause of systolic murmurs in cats. *J Vet Intern Med* **16**:547–552.

8 Haggstrom J, Kvart C, Hansson K (1995) Heart sounds and murmurs: changes related to severity of chronic valvular disease in the Cavalier King Charles Spaniel. *J Vet Intern Med* **9**:75–85.

7
Cardiomegaly

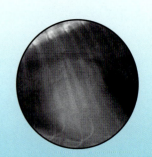

OVERVIEW

The term cardiomegaly is used to describe enlargement of the heart. The term is also applied when describing a large cardiac silhouette on radiographs. Apparent cardiomegaly (on radiographs) can occur when fluid or a mass lesion distends the pericardium, as well as when the heart itself is enlarged. Sometimes, excessive intrapericardial fat mimics the appearance of cardiomegaly, if the cardiac border is not seen as distinct from the fat density (see **37**, p.37).

Physical examination findings can sometimes suggest cardiomegaly. Caudal displacement of the precordial impulse, from left-sided or generalized cardiomegaly, may be detected by palpation. A more prominent right precordial impulse can be found with right-sided heart enlargement (see Chapter 2). A shift in the expected location of cardiac sounds may be discovered during auscultation in animals with marked cardiomegaly. However, a mass lesion in the thorax can also push the heart from its normal position, similarly displacing the palpated precordial impulse or location of heart sounds. Cardiac enlargement is also sometimes suggested by the appearance of ECG waveforms (see Chapter 4 and *Table 11*, p. 59 for enlargement criteria).

PATHOPHYSIOLOGY

Because cardiomegaly has many causes, a spectrum of pathophysiologic and morphologic changes can underlie the cardiac enlargement process. Cardiomegaly can be generalized to all chambers or involve only the left or right heart chambers, depending on the location and type of underlying lesion(s).

Enlargement of specific heart chambers is a consequence of chronically increased volume load, as with valvular insufficiencies or cardiac/vascular shunts (see Chapters 18, 19), or systolic pressure load, as with ventricular outflow obstructions or arterial hypertension (see Chapters 18, 23–25). The former leads to an eccentric (dilated) pattern of cardiac hypertrophy because of the regurgitant (or shunt) volume and activation of compensatory mechanisms

that increase vascular volume; the latter causes concentric hypertrophy, with increased wall thickening (see Chapter 1)[1]. Reduced systolic pump function, as with dilated cardiomyopathy (see Chapter 20) or a long-standing volume or pressure load, leads to chamber dilation as stroke volume diminishes and compensatory increases in total blood volume occur[1]. The heart also enlarges with idiopathic ventricular hypertrophy, as in hypertrophic cardiomyopathy (see Chapter 21), under the influence of excessive thyroid (or growth) hormone (**176–179**), or with sustained physical

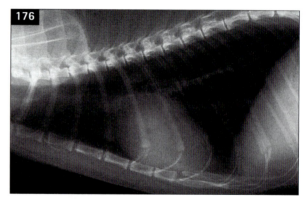

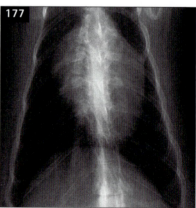

176–177 Lateral (**176**) and DV (**177**) radiographs from a 14-year-old-cat with chronic hyperthyroidism (T4 >244 nmol/l [19µg/dl]) showing generalized cardiomegaly (VHS = 8.6 v).

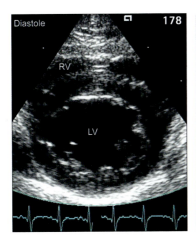 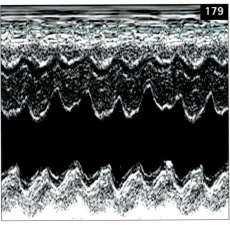

178–179 The 2-D echo of the LV in diastole (**178**) and the M-mode image (**179**) of the cat in **176** and **177** show left ventricular chamber enlargement (LV diastolic dimension = 18.4 mm) and vigorous motion consistent with a high output state. The LV wall (3.9 mm) and septal (4.2 mm) thicknesses were normal. Blood pressure was normal. LV = left ventricle; RV = right ventricle. **180** Diagram illustrating an approach for evaluating the patient with cardiomegaly.

training (physiologic hypertrophy, the 'athletic' heart)[2]. Hyperthyroidism alters myocardial protein synthesis and stimulates contractility by its direct effects and interactions with the sympathetic nervous system. Increased heart rate as well as reduced peripheral vascular resistance (from thyroid-induced vascular smooth muscle relaxation) further raise cardiac output[2–4]. Thyroid hormone also increases blood volume (and preload), as the renin-angiotensin-aldosterone system is activated in response to systemic vasodilation[4].

A cardiac mass lesion can enlarge or distort the heart by its physical presence, or by obstructing blood flow and causing secondary dilation or hypertrophy (see **522**, **523**, p.335). Chronic and profound bradycardia (such as from complete A-V block) leads to ventricular enlargement, as increases in preload and stroke volume become the prime determinants of cardiac output (CO = HR × SV). Cardiac enlargement can occur with chronic anemia, as reduced blood viscosity and peripheral vasodilation lead to a high cardiac output state[2, 3]. A large A-V fistula can also lead to cardiomegaly; flow through the fistula reduces total peripheral resistance and, with compensatory volume expansion, increases venous return and cardiac output[2, 3].

APPROACH TO THE PATIENT WITH CARDIOMEGALY

When cardiomegaly is suspected, other abnormalities that mimic it must be excluded (e.g. intrapericardial fluid or fat). Determination of the specific chamber(s) that are enlarged helps the clinician identify the underlying disease process. It is important to discern whether chamber dilation or increased wall thickness, or both, is present, and whether other related abnormalities exist. The decision to institute specific therapy in a patient with cardiomegaly must be based on an understanding of the underlying cause, its severity, and the related pathophysiology. *Table 20* and **180** (p. 100) outline an approach for evaluating the patient with cardiomegaly. *Table 6* (p. 37) lists some causes of an enlarged cardiac silhouette, as seen radiographically.

Table 20 An approach to the patient with suspected cardiomegaly.

1) Identify possible cardiomegaly from the physical examination (displacement of apex beat or heart sounds), radiographs (see Chapter 3), or enlargement criteria seen on electrocardiogram (see Chapter 4).

2) Evaluate chest radiographs for enlarged cardiac silhouette. Rule out:

   a) Positional shift of normal-sized heart (e.g. mass lesion, collapsed lung, diaphragmatic hernia, etc), increased intrapericardial fat, or PPDH.

   b) Generalized cardiomegaly (↑VHS) or specific chamber enlargement?

   c) Evidence for pulmonary infiltrates, pleural fluid, or other abnormalities?

3) If cardiac silhouette is enlarged, obtain echocardiogram to differentiate/detect pericardial effusion (or mass or PPDH), true chamber enlargement, mural or septal hypertrophy, valve morphology and function, ventricular function, other abnormalities.

4) If echo unavailable, use best clinical judgment (based on signalment, history, physical examination, and other test findings) to proceed.

5) Consider all findings when making final diagnosis and deciding whether specific therapy or additional tests are needed.

   VHS = vertebral heart score (see Chapter 3); PPDH = peritoneopericardial diaphragmatic hernia.

180

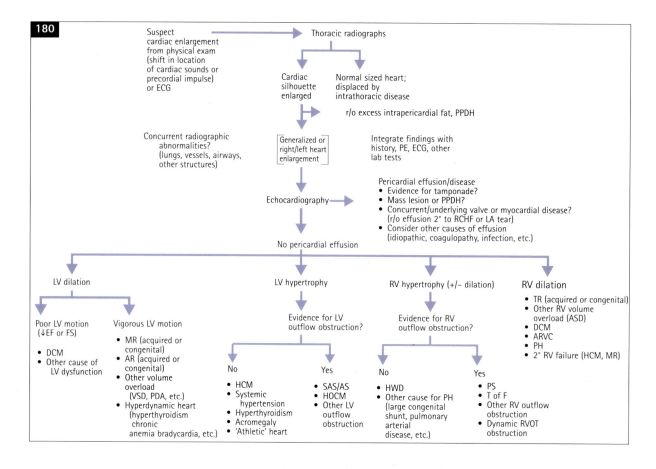

REFERENCES

1 Colucci WS, Braunwald E (2001) Pathophysiology of heart failure. In: *Heart Disease: A Textbook of Cardiovascular Medicine*, 6th edn. E Braunwald, DP Zipes, P Libby (eds). WB Saunders, Philadelphia, pp. 503–533.

2 Fox PR, Broussard JD, Peterson ME (1999) Hyperthyroidism and other high output states. In: *Textbook of Canine and Feline Cardiology*, 2nd edn. PR Fox, D Sisson, NS Moise (eds). WB Saunders, Philadephia, pp. 781–793.

3 Guyton AC, Hall JE (2000) *Textbook of Medical Physiology*, 10th edn. WB Saunders, Philadelphia, pp. 210–222.

4 Klein I, Ojamaa K (2001) Thyroid hormone and the cardiovascular system. *New Engl J Med* **344**:501–509.

8
Cough

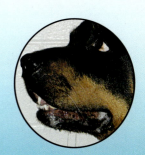

OVERVIEW

The cough reflex is a protective mechanism that helps clear the airways of secretions and foreign substances. Mechanical or chemical stimulation of receptors in the larynx, trachea, carina, and bronchi initiates the cough reflex[1]. Afferent impulses from the airway receptors travel mainly through the vagus nerves to the medulla, which triggers a sequence of events. An initial inspiration is followed by closure of the glottis; then, forceful contraction of the expiratory muscles sharply raises intrathoracic pressure; finally, the epiglottis and vocal folds suddenly open widely, allowing air to explode out of the lungs and carry irritant material toward the pharynx. The strong lung compression narrows the airways, further increasing airflow velocity[1, 2]. Coughing can occur voluntarily also. Persistent coughing is often a sign of disease.

PATHOPHYSIOLOGY

The cough reflex can be stimulated by the presence of foreign matter, accumulation of secretions or fluid within the airways, airway collapse or compression, and the effects of inhaled irritants or inflammatory mediators (*Table 21*)[2, 3]. Occasionally, coughing is associated with disease of the pleural, pericardial, diaphragmatic, mediastinal, or nasal tissues.

A cough is termed 'productive' when secretions (of mucus, edema fluid, exudate, or blood) are brought up. This feature may not be noticed by the owner because

---

Table 21 Common causes of coughing.

1) Airway disease/irritation:
   a) Pharyngitis, tonsillitis, laryngitis.
   b) Tracheobronchitis.
   c) Collapsing trachea or mainstem bronchus.
   d) Mainstem bronchus compression by enlarged left atrium or hilar lymphadenopathy.
   e) Airway foreign body.
   f) Airway mass lesion.
   g) Canine chronic bronchitis, bronchiectasis.
   h) Feline bronchial disease.
   i) Allergic bronchitis.
   j) *Oslerus osleri* infection (dog).
   k) Esophageal dysfunction.

2) Pulmonary disease:
   a) Edema (not usually associated with cough in cats).

   • Cardiogenic (high pulmonary venous pressure).
   • Noncardiogenic (e.g. increased capillary permeability, neurogenic, hypoproteinemia).
   b) Pneumonia:
   • Bacterial.
   • Aspiration.
   • Viral.
   • Fungal (e.g. *Blastomyces dermatitidis, Histoplasma capsulatum, Coccidioides immitis,* and *Cryptococcus neoformans* [dog and cat]).
   • Protozoal (e.g. *Toxoplasma gondii* [cat]; *Pneumocystis carinii* [dog]).
   c) Eosinophilic pulmonary disease.
   d) Neoplasia:
   • Primary.
   • Metastatic.

   e) Parasites:
   • Heartworms (*Dirofilaria immitis* [dog and cat]; *Angiostrongylus vasorum* [dog]).
   • Lungworms (e.g. *Paragonimus kellicotti* and *Capillaria aerophila,* [dog and cat]; *Aelurostrongylus abstrusus* [cat]; *Crenosoma vulpis* [dog]).
   • Larval migration (e.g. *Toxocara canis* and other intestinal parasites).

3) Other (uncommonly induce cough):
   a) Pleural, pericardial, diaphragmatic, mediastinal, or nasal diseases.
   b) ? Enalapril or other angiotensin converting enzyme inhibitors (related to bradykinin?).*

* Known to cause cough in people; occasional anecdotal association in dogs, but causal effect not proven.

dogs and cats usually do not expectorate these secretions. The cough may have a moist sound. Swallowing motions generally follow a productive cough. In some cases, retching or expectoration occurs. Conditions that stimulate a productive cough include bronchopneumonia, chronic bronchitis, bronchiectasis, pulmonary edema, and hemoptysis.

Hemoptysis is the coughing up of bloody foam or secretions. Although uncommon, it is most often associated with heartworm disease, other causes of pulmonary hypertension, or pulmonary neoplasia. Hemoptysis can also occur from a foreign body, mycotic infection, severe left-sided congestive heart failure (L-CHF), pulmonary thromboembolism, coagulopathy, or lung torsion.

A 'nonproductive' or 'dry' cough may be described as honking, or a 'goose-honk' sound. Minimal secretions are involved. Conditions that usually induce a dry cough include tracheal collapse, tracheobronchial irritation, mainstem bronchus compression (e.g. from LA enlargement or hilar lymphadenopathy), and allergic pulmonary disease. Early pulmonary edema or heartworm disease can also cause a nonproductive cough.

Coughing in cats is often associated with reactive airway disease, heartworm disease (see Chapter 24), or lungworms (see Table 21, p. 101). Lung parenchymal disease may not stimulate the cough reflex in cats, because cough receptors are lacking in their alveolar regions[4]. In contrast to dogs, cats with heart failure generally do not cough; however, an occasional cat with cardiogenic pulmonary edema (L-CHF) or pleural effusion has a history that includes coughing. Pharyngeal irritation, nasopharyngeal polyp, drainage of nasal/pharyngeal secretions into the larynx and trachea, and hairballs can also cause coughing as well as gagging sounds in cats.

APPROACH TO THE COUGHING PATIENT

It is important to differentiate coughing from gagging or retching or from other sounds the patient may make. Gagging or retching is often associated with upper gastrointestinal (GI) or pharyngeal disease, although animals sometimes retch at the end of a coughing episode. Expectorated mucous or foam that is bile tinged indicates vomitus rather than respiratory secretions.

When coughing is identified, it is helpful initially to determine whether airway irritation, L-CHF, or primary pulmonary disease is responsible (Table 22 and 181). More specific tests and therapy can then be pursued. The patient's signalment and history can help the clinician estimate the likelihood of conditions such as infectious disease, chronic airway disease or collapse, L-CHF, or heartworm disease. Diseases that involve the pulmonary parenchyma and interfere with normal lung function, including pulmonary edema, often cause reduced exercise tolerance as well as increased resting respiratory rate and effort. Sometimes, the cough interferes with sleep at night; this is classic but not pathognomonic for L-CHF. Cough can become worse with activity, especially in patients with L-CHF, collapsing trachea, inflammatory airway disease, heartworm disease, and other lung diseases. Primary airway disease is usually associated with normal resting respiratory rate and activity level, unless airway obstruction is present, although excitement, activity, and pulling against a collar or leash can provoke the cough. A productive cough in the early morning or after a nap can occur as airway secretions accumulated during sleep are cleared. Some diseases cause signs of both airway and lung parenchymal disease, including chronic bronchitis with secondary infection, neoplasia, and parasitic diseases.

Table 22 An approach to the coughing patient.

1) Determine if true cough:

  a) History, observation, physical examination.

  b) Rule out vomiting, gagging/retching, reverse sneeze, and so on.

2) Consider evidence for pulmonary parenchymal involvement or other concurrent disease:

  a) Signalment, history, physical examination, other findings (see text).

  b) Rule out primary airway cause or cardiopulmonary compromise.

  c) Abnormal respiratory rate, character or effort?

  d) Reduced exercise tolerance?

  e) Evidence for generalized disease process?

3) Evaluate chest radiographs (181).

4) Select other diagnostic tests as appropriate (see text):

  a) Consider all findings.

5) Treat based on underlying etiology:

  a) (Consider adjunctive antitussive therapy for persistent nonproductive cough.)

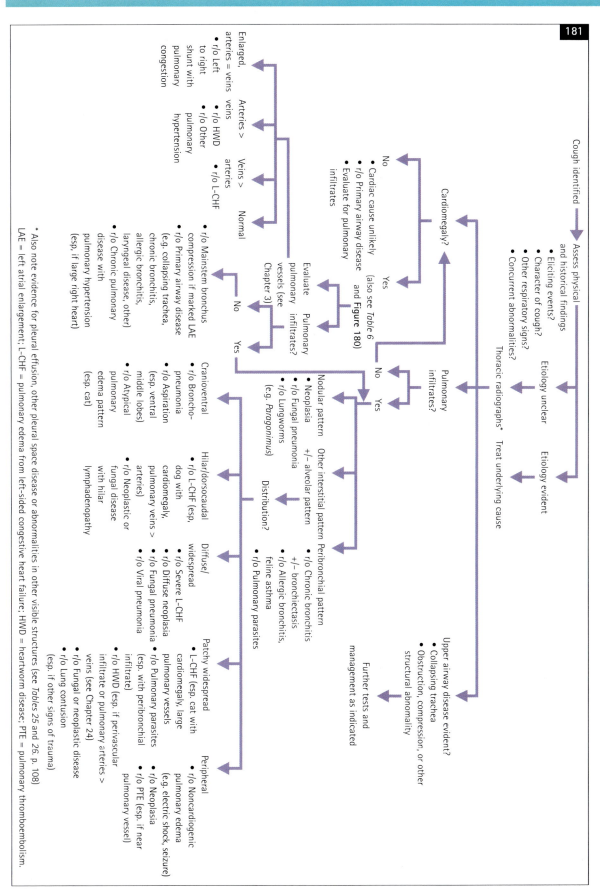

181 Diagram illustrating a diagnostic approach for evaluating the coughing patient.

The physical examination can also provide etiologic clues. The patient's demeanor and character of respirations (see Chapter 9) may help in localizing the disease process. Palpation of the cervical trachea may stimulate a cough in animals with collapsing trachea, but this maneuver can also provoke a cough when tracheal irritation from another cause of chronic coughing exists. Abnormal lung or heart sounds on auscultation may, or may not, be associated with the cause of the cough. For example, a coughing dog with a murmur of MR and pulmonary crackles may have L-CHF; however, the pulmonary crackles could be a manifestation of underlying chronic lung disease, with incidental MR. Alternatively, the cough may be secondary to chronic bronchitis, collapsing trachea, or mainstem bronchus compression from marked LA enlargement, rather than pulmonary edema.

Radiographs are an important diagnostic tool in most cases (**181**, p. 103). They should be evaluated for the presence, and pattern, of pulmonary infiltrates, cardiomegaly, including specific chamber enlargement criteria (see Chapter 3), evidence of large airway disease, and any pleural space or vascular abnormalities. Diagnosis of dynamic airway collapse may require fluoroscopy or comparison of inspiratory and expiratory films. If pulmonary edema is suspected based on the appearance and distribution of pulmonary infiltrates, especially with concurrent cardiomegaly, a diuretic trial and further cardiac assessment are indicated. If the animal is already being treated for heart failure of known cause,

intensification of therapy is warranted (see Chapter 16 and specific disease chapters).

Other diagnostic tests are indicated if the cause of the cough is unclear. The choice of these depends on the signalment, history, physical examination, and radiographic findings. Such tests might include a hemogram, serum biochemical profile, airway washings (tracheal wash or bronchoalveolar lavage), heartworm tests, fungal serology, fecal tests, bronchoscopy, lung biopsy, and others.

Treatment for the coughing patient should be directed at the underlying disease process whenever possible. An accurate diagnosis is obviously important; for example, it makes no sense to prescribe a cough suppressant or antibiotic for a dog coughing from L-CHF. Guidelines for managing heart failure can be found in Chapter 16 as well as in the chapters on specific heart diseases. Heartworm disease is discussed in Chapter 24. The reader is urged to consult other sources for current treatment recommendations for primary respiratory and airway diseases.

Antitussive therapy can be useful in selected cases; however, a productive cough is generally not suppressed, because it helps clear the airways. For persistent coughing that is not associated with infection or pulmonary edema, antitussive therapy can provide some relief to both patient and owner (*Table 23*). Such situations include dynamic large airway collapse and mainstem bronchus compression from marked LA enlargement when pulmonary edema is absent.

Table 23 Antitussive therapy.

Cough suppressants (for dogs only):	
Butorphanol	Dog: 0.5–1 mg/kg PO q6–12h
Hydrocodone bitartrate	Dog: 0.25 mg/kg PO q6–12h
Dextromethorphan	Dog: 1–2 mg/kg PO q6–8h
Bronchodilators:*	
Aminophylline	Dog: 11 mg/kg PO q8h
	Cat: 5 mg/kg PO q12h
Theophylline (long-acting)	Dog: 10–20 mg/kg PO q12h
	Cat: 25 mg/kg PO q24h (in evening)
Oxtriphylline elixir	Dog: 14 mg/kg PO q8h
	Cat: none
Terbutaline	Dog: 1.25–5 mg/dog PO q8–12h
	Cat: 1/8–1/4 of 2.5 mg tablet/cat PO q12h

* May be useful if bronchospasm is provoking cough.

REFERENCES

1 Lumb AB (2000) *Nunn's Applied Respiratory Physiology,* 5th edn. Butterworth Heinmann, Edinburgh, pp. 82–112.

2 Guyton AC, Hall JE (2000) *Textbook of Medical Physiology,* 10th edn. WB Saunders, Philadelphia, pp. 432–443.

3 Hawkins EC (2003) Clinical manifestations of lower respiratory tract disorders. In: *Small Animal Internal Medicine,* 3rd edn. RW Nelson, CG Couto (eds). Mosby, St. Louis, pp. 250–254.

4 Henik RA, Yeager AE (1994) Bronchopulmonary diseases. In: *The Cat: Diseases and Clinical Management,* 2nd edn. RG Sherding (ed). Churchill Livingstone, New York, pp. 979–1052.

9
Respiratory Difficulty

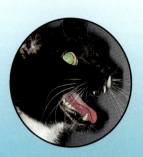

OVERVIEW

Normal respiration is characterized by quiet, active inspiration followed by passive expiration. Both phases are smooth and symmetrical[1]. The breath is generated by medullary neurons, but neural control of breathing also involves other brainstem centers, cervical vertebral segments, and the cerebral cortex. This allows involuntary rhythmic breathing, as well as involuntary nonrhythmic control (e.g. during swallowing) and voluntary control[2]. The diaphragm is the main inspiratory muscle. During contraction the diaphragmatic dome moves caudally, enlarging the thorax and creating the negative intrathoracic pressure that pulls air into the lungs[3]. The external intercostal muscles also help by moving the ribs cranially and outward during inspiration. Contraction of abductor muscles in the nares, pharynx, and larynx maximizes upper airway diameter to facilitate airflow during inspiration. During passive exhalation, elastic recoil of the lung and chest wall moves air out. Abdominal and internal intercostal muscles are also used for expiration; their contraction decreases thoracic size, thereby increasing intrathoracic pressure and forcing air out of the lungs[3].

The breathing rate is influenced by numerous factors such as exercise, ambient temperature, excitement, digestive tract filling, pregnancy and other causes of abdominal enlargement, and many diseases. Normal dogs and cats have resting (sleeping) respiratory rates of between 16 and 25 breaths/minute[1]. A general guideline of <30 breaths/minute is often used clinically.

Animals with respiratory difficulty usually have an increased effort and rate of breathing, among other signs (*Table 24*). Several descriptive terms are used:
- 'Tachypnea' is an increase in respiratory rate. Panting as a means of heat dissipation is normal in dogs; however, excessive panting or rapid shallow breathing can occur from respiratory compromise. Panting in cats is often a sign of

Table 24 Signs of hypoxemia.

1) Restlessness.
2) Anxiety.
3) ↑ Respiratory rate.
4) ↑ Respiratory effort.
5) Extended head and neck.
6) Orthopnea.
7) Pale grayish or cyanotic mucous membranes (unless marked anemia).
8) +/– Arrhythmias or tachycardia.
9) +/– Syncope.

respiratory compromise, although it can occur with stress and hyperthermia.
- 'Hyperpnea' is increased depth of breathing.
- 'Dyspnea', as used in human medicine, is the awareness of difficulty in breathing, breathlessness, or the sensation of air hunger; a number of mechanisms are thought to underlie this[4, 5]. In veterinary use the term is synonymous with labored breathing or respiratory distress.
- 'Orthopnea' refers to respiratory difficulty severe enough to cause the animal to assume a certain upright posture and resist other body positions. Dogs with orthopnea stand or sit with their elbows abducted, which allows full rib expansion, and their neck extended. They resist being positioned in lateral or dorsal recumbency (**182, 183**). Cats often crouch in a sternal or squatting position with their elbows abducted and neck extended; open-mouth breathing is usually a sign of severe respiratory distress (**184, 185**).

Animals with severe dyspnea are reluctant to eat or drink, or even swallow saliva. Some patients exhibit greater respiratory effort during inspiration or during expiration. Both phases are equally labored in others. The localization and pathophysiology of the

182 Respiratory distress in a 9-year-old male Doberman Pinscher with metastatic bronchoalveolar carcinoma and pulmonary thrombosis; PaO_2 = 47 mm Hg. Note the wide-based stance with head and neck extension (typical of orthopnea) and cyanotic tongue.

183 This 4-year-old Rottweiler with respiratory distress from bacterial pneumonia also exhibits head/neck extension; note the anxious expression and saliva drooling from the mouth.

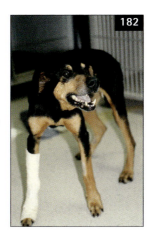
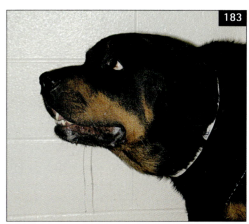

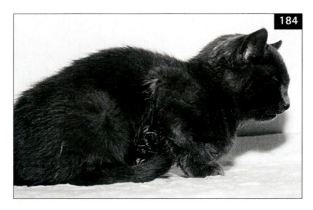
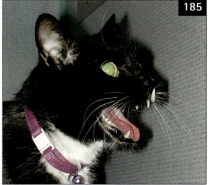

184 The crouched body position of this 4-month-old kitten with hypoxemia from Tetralogy of Fallot is typical for cats with orthopnea. Subtle open-mouth breathing is apparent.

185 Severe respiratory distress with open-mouth breathing in a 10-year-old cat with fulminant pulmonary edema from restrictive cardiomyopathy.

underlying disease process influence the pattern as well as the rate of breathing (see p. 110).

Disease at any level of the respiratory system, from the external nares to the pulmonary alveoli, or cardiovascular dysfunction commonly underlies respiratory difficulty[6–10]. Other diverse causes such as impaired blood oxygen-carrying capacity (e.g. anemia, hemoglobinopathy), pleural space disease, and disruption of thoracic cage integrity or respiratory muscle function also interfere with respiration (*Table 25*, p. 108)[7, 11].

PATHOPHYSIOLOGY

Inadequate blood oxygen (O_2) (hypoxemia) or excessive carbon dioxide (CO_2) (hypercarbia/hypercapnia) leads to respiratory distress. Ventilation is normally regulated reflexly in response to changes in the partial pressure of arterial carbon dioxide ($PaCO_2$), sensed by central and peripheral chemoreceptors. Central chemoreceptors (in the medulla) are highly sensitive to changes in cerebral spinal fluid pH, which is inversely related to $PaCO_2$. Small changes in alveolar pCO_2 affect ventilation. Hypoxia also affects the central respiratory center directly[12]. Peripheral chemoreceptors in the carotid bodies, located near the bifurcation of the common carotid arteries, and to a lesser extent the aortic bodies, respond more to low PaO_2 and reflexly stimulate ventilation; however, these chemoreceptors also respond to elevated $PaCO_2$, decreased pH, low perfusion rate, and increased temperature to raise the rate and depth of ventilation[12].

Besides chemoreceptor-mediated reflex effects on ventilation, other mechanisms influence ventilatory rate and depth. Dyspnea associated with pulmonary vascular congestion or thromboembolism (as well as the ventilatory response to exercise) may be mediated through C-fiber (nonmyelinated nerve) endings associated with the bronchial and pulmonary microcirculation (J-receptors)[12]. Primary central nervous system (CNS) disease occasionally causes abnormal regulation of respiratory rate or rhythm.

Table 25 Causes of respiratory difficulty.

1) Nasopharynx:

   a) Nasopharyngeal polyp.

   b) Rhinitis/sinusitis.

   c) Fungal infection (e.g. cryptococosis, aspergillosis).

   d) Neoplasia (e.g. lymphoma, carcinomas, mast cell tumor, fibrosarcoma).

   e) Other mass lesion (e.g. cyst, abscess).

   f) Foreign body.

   g) Nasopharyngeal stenosis.

   h) Brachycephalic airway abnormalities (e.g. stenotic nares, elongated soft palate).

2) Larynx:

   a) Unilateral or bilateral paralysis.

   b) Neoplasia (e.g. lymphoma, squamous cell carcimoma, adenocarcinoma).

   c) Granulomatous laryngitis.

   d) Abscess.

   e) Other mass lesion (e.g. cyst).

   f) Edema or laryngospasm.

   g) Foreign body.

   h) Trauma (hemorrhage, fractured cartilage, subcutaneous emphysema).

   i) Brachycephalic airway abnormalities (e.g. everted laryngeal saccules, laryngeal malformation).

3) Trachea:

   a) Collapse.

   b) Foreign body.

   c) Tracheal mass (neoplastic or non-neoplastic).

   d) Tracheal compression.

   e) Trauma.

   f) Brachycephalic airway abnormalities (e.g. hypoplastic trachea).

4) Bronchi:

   a) Chronic bronchitis/bronchiectasis (accumulation of secretions or exudate).

   b) Bronchospasm (e.g. asthma, inhaled irritant).

   c) Collapse.

5) Pulmonary parenchyma:

   a) Edema – cardiogenic (L-CHF: e.g. dilated cardiomyopathy [see Chapter 20], acquired mitral or aortic valve disease [see Chapter 19], feline myocardial disease [see Chapter 21], certain congenital heart defects [see Chapter 18]).

   b) Edema – noncardiogenic (neurogenic [e.g. seizures, electrocution], hypervolemia, smoke inhalation, near drowning, sepsis, severe hypoproteinemia, rapid lung expansion).

   c) Pneumonia (e.g. bacterial, fungal, aspiration, viral, protozoal).

   d) Fibrosis (e.g. from certain drugs, viral or other infections, dusts, and organic allergens).

   e) Parasites (e.g. *Aelurostrongylus* species, *Paragonimus* species).

   f) Pulmonary thromboemboli (see Chapters 15, 23).

   g) Heartworm disease (see Chapter 24).

   h) Neoplasia (primary or metastatic).

   i) Trauma (e.g. pulmonary contusion, traumatic cysts/bullae).

6) Pleural space:

   a) Hydrothorax: (modified) transudate – cardiogenic (R-CHF: e.g. dilated cardiomyopathy [see Chapter 20], acquired tricuspid valve disease [see Chapter 19], feline myocardial disease [see Chapter 21], pericardial disease [see Chapter 22], heartworm disease [see Chapter 24], certain congenital heart defects [see Chapter 18]).

   b) Hydrothorax: transudate/modified transudate – noncardiogenic (e.g. neoplasia [lymphoma, mesothelioma, thymoma], diaphragmatic hernia, lung lobe torsion, severe hypoproteinemia).

   c) Hydrothorax: nonseptic exudate (e.g. feline infectious peritonitis, neoplasia, chronic lung lobe torsion or diaphragmatic hernia, fungal infection).

   d) Chylothorax (e.g. feline myocardial disease [see Chapter 21], mediastinal lymphoma, trauma, lymphangiectasia, congenital lymphatic malformation, heartworm disease [see Chapter 24], cranial vena cava thrombosis [see Chapter 15]).

   e) Pyothorax (septic exudate; e.g. bite wound, systemic infection, migrating foreign body).

   f) Hemothorax (e.g. trauma, coagulopathy, neoplasia, lung lobe torsion).

   g) Pneumothorax (e.g. trauma, iatrogenic, *Paragonimus* infection, ruptured congenital lung cyst).

7) Diaphragm/thoracic cavity:

   a) Diaphragmatic hernia (e.g. traumatic, congenital peritoneopericardial [see Chapter 22]).

   b) Primary or metastatic neoplasia (including cranial mediastinal masses).

   c) Massive pericardial effusion (see Chapter 22).

8) Chest wall:

   a) Neuromuscular disease.

   b) Trauma (e.g. rib fractures, flail segment, muscle tears).

   c) Congenital pectus excavatum.

9) Other:

   a) Marked abdominal enlargement (e.g. ascites, gastric dilatation/volvulus, etc)

   b) Neurologic disease (e.g. coma, brainstem or high cervical injury)

   c) Drug-induced respiratory depression (e.g. sedative or anesthetic agents)

   d) ↓ O_2 carrying capacity (e.g. anemia, carbon monoxide toxicity/smoke inhalation, methemoglobinemia).

L-CHF = left-sided congestive heart failure;
R-CHF = right-sided congestive heart failure

HYPOXEMIA

Several abnormalities lead to hypoxemia (*Table 26*)[13]. These usually involve either alveolar hypoventilation, pulmonary ventilation/perfusion (V/Q) mismatch with venous admixture (shunt), anatomic right-to-left shunt, or a combination of these factors[7, 14]. Impaired alveolar gas diffusion or low O_2 content of inspired air are other causes of hypoxemia. In addition, tissue hypoxia can result from reduced blood O_2-carrying capacity (e.g. anemia or hemoglobinopathy), even with normal PaO_2.

When ventilation of pulmonary alveolar units is inadequate, not enough O_2 is available for absorption into alveolar capillaries and CO_2 is retained. Alveolar hypoventilation can occur from pleural space disease, multiple rib fractures with or without flail chest, respiratory muscle dysfunction or fatigue, severe upper airway obstruction, markedly increased small airway resistance, CNS disease with abnormal neural control of respiration, chest compression (e.g. tight bandage), or decreased lung elasticity (e.g. severe pulmonary fibrosis). Hypoventilation can also occur from the respiratory depressant effects of drugs used for sedation or anesthesia, as well as use of an excessively large breathing circuit during inhalation anesthesia, which functionally increases anatomical 'dead space'.

V/Q mismatch occurs with relative overperfusion of poorly or nonventilated lung regions or by ventilation of poorly perfused regions. Pulmonary arterioles normally constrict in response to low O_2 levels. Such vasoconstriction shifts blood flow from poorly ventilated regions preferentially toward well ventilated areas, which minimizes V/Q mismatch. Accumulation of alveolar fluid or exudate and bronchoconstriction, as well as the degree of hypoxic vasoconstriction, impact the balance of ventilation to perfusion. Inflammatory mediators associated with pneumonia or other lung disease may interfere with hypoxic vasoconstriction and contribute to greater V/Q abnormality. V/Q mismatch occurs with pulmonary edema, pulmonary interstitial disease and fibrosis, airway obstruction with partial lung collapse, and lung collapse related to pleural space disease, diaphragmatic hernia, and multiple rib fractures.

When alveoli collapse or fill with fluid or exudate, gas exchange ceases in those units. Deoxygenated blood flowing through adjacent pulmonary capillaries functionally creates an area of A-V shunt or 'venous admixture'. Alveolar flooding from severe pulmonary edema and pulmonary consolidation from pneumonia are common causes of functional intrapulmonary A-V shunt. True anatomic shunts, such as a pulmonary A-V fistula or right-to-left shunting cardiac malformation or reverse PDA, also cause hypoxemia.

Diffusion impairment occurs when alveolar capillary wall thickening prevents rapid equilibration between capillary blood and alveolar gas. It is thought to be an uncommon cause of hypoxemia in dogs and cats[7].

Hypoxemia causes visible cyanosis when desaturated hemoglobin exceeds 5 g/dl (see Chapter 2 and *Table 3*, p. 28). Oral mucous membranes appear grayish ('muddy') or bluish. In animals with a normal PCV, cyanosis usually indicates severe hypoxemia (PaO_2 <45–50 mm Hg)[7, 15]. Polycythemic animals may appear cyanotic, with less severe hypoxemia by virtue of their greater hemoglobin content. Anemic animals may be severely hypoxemic without cyanosis. Hypoxemia and cyanosis are difficult to detect with carbon monoxide toxicity or methemoglobinemia because mucous membrane color is altered; even with a normal PaO_2, total blood O_2 content is reduced[16]. 'Central' cyanosis is associated with generalized hypoxemia; 'peripheral' cyanosis refers to local hemoglobin desaturation caused by poor peripheral circulation (as with arterial thromboembolism).

PULMONARY EDEMA

Pulmonary edema, an increase in pulmonary extravascular water, occurs when capillary transudation or exudation exceeds pulmonary lymphatic drainage capacity. Usually an imbalance in Starling's forces (see Chapter 1) underlies pulmonary edema formation[17]. The most common mechanism is increased pulmonary capillary hydrostatic pressure, which results from high pulmonary venous pressure (e.g. L-CHF), hypervolemia, or pulmonary overcirculation (e.g. left-to-right shunting cardiac defects). Another mechanism is increased capillary permeability, which occurs with diseases that directly or indirectly injure the capillary membrane. Leakage of albumin and other large molecules into the alveoli and interstitium causes edema fluid with a protein content similar to plasma. Large increases in pulmonary capillary pressure (e.g. to 30–50 mm Hg) can also create gaps in the membrane ('stress failure'), which allow protein leakage[17]. Low plasma osmotic pressure from severe hypoalbuminemia (~10 g/l [~1 g/dl] or less) promotes fluid transudation out of the capillaries. Moderate hypoalbuminemia magnifies the tendency for edema formation from other mechanisms. Pulmonary lymphatic obstruction or high lymphatic pressure secondary to high systemic venous pressure will also promote pulmonary edema formation. Neurogenic pulmonary edema is thought to result from a surge in

---

Table 26 Causes of hypoxemia.

1) Alveolar hypoventilation.
2) Ventilation/perfusion (V/Q) mismatch.
3) Shunt.
4) ↓ Inspired O_2 concentration (F_IO_2).
5) Diffusion impairment.
6) Abnormal hemoglobin.

circulating epinephrine or a neural response that causes acute constriction of pulmonary venous sphincters and high pulmonary venous pressure[17]. Pulmonary edema can also develop with rapid reexpansion of collapsed lung tissue, probably from increased capillary permeability. High-altitude pulmonary edema, of unclear mechanism, is also recognized.

Overt pulmonary edema is presumably preceded by a 'prodromal' stage, where increased lymph flow maintains a normal amount of extravascular fluid. The progression of pulmonary edema severity has been described in four stages[17]:

- In stage 1 (increased interstitial fluid), distended lymphatics are seen around adjacent bronchi and pulmonary arteries. Gas exchange is well preserved and physical signs minimal, although mild dyspnea with exercise may occur.
- In stage 2, interstitial edema accumulates along portions of alveolar septa and between adjacent alveoli, sometimes described as 'crescentic filling' of alveoli. Increased respiratory effort may be noted at rest.
- Stage 3 (alveolar flooding) involves 'quantal' alveolar flooding, where some units are totally fluid filled and others are clear or show only crescentic filling, especially in dependent lung regions. Blood flow past flooded alveoli creates venous admixture (shunt), eventually leading to hypoxemia and increased alveolar–arterial O_2 gradient. Pulmonary crackles are heard on inspiration, especially in dependent regions.
- Stage 4 occurs when froth enters the airways and effectively stops gas exchange[17].

PLEURAL EFFUSION

Many diseases cause pleural fluid accumulation[18]. As with tissue edema formation, effusion usually results from an imbalance of Starling's forces: increased systemic capillary hydrostatic pressure or permeability, reduced lymphatic drainage, or low capillary oncotic pressure. Elevated right heart filling pressure increases systemic venous and capillary pressures, causing greater transudation into the pleural space as well as the peritoneal and sometimes pericardial spaces. This can occur with any disease that raises right heart filling pressure, including primary heart disease, pericardial disease, intracardiac mass lesions, and pulmonary hypertension, or that obstructs venous inflow to the heart.

Fluid appearance, protein concentration, and cell content typify different effusions (*Table 27*). The character of the pleural fluid depends on the underlying mechanism[11]. Because the mediastinum is fenestrated in dogs and cats, pleural effusion is usually bilateral. The volume of fluid as well as how rapidly it accumulates influences the degree of respiratory compromise.

PATTERNS OF BREATHING

The patient's respiratory rate and character can provide clues to the underlying disease process. Reduced lung compliance produces a 'restrictive' breathing pattern, characterized by more rapid and shallow breaths. This breathing pattern minimizes the work of ventilating stiffer lungs[6]. Exhalation or both phases of respiration may appear labored. Pulmonary edema, other interstitial or infiltrative disease, and pulmonary fibrosis produce this pattern. Such diseases reduce the area available for gas exchange as well as decrease compliance. Pulmonary crackles (see below) are often heard on inspiration; these can be especially loud with fibrosis. Partial lung collapse from pleural fluid accumulation or other pleural space abnormalities also decrease lung compliance. With large volume pleural effusion, inspiration often becomes labored and abdominal effort pronounced.

An 'obstructive' breathing pattern is associated with airway narrowing. Slower, deeper breathing reduces frictional resistance and the work of breathing[6]. However, the breathing rate may be normal or increased with peripheral airway obstruction or from the effects of irritant receptors in the airways[6]. The location of narrowing determines which phase of respiration is more labored and (often) prolonged. Expiratory difficulty is characteristic of lower airway obstruction, such as with bronchial narrowing (bronchospasm, secretions, thickened walls) and intrathoracic tracheal or mainstem bronchial collapse. Wheezing sounds may be heard on exhalation. 'Air trapping' in peripheral lung regions is common with obstructive bronchial disease. Some animals with chronic lower airway obstruction have an expiratory heave or grunt. Inspiratory difficulty, with slow or labored inspiration, is generally associated with upper airway obstruction, including nasal disease, laryngeal/pharyngeal obstruction, intratracheal mass lesions, and cervical tracheal collapse. Abnormal inspiratory sounds may be apparent without a stethoscope, especially stridor or stertor (see below).

Tachypnea and hyperpnea are not always related to hypoxemia or abnormalities of pulmonary mechanics. Hypercarbia and acidosis cause hyperpnea as an attempt to blow off CO_2. This may be interpreted as dyspnea. CNS injury (e.g. infection, neoplasia, vascular accident, or trauma) can produce an abnormal rate or character of ventilation.

RESPIRATORY SOUNDS

Pulmonary auscultation may help in localizing the disease process. Normal lung ('breath' or 'bronchovesicular') sounds are created by turbulent air movement through major airways and related tissue vibrations[19, 20]. These sounds are similar to wind blowing gently through trees. They are loudest over the trachea and may be barely audible over

Table 27 Pleural effusions.

Type	Appearance	Protein	Nucleated cells	Predominant cells	Common cause
Pure transudate	Clear	<30 g/l (<3 g/dl)	<1,000/µl	M, L, mesothel.	↓ capillary oncotic P (hypoalbuminemia)
Modified transudate	Slightly turbid; amber/pinkish	up to 35 g/l (<3.5 g/dl)	to 5,000/µl	M, L, mesothel., PMN	↑ capillary hydrostatic P (R-CHF, ↓ lymph drainage)
Exudate	Turbid to opaque; amber/pink/white	>30 g/l (>3 g/dl)	>5,000/µl	PMN, M, L, E (degenerate PMN +/− bacteria if septic)	↑ capillary permeability (septic or nonseptic inflammation)
Hemorrhage	Red-tinged to frank blood	Similar to peripheral blood	Variable	RBC, PMN, M	Vascular disruption (trauma, inflammation, coagulopathy)
Chyle	Turbid to milky white or pink	Variable	~5,000–10,000/µl	Mature L, M, PMN	↓ lymphatic drainage (lymphatic obstruction or rupture, ↑ systemic venous P)

E = eosinophils; L = lymphocytes; M = macrophages; mesothel = mesothelial cells; PMN = neutrophils; RBC = red blood cells.

the lung periphery. The intensity of normal breath sounds increases when airflow rate and turbulence are greater (e.g. with panting or excitement). Breath sounds are also louder in thin chested animals because of better sound transmission[19]. Increased breath sounds may be heard in animals with pneumonia, airway obstruction, and, sometimes, pleural effusion[19, 21]. Lung sounds are muffled or absent over areas of pneumothorax or solid tissue (e.g. mass, diaphragmatic hernia). Breath sounds may be difficult to hear in normal cats and in animals with shallow respirations, and with obesity, emphysema, hyperinflation, or pleural effusion.

Abnormal ('adventitious') lung sounds are superimposed on normal breath sounds and are usually loudest over the area of disease[19]. Abnormal sounds are categorized as continuous (wheezes) or noncontinuous (crackles). Their location and the phase of respiration when heard should be noted. Pulmonary crackles (sometimes called rales) are intermittent and discrete nonmusical sounds. They are usually caused by the sudden equalization of airway pressure as small airways that are collapsed, or partially filled with fluid or secretions, 'pop' open. They are usually heard during inspiration and in dependent lung regions[19]. The sound can be analogous to that created by rolling a few hairs between thumb and forefinger next to one's ear, by crumpling cellophane, or by separating a thin strip of Velcro. Pulmonary crackles are associated with interstitial diseases such as pulmonary edema, pneumonia, and fibrosis.

Wheezes, sometimes called rhonchi, are musical or whistling sounds that occur when partial obstruction of airways leads to audible oscillation of the airway walls. Wheezes usually occur during expiration. Bronchoconstriction, bronchial wall thickening, secretions, lower airway foreign body or mass lesions, and dynamic or external airway compression may cause expiratory wheezes. Rigid tracheal or main bronchus narrowing may create inspiratory wheezes.

Inspiratory 'stridor' is a harsh, high-pitched continuous sound caused by laryngeal or upper tracheal obstruction. Noises originating from the upper airways such as purring, stridor, stertor (snoring, snorting sounds occurring with nasal or pharyngeal disease), and vocalizations are easily referred to the thorax. Auscultation over the trachea and thoracic inlet helps the clinician differentiate these from sounds originating lower in the respiratory system.

APPROACH TO THE PATIENT WITH RESPIRATORY DIFFICULTY

The severity of the animal's respiratory compromise as well as surrounding circumstances influences the clinician's approach. Care must be taken not to increase patient distress. Brief observation before the patient is handled, with or without a cursory physical examination (including pulse rate and chest auscultation) may be all that is possible initially. A severely dyspneic animal should be given supplemental O_2 immediately; full examination and other testing can follow when the patient is more stable (186). Various methods for O_2 administration are described, including an O_2 cage or chamber, a face mask, or holding the O_2 tubing near the nose/mouth[22, 23]. While 100% O_2 is usually given initially, supplementation for more than a few hours should be at 40% or less because of the risk of O_2 toxicity[23]. A nasal cannula is useful for more long-term O_2 administration. As long as undue patient stress can be avoided, placing an IV catheter as soon as possible allows for initial blood tests (e.g. PCV, TP, blood smear, BUN, glucose) and provides access for emergency drugs and fluids.

Observation of the patient's rate and character of respirations, including whether inspiration or expiration is more labored (*Table 28* and see above), attitude and level of alertness, mucous membrane color, general body condition, and evidence for trauma or other external abnormalities can be done with minimal or no physical contact. Most dyspneic animals have respiratory rates >50–60 breaths/minute. Rates are slower with airway obstruction or large volume pleural effusion. Overly stressed and anxious animals may benefit from sedation (e.g. acepromazine

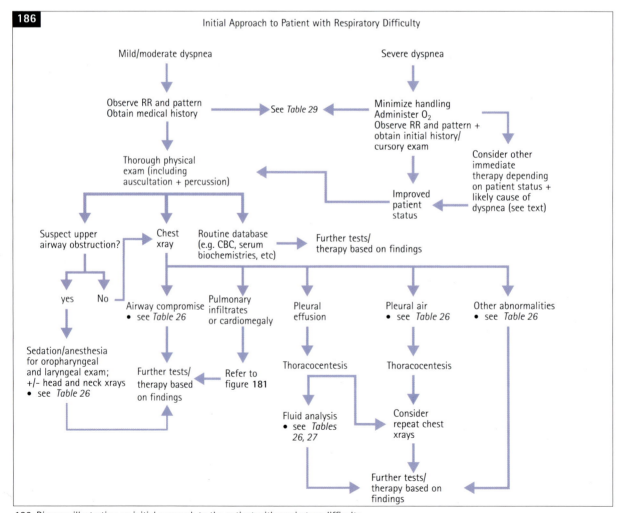

186 Diagram illustrating an initial approach to the patient with respiratory difficulty.

Table 28 Respiratory signs by disease localization*.

1) Nasopharynx:
  a) Stertor.
  b) Open-mouth breathing.
  c) Nasal discharge.
  d) Cough.
  e) Gagging/retching.
2) Larynx:
  a) Stridor.
  b) Inspiratory difficulty.
  c) Cough.
  d) Change in voice or bark.
3) Trachea:
  a) Inspiratory difficulty (cervical trachea).
  b) Expiratory difficulty (intrathoracic trachea).
  c) Mixed inspiratory and expiratory difficulty (especially with fixed obstruction).
  d) Cough.
	4) Lower airways/bronchi:
	  a) Expiratory difficulty.
	  b) Cough.
	  c) Wheezes.
	5) Pulmonary parenchyma:
	  a) Tachypnea.
	  b) Mixed inspiratory and expiratory difficulty.
	  c) Pulmonary crackles (especially end inspiratory).
	  d) Areas of ↑ or ↓ breath sounds.
	6) Pleural space/thoracic cavity:
	  a) Tachypnea or slower labored breathing.
	  b) Areas of muffled lung sounds.
	  c) Areas of hypo- or hyperresonance on percussion.
	7) Chest wall/other:
	  a) ↓ Chest wall excursion.
	  b) Abnormal chest wall appearance or motion.

*Cyanosis may occur with any disease causing >50 g/l (>5 g/dl) desaturated hemoglobin.

maleate [0.025–0.1 mg/kg IV or IM] or butorphanol tartrate [0.1–0.2 mg/kg IV). A complete medical history should be obtained as soon as possible.

Initial therapy in addition to O_2 supplementation is sometimes warranted before diagnostic tests can be done safely. Depending on the clinician's judgment as to the likely cause of the dyspnea, this might include furosemide and a vasodilator (for suspected pulmonary edema [see Chapter 16]); bronchodilators (for suspected bronchospasm, plus corticosteroid for noninfectious inflammatory causes); thoracocentesis (for suspected pleural effusion or pneumothorax); or sedation/anesthesia for pharyngeal/laryngeal inspection and intubation or for emergency tracheostomy for suspected upper airway obstruction[7, 24]. Ventilatory support may be needed in some cases[25]. (See references for further information on these techniques.)

A complete physical examination should be done as soon as is safely possible (see Chapters 2, 6, 10, and 13 for further details on aspects of cardiovascular examination). Besides the respiratory abnormalities, signs of other organ system disease may be apparent, such as a cardiac murmur, gallop sound, or arrhythmia; neurologic deficits; ocular abnormality; a palpable mass; organomegaly; or evidence for abnormal fluid accumulation. Careful pulmonary auscultation is important (see p. 110). Chest percussion may reveal areas of increased (air) or decreased (fluid/solid tissue) resonance of the thorax.

Body temperature elevation can occur from increased respiratory effort and anxiety, as well as from infectious, inflammatory, or neoplastic disease. Reduced chest compressibility in cats may indicate a cranial mediastinal mass or large pleural effusion, but geriatric cats normally have reduced chest compliance.

Thoracic radiographs are done as soon as the animal's breathing has stabilized[26–29]. The DV rather than the VD view is usually less stressful for patients with respiratory difficulty. Both left and right lateral views are helpful if unilateral disease is suspected. Radiographs of the upper cervical and nasopharyngeal regions may be useful if signs suggest upper airway disease, but direct visual examination is usually needed. Pleural fluid or air of more than minimal volume should be removed by thoracocentesis before additional testing. Thoracic radiographs taken again after full lung expansion usually yield more diagnostic information.

Additional diagnostic testing is guided by patient history, observation, physical abnormalities, and radiographic findings. This might include direct nasopharyngeal and/or laryngeal examination, CBC, serum biochemistries, pleural fluid analysis, echocardiography (see Chapter 5), electrocardiography (see Chapter 4), pulse oximetry or arterial blood gas analysis, capnography, fungal or heartworm serologic tests, lymph node aspirates, coagulation profile, fecal tests, bronchoscopy, bronchoalveolar lavage, pulmonary fine needle aspiration or biopsy, CT scan, thoracoscopy, pulmonary function testing, and pulmonary or ventilation scintigraphy.

Pulse oximetry is useful as a noninvasive means of estimating hemoglobin saturation and monitoring the animal's response to O_2 administration, although it will not differentiate partial pressure of O_2 in arterial blood (PaO_2) gradations above 100 mm Hg[30, 31]. For example, in a patient with normal lung function breathing 100% O_2, PaO_2 is 500 mm Hg yet hemoglobin saturation is still 100%. Approximate correlation of selected hemoglobin saturation values with the PaO_2, based on the normal hemoglobin dissociation curve, are listed in *Table 29*. However, pulse oximetry does not indicate if hypoventilation (hypercarbia) is the cause of the hypoxemia. Furthermore, the technique can be inaccurate, especially when the patient is poorly perfused, moving, or has deep pigmentation[15, 30, 31].

Arterial blood gas analysis will allow differentiation of alveolar hypoventilation from other causes of hypoxemia (*Table 29*), verify the need for O_2 supplementation, and monitor its effectiveness[7, 32–35];

however, the stress of arterial puncture and availability of rapid analysis capability must be considered (*Table 30*). Venous partial pressure of O_2 (PvO_2) does not reflect pulmonary function, but can provide a rough estimate of whether tissue oxygenation is adequate[15]. When obtained from a central vein, PvO_2 <30 mm Hg suggests either decreased O_2 delivery to the tissues or an increased O_2 consumption. Venous PCO_2 is usually 3–6 mm Hg higher than arterial PCO_2; this can provide an estimate of ventilatory status[15].

Calculation of the A–a O_2 gradient can help in disease assessment (*Table 29*). In the normal lung, the partial pressure of O_2 in the alveolus (PAO_2) should equal that in the pulmonary capillary and, therefore, in arterial blood (PaO_2). Higher than normal gradients occur with V/Q mismatch, shunt, and impaired gas diffusion. The ratio of PaO_2 to the fraction of inspired O_2 (F_IO_2) also provides a rough estimate of lung function (*Table 29*)[15, 36, 37].

Specific therapy depends on the etiology and pathophysiology involved. However, general principles apply to all cases: remove or minimize any airway

---

Table 29 Assessment of hypoxemia.

Pulse oximetry

Correlation of hemoglobin saturation with PaO_2:

Hemoglobin saturation (%)	PaO_2 (mm Hg)
99–100	>100
96	80
91	60

Arterial blood gas analysis

Normal values (room air):

PaO_2 = 85–100 mm Hg
$PaCO_2$ = 35–45 mm Hg
pH = 7.35–7.45
HCO_3 = 21–27 mmol/l

O_2 supplementation recommended if PaO_2 < 60(–80) mm Hg (or hemoglobin saturation <92%), or if signs of hypoxemia are evident. O_2 supplementation of minimal help with hypoventilation (unless assisted ventilation provided), pleural space disease, or anatomic shunt as the cause of hypoxemia.

Assisted ventilation recommended if $PaCO_2$ is persistently > 45 mm Hg (indicates alveolar hypoventilation) after O_2 supplementation, and airway obstructive or anesthesia-related causes are excluded.

Alveolar-arterial (A-a) O_2 gradient

A-a gradient = PAO_2 - PaO_2
$\qquad PAO_2 = F_IO_2 (P_B - P_{H2O}) - PaCO_2/R$

A-a gradient (mm Hg; on room air at sea level) = (150 – [$PaCO_2/0.8$]) – PaO_2

<10–15 is normal
>15 indicates compromised ability of lung to oxygenate blood
>30 indicates severely impaired gas exchange

↑ A-a gradient occurs with V/Q mismatch, shunt, diffusion impairment.
Hypoxemia with normal A-a gradient is associated with hypoventilation (hypercapnia) or ↓ inspired O_2.

PaO_2:F_IO_2 ratio

Allows quick estimation of oxygenation, but is less accurate than A-a gradient because $PaCO_2$ is not considered.

PaO_2:F_IO_2 ratio and lung function:
$\qquad$ 500 is normal
$\qquad$ 300–500 indicates mild disease
$\qquad$ 200–300 indicates moderate disease
$\qquad$ <200 indicates severe disease

F_IO_2(%) × 5 = approximate PaO_2 (assuming normal lung function in animal at sea level):

F_IO_2 (%)	PaO_2 (mm Hg)
0.2 (room air)	100
1.0 (100% O_2)	500

F_IO_2 = fraction of inspired O_2; PAO_2 = partial pressure of O_2 in alveolar air; PaO_2 = partial pressure of O_2 in arterial blood; P_B = barometric pressure; $PaCO_2$ = partial pressure of CO_2 in arterial blood; P_{H2O} = partial pressure of water; R = respiratory quotient (assumed to be 0.8 for fasting animal).

Table 30 Arterial blood sample acquisition.

1) **Supplies.** 25 gauge needle; 3 cc syringe; heparin (1,000 U/ml); rubber blood tube stopper or cork; clippers; surgical scrub solution and alcohol.

2) **Preparation.** Attach the needle to the syringe. Heparinize both by drawing heparin into the syringe then expelling it back into its bottle, leaving heparin only in the needle hub. Choose the arterial puncture site: the femoral artery is used most often, but the dorsal pedal artery is an alternative, especially if there is difficulty accessing the femoral artery or if restraint in lateral recumbency would exacerbate respiratory distress. At least one assistant will be needed to help with restraint and positioning.

3) **Femoral artery puncture.** Position the animal in lateral recumbency. Extend the lower hindlimb and abduct and flex the upper hindlimb to expose the inguinal area. Lift the prepuce or caudal mammary tissue if necessary to gain adequate access to the femoral artery region. Clip hair from the puncture site and surgically scrub the area. Palpate for the arterial pulse, then position the artery between the tips of the first two fingers of the free hand. Position the prepared needle/syringe at a 60–90° angle to the skin. Hold the syringe at the plunger end so that it is possible to pull back on the plunger without having to reposition the hand (and risk moving the syringe and needle). Slowly

insert the needle into the artery through the skin between the fingertips while watching for a flash of bright red blood in the needle hub. It may help to apply a tiny amount of pull on the plunger after the needle penetrates the skin. Aspirate 1–1.5 ml of blood. Withdraw the needle and immediately apply direct pressure to the puncture site for at least 5 minutes. Immediately after withdrawing the needle, hold the syringe/needle upright to expel all air bubbles, then insert the needle into the rubber stopper or cork. Place on ice for transport to the lab.

4) **Dorsal pedal artery puncture.** Position animal with the hindlimbs to one side in sternal (or lateral) recumbency. Extend and stabilize the lower hindlimb. Palpate for the arterial pulse along the dorsal and proximal metatarsal area (slightly medial to midline) to locate the puncture site. Clip hair from the puncture site and surgically scrub the area. Proceed as for femoral artery puncture, except hold the syringe at a 15–30° angle to the skin (more parallel).

---

obstruction, promote full lung expansion by removing pleural air or fluid, and improve oxygenation using supplemental O_2 and assisted ventilation if necessary (see references for additional recommendations and details)[15, 25, 38, 39]. Guidelines for managing patients with heart failure can be found in Chapter 16 and in specific chapters related to the underlying cardiac disease. Reference citations and other appropriate sources should be consulted for further information on diagnosis and management of the many noncardiac diseases that cause respiratory difficulty.

REFERENCES

1 Reece WO (1993) Respiration in mammals. In: *Duke's Physiology of Domestic Animals*, 11th edn. MJ Swenson, WO Reece (eds). Cornell University Press, Ithaca, pp. 263–293.

2 Campbell VL, Perkowski SZ (2004) Hypoventilation. In: *Textbook of Respiratory Disease in Dogs and Cats*, LG King (ed). Elsevier Saunders, St. Louis, pp. 53–61.

3 Robinson NE (2002) Overview of respiratory function: ventilation of the lung. In: *Textbook of Veterinary Physiology*, 3rd edn. JG Cunningham (ed). WB Saunders, Philadelphia, pp. 468–477.

4 Lumb AB (2000) Ventilatory failure. In: *Nunn's Applied Respiratory Physiology*, 5th edn. Butterworth Heinemann, Edinburgh, pp. 513–524.

5 Manning HL, Schwartzstein RM (1995) Pathophysiology of dyspnea. *New Engl J Med* 333:1547–1553.

6 Henik RA, Yeager AE (1940 Bronchopulmonary diseases. In: *The Cat: Diseases and Clinical Management*. RG Sherding (ed). Churchill Livingstone, New York, pp. 979–1052.

7 Forrester SD, Moon ML, Jacobson JD (2001) Diagnostic evaluation of dogs and cats with respiratory distress. *Compend Cont Educ Pract Vet* 23:56–68.

8 Griffon DJ (2000) Upper airway obstruction in cats: diagnosis and treatment. *Compend Cont Educ Pract Vet* 22:897–907.

9 Koch DA, Arnold S, Hubler M *et al.* (2003) Brachycephalic syndrome in dogs. *Compend Cont Educ Pract Vet* 25:48–54.

10 Hunt GB, Perkins MC, Foster SF *et al.* (2002) Nasopharyngeal disorders of dogs and cats: a review and retrospective study. *Compend Cont Educ Pract Vet* 24:184–199.

11 Cowell RL, Tyler RD, Meinkoth JH (1999) Abdominal and thoracic fluid. In: *Diagnostic Cytology and Hematology of the Dog and Cat*, 2nd edn. RL Cowell, RD Tyler, JH Meinkoth (eds). Mosby, St. Louis, pp. 142–158.

12 Lumb AB (2000). Control of breathing. In: *Nunn's Applied Respiratory Physiology*, 5th edn. Butterworth Heinemann, Edinburgh, pp. 82–112.

13 West JB (2003) *Pulmonary Pathophysiology*, 6th edn. Lippincott, Williams & Wilkins, Philadelphia, pp. 17–34.

14 Lumb AB. Distribution of pulmonary ventilation and perfusion. In: *Nunn's Applied Respiratory Physiology*, 5th edn. Butterworth Heinemann, Edinburgh, pp. 163–199.

15 Clare M, Hopper K (2005) Mechanical ventilation: indications, goals, and prognosis. *Compend Cont Educ Pract Vet* 27:195–207.

16 Lee JA, Drobatz KJ (2004) Respiratory distress and cyanosis in dogs. In: *Textbook of Respiratory Disease in Dogs and Cats*. LG King (ed). Elsevier Saunders, St. Louis, pp. 1–12.

17 Lumb AB (2000) Pulmonary vascular disease. In: *Nunn's Applied Respiratory Physiology*, 5th edn. Butterworth Heinemann, Edinburgh, pp. 541–558.

18 Mellanby RJ, Villiers E, Herrtage ME (2002) Canine pleural and mediastinal effusions: a retrospective study of 81 cases. *J Small Anim Pract* 43:447–451.

19 Roudebush P (1982) Lung sounds. *J Am Vet Med Assoc* 181:122–126.

20 Kotlikoff MI, Gillespie JR (1983) Lung sounds in veterinary medicine. Part I: Terminology and mechanisms of sound production. *Compend Cont Educ Pract Vet* 5:634–639.

21 Kotlikoff MI, Gillespie JR (1984) Lung sounds in veterinary medicine. Part II: Deriving clinical information from lung sounds. *Compend Cont Educ Pract Vet* 6:462–467.

22 Crowe DT (2003) Supplemental oxygen therapy in critically ill or injured patients. *Vet Med* 98:935–953.

23 Tseng LW, Drobatz KJ (2004) Oxygen supplementation and humidification. In: *Textbook of Respiratory Disease in Dogs and Cats*. LG King (ed). Elsevier Saunders, St. Louis, pp. 205–213.

24 Crowe DT (2003) Rapid sequence intubation and surgical intervention in respiratory emergencies. *Vet Med* 98:954–968.

25 Clare M, Hopper K (2005) Mechanical ventilation: ventilator settings, patient management, and nursing care. *Compend Cont Educ Pract Vet* 27:256–268.

26 Mattoon JS, Drost WT (2004) Obtaining nasal radiographs in small animals. *Vet Med* 99:34–45.

27 Mattoon JS, Drost WT (2004) Pharyngeal and laryngeal radiography in small animals. *Vet Med* 99:50–70.

28 Mattoon JS, Drost WT (2004) Radiographing the trachea in small animals. *Vet Med* 99:72–83.

29 Nycamp SG, Scrivani PV, Dykes NL (2002) Radiographic signs of pulmonary disease: an alternative approach. *Compend Cont Educ Pract Vet* 24:25–35.

30 Grosenbaugh DA, Muir WW (1998) Accuracy of noninvasive oxyhemoglobin saturation, end-tidal carbon dioxide concentration, and blood pressure monitoring during experimentally induced hypoxemia, hypotension, or hypertension in anesthetized dogs. *Am J Vet Res* 59:205–212.

31 Matthews NS, Hartke S, Allen JC Jr (2003) An evaluation of pulse oximeters in dogs, cats, and horses. *Vet Anaesth Analg* 30:3–14.

32 Proulx J (1999) Respiratory monitoring: arterial blood gas analysis, pulse oximetry, and end-tidal carbon dioxide analysis. *Clin Tech Small Anim Pract* 14:227–230.

33 Camps-Palau MA, Marks SL, Cornick JL (1999) Small animal oxygen therapy. *Compend Cont Educ Pract Vet* 21:587–598.

34 Shiroshita Y, Tanaka R, Shibazaki A et al. (1999) Accuracy of a portable blood gas analyzer incorporating optodes for canine blood. *J Vet Intern Med* 13:597–600.

35 Hawkins EC (2003) Diagnostic tests for the lower respiratory tract. In: *Small Animal Internal Medicine*, 3rd edn. RW Nelson, CG Couto (eds.) Mosby, St. Louis, pp. 255–286.

36 Powell LL (2002) Causes of respiratory failure. *Vet Clin North Am: Small Anim Pract* 32:1049–1058.

37 Manning AM (2002) Oxygen therapy and toxicity. *Vet Clin North Am: Small Anim Pract* 32:1005–1020.

38 Haskins SC, King LG (2004) Positive pressure ventilation. In: *Textbook of Respiratory Disease in Dogs and Cats*. LG King (ed). Elsevier Saunders, St. Louis, pp. 217–229.

39 Haskins SC (2004) Interpretation of blood gas measurements. In: *Textbook of Respiratory Disease in Dogs and Cats*. LG King (ed). Elsevier Saunders, St. Louis, pp. 181–193.

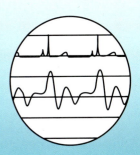

10
Jugular Vein Distension or Pulsations

OVERVIEW

Jugular veins distend when pressure within rises. The jugular veins are normally not distended when the animal is standing with its head in a normal position and its jaw parallel to the floor. Persistent jugular vein distension when the head is erect is most often associated with R-CHF (**187, 188**). Lesions that obstruct venous flow from the external jugular veins to the heart are less commonly responsible (*Table 31*). Because of the effects of gravity, jugular veins normally distend when the head is lowered below the level of the RA.

Fluctuations in atrial pressure occur during the cardiac cycle related to filling, emptying, and contraction (see Chapter 1 and **14**, p. 19)[1]. Because no valves lie between the RA and the jugular veins, these

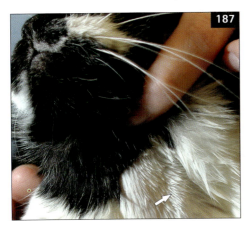

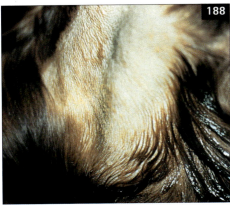

187, 188 (187) Right-sided heart failure secondary to tricuspid valve dysplasia caused marked jugular vein distension in this cat. (188) Image of a greatly distended jugular vein from an 11-year-old Irish Setter with heart failure from dilated cardiomyopathy.

Table 31 Causes of jugular vein distension/pulsation.

1) Distension:
  a) Cranial vena cava/jugular vein obstruction:
    ■ Cranial mediastinal mass.
    ■ Thrombosis.
  b) Right atrial mass with inflow obstruction.
  c) Pericardial effusion with tamponade.
  d) Dilated cardiomyopathy.

2) Pulsation +/- distension (with elevated mean RA pressure/R-CHF):
  a) Tricuspid insufficiency:
    ■ Degenerative AV valve disease.
    ■ Cardiomyopathy.
    ■ Congenital tricuspid dysplasia.
    ■ Secondary to disease causing systolic RV pressure overload (e.g. heartworm disease, other causes of pulmonary hypertension, pulmonic stenosis, tetralogy of Fallot).
  b) RV hypertrophy/increased stiffness:
    ■ Pulmonic stenosis.
    ■ Tetralogy of Fallot.
    ■ Other RV outflow obstruction.
    ■ Heartworm disease.
    ■ Pulmonary hypertension from other cause.
  c) Arrhythmia causing AV dissociation:
    ■ Complete (3rd degree) AV block.
    ■ Ventricular premature contractions.
  d) Pericardial effusion with tamponade.
  e) Constrictive pericarditis.
  f) Hypervolemia.

pressure fluctuations reflect backward along the great veins and are sometimes visible as pulsations in the jugular veins[1]. In the standing normal animal, jugular pulsations do not extend higher than one third of the way up the neck from the thoracic inlet, at about the point of the shoulder. Jugular pulsations visible higher on the neck indicate increased amplitude RA pressure waves and often increased mean RA pressure as well. Jugular pulsations must be differentiated from tissue motion caused by the pulsation of the underlying carotid arteries (see Chapter 2, p. 28). Carotid pulse transmission is more likely to be seen in thin or excited animals.

PATHOPHYSIOLOGY

Right heart filling pressure and, therefore, CVP directly influence the degree of jugular vein filling. As long as there is no obstructive lesion between the jugular vein(s) and the RA, the appearance of the jugular veins provides an indication of right heart filling pressure. CVP is functionally coupled with cardiac output. Conditions that decrease cardiac output lead to a rise in CVP[2]. Intrathoracic pressure fluctuation during the respiratory cycle also influences CVP. During inspiration there is a decrease in CVP, which tends to collapse the jugular veins; however, during this time there is also increased venous return and cardiac filling, so any visible pulsations are amplified[1, 3]. Venous distension secondary to high RA pressure is often accompanied by visible pulsations (see below). Jugular vein distension without pulsation occurs with diseases that restrict or obstruct blood flow through the cranial vena cava or proximal jugular veins, as well as with obstruction to venous inflow within the RA. Jugular pulsations may be minimal with impaired RA filling (e.g. cardiac tamponade) or contractility failure (e.g. dilated cardiomyopathy).

Jugular pulse waves are related to atrial contraction and filling (see **14**, p.19). When RA pressure is elevated or when atrial ('a') or ventricular ('v') contraction waves are accentuated, the atrial pressure waves are more likely to reflect backward a greater distance and be visible higher on the jugular veins. Visible pulsations occur with several abnormalities. Tricuspid insufficiency causes a jugular pulse after the first heart sound, as blood regurgitates backward into the RA during ventricular contraction. The 'v' wave on the atrial pressure trace is magnified as pressure is reflected backward toward the jugular veins (**189**). With severe tricuspid insufficiency, there is fusion of the 'c' and 'v' waves and loss of the 'x' descent on the RA pressure curve.

Jugular pulsations that originate during atrial contraction, just before the first heart sound, occur with diseases that cause RV hypertrophy, increased stiffness, or restriction because greater atrial pressure generation is required for ventricular filling. Pressure is reflected backward during the accentuated 'a' wave (**190**).

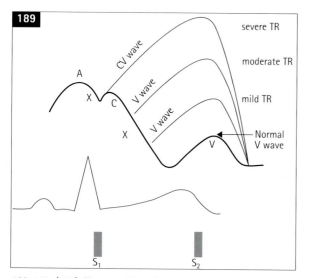

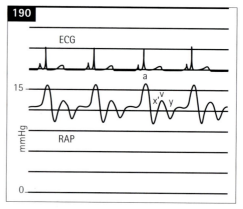

189, 190 (189) Diagram of the effects of tricuspid insufficiency on the jugular pulse wave. The timing of the waveform is shown against a depiction of ECG and heart sounds. The normal waveform is in red. The 'A' wave results from venous distension associated with atrial contraction. The 'X' descent occurs with atrial relaxation and descent of the atrial floor during ventricular contraction. The 'C' wave occurs during ventricular contraction at the time of the carotid pulse. The 'V' wave results from atrial filling during ventricular systole. The 'X' descent relates to the decrease in atrial pressure when the tricuspid valve opens and ventricular filling occurs. As the severity of TR increases, the 'X' descent becomes minimized and the 'CV' wave predominates. TR = tricuspid regurgitation. (From Braunwald E, Perloff JK (2001) Physical examination of the heart and circulation. In *Heart Diseases: A Textbook of Cardiovascular Medicine* (6th edn). (eds E Braunwald, DP Zipes, P Libby) WB Saunders, Philadelphia, p. 49, with permission.) (190) Right atrial pressure (RAP) trace from a 5-year-old male Bulldog with pulmonic stenosis and signs of right-sided heart failure. Jugular distension and pulsation were evident clinically. Overall RAP is elevated (mean ~13 mm Hg) and the 'a' wave is especially prominent (>15 mm Hg), which is consistent with increased stiffness of the hypertrophied right ventricle.

Cardiac arrhythmias that cause dissociation of atrial and ventricular contractions are associated with intermittent, bounding jugular pulse waves. These so-called cannon 'a' waves occur when the atria contract against closed AV valves, causing retrograde blood flow toward the vena cavae and jugular veins[1]. Complete (3rd degree) AV block with a ventricular escape rhythm is the most common cause.

APPROACH TO THE PATIENT WITH JUGULAR VEIN DISTENSION/PULSATIONS

Identification of a jugular vein abnormality provides clues to the underlying disease process. Remembering to examine the jugular veins is the first step. Evaluation is done with the patient in a normal upright posture and a horizontal head position.

The veins should empty quickly after release of manual compression at the thoracic inlet. Whether abnormal distension, pulsation, or both is present and whether both veins are equally involved are considerations. Pulse waves arising from the carotid arteries, especially in anxious animals, must be differentiated from true jugular pulsations (see Chapter 2, p. 28). A careful history and complete physical examination are important to detect evidence of heart disease or other potential underlying cause (191).

The hepatojugular reflux test is a provocative maneuver that will magnify jugular distension and pulsation in patients with equivocal findings. A positive test most often suggests RV hypertrophy, impaired filling, or tricuspid regurgitation. (See Chapter 2 and 21, p. 29 for a description of the technique.)

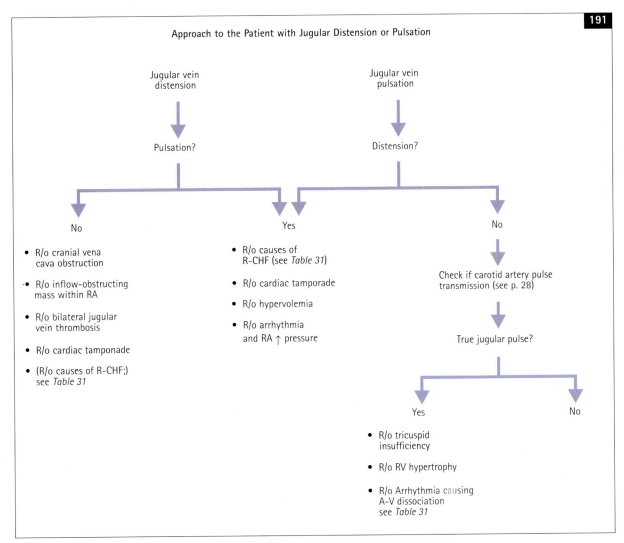

191 Diagram of an approach to the patient with jugular distension/pulsation.

CENTRAL VENOUS PRESSURE

Measurement of CVP is done when needed to verify high systemic venous pressure or to monitor right heart filling pressure during fluid therapy in certain patients. CVP is influenced by intravascular volume, venous compliance, and cardiac function. Right-sided heart failure and pericardial disease increase CVP to the extent that right heart filling pressure increases. CVP measurement helps differentiate these abnormalities from other causes of pleural or peritoneal effusion. However, large volume (e.g. >20 ml/kg body weight) pleural effusion can increase intrapleural pressure and compress the heart to the point where cardiac filling is impaired. This can raise CVP even in the absence of cardiac disease[4]; therefore, in patients with moderate to large pleural effusions, CVP should be measured after thoracocentesis. CVP is sometimes used to monitor critical patients receiving large volume fluid infusions; however, the CVP is not an accurate reflection of left heart filling pressure and as such is not reliable for monitoring treatment of cardiogenic pulmonary edema. CVP in normal dogs and cats is usually between 0 and 8 (up to 10) cm H_2O; fluctuations that parallel intrapleural pressure changes occur during respiration.

To measure CVP, a large bore jugular catheter that extends into or close to the RA is placed aseptically and connected via extension tubing and a three-way stopcock to a fluid administration set. A water manometer is attached to the stopcock and positioned vertically, with the stopcock (representing 0 cm H_2O) located at the same horizontal level as the patient's RA. The stopcock is turned off to the animal, allowing the manometer to fill with crystalloid fluid; then the stopcock is turned off to the fluid reservoir to allow equilibration of the fluid column in the manometer with the animal's CVP. Repeated measurements will be more consistent when taken with the animal and manometer in the same position and during the expiratory phase of respiration. Small fluctuations of the fluid meniscus within the manometer occur with the heartbeat; slightly larger movement is associated with respiration. Marked change in the height of the fluid column associated with the heartbeat suggests either severe tricuspid insufficiency or that the catheter tip is within the right ventricle.

REFERENCES

1 Braunwald E, Perloff JK (2001) Physical examination of the heart and circulation. In: *Heart Disease: A Textbook of Cardiovascular Medicine*, 6th edn. E Braunwald, DP Zipes, P Libby (eds). WB Saunders, Philadelphia, pp. 45–81.

2 Berne RM, Levy MN (1997) *Cardiovascular Physiology*, 7th edn. Mosby, St. Louis, pp. 204–211.

3 Sisson D, Ettinger SJ (1999) The physical examination. In: *Textbook of Canine and Feline Cardiology*, 2nd edn. PR Fox, D Sisson, NS Moise (eds). WB Saunders, Philadephia, pp. 46–64.

4 Gookin JL, Atkins CE (1999) Evaluation of the effect of pleural effusion on central venous pressure in cats. *J Vet Intern Med* 13:561–563.

11
Abdominal Distension

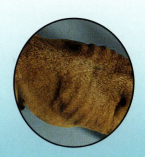

OVERVIEW

The abdomen becomes distended when there is marked enlargement of an intraabdominal organ, when a large mass lesion develops, or when free peritoneal fluid accumulates (*Table 32*, p. 122). Abdominal distension is usually a sign of an underlying disease process, unless caused by pregnancy or obesity. The peritoneal cavity is lined by a serous membrane of mesothelial cells (parietal layer), which also extends to cover the abdominal organs and the associated vasculature and connective tissue (visceral layer). This membrane allows absorption and transudation of fluid, and can serve a protective function (e.g. by walling-off an area of infection). The space between the parietal and visceral peritoneal layers normally contains very little free fluid. Several disease processes cause excessive abdominal fluid (effusion) to accumulate. Abdominal fluid characterized as a transudate, modified trandudate, or chyle is known as ascites (see *Table 27*, p. 111 for fluid classification guidelines)[1]. As a manifestation of cardiovascular disease, ascites is associated with right-sided or biventricular congestive failure, or impaired venous inflow to the right heart (**192**, **193**). An exudative abdominal effusion, either septic or nonseptic, is characteristic of an inflammatory process involving all or part of the peritoneal cavity (peritonitis)[1].

Regardless of the cause, abdominal enlargement tends to push the diaphragm cranially, and it can interfere with respiration. Massive enlargement, as with large volume ascites, can cause respiratory distress. Abdominal enlargement may be associated with pain, especially when inflammation of the peritoneum or other intraabdominal structure is present.

PATHOPHYSIOLOGY

ABDOMINAL EFFUSIONS

Peritoneal effusion usually results from an imbalance of Starling's forces (see Chapter 1), similar to the formation of pleural effusion. An increase in systemic venous hydrostatic pressure or portal pressure is a common cause. Increased capillary endothelial

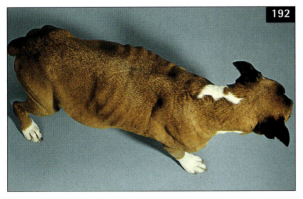

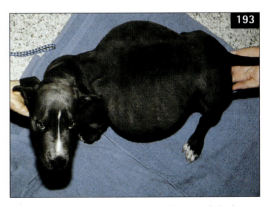

192, 193 (**192**) Top down view of an older male Boxer with ascites secondary to cardiac tamponade, associated with an aortic body tumor. Note the poor body condition (easily visible ribs and iliac crests) in contrast to the distended abdomen. (**193**) Massive ascites in a 5-month-old male Pit Bull Terrier with cor triatriatum dexter (see also figures **358–364**, pp. 256, 257).

Table 32 Causes of abdominal distension.

1) Free peritoneal fluid:

   a) Pure transudate:

   - Hypoalbuminemia (e.g. glomerulopathy/nephrotic syndrome, protein-losing enteropathy, intestinal malabsorption or maldigestion, heavy parasitism, liver failure, starvation).

   b) Modified transudate:

   - R-CHF:
     - Tricuspid valve insufficiency (see Chapters 18, 19).
     - Dilated cardiomyopathy (see Chapter 20).
     - Pericardial disease (effusion/tamponade or restrictive; see Chapter 22).
     - Heartworm disease (see Chapter 24).
     - Pulmonic stenosis (see Chapter 18).
     - Intracardiac tumor (see Chapter 22).
   - Caudal vena caval obstruction:
     - Cor triatriatum dexter (see Chapter 18).
     - CaVC obstruction (e.g. thrombus, pheochromocytoma, external compression).
   - Hepatic vein obstruction/thrombosis:
     - Hepatic cirrhosis.
     - Other causes of portal hypertension.
     - Neoplasia (liver, lymphoma, other).
     - Carcinomatosis.
     - Mesothelioma.

   c) Chyle:

   - Traumatic rupture of major lymph channel.
   - Neoplastic obstruction of lymphatics (e.g. lymphoma involving lymph channels, other neoplasia).
   - Intestinal lymphangiectasia.
   - Intestinal obstruction with rupture of lymphatics.
   - Thoracic duct ligation/obstruction.
   - R-CHF (uncommon; see modified transudate, above).

   d) Hemorrhage:

   - Hemangiosarcoma or other neoplasm (e.g. spleen, other sites).
   - Coagulopathy/anticoagulant toxicity.
   - Trauma.

   e) Nonseptic exudate:

   - Ruptured bladder/uroperitoneum.
   - Gall bladder or bile duct tear/bile peritonitis.
   - Pancreatitis.
   - Neoplasia.
   - Parasitic peritonitis (e.g. *Mesocestoides* species).
   - Feline infectious peritonitis (coronavirus).
   - Steatitis (cats).

   f) Septic exudate:

   - Perforated bowel.
   - Devitalized intestinal wall (e.g. ischemia, intussusception, thrombosis).
   - Pyometra/uterine rupture.
   - Other septic peritonitis (including *Actinomyces* or *Nocardia* species infection).

2) Organ/soft tissue enlargement:

   a) Gastric distention:

   - Gastric dilatation +/− volvulus.
   - Aerophagia.
   - Pyloric obstruction.

   b) Intestinal distension:

   - Ileus.
   - Intestinal obstruction.
   - Obstipation/megacolon.

   c) Hepatomegaly:

   - Venous congestion (e.g. R-CHF, caudal caval obstruction).
   - Neoplastic infiltration.
   - Hyperadrenocorticism.
   - Hepatic lipidosis.

   d) Splenomegaly:

   - Venous congestion (e.g. from torsion).
   - Neoplastic infiltration.
   - Infection (e.g. *Rickettsia* species).

   e) Fat.

   f) Pregnancy.

   g) Pyometra.

   h) Renomegaly:

   - Ureteral obstruction.
   - Neoplastic infiltration.
   - Cyst.

   i) Tumor (e.g. of spleen, liver, lymph nodes, intestine, ovary, retained testicle, other organ).

   j) Chronic urinary bladder distension:

   - Urethral obstruction.
   - Neurologic dysfunction.

   k) Obstipation/megacolon.

3) Marked abdominal muscle weakness:

   a) Hyperadrenocorticism.

permeability (from inflammation or other vascular disruption) or low capillary colloid oncotic pressure (from hypoalbuminemia) are other mechanisms affecting transcapillary fluid movement. Obstruction in the lymphatic drainage system also promotes peritoneal effusion accumulation.

Ascites caused by high venous and, therefore, capillary hydrostatic pressure is categorized according to the location of the pathology. 'Posthepatic' or 'postsinusoidal' ascites occurs when blood flow is restricted or obstructed between the hepatic vein and the RV. Excessive fluid (lymph) formation occurs mainly in hepatic sinusoids and fluid then diffuses across the liver capsule. This fluid is typically a modified transudate. Posthepatic ascites is usually secondary to R-CHF or cardiac tamponade. Uncommon causes include CaVC or hepatic venous obstruction (e.g. thrombus, tumor infiltration, or intravascular fibrous obstruction) and RA inflow obstruction (e.g. an intracardiac tumor or congenital cor triatriatum dexter; see Chapter 22 and Chapter 18). The term 'Budd–Chiari-like syndrome' has been used to describe postsinusoidal portal hypertension and ascites that result from such caudal caval or RA inflow obstructions[2, 3]. External CaVC compression by a mass lesion or diaphragmatic hernia can also lead to posthepatic ascites. In general, dogs are more likely to develop ascites as a manifestation of R-CHF than cats; however, heart failure-induced ascites in cats does occur, especially with dilated, restrictive, and arrhythmogenic RV forms of cardiomyopathy, as well as congenital malformations involving the right heart and pericardial disease[4]. When ascites is secondary to heart failure, jugular vein distension and pulsation are usually evident because central venous pressure is high. Hepatomegaly also develops from passive venous congestion.

So-called 'hepatic' ascites, caused by primary liver disease, can be either a transudate or modified transudate. The mechanism largely involves portal hypertension, although other mechanisms may also be involved, especially with hepatic cirrhosis[1]. 'Prehepatic' ascites develops when blood flow is restricted at the level of the portal vein; excess fluid transudation from the intestinal serosa leads to increased lymph formation. This fluid is usually lower in protein than posthepatic ascites[1]. Prehepatic causes of ascites are relatively uncommon because collateral portosystemic shunting often develops as portal pressure rises, thus reducing portal hypertension.

Effusions classified as pure transudates are most likely with severe hypoalbuminemia. Protein-losing glomerulopathy and enteropathy are common causes.

Chylous abdominal effusion contains intestinal lymph with a high lipid content. Causes of lymphatic disruption and leakage include neoplasia, trauma, infection, and, occasionally, congestion associated with R-CHF[5]. Neoplastic infiltration of the abdominal serosa can produce a modified transudate or an exudate related to inflammation and capillary obstruction. Increased capillary permeability as well as inflammatory cell recruitment occur from the effects of inflammatory mediators. Nonseptic exudates are also caused by the presence of bile or urine in the abdominal cavity. Traumatic rupture of the gallbladder or a biliary duct leads to bile peritonitis. A tear in the bladder or ureter results in uroabdomen. Feline infectious peritonitis is an important cause of nonseptic, exudative abdominal effusion in cats. Septic exudates are usually caused by bacterial infection. Sources can include intestinal perforation or devitalization, extension from infection or abcess in adjacent tissues, surgical contamination or wound dehiscence, and injury related to abdominal trauma (blunt or sharp)[6]. Bleeding into the peritoneal cavity (hemoabdomen) occurs from trauma, coagulopathy (e.g. rodenticide toxicity), or neoplastic invasion, especially with hemangiosarcoma of the spleen or liver.

During peritoneal effusion formation from any cause, fluid is redistributed out of the vascular space into the peritoneal cavity. The reduction in effective plasma volume stimulates compensatory mechanisms (e.g. the renin-angiotensin-aldosterone system and antidiuretic hormone release) to expand total body water and sodium (see Chapter 1)[1].

OTHER CAUSES OF ABDOMINAL DISTENSION

Marked organomegaly can cause abdominal distension. Pregnancy must be considered in the intact female. Excessive fat accumulation is responsible in some individuals. The stomach or intestines can distend greatly with gas or fluid. Examples include aerophagia, usually secondary to respiratory distress; gastric dilatation, with or without volvulus; ileus; or bowel obstruction. Obstipation, especially in cats with megacolon, can enlarge the abdomen. Similarly, urinary bladder dilation from chronic urethral obstruction or neurologic dysfunction, or renomegaly secondary to ureteral obstruction, may underlie abdominal distension. Chronic venous congestion will enlarge the liver (e.g. with chronic R-CHF or CaCV obstruction) or spleen (e.g. with splenic torsion).

Diffuse or localized neoplastic infiltration also causes generalized organ enlargement. Common examples are hemangiosarcoma of the spleen or liver, lymphoma, or primary liver cancers. Discrete mass lesions may be neoplastic or inflammatory in nature.

Abdominal distension in animals with hyperadrenocorticism is associated with weakness of the abdominal wall muscles as well as hepatomegaly.

Abdominal enlargement is often a slow process; it may be interpreted by the owner simply as weight gain. Exceptions include traumatic intraabdominal hemorrhage, ruptured bladder, or gastric dilatation/volvulus. Decreased activity and exercise tolerance, reduced appetite, and increased respiratory rate often accompany abdominal distension of any cause, as ventilation becomes restricted by cranial displacement of the diaphragm.

APPROACH TO THE PATIENT WITH ABDOMINAL DISTENSION

A complete history and a careful physical examination may reveal the likely cause, especially if signs of heart disease or other abnormalities are found. Initial diagnostic questions relate to whether the distension is due to peritoneal fluid accumulation, organomegaly, a mass lesion, or a combination (194). Pregnancy should be ruled out in the intact female.

Organomegaly, larger mass lesions, and free peritoneal fluid can usually be detected by abdominal palpation. Small amounts of fluid tend to make the intestines feel slippery as they pass under the examiner's fingers during palpation. A larger volume of ascites will cause a fluid wave during abdominal ballottement. To test for this, the palm of one hand is placed on one side of the abdomen and the other side of the abdomen is tapped sharply with the fingertips of the opposite hand. A fluid wave can be felt against the palm when moderate to large volume ascites is present.

Animals with ascites caused by heart failure generally have concurrent jugular vein distension and/or pulsation, unless vascular volume has been reduced by diuretic therapy. A murmur, gallop sound, or arrhythmia is also common. Muffled heart sounds are typical of a large pericardial effusion. Abdominal tenderness is usually evident with peritonitis, and is sometimes present with noninflammatory causes of ascites. Poor body condition is common with chronic R-CHF and neoplastic disease, as well as with causes of hypoalbuminemia.

Abdominal radiographs are useful for delineating organomegaly and mass lesions; however, free peritoneal fluid produces a hazy, 'ground glass' appearance that obscures serosal margins. Abdominocentesis prior to radiography is recommended with moderate to large volume peritoneal effusions to improve radiographic visualization. Nevertheless, gas-filled bowel loops, displacement of other organs by a large mass lesion, or free abdominal gas associated with peritonitis can still be appreciated.

A sample of fluid obtained during abdominocentesis should be saved in sterile serum (clot) and EDTA tubes for biochemical and cytologic analysis and, possibly, culture (see *Table 27*, p. 111 for fluid descriptions).

Abdominal ultrasonography is used to further evaluate radiographically normal organs and abnormal structures. Changes in echogenicity or shape/size of specific organs, mass lesions, vascular abnormalities, and small volumes of peritoneal effusion can be detected. Ultrasound-guided needle biopsy or aspiration can be performed.

Diagnostic testing should also include CBC, serum biochemical profile, and urinalysis. Depending on the initial results, further diagnostic evaluation might include thoracic radiographs, echocardiography, electrocardiography, heartworm testing, evaluation of the coagulation cascade, endocrine testing (e.g. for hyperadrenocorticism), CT or MRI scans, surgical exploration and biopsy, cultures, or lymph node aspirate/biopsy.

Specific therapy is based on the underlying diagnosis. For patients with ascites, diuretic therapy may or may not be helpful, so it is important to identify the underlying cause. Therapy for heart failure is outlined in Chapter 16; (see also other chapters in this text relevant to causes of R-CHF). Because large volume ascites can impede respiration, periodic removal of enough fluid to relieve patient discomfort and improve ventilation is advised, no matter what the etiology. Repeatedly draining the abdomen completely is not recommended.

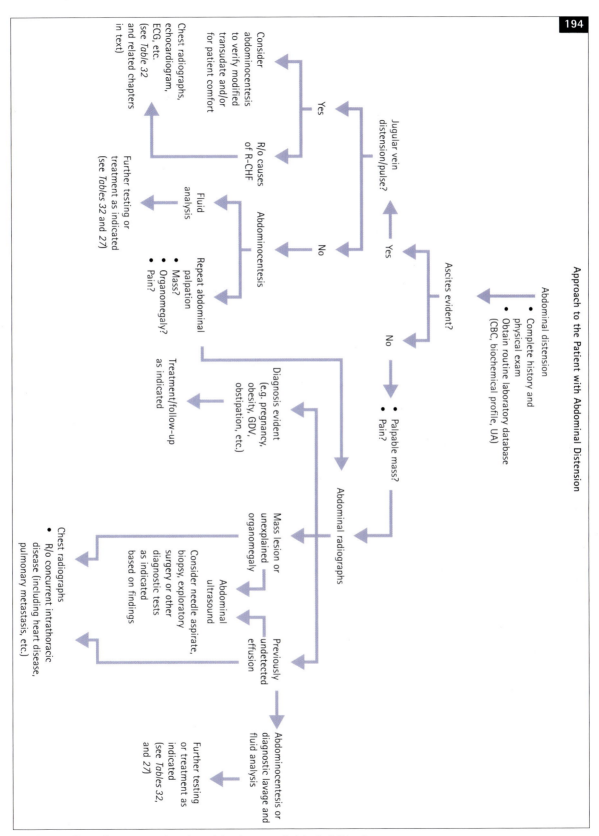

194 Diagram illustrating an approach to determining the cause of abdominal distension.

REFERENCES

1 Kruth SA (2005) Abdominal distention, ascites, and peritonitis. In: *Textbook of Veterinary Internal Medicine*, 6th edn. SJ Ettinger, EC Feldman (eds). WB Saunders, Philadelphia, pp. 150–153.

2 Grooters AM, Smeak DD (1995) Budd–Chiari-like syndromes in dogs. In: *Current Veterinary Therapy XII.* JD Bonagura (ed). WB Saunders, Philadelphia, pp. 876–879.

3 Cave TA, Martineau H, Dickie A *et al.* (2002) Idiopathic hepatic veno-occlusive disease causing Budd-Chiari-like syndrome in a cat. *J Small Anim Pract* **43:**411–415.

4 Wright KN, Gompf RE, DeNovo RC (1999) Peritoneal effusion in cats: 65 cases (1981–1997). *J Am Vet Med Assoc* **214:**375–381.

5 Gores BR, Berg J, Carpenter JL *et al.* (1994) Chylous ascites in cats: nine cases (1978–1993). *J Am Vet Med Assoc* **205:**1161–1164.

6 Hosgood G, Salisbury SK (1988) Generalized peritonitis in dogs: 50 cases (1975–1986). *J Am Vet Med Assoc* **193:**1448–1450.

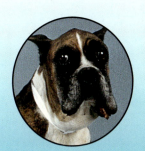

12
Subcutaneous Edema

OVERVIEW

Subcutaneous edema is an abnormal increase in the amount of interstitial fluid within the superficial tissues. The relationship between hydrostatic and oncotic pressures across the capillary membrane (Starling's forces; see Chapter 1) defines the movement of fluid between the interstitial space and the vascular compartment. Fluid filtration into the interstitium is, on average, greater on the arterial side of the capillary because of higher intravascular hydrostatic pressure. However, greater absorption at the venous side, related to oncotic and lower hydrostatic pressure effects, along with lymphatic uptake of interstitial fluid, normally maintains a slightly negative interstitial pressure and a minimal amount of interstitial fluid[1, 2].

PATHOPHYSIOLOGY

Tissue edema develops when the balance of Starling's forces or lymphatic function is disrupted. This can occur with low capillary oncotic pressure, mainly from hypoalbuminemia; abnormal capillary permeability, as with inflammation; lymphatic obstruction; or increased capillary hydrostatic pressure[1, 2].

The effects of gravity cause tissue edema to be more prominent in dependent areas of the body. Subcutaneous edema may be noticeable only along the ventral trunk, under the mandible, or in the lower limbs or paws (195, 196). Edema that is not associated with inflammatory lesions causes nonpainful swelling. When digital pressure is applied firmly to edematous superficial tissue, an indentation is often left behind as interstitial fluid is displaced (196). This is known as 'pitting edema'. The finger-shaped depression persists for a time until interstitial fluid is redistributed back into the area.

Subcutaneous edema is usually associated with either regional lymphatic or venous obstruction, profound hypoalbuminemia, or with vasculitis and local tissue injury (Table 33, p. 128). Subcutaneous edema in dogs and cats is an uncommon feature of congestive heart failure. Although it is observed in some cases, increased capillary hydrostatic pressure secondary to high cardiac filling pressure most often causes either pulmonary edema (with LV failure) or body cavity effusion (with RV or biventricular failure). Localized venous obstruction or compression (e.g.

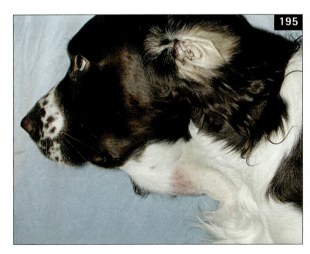

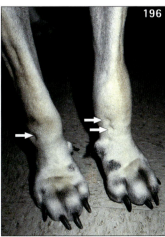

195, 196 (195) Submandibular edema is evident in a 2-year-old male English Springer Spaniel with vasculitis. Edema was also seen along the ventral trunk and lower limbs. (196) Pitting edema in the distal forelimbs of a Great Dane with CHF from AV valve insufficiency and myocardial failure. Arrows indicate indentations created by digital pressure.

Table 33 Causes of subcutaneous edema.

1) Low capillary oncotic pressure:

  a) Hypoalbuminemia (e.g. protein-losing glomerulopathy [nephrotic syndrome], protein-losing enteropathy, intestinal malabsorption or maldigestion, parasites, reduced hepatic production, starvation, exudative skin lesions).

2) High capillary hydrostatic pressure:

  a) Venous thrombosis.

  b) Tissue constriction or compression (e.g. rubber band, mass lesion).

  c) R-CHF (see *Table 32* for causes).

  d) A-V fistula.

  e) Overhydration (IV fluid administration).

3) Reduced lymphatic uptake:

  a) Lymphatic obstruction (lymphoma, other neoplasm that causes lymphatic infiltration or compression).

  b) Congenital lymphatic dysplasia.

4) Increased capillary permeability:

  a) Vasculitis (e.g. immune-mediated; infectious [rickettsial, ehrlichial, infectious canine hepatitis, other], drug-induced).

  b) Thrombophlebitis.

  c) Local tissue infection/inflammation.

  d) Anaphylaxis (e.g. secondary to spider bite, insect sting, drug reaction).

thrombosis or a mass lesion) is more likely to cause subcutaneous edema from high capillary hydrostatic pressure. Although uncommon, a peripheral A-V fistula can cause tissue edema by increasing local venous (and capillary) pressure related to high flow; venous dilation and tortuosity occur as well[3].

Compression of the cranial vena cava, usually related to a cranial mediastinal mass, or complete cranial caval thrombosis leads to the so-called 'cranial caval syndrome' (**197–199**). This is characterized by bilaterally symmetric edema of the head, neck, and forelimbs. Pleural effusion is also common in these cases. Cranial mediastinal lymphoma and thymoma are the most common neoplastic causes of cranial caval syndrome. Caval thrombosis has been associated with diseases that induce a hypercoaguable state (e.g. immune-mediated thrombocytopenia or hemolytic anemia, sepsis, nephrotic syndrome, and some neoplasia) in conjunction with central venous catheter placement[4]. Neoplastic obstruction of venous and lymphatic flow within the pelvic inlet can cause bilaterally symmetric edema of the hindlimbs.

Myxedema is a rare manifestation of hypothyroidism that is characterized by nonpitting thickening of the skin, especially the forehead, eyelids, and cheeks. Tissue swelling in this condition is related to hyaluronic acid deposition in the dermis, rather than subcutaneous edema[5].

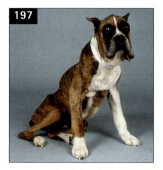 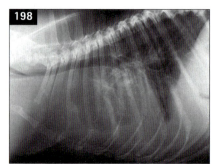 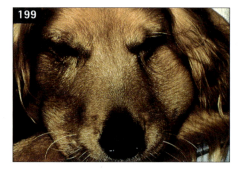

197–199 (197) Cranial caval syndrome in a 7-year-old male Boxer with cranial mediastinal lymphoma. The head, neck, and forelimbs are swollen from subcutaneous edema, but muscle wasting is evident in the caudal body. (198) Lateral thoracic radiograph from the dog in **197**. Increased soft tissue opacity cranial to the heart and dorsal tracheal displacement caused by the tumor are apparent, despite the presence of pleural effusion. (199) Marked facial edema is seen in this Golden Retriever with thrombosis of the cranial vena cava. (Courtesy Dr CJ Baldwin.)

APPROACH TO THE PATIENT WITH SUBCUTANEOUS EDEMA

The history and physical examination may provide important information as to the cause of superficial edema. Whether the edema is localized to one limb or region or is generalized throughout the body should be noted (200). Nonpainful pitting edema is more likely with an underlying mechanism related to high capillary hydrostatic pressure, hypoalbuminemia, or lymphatic obstruction. Painful swelling that is warmer than surrounding tissue is more likely associated with

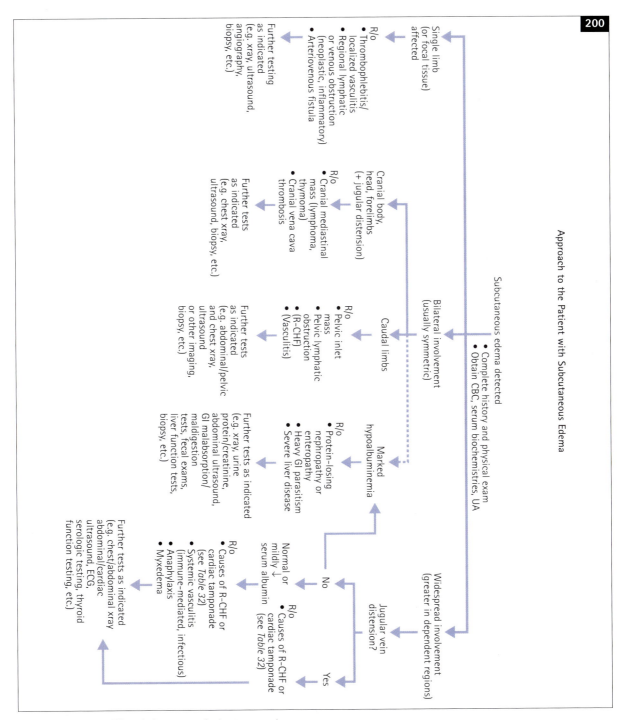

200 An approach to differentiating causes of subcutaneous edema.

increased capillary permeability (e.g. inflammation or infection). Warm swelling is also reported with A-V fistulas. Other signs of disease are usually evident and help guide diagnostic test selection.

A routine laboratory database (hemogram, serum biochemical profile, urinalysis) will reveal hypoalbuminemia, evidence for inflammation, and many other abnormal parameters. Thoracic and abdominal radiographs help identify other areas of fluid accumulation, mass lesions, and organomegaly. Additional testing that may be useful includes regional lymph node aspirates/biopsy, ultrasonography of the areas affected and related to venous/lymphatic drainage, echocardiography, serologic tests (e.g. for infectious agents, heartworm disease), and angiography. Although some patients may benefit from diuretic use, specific therapy depends on the underlying cause.

REFERENCES

1 Raffe MR, Roberts J (2005) Edema. In: *Textbook of Veterinary Internal Medicine*, 6th edn. SJ Ettinger, EC Feldman (eds). WB Saunders, Philadelphia, pp. 70–72.

2 Berne RM, Levy MN (1997) *Cardiovascular Physiology*, 7th edn. Mosby, St. Louis, pp. 153–170.

3 Bouayad H, Feeney DA, Lipowitz AJ *et al.* (1986) Peripheral acquired arteriovenous fistula: a report of four cases and literature review. *J Am Anim Hosp Assoc* **23**:205–211.

4 Palmer KG, King LG, Van Winkle TJ (1998) Clinical manifestations and associated disease syndromes in dogs with cranial vena cava thrombosis: 17 cases (1989–1996). *J Am Vet Med Assoc* **213**:220–224.

5 Doliger S, Delverdier M, More J *et al.* (1995) Histochemical study of cutaneous mucins in hypothyroid dogs. *Vet Pathol* **32**:628–634.

13
Abnormal Heart Rate or Rhythm

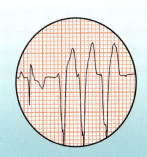

OVERVIEW

This clinical problem can pertain to heartbeats originating from ectopic foci (outside the sinus node), abnormal intracardiac conduction, or even to heart rhythms of normal (sinus) origin but inappropriate or unexpected rate. Cardiac arrhythmias occur for many reasons. While some arrhythmias are of no clinical consequence, others cause weakness, syncope, or sudden death, especially in animals with underlying disease. An arrhythmia may be suspected from the animal's history or identified on physical examination. An accurate ECG diagnosis is important (*Table 34* and see Chapter 4). The clinical context of the arrhythmia, and whether it is of hemodynamic significance, are also important. Some arrhythmias are benign and do not require treatment. However, therapy (see Chapter 17) is indicated for arrhythmias associated with clinical signs or a disease known to pose increased risk for sudden arrhythmic death.

The factors that control sinus node rate and sympathetic and vagal neural activity, as well as circulating cathecholamines, are strongly influenced by conditions outside the heart. Sinus tachycardia reflects increased sympathetic tone associated with underlying physiologic or pathologic conditions, or drug-induced vagal blockade (see *Table 10*, p. 52). Abnormally slow sinus rhythms may indicate high vagal tone (usually from noncardiac conditions) or primary sinus node disease (see *Table 10*, p. 52 and 75, 76, p. 51). Slow sinus rhythm, or arrhythmia, can be a normal finding, especially in athletic dogs. Chronic pulmonary disease is often associated with pronounced respiratory sinus arrhythmia.

Table 34 Guide for ECG interpretation.

1) Determine the heart rate. Is it too fast, too slow, or normal? (See *Table 9*, p. 50)

2) Is the rhythm regular or irregular?

3) Is sinus rhythm present (with or without other abnormalities), or are there no consistent P-QRS-T relationships?

4) Are all P waves followed by a QRS and all QRS complexes preceded by a P wave?

5) If premature (early) complexes are present, do they look the same as sinus QRS complexes, implying atrial or junctional (supraventricular) origin, or are they wide and of different configuration than sinus complexes, implying a ventricular origin or, possibly, abnormal (aberrant) ventricular conduction of a supraventricular complex (e.g. bundle branch block pattern)?

6) Are premature QRS complexes preceded by an abnormal P wave (suggesting atrial origin)?

7) Are there baseline undulations instead of clear and consistent P waves, with a rapid, irregular QRS occurrence (compatible with atrial fibrillation)?

8) Are there long pauses in the underlying rhythm before an abnormal complex occurs (escape beat)?

9) Is an intermittent AV conduction disturbance present?

10) Is there no consistent relation between P waves and QRS complexes, with a slow and regular QRS occurrence (implying complete AV block with ventricular escape rhythm)?

11) For sinus and supraventricular complexes, is the mean electrical axis normal? (See Chapter 4, p. 60)

12) Are all measurements and waveform durations within normal limits? (See *Table 9*, p. 50)

PATHOPHYSIOLOGY

Multiple factors underlie the development of cardiac rhythm disturbances. In general, underlying mechanisms are categorized as disorders of impulse formation, disorders of impulse conduction, or combinations of both[1-3]; however, identifying the specific mechanism for an arrhythmia in the individual patient is often problematic. Disorders of impulse formation can include an inappropriate sinus node rate for the patient's physiologic needs, discharge from ectopic (subsidiary) pacemaker cells that normally are overdrive suppressed (enhanced normal automaticity), or spontaneous discharge (abnormal automaticity) from cells that normally have no pacemaker activity (e.g. myocardial cells injured by ischemia). Triggered activity is a form of abnormal automaticity, where membrane oscillations following an action potential (afterdepolarizations) are strong enough to reach threshold potential and trigger another action potential. These oscillations can occur before full repolarization is reached (early afterdepolarizations [EADs]) or after repolarization (delayed afterdepolarizations [DADs]). Catecholamines can increase both types. Conditions that prolong action potential duration, digitalis, and other drugs have also been shown to increase afterdepolarizations and provoke arrhythmias[1, 4].

Disorders of impulse conduction can cause bradyarrhythmias when conduction fails in the AV node, atria, or SA node, causing asystole or a slow escape rhythm. Disorders of impulse conduction can also cause tachyarrhythmias when reentry (reentrant excitation, circus movement, reciprocating tachycardia) occurs. Reentry involves an area where conduction is blocked or delayed, but which recovers excitability in time to transmit the depolarizing wave back around so that tissue that had been previously depolarized becomes activated again. Reentry can occur within defined anatomic pathways (anatomic reentry) or because of functional electrophysiologic changes in adjacent tissues (functional reentry)[1]. Many clinical arrhythmias are caused by reentry, including AF, VF, many atrial and ventricular tachycardias, and AV reciprocating tachycardia (see Chapter 4).

Changes in normal cellular conduction properties or automaticity caused by cardiac structural or physiologic remodeling can predispose to arrhythmia development, even when overt cardiac disease is absent. Genetic factors and environmental stresses can contribute to this. Additional triggering (e.g. premature stimulus or abrupt change in heart rate) and/or modulating factors (e.g. changes in autonomic tone, circulating catecholamines, ischemia, or electrolyte disturbances) also appear necessary to provoke and sustain rhythm disturbances. For example, anger and aggressive behavior have been associated with

increased susceptibility to arrhythmias and sudden arrhythmic death in both dogs and people, especially when coronary blood flow is compromised[5, 6].

The clinical context is important, because some diseases are associated with higher risk for sudden arrhythmic death, in particular dilated cardiomyopathy, especially in Doberman Pinschers, and arrhythmogenic right ventricular cardiomyopathy in Boxers (see Chapter 20 and **91, 94**, pp. 55, 56). Diseases that cause marked myocardial concentric hypertrophy with consequent subendocardial ischemia and fibrosis also have a higher rate of sudden death (e.g. subaortic stenosis [see Chapter 18]). An inherited disorder of cardiac autonomic maturation predisposing to sudden death is also described in young German Shepherd Dogs[7].

In previously healthy animals, the ventricular ectopy common after thoracic trauma (see Chapter 20, p. 295 and **97**, p. 57) generally resolves without therapy. Occasional VPCs have also been identified in healthy animals[8, 9]. However, arrhythmias that compromise cardiac output, arterial blood pressure, and coronary perfusion can promote myocardial ischemia, deterioration of cardiac pump function, and, sometimes, sudden death (see **98, 99**, p. 57). These arrhythmias tend to be either very rapid (e.g. sustained ventricular or supraventricular tachyarrhythmias) or very slow (e.g. advanced AV block with a slow or unstable ventricular escape rhythm). Rapid sustained tachycardia of either supraventricular or ventricular origin reduces cardiac output acutely, and eventually leads to myocardial dysfunction and CHF (see Chapter 20, p. 292)[10, 11].

An abnormally or unexpectedly rapid heart rate for the clinical context can be caused by sinus tachycardia or an ectopic tachyarrhythmia. Sinus tachycardia is a rhythm with regular QRS intervals. Sustained tachycardias originating either in atrial or AV junctional tissues (supraventricular) or from a ventricular focus also tend to have regular RR intervals once they become established. Rapid irregular rhythms can result from intermittent premature ectopic beats or (paroxysmal) tachycardias that interrupt underlying sinus rhythm, AF, or atrial tachycardia with variable (physiologic) AV block. Characteristics helpful in differentiating these rhythms on ECG are described in Chapter 4, p. 51.

VPCs occur with disorders that affect cardiac tissue either directly or indirectly through neurohormonal effects (*Table 35*). CNS disease can cause ventricular or supraventricular arrhythmias via abnormal neural effects on the heart (brain–heart syndrome)[12]. Supraventricular tachyarrhythmias are also caused by various mechanisms (see Chapter 4, p. 53). Atrial enlargement is often present. Heart diseases commonly associated with supraventricular tachyarrhythmias include chronic mitral or tricuspid

Table 35 Factors predisposing to arrhythmias.

1) Supraventricular arrhythmias:

a) Cardiac:

- Mitral or tricuspid insufficiency.
- Dilated cardiomyopathy.
- Hypertrophic cardiomyopathy.
- Restrictive cardiomyopathy.
- Cardiac neoplasia.
- Congenital malformation.
- Accessory AV nodal bypass tract(s).
- Myocardial fibrosis.
- High sympathetic tone.
- Digitalis glycosides.
- Other drugs (anesthetic agents, bronchodilators).
- Ischemia.
- Intraatrial catheter placement.

b) Extracardiac:

- Catecholamines.
- Electrolyte imbalances.
- Acidosis/alkalosis.
- Hypoxia.
- Thyrotoxicosis.
- Severe anemia.
- Electric shock.
- Thoracic surgery.

2) Ventricular arrhythmias:

a) Cardiac:

- Congestive heart failure.
- Cardiomyopathy, especially Doberman Pinschers and Boxers.
- Myocarditis.
- Pericarditis.
- Degenerative valvular disease with myocardial fibrosis.
- Ischemia.
- Trauma.
- Cardiac neoplasia.
- Heartworm disease.
- Congenital heart disease.
- Ventricular dilation.
- Mechanical stimulation (intracardiac catheter, pacing wire).
- Drugs (digitalis, sympathomimetics, anesthetics, tranquilizers, anticholinergics, antiarrhythmics).

b) Extracardiac:

- Hypoxia.
- Electrolyte imbalances (especially K^+).
- Acidosis/alkalosis.
- Thyrotoxicosis.
- Hypothermia.
- Fever.
- Sepsis/toxemia.
- Trauma (thoracic or abdominal).
- Gastric dilatation/volvulus.
- Splenic mass or splenectomy.
- Hemangiosarcoma.
- Pulmonary disease.
- Uremia.
- Pancreatitis.
- Pheochromocytoma.
- Other endocrine diseases (diabetes mellitus, Addison's disease, hypothyroidism).
- High sympathetic tone (pain, anxiety, fever).
- Central nervous system disease (increases in sympathetic or vagal stimulation).
- Electric shock.

valve degeneration with regurgitation, dilated cardiomyopathy, congenital malformations, and hypertrophic or restrictive cardiomyopathy in cats. Other factors also may predispose to atrial tachyarrhythmias (*Table 35*).

AF in cats and dogs most often occurs when atrial enlargement is marked (see **87, 88**, pp. 54, 55 and Chapter 17 p. 205)[13, 14]. Clinical heart failure is common in affected animals, especially when the ventricular response rate is uncontrolled (high). A rapid as well as irregular ventricular activation rate allows little time for ventricular filling. Stroke volume is further compromised because the contribution of atrial contraction to ventricular filling ('atrial kick'), which is especially important at faster heart rates, is lost. Consequently, cardiac output can decrease considerably when AF develops, especially if myocardial function is poor. AF with a slow

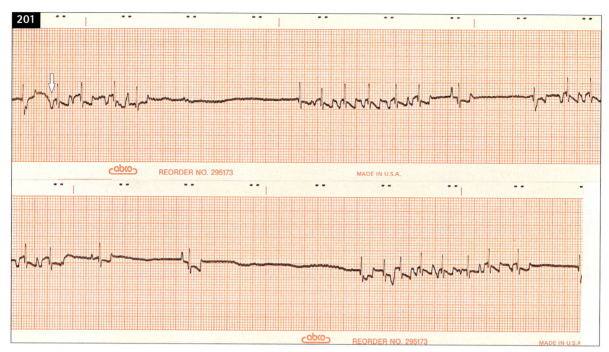

201 Lead II rhythm strip from an 11-year-old spayed female Miniature Schnauzer with sick sinus syndrome and paroxysmal atrial tachycardia (bradycardia–tachycardia syndrome). The dog had experienced multiple episodes of syncope. An escape complex is seen at the top left, followed by 3 atrial premature complexes (note negative P' waves; arrow) and a sinus complex. A period of sinus arrest is interrupted by a junctional escape complex, then another paroxysm of atrial tachycardia, then a single sinus complex. The remainder of the ECG is similar. Top and bottom strips are continuous; 25 mm/sec, 1 cm = 1 mV.

ventricular response rate may be an incidental finding in some large or giant breed dogs without cardiomegaly or other evidence of heart disease (lone AF), although some of these dogs later develop myocardial dysfunction.

An inappropriately slow heart rate can be caused by excessive vagal tone, sinus node disease, or conduction block in the AV node or the bundle of His (see **100–105**, pp. 57, 58). Most animals with bradycardia have irregular RR intervals; the mechanism may be excessive, but variable vagal tone (e.g. sinus bradyarrhythmia), intermittent sinus arrest (e.g. sick sinus syndrome), inconsistent AV conduction (2nd degree AV block [see Chapter 4, p. 58]), or hyperkalemia (e.g. slow sinoventricular rhythm [see Chapter 4, p. 64]). A regular, slow heart rhythm could relate to a regular sinus bradycardia, but more often it is caused by an ectopic escape rhythm that arises because complete (3rd degree) AV block, sinus arrest, or atrial standstill has occurred (see Chapter 4, p. 57).

Diseases that have been associated with AV conduction disturbances include bacterial endocarditis (of the aortic valve), hypertrophic cardiomyopathy, infiltrative myocardial disease, and myocarditis.

Idiopathic heart (AV) block may occur in middle-aged to older dogs; congenital 3rd degree AV block has also been seen in dogs. Symptomatic AV block is less common in cats. Cases have been associated with various myocardial or other structural heart diseases, although heart block is sometimes found in older cats without detectable organic heart disease[15].

The 'sick sinus syndrome' is a condition of erratic sinoatrial function characterized by episodic weakness, syncope, and Stokes–Adams seizures. There is geographic variation in the breeds most commonly affected. The syndrome is most prevalent in older female Miniature Schnauzers in the US, and in West Highland White Terriers in the UK. It also occurs in Dachshunds, Cocker Spaniels, Pugs, and mixed-breed dogs. Sick sinus syndrome is extremely rare in cats. Affected dogs have episodes of marked sinus bradycardia with sinus arrest (or sinoatrial block). Abnormalities of the AV conduction system may coexist, with depression of subsidiary pacemaker activity and prolonged periods of asystole. Some affected dogs also have paroxysmal supraventricular tachyarrhythmias, prompting the name 'bradycardia–tachycardia syndrome' (**201**). Premature complexes may be followed by long

Table 36 Differential diagnoses for common heart rate and rhythm disturbances.

1) Rapid, irregular rhythms:

    a) Ventricular premature contractions.

    b) Paroxysmal ventricular tachycardia.

    c) Atrial fibrillation or flutter.

    d) Atrial or supraventricular premature contractions.

    e) Paroxysmal atrial or supraventricular tachycardia.

2) Rapid, regular rhythms:

    a) Sinus tachycardia.

    b) Sustained supraventricular tachycardia (atrial, AV reciprocating, or junctional origin).

    c) Sustained ventricular tachycardia.

3) Slow, irregular rhythms:

    a) Sinus bradyarrhythmia.

    b) Sinus arrest.

    c) Sick sinus syndrome (sometimes also with paroxysmal supraventricular tachycardia and premature beats [bradycardia–tachycardia syndrome]).

    d) Sinoventricular rhythm (hyperkalemia).

    e) 2nd degree AV block.

4) Slow, regular rhythms:

    a) Sinus bradycardia.

    b) Complete (3rd degree) AV block with ventricular escape rhythm.

    c) Sinoventricular rhythm (hyperkalemia).

    d) Atrial standstill with junctional or ventricular escape rhythm.

pauses before sinus node activity resumes, indicating prolonged sinus node recovery time. Intermittent periods of accelerated junctional rhythms and variable junctional or ventricular escape rhythms may also occur. Clinical signs most often result from bradycardia and sinus arrest, but weakness from paroxysmal tachycardia is possible. Signs can mimic neurologic- or metabolic-induced seizure activity. Concurrent degenerative AV valve disease is common in these older, small breed dogs. Congestive heart failure, if present, is usually related to AV valve insufficiency, although the arrhythmias may be a complicating factor. ECG abnormalities are often pronounced in dogs with long-standing sick sinus syndrome. However, in some dogs, the resting ECG may be normal; ambulatory ECG or prolonged visual ECG monitoring can help establish a definitive diagnosis.

Hyperkalemia (see Chapter 4, p. 64 and **114–117**, p. 64) should be ruled out when P waves are absent or hard to see and heart rate is somewhat slow. Persistent atrial standstill is another arrhythmia characterized by lack of effective atrial electrical activity (i.e. no P waves and a flat baseline) in which a junctional or ventricular escape rhythm controls the heart. This bradyarrhythmia is rare in dogs and extremely rare in cats; most cases have occurred in English Springer Spaniels with muscular dystrophy of the fascioscapulohumeral type, although infiltrative and inflammatory diseases of the atrial myocardium can also result in atrial standstill[16]. Because organic disease of the atrial myocardium may also involve the ventricular myocardium, persistent atrial standstill may be a harbinger of a serious and progressive cardiac disorder.

APPROACH TO THE PATIENT WITH ABNORMAL HEART RATE OR RHYTHM

Cardiac arrhythmias in an individual animal often occur inconsistently and are influenced by drug therapy, prevailing autonomic tone, baroreceptor reflexes, and variations in heart rate, as well as underlying disease. Many clinical abnormalities have been associated with cardiac arrhythmias (*Table 35*). A history that includes episodic weakness, syncope (see Chapter 14), or worsening of previously compensated CHF raises suspicion that the patient may have a serious cardiac arrhythmia, even when heart rate and rhythm are normal on initial evaluation (**202**, p. 136).

The physical examination may reveal an excessively fast or slow heart rate, with or without abnormal irregularity. Common arrhythmias according to a clinical description of the heartbeat are listed in *Table 36*. Arterial pulses of variable timing or intensity or pulse deficits (see Chapter 2) may be detected during examination. Likewise, the heart sounds may vary in intensity as well as regularity. Rapid AF and premature contractions of any origin often cause pulse deficits. VPCs can cause audible splitting of the heart sounds because of asynchronous ventricular activation. Ventricular and supraventricular tachycardias and AF cause more severe hemodynamic compromise than do isolated premature contractions. However, frequent premature contractions and paroxysmal tachycardias can compromise ventricular filling, especially if underlying heart disease exists. Poor cardiac output and hypotension can cause weakness, lethargy, pallor, slow capillary refill time, exercise intolerance, syncope, dyspnea, prerenal azotemia,

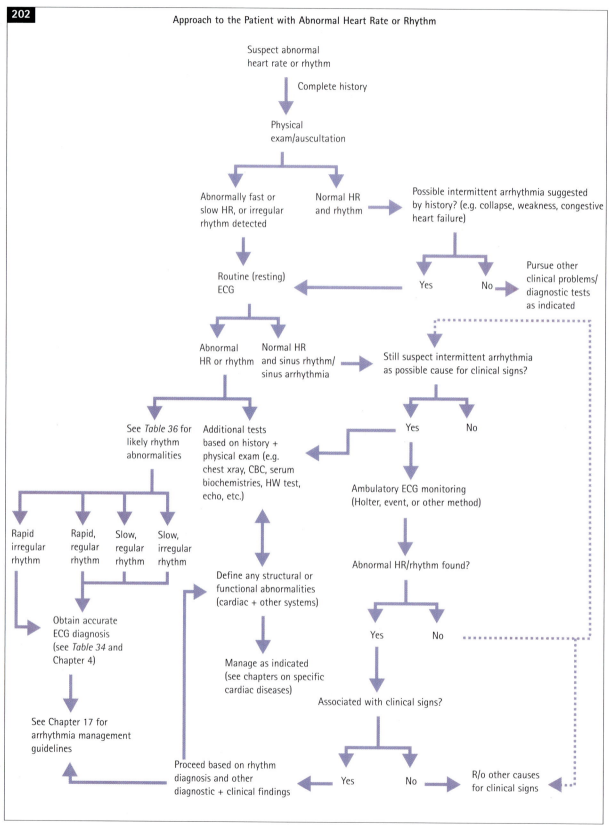

202 Diagram of an approach to the patient with abnormal heart rate or rhythm.

worsening rhythm disturbances, and, sometimes, altered mentation, seizure activity, and sudden death.

Irregular heart rhythms are common; an ECG is important for differentiating abnormal rhythms and, sometimes, sinus arrhythmia as well. While a routine (resting) ECG documents arrhythmias present during the recording period, it provides only a glimpse of the cardiac rhythms occurring over the course of a day. Since arrhythmias can have marked variation in frequency and severity over time, potentially critical arrhythmias can easily be missed. For this reason, Holter monitoring or other forms of extended ECG acquisition are useful in assessing the severity and frequency of arrhythmias, and for monitoring treatment efficacy (see Chapter 14, p. 142).

Differentiation of sustained supraventricular tachycardia from sinus tachycardia is sometimes difficult, but it is important because specific antiarrhythmic drug therapy is indicated for the former (see Chapter 17, p. 202). The heart rate with supraventricular tachycardia is often >300 beats/minute, but it is rare for the sinus rate to be this rapid. Usually, the QRS configuration is normal (narrow and upright in lead II). However, if an intraventricular conduction disturbance is present (see **106–108**, p. 59), supraventricular tachycardia may look like ventricular tachycardia on ECG. For sinus tachycardia, alleviation of the underlying cause and administration of IV fluids to reverse hypotension (in animals without edema) should allow sympathetic tone and sinus rate to decrease.

In most cases with sinus bradycardia, the heart rate increases in response to exercise or atropine administration, and no clinical signs are apparent. Symptomatic dogs usually have a heart rate slower than 50 beats/minute and/or pronounced underlying disease. Because sinus bradycardia or bradyarrhythmia is quite rare in cats, a search for underlying cardiac or systemic disease (e.g. hyperkalemia) is warranted in any cat with a slow heart rate. High-grade 2nd degree AV block (many blocked P waves) and complete (3rd degree) heart block usually produce signs of low cardiac output (e.g. lethargy, exercise intolerance, weakness, or syncope), especially in dogs. These signs become severe when the heart rate is consistently <40 beats/minute. CHF develops subsequent to chronic bradycardia in some dogs, especially if other cardiac disease is present.

An atropine challenge test (see Chapter 17, p. 210) is done in dogs with persistent bradycardia or AV block to determine the degree of vagal influence on the arrhythmia. The normal response is an increase in heart rate of 150%, or to >130–150 beats/minute, or return of AV conduction. Dogs with sick sinus syndrome generally have a subnormal response. Those with 3rd degree AV block rarely regain normal conduction, although the P wave (sinus) rate generally increases.

Some rhythm abnormalities do not require therapy, whereas others demand immediate aggressive treatment (see Chapter 17). Close patient monitoring is especially important in animals with more serious arrhythmias. Treatment decisions are based on consideration of the origin (supraventricular or ventricular), timing (premature or escape), frequency, and complexity of the rhythm disturbance, as well as the clinical context. Arrhythmias generally considered benign include infrequent premature beats and occasional blocked P waves. Post-traumatic accelerated idioventricular rhythm or slow, monomorphic ventricular tachycardia in dogs with otherwise normal cardiac function usually disappears without antiarrhythmic therapy after a few days. Correcting underlying hypoxia, electrolyte or acid-base imbalances, abnormal hormone concentrations (e.g. thyroid), or discontinuing certain drugs can be important for arrhythmia control.

REFERENCES

1 Rubart M, Zipes DP (2001) Genesis of cardiac arrhythmias: electrophysiological considerations. In: *Heart Disease: A Textbook of Cardiovascular Medicine*, 6th edn. E Braunwald, DP Zipes, Libby P (eds). WB Saunders, Phildelphia, pp. 659–699.

2 Dangman KH (1999) Electrophysiologic mechanisms for arrhythmias. In: *Textbook of Canine and Feline Cardiology*, 2nd edn. PR Fox, D Sisson, NS Moise (eds). WB Saunders, Philadelphia, pp. 291–305.

3 Moise NS (1999). Diagnosis and management of canine arrhythmias. In: *Textbook of Canine and Feline Cardiology*, 2nd edn. PR Fox, D Sisson, NS Moise (eds). WB Saunders, Philadelphia, pp. 331–385.

4 Viskin S (1999) Long QT syndromes and torsade de pointes. *Lancet* 354:1625–1633.

5 Pinson DM (1997) Myocardial necrosis and sudden death after an episode of aggressive behavior in a dog. *J Am Vet Med Assoc* 211:1371–1372.

6 Brodsky MA, Sato DA, Iseri LT *et al.* (1987) Ventricular tachyarrhythmia associated with psychological stress. *J Am Med Assoc* 257:2064–2067.

7 Mosie NS, Gilmour RF, Riccio ML *et al.* (1997) Diagnosis of inherited ventricular tachycardia in German Shepherd Dogs. *J Am Vet Med Assoc* 210:403–410.

8 Meurs KM, Spier AW, Wright NA *et al.* (2001) Use of ambulatory electrocardiography for detection of ventricular premature complexes in healthy dogs. *J Am Vet Med Assoc* 218:1291–1292.

9 Ware WA (1999) Twenty-four-hour ambulatory electrocardiography in dogs and cats. *J Vet Intern Med* 13:175–180.

10 Zupen I, Rakovec P, Budihna N *et al.* (1996) Tachycardia induced cardiomyopathy in dogs: relation between chronic supraventricular and chronic ventricular tachycardia. *Int J Cardiol* 56:75–81.

11 Wright KN, Mehdirad AA, Giacobbe P *et al.* (1999) Radiofrequency catheter ablation of atrioventricular accessory pathways in 3 dogs with subsequent resolution of tachycardia-induced cardiomyopathy. *J Vet Intern Med* 13:361–371.

12 Samuels MA (1993) Neurally induced cardiac damage. *Neurocardiology* 11:273–291.

13 Cote E, Harpster NK, Laste NJ *et al.* (2004) Atrial fibrillation in cats: 50 cases (1979–2002). *J Am Vet Med Assoc* 225:256–260.

14 Guglielmini C, Chetboul V, Pietra M *et al.* (2000) Influence of left atrial enlargement and body weight on the development of atrial fibrillation: retrospective study on 205 dogs. *Vet J* 160:235–241.

15 Kellum HB, Stepien RL (2006) Third-degree atrioventricular block in 21 cats. *J Vet Intern Med* 20:97–103.

16 Miller MS, Tilley LP, Atkins CE (1992) Persistent atrial standstill (atrioventricular muscular dystrophy). In: *Current Veterinary Therapy XI*. RW Kirk, JD Bonagura (eds). WB Saunders, Philadelphia, pp. 786–791.

14
Syncope or Intermittent Collapse

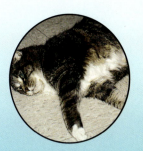

OVERVIEW

Syncope is a sudden, transient loss of consciousness associated with loss of postural tone (collapse). Syncope results from an abrupt decrease in cerebral perfusion or essential substrate delivery[1, 2]. It can be difficult to differentiate syncope from seizure activity or transient weakness episodes, as well as identify the underlying cause of syncope in an individual.

During a syncopal event, the animal usually collapses into lateral recumbency (203, 204). Stiffening of the limbs, opisthotonic posture, micturition, and vocalization are common, but facial fits, persistent tonic/clonic motion, defecation, a prodromal aura, (postictal) dementia, and neurologic deficits are not usually associated with cardiovascular syncope; however, profound hypotension or asystole can cause hypoxic 'convulsive syncope', with seizure-like activity or twitching[3, 4]. Convulsive syncopal episodes are preceded by loss of muscle tone; however, seizure activity caused by underlying neurologic disease is usually preceded by atypical limb or facial movement or staring spells before the loss of postural tone[3]. Presyncope, where reduced brain perfusion, or substrate delivery, is not severe enough to cause unconsciousness, may appear as transient 'wobbliness' or weakness, especially in the hindlimbs.

PATHOPHYSIOLOGY

Many diseases can cause syncope (*Table 37*, p. 140). Mechanisms underlying syncope usually involve either acutely reduced cardiac output (often related to arrhythmias, decreased cardiac filling), outflow obstruction, hypoxia or hypoglycemia with normal cerebral blood flow, or decreased vascular resistance related to neurocardiogenic reflexes. A fall in cardiac output or vascular resistance reduces mean arterial pressure and, consequently, cerebral perfusion. Syncope occurs when cerebral blood flow falls below a critical level (30–50% of normal in people[3]). Reduced cerebral blood flow can also result from cerebrovascular or other intracranial disease. Some

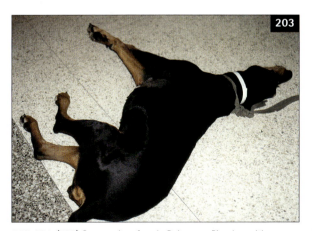
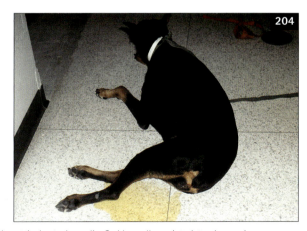

203-204 (203) Syncope in a female Doberman Pinscher with paroxysmal ventricular tachycardia. Sudden collapse into lateral recumbency was followed immediately by extension and stiffening of the forelimbs and neck. (From Ware WA (2003) The cardiovascular examination. In *Small Animal Internal Medicine* (3rd edn). (eds RW Nelson, CG Couto) Mosby, St Louis, p. 3, with permission.) (204) The dog lost bladder control, but regained consciousness within about a minute.

Table 37 Potential causes of syncope.

1) Cardiovascular:

  a) Arrhythmias (see Chapters 4, 13, 17):

    ■ Tachyarrhythmias:

      • Ventricular tachyarrhythmias.

      • Supraventricular (atrial or AV junctional) tachyarrhythmias.

      • Atrial fibrillation.

    ■ Bradyarrhythmias:

      • Sinus node dysfunction - sick sinus syndrome.

      • Atrial standstill.

      • High grade AV blocks (2nd degree, 3rd degree).

  b) Impaired forward cardiac output:

    ■ Myocardial failure (see Chapter 20):

      • Dilated cardiomyopathy.

      • Myocardial infarction or inflammation.

    ■ Severe valvular insufficiency (see Chapters 18, 19):

  c) Impaired cardiac filling:

    ■ Hypertrophic cardiomyopathy (see Chapter 21).

    ■ Restrictive cardiomyopathy (see Chapter 21).

    ■ Cardiac tamponade (see Chapter 22).

    ■ Constrictive pericarditis (see Chapter 22).

    ■ Intracardiac tumor (see Chapter 22).

  d) Cardiac outflow obstruction:

    ■ (Sub)aortic stenosis (see Chapter 18).

    ■ Hypertrophic obstructive cardiomyopathy (see Chapter 21).

    ■ Intracardiac tumor or thrombus.

    ■ Pulmonic stenosis (see Chapter 18).

    ■ Pulmonary hypertension (including heartworm disease; see Chapters 23, 24).

    ■ Pulmonary thromboembolism (see Chapters 15, 23).

  e) Cyanotic heart disease (right-to-left shunts; see Chapter 18):

    ■ Tetralogy of Fallot.

    ■ Eisenmengers physiology ('reversed' ASD, VSD, or PDA).

2) Noncardiac:

  a) Neurologic:

    ■ Cerebrovascular disease or thromboembolism.

    ■ Brain tumor.

    ■ (Seizures).

    ■ (Narcolepsy/cataplexy).

  b) Metabolic and hematologic:

    ■ Acute hemorrhage (external or internal).

    ■ Anemia (e.g., hemolysis, chronic blood loss, bone marrow suppression).

    ■ Diseases causing hypoxemia (e.g. primary respiratory or pleural space disease, right-to-left shunts, hemoglobin abnormalities).

    ■ Hypoglycemia (e.g., insulinoma, other neoplasia, insulin overdose, idiopathic [puppies, toy breeds], sepsis, liver failure).

3) Reflex:

  a) Neurocardiogenic (vasovagal).

  b) Situational:

    ■ Cough.

    ■ Micturition, defecation.

  c) Carotid sinus hypersensitivity.

4) Primary and secondary autonomic failure syndromes (reported in people).

---

cases of syncope may involve multiple mechanisms. For example, syncope associated with subaortic stenosis may relate to LV outflow obstruction, arrhythmias, and also neurocardiogenic reflex mechanisms (see Chapter 18)[1].

Syncope in dogs and cats is often associated with excitement or exertion, when the demand for cardiac output and oxygenation is increased[2, 5–7]. Cardiac arrhythmias, as well as organic heart disease, are commonly involved. Tachyarrhythmias, such as paroxysmal ventricular or supraventricular tachycardias and atrial fibrillation (see Chapters 4 and 13), can markedly reduce cardiac output by compromising ventricular filling time and stroke volume (CO = HR × SV). Bradyarrhythmias (e.g. complete AV block, sinus arrest) can profoundly reduce heart rate and, therefore, cardiac output (205–207). Underlying cardiac functional or structural abnormalities exacerbate the negative effect of arrhythmias on cardiac output. Even when the heart rhythm is normal, diseases that cause poor myocardial contractility, impaired filling, or outflow obstruction may prevent sufficient rise in cardiac output to meet increased demand during activity or excitement[2, 8–10].

In animals with normal cardiac output, insufficient cerebral oxygen delivery can occur when blood oxygenation is impaired, as with right-to-left shunts, anemia, or severe pulmonary disease[2]. Hypoglycemia can also precipitate syncope, especially with exertion, although weakness and seizures are more common manifestations[2, 11]. Diseases that increase intracranial pressure can cause inadequate

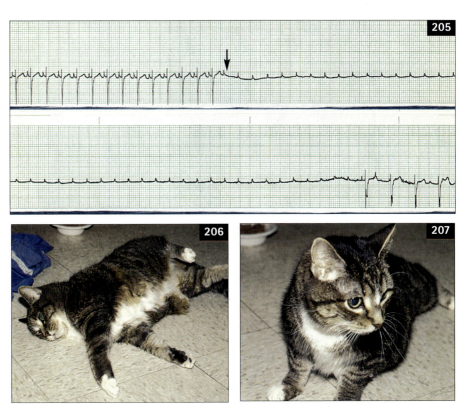

205–207 (205) Continuous lead II ECG strip recorded from an 18-year-old spayed female DSH cat. Sinus rhythm is seen at the top left, although intraventricular conduction is abnormal (QRS shows right bundle branch block pattern). The onset of conduction failure in the left bundle branch and/or AV node caused complete heart block (arrow). Only P waves are seen during the ventricular asystole that follows (~12 seconds duration); syncope was observed during this time. A ventricular escape rhythm finally appears (bottom right). 25 mm/sec; 1 cm = 1 mV.
(206) After a few seconds of unsteadiness, syncope occured in the cat in 205. The limbs were stiff but twitched briefly. (207) After several seconds, the cat regained consciousness and righted herself, then walked away normally.

blood flow to the brain by reducing cerebral perfusion pressure and compressing intracranial vessels: blood flow = perfusion pressure/vascular resistance; perfusion pressure = MAP – intracranial pressure[2]. Cerebrovascular disease can critically reduce cerebral blood flow either by vascular obstruction or rupture.

Neurocardiogenic reflex mechanisms appear to cause syncope in some animals, but this is much less common than in people[2, 12, 13]. Quadrupedal, rather than upright, posture makes animals less susceptible to gravitational effects on the circulation and orthostatic hypotension. Neurocardiogenic (previously called vasovagal) syncope is not well-documented in animals, but syncope that occurs during sudden bradycardia after a burst of sinus tachycardia has been observed in a number of dogs, especially small breed dogs with advanced AV valve disease; excitement often precipitates such an episode. Doberman Pinschers and Boxers may experience a similar syndrome[7]. Whether and to what degree hypotension occurs in these dogs is unknown because of the difficulty in documenting blood pressure during the syncopal episode. It is suspected that an acute sympathetic surge induced by excitement or exercise provokes a strong reflex vagal response that results in bradycardia as well as hypotension. Activation of ventricular mechanoreceptors by forceful contractions, especially when ventricular filling is reduced, may play a role. The resulting surge in afferent neural traffic is thought to mimic that associated with hypertension, stimulating a paradoxical brainstem response of sympathetic withdrawal and vagal activation[12]. Syncope in dogs with pheochromocytoma may represent a neurocardiogenic response to surges in sympathetic activity. It is also possible that neurocardiogenic mechanisms may be involved in animals with anemia and syncope.

Syncope precipitated by coughing (cough syncope, 'cough-drop') is a form of situational syncope (Table 37) that occurs more often in dogs with brachycephalic conformation, underlying airway disease or collapse, or with chronic mitral regurgitation and marked LA enlargement. Coughing transiently increases intrathoracic pressure, which reduces venous return to the heart, and intracranial pressure, which reduces cerebral perfusion pressure. The fall in cardiac output and cerebral perfusion pressure can reduce cerebral blood flow below the level needed to maintain consciousness. Coughing can also reflexly stimulate vagally-mediated bradycardia and vasodilation, which can contribute to hypotension and syncope[2].

The true incidence of syncope in dogs and cats is unknown; however, a large database survey over a 10-year period (Veterinary Medical Database, Purdue University, January 1990 to December 1999) found 0.15% of all dogs and 0.03% of cats within the database were given a diagnostic code for syncope[14]. While syncope may be underreported, this low prevalence in dogs and cats compared with people (estimated as high as 30–50%)[1, 15] suggests that neurocardiogenic syncope, especially orthostatic hypotension, is rare in quadrupeds. Syncope occurs more frequently in older animals and is often associated with cardiac and, to a lesser extent, other disease. According to the database survey described above, about two thirds of the dogs with syncope also had a cardiac disease and/or arrhythmia[14]. Less frequently, respiratory diseases, anemia, or various other metabolic, neoplastic, or neurologic conditions were concurrently diagnosed in these dogs with syncope. Similarly, about two thirds of cats with syncope were noted to have myocardial disease and/or an arrhythmia[14].

APPROACH TO THE PATIENT WITH SYNCOPE OR INTERMITTENT COLLAPSE

The clinical history and physical examination often give clues to the underlying cause of episodic collapse (208)[1, 2, 13]. Detailed description of the episodes themselves, as well as preceding events, prodromal signs, and the animal's mentation and behavior after the event, can be helpful in differentiating cardiovascular syncope from seizure activity or other causes of collapse. Other information to be collected includes the number and frequency of previous events, whether the patient has had signs of cardiopulmonary or other systemic disease, what medications the animal is taking, and whether there has been collapse or sudden death in related animals. The physical examination should evaluate all body systems thoroughly, with particular focus on the cardiovascular (see Chapter 2), nervous, and respiratory systems.

A routine database of CBC, biochemical profile, urinalysis, heartworm test, and arterial blood pressure measurement should be done. Although these tests are often normal, contributory underlying disease may be revealed. Endocrine tests (e.g. for adrenal or thyroid function) may be useful in some cases. A baseline ECG

is recommended. Although a resting ECG may be nondiagnostic, it may suggest underlying cardiac enlargement, conduction abnormalities, or arrhythmia that could contribute to syncope. Thoracic radiographs are taken to evaluate the lungs, pleural space, mediastinum and pulmonary vasculature, as well as the cardiac size and shape. Suspicion for an underlying cardiac cause for syncope is usually generated by the combination of history, physical examination, the ECG, and thoracic radiographs. Echocardiography can confirm the presence and severity of cardiac structural or functional abnormalities that could lead to syncope or be risk factors for arrhythmias.

Ambulatory ECG monitoring (e.g. with a Holter or event monitor) can help identify or exclude cardiac arrhythmias as a cause for syncope in some animals[1, 4, 6, 13, 16]. The reported diagnostic yield, both positive and negative results, has ranged from 42–85%[5, 6, 16]. Event monitors, which are generally worn for a 1–2 week period, have a higher diagnostic yield than Holter monitors, especially in animals with structural heart disease[1, 5, 13]. A syncopal episode must occur during monitoring to make a definitive diagnosis. While a brady- or tachyarrhythmia may underlie the syncopal event, in many cases cardiac arrhythmia can be excluded as the precipitating cause. Arrhythmias often occur without clinical signs; not all arrhythmias cause sufficient hemodynamic compromise to induce syncope or weakness[5, 6, 13, 17–20]. Twenty four- (to 48) hour Holter monitoring is most likely to be diagnostic in animals with multiple syncopal episodes over a short period of time, although the frequency of syncope does not predict the likelihood of an event during Holter monitoring[6]. Holter monitoring is useful for quantifying the type and severity of arrhythmias, for identifying arrhythmias in asymptomatic patients, and for assessing antiarrhythmic drug efficacy. Continuous loop event monitors allow a longer monitoring period than Holter monitors and are better suited for patients with infrequent symptoms[5, 13, 16, 21]. These digital loop recorders monitor heart rhythm continuously; when activated, the ECG is saved into memory for a brief period prior to and following activation. The ECG data are then transmitted by telephone for printing and interpretation. The disadvantages of event monitors are that they do not record potentially significant arrhythmias unless activated, and they do not quantify the frequency of arrhythmias. Implantable loop recorders (Reveal, Medtronic) have also been used in veterinary patients with recurrent but infrequent and unexplained syncope[22]. These subcutaneously implanted devices must be activated at the onset of symptoms in order to save ECG data. They can be

208

Approach to the Patient with Intermittent Collapse or Syncope

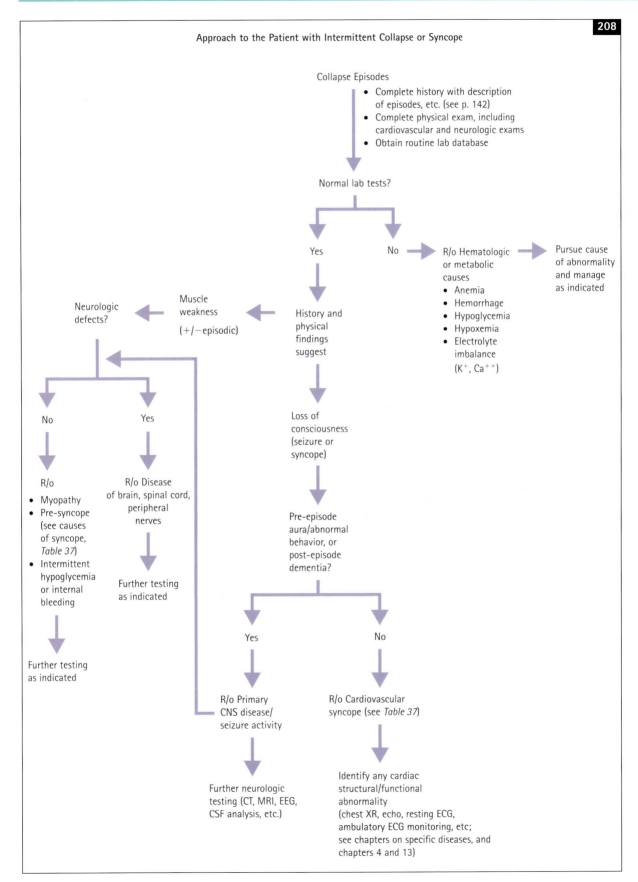

Collapse Episodes

- Complete history with description of episodes, etc. (see p. 142)
- Complete physical exam, including cardiovascular and neurologic exams
- Obtain routine lab database

Normal lab tests?

Yes / No

No → R/o Hematologic or metabolic causes
- Anemia
- Hemorrhage
- Hypoglycemia
- Hypoxemia
- Electrolyte imbalance (K^+, Ca^{++})
→ Pursue cause of abnormality and manage as indicated

Yes → History and physical findings suggest

Muscle weakness (+/−episodic)

Neurologic defects?

No → R/o
- Myopathy
- Pre-syncope (see causes of syncope, Table 37)
- Intermittent hypoglycemia or internal bleeding
→ Further testing as indicated

Yes → R/o Disease of brain, spinal cord, peripheral nerves
→ Further testing as indicated

Loss of consciousness (seizure or syncope)

Pre-episode aura/abnormal behavior, or post-episode dementia?

Yes → R/o Primary CNS disease/ seizure activity → Further neurologic testing (CT, MRI, EEG, CSF analysis, etc.)

No → R/o Cardiovascular syncope (see Table 37) → Identify any cardiac structural/functional abnormality (chest XR, echo, resting ECG, ambulatory ECG monitoring, etc; see chapters on specific diseases, and chapters 4 and 13)

191 Diagram of an approach to the patient with intermittent collapse or syncope.

worn for many months but cannot be downloaded transtelephonically.

When signs of neurologic disease are present, an EEG, CT of the head, or other neurologic testing may be helpful. However, without a history typical for seizures (e.g. tonic/clonic movement, postictal confusion) or an abnormal neurologic examination, the diagnostic yield of these tests is likely to be low[1, 13].

Therapy is aimed at managing underlying disease and avoiding precipitating factors, such as exertion or environmental stressors, as far as possible. This may include instituting or adjusting medications for heart failure (see Chapter 16) or hypertension (see Chapter 25), correcting anemia, or treating respiratory or metabolic diseases. When an arrhythmia appears to be the cause, appropriate antiarrhythmic drug therapy or pacing is indicated (see Chapter 17), but pacing is unlikely to modulate hypotension caused by neurocardiogenic syncope. Several strategies have been tried to manage suspected neurocardiogenic syncope. Beta-blockers can be used as a means to blunt the initiating sympathetically-induced tachycardia and/or vigorous ventricular contraction, but exacerbation of bradycardia can be a concern. Other strategies that have been effective anecdotally include theophylline or aminophylline, starting with a low dose and titrating up to effect, or low-dose digoxin in animals with AV valve disease.

REFERENCES

1 Schnipper JL, Kapoor WN (2001) Diagnostic evaluation and management of patients with syncope. *Med Clin N Amer* 85:423–456.

2 Davidow EB, Proulx J, Woodfield JA (2001) Syncope: pathophysiology and differential diagnosis. *Compend Cont Educ Pract Vet* 23:608–620.

3 Johnsrude CL (2000) Current approach to pediatric syncope. *Pediatr Cardiol* 21:522–531.

4 Heaven DJ, Sutton R (2000) Syncope. *Crit Care Med* 28:N116–N120.

5 Bright JM, Cali JV (2000) Clinical usefulness of cardiac event recording in dogs and cats examined because of syncope, episodic collapse, or intermittent weakness: 60 cases (1997–1999). *J Am Vet Med Assoc* 216:1110–1114.

6 Miller RH, Lehmkuhl LB, Bonagura JD *et al.* (1999) Retrospective analysis of the clinical utility of ambulatory electrocardiographic (Holter) recordings in syncopal dogs: 44 cases (1991–1995). *J Vet Intern Med* 13:111–122.

7 Calvert CA, Jacobs GJ, Pickus CW (1996) Bradycardia-associated episodic weakness, syncope, and aborted sudden death in cardiomyopathic Doberman Pinschers. *J Vet Intern Med* 10:88–93.

8 Ware WA, Hopper DL (1999) Cardiac tumors in dogs: 1982–1995. *J Vet Intern Med* 13:95–103.

9 Fingland RB, Bonagura JD, Myer W (1985) Pulmonic stenosis in the dog: 29 cases (1975–1984). *J Am Vet Med Assoc* 189:218–226.

10 Johnson L, Boon J, Orton EC (1999) Clinical characteristics of 53 dogs with Doppler-derived evidence of pulmonary hypertension: 1992–1996. *J Vet Intern Med* 13:440–447.

11 Flie MS, Zerbe C (1995) Insulinoma in dogs, cats, and ferrets. *Compend Cont Educ Pract Vet* 17:51–60.

12 Grubb BP (1999) Pathophysiology and differential diagnosis of neurocardiogenic syncope. *Am J Cardiol* 84:3Q–9Q.

13 Arthur W, Kaye GC (2001) Current investigations used to assess syncope. *Postgrad Med J* 77:20–23.

14 Ware WA (2002) Syncope. In: *Proceedings of the 26th Annual OSU/Waltham Symposium,* Columbus.

15 Cunningham R, Mikhail MG (2001) Management of patients with syncope and cardiac arrhythmias in an emergency department observation unit. *Emergency Med Clin N Amer* 19:105–121.

16 Goodwin J (1998) Holter monitoring and cardiac event recording. Advances in cardiovascular diagnostics and therapy. *Vet Clin North Am: Small Anim Pract* 28:1391–1407.

17 Meurs KM, Spier AW, Wright NA *et al.* (2001) Use of ambulatory electrocardiography for detection of ventricular premature complexes in healthy dogs. *J Am Vet Med Assoc* 218:1291–1292.

18 Ware WA (1999) Twenty-four-hour ambulatory electrocardiography in normal cats. *J Vet Intern Med* 13:175–180.

19 Meurs KM, Spier AW, Wright NA *et al.* (2001) Comparison of in-hospital versus 24-hour ambulatory electrocardiography for detection of ventricular premature complexes in mature Boxers. *J Am Vet Med Assoc* 218:222–224.

20 Calvert CA, Jacobs GJ, Pickus CW *et al.* (2000) Result of ambulatory electrocardiography in overtly healthy Doberman Pinschers with echocardiographic abnormalities. *J Am Vet Med Assoc* 217:1328–1332.

21 Cote E, Richter K, Charuvastra E (1999) Event-based cardiac monitoring in small animal practice. *Compend Cont Educ Pract Vet* 21:1025–1033.

22 Willis R, McLeod K, Cusak J *et al.* (2003) Use of an implantable loop recorder to investigate syncope in a cat. *J Small Anim Pract* 44:181–183.

15
Thromboembolic Disease

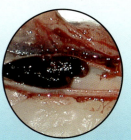

OVERVIEW

Thromboembolic (TE) disease can result when normal hemostatic mechanisms are disturbed. A thrombus is a locally formed (*in situ*) clot or aggregation of platelets and other blood elements that partially or completely obstructs blood flow either in a vessel or in the heart. An embolus is a clot or other aggregate that breaks away from its origination site and is carried by blood flow until it lodges in a smaller vessel[1]. Any part of the body may be affected, but most clinically recognized TE events involve the distal aorta, pulmonary arteries, heart, or cranial vena cava. Both emboli and thrombi occur concurrently in some individuals.

The clinical sequelae of thromboemboli depend mainly on the size and location of the clot(s), which determine how much compromise occurs and in which organs/tissues. Thromboemboli can cause acute and profound clinical signs or subclinical tissue damage that ultimately leads to varying degrees of pathology. TE disease is sometimes suspected antemortem, but in other cases is discovered at necropsy (or not at all).

When a thrombus forms, the fibrinolytic system immediately begins to break it down. Normally, contraction and complete dissolution of the clot soon follow, but if hemostatic and fibrinolytic processes are deranged, the clot may persist and become more extensive. Over time, persistent clots usually organize and eventually recanalize.

THE HEMOSTATIC PROCESS

Normal hemostasis depends on the interplay among the different factors that promote coagulation, inhibit coagulation, and promote fibrinolysis. A proper balance of these factors maintains blood fluidity while minimizing loss when vessels are damaged. Tissue injury, inflammation, and other situations can disturb this balance. In general, conditions that cause vascular endothelial damage, blood stasis, or hypercoagulability (including impaired fibrinolysis) promote TE disease.

The hemostatic process involves platelets, the vascular endothelium, proteins of the coagulation cascade, and the fibrinolytic system. Injury to the vascular endothelium quickly induces several reactions that cause vasoconstriction, hemostatic plug formation, and attempts at vascular repair (**209**). This is the normal hemostatic mechanism to prevent blood loss.

Intact vascular endothelial cells secrete substances that help prevent inappropriate thrombosis and participate in vasoregulation[1]. Damaged endothelial cells promote thrombus formation. While this reduces blood loss in the event of vascular laceration, in other settings TE disease can result. Endothelial damage contributes to thrombus formation in several ways. Injured endothelial cells release endothelin, which promotes vasoconstriction and decreases local blood flow. Exposed subendothelial collagen and other substances stimulate platelet adherence and aggregation. Injured endothelial cells also release tissue factor (thromboplastin), which activates the extrinsic pathway of the coagulation cascade[1-3].

Platelets adhere to damaged endothelial cells and underlying tissue. The initial attachment is strengthened by interactions with von Willebrand's factor, glycoprotein receptors, and fibrinogen. After platelets adhere they undergo activation, with expression of surface glycoprotein (gp) IIb/IIIa receptors. Fibrinogen binds to these receptors during the process of platelet aggregation. Activated platelets synthesize thromboxane A_2 and platelet-activating factor, as well as release a number of substances from intracytoplasmic granules that stimulate platelet aggregation (**209**, p. 146)[1,4]. Platelet aggregation, via linkage with fibrinogen, is the third step in primary platelet plug formation (primary hemostasis). The platelet plug becomes stabilized as platelets contract and fibrinogen is converted to fibrin through the action of thrombin (factor IIa), produced by the coagulation cascade.

The coagulation cascade consists of the sequential activation of a series of serine proteases (209). The cascade has two arms (intrinsic and extrinsic pathways) that feed into the common pathway to produce thrombin. Thrombin mediates the conversion of fibrinogen into fibrin to stabilize

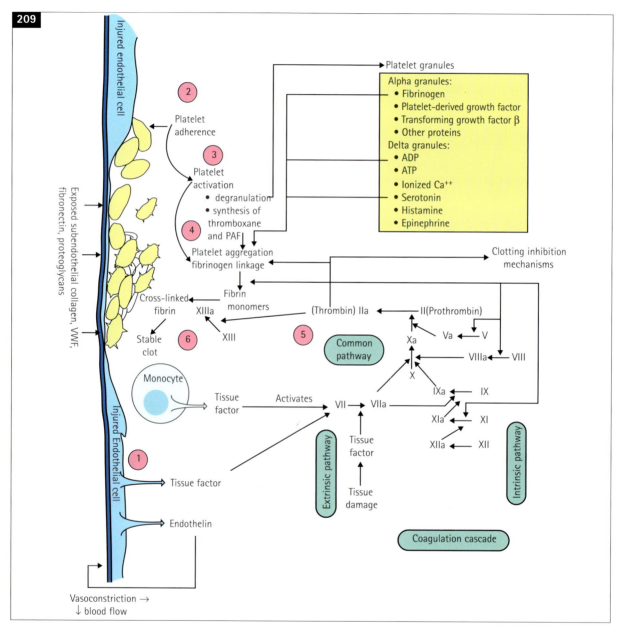

209 Schematic diagram summarizing major events in the hemostatic process. 1) Endothelial injury initiates clotting by: a) exposing collagen and other substances that promote platelet adherence; b) releasing tissue factor to activate the coagulation cascade; and c) stimulating vasoconstriction (via endothelin release), which slows local blood flow. 2) Platelets adhere to the injured area, then 3) platelets become activated to release their granule contents and increase thromboxane and PAF synthesis; 4) these substances promote platelet aggregation via linkage with fibrinogen. 5) Thrombin, produced by the coagulation cascade, further promotes platelet aggregation and helps stabilize the clot by cleaving fibrinogen to fibrin. Thrombin also stimulates activation of the coagulation cascade as well as clot inhibiting mechanisms. 6) Final clot stabilization occurs as thrombin-activated factor XIIIa catalyzes cross-linkage of fibrin monomers into insoluble fibrin. Activated clotting factors are designated by 'a' following their Roman numeral. ADP = adenosine diphosphate; ATP = adenosine triphosphate; PAF = platelet activating factor; vWF = von Willebrand's factor.

the clot (secondary hemostasis) and it is also important in sustaining the coagulation process via interaction with the intrinsic pathway. The activation processes that occur within the coagulation cascade require a substrate and a cofactor as well as the coagulation factors themselves. Usually, the substrate is the platelet phospholipid layer, with ionized calcium as the cofactor. This tends to limit clot formation to the area near activated platelets[1]. Tissue factor, released from monocytes and damaged cells, stimulates the extrinsic pathway by activating factor VII. The intrinsic pathway amplifies the process and also modulates fibrinolysis. Thrombin converts fibrinogen into fibrin monomers. These polymerize to soluble fibrin, which then is cross-linked by the action of thrombin-activated factor XIII. This now insoluble fibrin stabilizes the clot. Thrombin also stimulates further platelet aggregation, as well as contributing to negative feedback inhibition of clotting by interacting with thrombomodulin, protein C and S, and antithrombin III[1].

FIBRINOLYSIS

Once a thrombus forms, several mechanisms limit the extent of the clot and promote its breakdown. Thrombolysis requires plasmin. Its inactive precursor, plasminogen, is converted to plasmin by tissue plasminogen activator (t-PA) when fibrin is present. During coagulation cascade activation, endothelial cells simultaneously release t-PA[5]. Other substances also act as plasminogen activators, including urokinase, bradykinen, kallikrein, and factor VII. Plasmin degrades fibrinogen and soluble (noncross-linked) fibrin to yield fibrinogen/fibrin degradation products (FDPs). Plasmin also cleaves cross-linked fibrin in stabilized clots into large fragments (x-oligomers) that are further broken down into D-dimers and other fragments. D-dimers are produced only with active coagulation and subsequent fibrinolysis[6, 7]. There are also negative feedback constraints on fibrinolysis (e.g. plasminogen activator inhibitors, alpha$_2$-antiplasmin, thrombin-activated fibrinolytic factor). Defective fibrinolysis is thought to play a role in pathologic thrombosis.

MECHANISMS OPPOSING THROMBOSIS

Inhibition of platelet adherence and activation is important in preventing primary platelet plug formation. In addition, there are three main mechanisms that limit thrombus formation: antithrombin III, protein C, and the fibrinolytic system. Malfunction of one or more of these systems promotes thrombosis.

Intact endothelium normally produces factors with antiplatelet, anticoagulant, and also fibrinolytic effects. Antiplatelet substances include nitric oxide, prostacyclin, and adenosine diphosphatase (ADPase). Nitric oxide inhibits platelet activation and promotes local vasodilation[8]. Prostacyclin also inhibits platelet activation and aggregation, while mediating vascular smooth muscle relaxation. Endothelial prostacyclin synthesis is stimulated by thrombin, bradykinin, and histamine. ADPase, on the endothelial surface, degrades ADP released from activated platelets, preventing ADP-induced platelet aggregation[1, 3]. Anticoagulant substances synthesized by intact endothelium include thrombomodulin, protein S, heparan sulfate, and tissue factor pathway inhibitor (TFPI). Thrombomodulin binds thrombin at the cell surface, inhibiting its procoagulant effect; thrombomodulin is recycled after the thrombin is degraded within the cell. Thrombomodulin also binds factor Xa, which inhibits prothrombin activation, and enhances protein C activation by thrombin. Endothelial-produced protein S enhances the action of protein C. Heparan sulfate acts as a cofactor to AT III to inactivate several coagulation factors (IXa, Xa, XIa, XIIa). TFPI, a protease inhibitor, is synthesized mainly by the liver but also by endothelial cells, especially when inflammation is present. TFPI, combined with factor Xa, inhibits the tissue factor-factor VIIa complex to block the extrinsic coagulation pathway. The endothelium contributes to fibrinolysis by producing t-PA[1].

AT III is a small (up to 65,000 daltons) alpha$_2$-globulin produced by the liver. It is responsible for most of the anticoagulant effect of plasma[9]. AT III binds and inactivates thrombin, factors IXa, Xa, XIa and XIIa, and kallikrein. This process is accelerated by cofactors (e.g. heparan sulfate and heparin)[1].

Protein C is a vitamin K-dependent glycoprotein involved in countering thrombosis. It is converted to its active form by thrombin. Activation is accelerated on vascular surfaces by the cofactor thrombomodulin. Protein S, another vitamin K-dependent protein, also acts as a cofactor. When activated by the thrombin–thrombomodulin complex, protein C, with protein S, acts as an anticoagulant and profibrinolytic. It inhibits thrombin generation by inactivating factors Va and VIIIa, and stimulates fibrinolysis by inhibiting plasminogen activator inhibitor type 1 (PAI-1). Deficiency of protein C may occur with neoplastic, infectious or other disease, but this is not yet clear in dogs and cats.

PATHOPHYSIOLOGY

MECHANISMS OF PATHOLOGIC THROMBOSIS

TE disease is more likely when changes in normal hemostatic processes create conditions that favor clot formation or impair thrombolysis. Three general situations, the so-called Virchow's triad, promote pathologic thrombosis: abnormal endothelial structure or function; slowed or static blood flow; and a hypercoagulable state, either from increased procoagulant substances or decreased anticoagulant or fibrinolytic substances[1, 10]. A number of common diseases produce such conditions (Table 38)[3, 11–19].

Vascular endothelial integrity is highly important. Diseases that induce severe or widespread endothelial injury also cause loss of normal endothelial antiplatelet, anticoagulant, and fibrinolytic functions. Increased coagulability and platelet activation favor pathologic thrombosis. Injured endothelium also produces tissue factor as well as antifibrinolytic factors, such as PAI-1. Subendothelial tissue, exposed because of endothelial cell damage, promotes thrombosis by acting as a substrate for clot formation and stimulating platelet adherence and aggregation[1, 3, 13, 19]. Systemic release of inflammatory cytokines (e.g. tumor necrosis factor [TNF], various interleukins, platelet activating factor, nitric oxide) can cause widespread endothelial injury[19, 20]. This occurs with sepsis and, probably, with other systemic inflammatory conditions as well. Neoplastic invasion, vascular disruption from other disease, and postischemic injury also induce endothelial damage[19]. Primary vascular disease as an underlying cause is suggested in Cavalier King Charles Spaniels by a genetic predisposition to femoral artery thrombosis[21].

Mechanical trauma to the vascular endothelium (e.g. catheterization) can also precipitate TE disease, especially when other predisposing conditions exist. Pulmonary artery endothelial injury from heartworm disease (HWD) is well known (see Chapter 24). The inflammatory reaction to dead worms and worm fragments exacerbates the endothelial damage and prothrombotic conditions.

Stagnant blood flow promotes thrombosis by impeding the dilution and clearance of coagulation factors. A low level of systemic coagulation factor activation normally occurs, but adequate blood flow rapidly disperses the activated factors. This dilution, along with hepatic clearance of activated factors and the normal anticoagulation mechanisms, usually prevents thrombus formation. Blood stasis negates such protections against thrombosis. Poor flow can promote local tissue hypoxia and endothelial injury as well. Abnormal turbulence has also been associated with thrombus formation. Turbulence can mechanically injure the endothelial surface. Heart diseases that cause low intracardiac flow velocity or increased turbulence can create prothrombotic conditions. Other diseases that produce localized blood stasis may similarly create conditions favoring thrombosis. This includes circulatory shock and prolonged recumbency. Hyperviscosity syndromes increase resistance to blood flow and so can reduce flow velocity.

Table 38 Diseases associated with conditions favorable for thromboembolism formation.

1) Endothelial disruption:
   a) Sepsis.
   b) Systemic inflammatory disease.
   c) Heartworm disease.
   d) Neoplasia.
   e) Massive trauma.
   f) Shock.
   g) Intravenous catheterization.
   h) Injection of irritant substance.
   i) Reperfusion injury.
   j) Atherosclerosis.
   k) Arteriosclerosis.
   l) Hyperhomocysteinemia.
2) Abnormal blood flow:
   a) Vascular obstruction (e.g. mass lesion, adult heartworms, catheter or other device).
   b) Heart disease.
   c) Cardiomyopathy (especially in cats).
   d) Endocarditis.
   e) Congestive heart failure.
   f) Shock.
   g) Hypovolemia/dehydration.
   h) Prolonged recumbency.
   i) Hyperviscosity (e.g. polycythemia, leukemia, hyperglobulinemia).
   j) Hypoviscosity (anemia).
   k) Anatomic abnormality (e.g. aneurysm, A-V fistula).
3) Increased coagulability:
   a) Glomerular disease/protein-losing nephropathy.
   b) Hyperadrenocorticism.
   c) Immune-mediated hemolytic anemia (+/– thrombocytopenia).
   d) Pancreatitis.
   e) Protein-losing enteropathy.
   f) Sepsis/infection.
   g) Neoplasia.
   h) Disseminated intravascular coagulation.
   i) Heart disease.

Hypercoagulability develops secondary to various systemic diseases in dogs and cats. Multiple mechanisms are probably involved[1]; however, thrombus formation in these animals may also require altered endothelial integrity or blood flow characteristics. AT III deficiency is the most common cause of hypercoagulability[19]. Excessive loss, increased consumption, or possibly inadequate hepatic synthesis leads to AT III deficiency. Inadequate amount or function of proteins C and S may occur in animals with hypercoagulability associated with malignancy, disseminated intravascular coagulation (DIC), and other conditions, as it does in some people[1]. Reduced protein C and AT III activities, as well as evidence for DIC, have been shown in dogs with sepsis[22].

Excessive platelet activation and aggregability can contribute to a hypercoagulable state. Increased platelet aggregability has been associated with neoplasia, some heart diseases, diabetes mellitus, and nephrotic syndrome in some animals[1, 19, 23–25]. Thrombocytosis alone, without an increase in platelet aggregability, is not thought to create greater risk for thrombosis[26].

Defective fibrinolysis can promote pathologic thrombosis by preventing efficient breakdown of physiologic clots. Reduced levels of fibrinolytic substances (e.g. t-PA, plasminogen, urokinase) or increased amounts of plasminogen activator inhibitors, which reduce conversion of plasminogen to plasmin, are implicated[1]. PAI-1 is the major inhibitor of the fibrinolytic system. Most PAI-1 is produced by macrophages. Systemic inflammation stimulates its synthesis (as well as that of alpha$_2$-antiplasmin and thrombin-activated fibrinolytic factor) through the effects of various cytokines[1].

THROMBOEMBOLISIM AND COMMON DISEASE CONDITIONS

Conditions that induce a systemic inflammatory response promote TE disease in multiple ways. Various proinflammatory cytokines, such as TNF and interleukins, cause endothelial damage, induce tissue factor expression on monocytes and endothelial cells, and inhibit anticoagulant mechanisms (e.g. protein C, TFPI, AT III), among other effects[27]. Pancreatitis, shock, trauma, sepsis, neoplasia, severe hepatopathy, heatstroke, immune-mediated disease, and other conditions can lead to gross thrombosis as well as DIC[28, 29]. DIC involves massive activation of thrombin and plasmin, with generalized consumption of coagulation factors and platelets. DIC produces extensive thrombosis as well as hemorrhage in the microcirculation, resulting in widespread tissue ischemia and multiorgan failure.

Protein-losing nephropathy, from glomerulonephritis, renal amyloid deposition, or hypertensive injury, can cause marked AT III deficiency. Because of its small size, AT III is lost through damaged glomeruli more easily than most procoagulant proteins. This predisposes to thrombosis[10, 30]. Protein-losing enteropathies also cause AT III deficiency, but concurrent loss of larger proteins tends to maintain a balance between procoagulant and anticoagulant factors in many cases[30]. Other factors that may contribute to TE disease in animals with protein-losing nephropathies include increased thromboxane and fibrinogen concentrations, as well as enhanced platelet aggregability associated with hypoalbuminemia and hypercholesterolemia[19]. Thrombosis has also been associated with chronic interstitial nephritis and acute tubular necrosis. The mechanism may relate to endothelial damage from uremic toxins or possibly to altered coagulability, although this is unclear. Other predisposing conditions may be involved[10].

Thrombosis associated with immune-mediated hemolytic anemia (IMHA) is also thought to be multifactorial, with the systemic inflammatory (immune-mediated) response playing a large role[31]. Thrombocytopenia, elevated bilirubin, and hypoalbuminemia have been identified as risk factors for thromboembolism. These may reflect the severity of disease or may contribute to hypercoagulability or increased platelet aggregability[31]. DIC is common with this disease. The potential role of high-dose corticosteroid therapy in pathologic thrombosis is unclear. Although most often considered idiopathic, IMHA can develop secondary to systemic lupus erythematosis, neoplasia, and blood parasites. These diseases exacerbate conditions favoring thrombosis. Pulmonary TE disease appears to be most common with IMHA, but other sites are also affected.

TE disease occurs in some dogs with spontaneous hyperadrenocorticism. This endocrinopathy has been associated with decreased fibrinolysis, from increased PAI activity, and elevated levels of several coagulation factors[10, 17, 19, 32]. Renal glomerular damage, associated with hypertension in some of these cases, can promote AT III loss. TE disease has occurred in animals given exogenous corticosteroids. Other predisposing factors are usually concurrent in these cases as well[10, 33]. Diabetes mellitus is occasionally associated with TE disease in dogs. Platelet hyperaggregability and possibly hypofibrinolysis are thought to be involved.

Cats with myocardial disease (see Chapter 21) are at risk for intracardiac thrombus formation and subsequent arterial embolization[19]. LA thrombi are often found in cats with cardiomyopathy during echocardiography or at necropsy[34]. Marked LA enlargement may magnify the risk, but this is controversial. The mechanisms involved probably relate to poor intracardiac blood flow, especially within the LA, altered blood coagulability, local tissue or blood vessel injury, or a combination of these[34–37]. Increased platelet reactivity occurs in some of these cats[25, 38, 39]. Abnormal turbulence may be a factor when MR occurs. DIC can accompany thromboembolism. Some cats with TE disease have decreased plasma arginine and vitamin B_6 and B_{12} concentrations; hyperhomocysteinemia may be a factor in some[40]. Hyperhomocysteinemia and low plasma vitamin B are risk factors for thromboembolism in people. It is not known if hypercoagulability induced by a genetic abnormality exists in some cats, as occurs in people[35].

SYSTEMIC ARTERIAL TE DISEASE

The most common cause for arterial TE disease in cats is cardiomyopathy, of any type (see Chapter 21)[35, 37, 41]. Thrombi initially form in the left heart and can become quite large. Although some remain in the heart, usually the LA appendage, others embolize to the distal aorta or, less often, other sites (**210**). Hyperthyroidism may be a risk factor for TE in cats independent of its cardiac effects[41]. Neoplastic and systemic inflammatory disease occasionally underlie systemic thromboemboli in cats[35]. No cause is identified in some cases.

Arterial TE disease in dogs is relatively uncommon compared with cats (**211**). It has been associated with many conditions, including protein-losing nephropathies, hyperadrenocorticism, neoplasia, chronic interstitial nephritis, dirofilariasis, hypothyroidism, gastric dilatation-volvulus, pancreatitis, and a number of CV diseases[10, 42, 43]. Often, more than one potential association exists concurrently. Kidney disease was involved in about half of the cases in one report[10]. Vegetative endocarditis is the most common CV disease associated with systemic TE. Other CV associations include PDA (surgical ligation site), dilated cardiomyopathy, myocardial infarction, arteritis, aortic intimal fibrosis, atherosclerosis, aortic dissection, granulomatous inflammatory erosion into the LA, and other thrombi in the left heart[10, 42, 44–46]. TE disease as a rare complication of A-V fistulae may develop secondary to venous stasis related to distal venous hypertension. Atherosclerosis is an important risk factor for arterial thromboembolism in people. Although atherosclerosis is uncommon in dogs, it has been associated with TE disease in this species as well[10, 46]. Endothelial disruption in areas of atherosclerotic plaque, hypercholesterolemia, increased PAI-1, and possibly other mechanisms are thought to be involved in thrombus formation[46]. Atherosclerosis can develop with profound hypothyroidism, hypercholesterolemia, and hyperlipidemia. The aorta as well as coronary and other medium to large arteries are affected.

Myocardial and cerebral infarctions occur in some cases, and there is a high rate of interstitial myocardial fibrosis in affected dogs. Vasculitis related to infectious, inflammatory, immune-mediated, or toxic disease can occasionally underlie

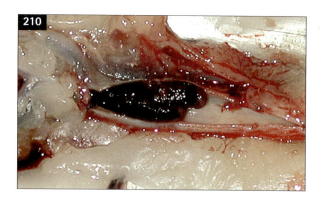

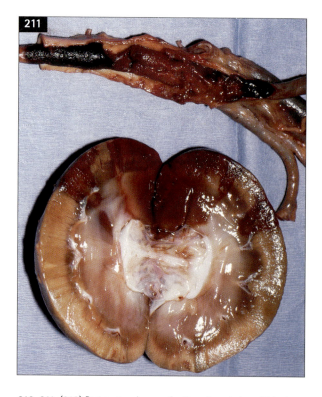

210, 211 (210) Postmortem image of a thromboembolus within the opened distal aorta of a male DSH cat with LA enlargement and CHF secondary to mitral valve dysplasia and subaortic stenosis. (211) Section of the caudal aorta and iliac arteries (top) filled with a long thromboembolus, and left kidney showing a large infarcted (dark) area. From a dog with multiple TE events originating from thrombi formed at an inflammatory erosion into the dorsal LA associated with mycotic infection of the hilar lymph node.

TE events. Arteritis of immune-mediated pathogenesis is described in some young Beagles and other dogs. Inflammation and necrosis affect small to medium-sized arteries and are associated with thrombosis[47].

Systemic arterial emboli usually lodge at the aortic trifurcation (so-called 'saddle thrombus'), but iliac, femoral, renal, brachial, and other arteries can be affected, depending on embolus size and flow path[15, 48]. Some small emboli are clinically 'silent'. Emboli can originate from within the heart or an upstream vascular site; they may consist of only blood elements or contain neoplastic cells or infectious organisms. Emboli can also form from fat, tissue fragments, gas, or parasites. Pulmonary thromboemboli and intracardiac or venous thrombi can exist concurrently with arterial thromboemboli. In situ thrombosis causes arterial occlusion in some cases.

In addition to obstructing flow in the affected artery, thromboemboli release vasoactive substances (e.g. thromboxane A_2 and serotonin). These induce vasoconstriction and compromise collateral blood flow development around the obstructed vessel[19, 35, 48]. The resulting tissue ischemia causes further damage and inflammation. An ischemic neuromyopathy occurs in the affected limb(s), with peripheral nerve dysfunction and degeneration as well as pathologic changes in associated muscle tissue.

Coronary artery thromboembolism causes myocardial ischemia and infarction. Infective endocarditis, neoplasia that involves the heart directly or by neoplastic emboli, coronary atherosclerosis, dilated cardiomyopathy, degenerative mitral valve disease with congestive heart failure, and coronary vasculitis are reported causes[32, 49]. In other dogs, coronary TE events have occurred with severe renal disease, IMHA, exogenous corticosteroids or hyperadrenocorticism, and acute pancreatic necrosis. Such cases often have TE lesions in other locations as well[32, 49]. Coronary thromboembolism with myocardial necrosis has occurred in cats with cardiac disease, especially severe hypertrophic cardiomyopathy or infective endocarditis, as well as from carcinoma emboli[32, 49].

PULMONARY ARTERIAL TE DISEASE

Pulmonary thromboemboli (212) in dogs are associated with HWD, other heart diseases, IMHA, neoplasia, DIC, sepsis, hyperadrenocorticism, nephrotic syndrome, pancreatitis, trauma, hypothyroidism, and RA thrombus related to infection[11, 12, 33, 50–54]. Deep vein thrombosis, the main cause of pulmonary thromboembolism in people, is not a clinical problem in dogs and cats[54]. Pulmonary TE disease also occurs in cats with a variety of systemic and inflammatory disorders. These have included neoplasia, HWD, anemia (probably immune-mediated), pancreatitis,

glomerulonephritis, encephalitis, pneumonia, heart disease, sepsis, glucocorticoid administration, protein-losing enteropathy, and hepatic lipidosis[55–57]. Pulmonary TE disease appears to be rare in cats compared with dogs, except in those with HWD. Although most affected cats have respiratory signs before death or euthanasia, diagnosis has usually been made post mortem[55–57].

VENOUS THROMBOSIS

Thrombosis in large veins is more likely to be clinically evident than thrombosis in small vessels. Cranial vena caval thrombosis has been associated with IMHA and/or immune-mediated thrombocytopenia, sepsis, neoplasia, protein-losing nephropathies, mycotic disease, heart disease, and glucocorticoid therapy (especially with systemic inflammatory disease) in dogs[13, 14]. Most cases have more than one predisposing factor. An indwelling jugular catheter increases the risk for cranial caval thrombosis, probably by causing vascular endothelial damage or laminar flow disruption, or by acting as a nidus for clot formation.

Portal vein thrombosis, along with DIC, has occurred with pancreatitis and pancreatic necrosis in dogs[58]. Peritonitis, neoplasia, hepatitis, PLN, IMHA, and vasculitis have also been diagnosed occasionally in dogs with portal thrombosis[58–60].

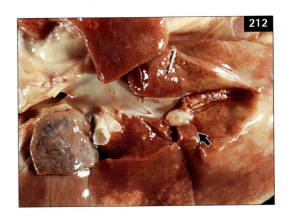

212 Postmortem image showing the opened left pulmonary artery, obstructed by a thromboembolus (arrow), from a 5-year-old male Dachshund with IMHA. The main pulmonary artery is to the left; the left auricular appendage and a portion of the dorsal left ventricle are seen in the lower left corner of the image.

APPROACH TO THE PATIENT WITH TE DISEASE

CLINICAL PRESENTATION

Clinical manifestations of TE disease depend on the type and location of vessels obstructed, the duration and degree of vascular obstruction, the extent of tissue damage, and any related complications. Most reported cases involve clots in the distal aorta, heart, brachial or other large systemic artery, pulmonary arteries, cranial vena cava, or portal vein. Multiple sites are affected in some animals. An index of suspicion for TE disease is important for antemortem diagnosis, and is based on the patient's history, physical findings, and concurrent disease(s).

Arterial TE disease in cats usually causes acute and dramatic clinical signs secondary to tissue ischemia. Male cats are at higher risk for thromboembolism, but this gender bias appears related to the prevalence of hypertrophic cardiomyopathy[15, 41, 61, 62]. Distal aortic embolization occurs in most cases (**213–215**). Acute hindlimb paresis without palpable femoral pulses is typical. Common clinical findings are summarized in *Table 39*.

Signs of pain and poor systemic perfusion are usually present. Hypothermia and azotemia are common, even when a site other than the distal aorta is affected[41]. A cardiac murmur, gallop sound, or

---

Table 39 Common clinical findings in cats with arterial thromboembolism.

1) Acute limb paresis:
   a) Posterior paresis.
   b) Monoparesis.
   c) ± Intermittent claudication.
2) Characteristics of affected limb(s):
   a) Painful.
   b) Cool distal limbs.
   c) Pale footpads.
   d) Cyanotic nailbeds.
   e) Absent arterial pulse.
   f) Contracture of affected muscles, especially gastrocnemius and cranial tibial.
3) Tachypnea/dyspnea (rule out pain or congestive heart failure).
4) Vocalization (pain and distress).
5) Hypothermia.
6) Signs of heart disease (not always present):
   a) Systolic murmur.

b) Gallop sounds.
c) Arrhythmias.
d) Cardiomegaly.
e) Anorexia.
f) Lethargy/weakness.
7) Signs of congestive heart failure (not always present):
   a) Pulmonary edema.
   b) Pleural effusion.
8) Hematologic and biochemical abnormalities:
   a) Azotemia (prerenal or renal).
   b) Increased alanine aminotransferase activity.
   c) Increased aspartate aminotransferase activity.
   d) Increased lactate dehydrogenase activity.
   e) Increased creatine phosphokinase activity.
   f) Hyperglycemia (stress).
   g) Lymphopenia (stress).
   h) Disseminated intravascular coagulation.

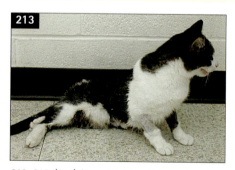
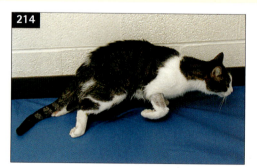
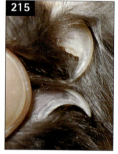

213–215 (213) Acute caudal aortic thromboembolism caused respiratory distress and panting as well as posterior paresis in this 4-year-old male DSH cat with restrictive cardiomyopathy. (214) The cat could ambulate with difficulty by shifting its weight to the forelimbs and dragging the hindlimbs and tail. (215) A cyanotic hindlimb nail bed (lower) from another cat with caudal aortic thromboembolism is compared with the pink nail bed (upper) of a forelimb.

arrhythmia is often noted, but these signs are not always evident even with underlying heart disease. Clinical signs of heart disease prior to the TE event are often absent[41]. Tachypnea and open-mouth breathing frequently occur with acute arterial embolization, despite the absence of overt CHF in many cats. This may represent a pain response, although it could be related to increased pulmonary venous pressure[41]. Because it is important to determine if CHF underlies the acute respiratory signs, thoracic radiographs should be taken as soon as possible. Motor function in the lower limbs is minimal to absent in most cases, although the cat is usually able to flex and extend the hips. Sensation to the lower limbs is poor. One side may show greater deficits than the other. Emboli are occasionally small enough to lodge more distally in only one limb, which causes paresis of the lower limb alone. Embolization of a brachial artery produces forelimb monoparesis. Intermittent claudication (see below) occurs rarely. Thromboemboli within the renal, mesenteric, or pulmonary arterial circulation may result in failure of these organs and death. Emboli to the brain could induce seizures or various neurologic deficits.

Arterial thromboembolism in dogs appears to have no age, breed, or sex predilections[10]. Most dogs with arterial (usually distal aortic) thromboemboli have some clinical signs from 1–8 weeks before presentation. Less than a quarter of cases have peracute paralysis without prior signs of lameness, as usually occurs in cats[10]. Most dogs are presented for signs related to the TE event. These include pain, hindlimb paresis, lameness or weakness, which may be progressive or intermittent, and chewing or hypersensitivity of the affected limb(s) or lumbar area. About half of the dogs are presented with sudden paralysis, but this is often preceded by a variable period of lameness[10]. Intermittent claudication, common in people with peripheral occlusive vascular disease, can be a manifestation of distal aortic TE disease[45]. This involves pain, weakness, and lameness that develop during exercise. These signs intensify until walking becomes impossible, then disappear with rest. Inadequate perfusion during exercise leads to lactic acid accumulation and cramping. Physical findings in dogs with aortic thromboembolism are similar to those in cats, including absent or weak femoral pulses, cool extremities, hindlimb pain, loss of sensation in the digits, hyperesthesia, cyanotic nailbeds, and neuromuscular dysfunction[10]. Occasionally, the brachial or other artery is embolized (216, 217). TE disease involving an abdominal organ causes abdominal pain, along with clinical and laboratory evidence of damage to the affected organ.

Coronary artery thromboembolism is likely to be associated with arrhythmias, as well as ST segment and T wave changes on ECG. Ventricular, or other, tachyarrhythmias are common, but if the AV nodal area is injured, conduction block can result[32]. Clinical signs of acute myocardial infarction/necrosis mimic those of pulmonary TE disease; these include weakness, dyspnea, and collapse[49]. Dyspnea may develop from underlying pulmonary disease or left-sided heart failure, depending on the underlying disease and degree of myocardial dysfunction. Some animals with respiratory distress have no radiographically evident pulmonary infiltrates. Increased pulmonary venous pressure before overt edema develops (from acute myocardial dysfunction) or concurrent pulmonary emboli are potential causes. Other findings in animals with myocardial necrosis include sudden death, tachycardia, weak pulses, increased lung sounds or crackles, cough, cardiac murmur, hyperthermia or, sometimes, hypothermia, and, less commonly, gastrointestinal signs[49]. Signs of other systemic disease can be concurrent. Acute ischemic myocardial injury causing sudden death may not be detectable on routine histopathology[31].

Pulmonary TE disease (see also Chapter 23) has no apparent age or sex predilection in dogs or cats[54, 55]. Classically, pulmonary TE disease causes dyspnea or tachypnea, but this is not evident in all cases[11, 50, 54]. Increased lung sounds, a cardiac murmur, and hepatosplenomegaly are also reported in many affected dogs[54]. Hypoxia develops mainly from V/Q mismatch related to aeration of nonperfused lung[19, 54].

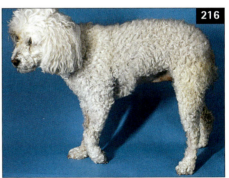

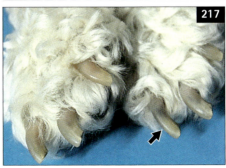

216, 217 (216) This 6-year-old female Poodle developed acute paresis of the left forelimb because of a TE event soon after surgery for cystotomy. The dog recovered normal function after supportive therapy. (217) Cyanosis of the left forepaw is seen best on the nail of the 3rd digit (arrow); the normal pink right forepaw is to the left of the image.

Unexplained respiratory distress with a high A-a gradient should generate suspicion for pulmonary TE disease. Chest pain and hemoptysis are typical signs in people, but not usually recognized in animals[54].

Systemic venous thrombosis produces signs related to increased venous pressure upstream from the obstruction. Thrombosis of the cranial vena cava leads to the cranial caval syndrome (see Chapter 12 and **199**, p. 128). Pleural effusion occurs commonly. This effusion is often chylous because lymph flow from the thoracic duct into the cranial vena cava is also impaired. Palpable thrombosis extends into the jugular veins in some cases. Because vena caval obstruction reduces pulmonary blood flow and left heart filling, signs of poor cardiac output are common.

LABORATORY TESTS

Results of routine laboratory tests depend largely on the disease process underlying the TE event(s). Systemic arterial TE disease also produces elevated muscle enzyme concentrations from skeletal muscle ischemia and necrosis. Aspartate aminotransferase (AST) and alanine aminotransferase (ALT) activities rise soon after the TE event. Widespread muscle injury also causes increased lactate dehydrogenase and creatine kinase (CK) activities[10]. Azotemia is common with arterial thromboembolism, especially in cats. This can be prerenal from poor systemic perfusion or dehydration, primary renal from embolization of the renal arteries or preexisting kidney disease, or a combination of both. Metabolic acidosis, DIC, electrolyte abnormalities, especially low serum sodium, calcium, and potassium, and elevated phosphorus, are common in cats, as is stress hyperglycemia. Hyperkalemia can develop secondary to ischemic muscle damage and reperfusion[15, 41, 61].

Myocardial damage from coronary artery embolization increases circulating cardiac troponin levels. Increased AST activity has been reported with myocardial necrosis[49]. Total CK and ALT are variably increased within a few hours of injury; elevated cardiac-specific isoenzyme of CK (CK-MB) is expected but not usually measured in animals[49]. Values peak in 6–12 hours then return to normal within 1–2 days. Continued increase indicates ongoing injury. Other laboratory parameters reflect underlying disease, as is the case with pulmonary TE disease and venous thrombosis. Leukocytosis and increased liver enzymes have been noted commonly with pulmonary thromboembolism and thrombocytopenia with cranial caval thrombosis[13].

Routine coagulation test results are variable with TE disease. Levels of FDPs may be increased, but this can occur with inflammatory disease and is not specific for a TE event or DIC[19]. Cats with arterial TE disease usually have normal coagulation profiles[35]. Coagulation test results are more variable in dogs with systemic arterial, including coronary, and pulmonary

TE disease. Prolonged coagulation times and thrombocytopenia consistent with DIC are reported in many cases, but results are normal in some dogs[10, 49]. However, many conditions that underlie TE disease are also associated with DIC. Coagulation profile results have usually been normal with cranial vena cava thrombosis. Shortened coagulation (prothrombin, activated partial thromboplastin, and thrombin) times have not been correlated with thrombosis[19].

D-dimer assays provide a more specific indicator of clot breakdown than FDPs in dogs[5, 7, 63, 64]. D-dimers are degradation products specific to cross-linked fibrin. FDP assays do not discriminate between breakdown of fibrinogen and stable clots and are not sensitive enough to detect thromboemboli. D-dimer concentrations are elevated with TE disease, with higher concentrations more specific for thromboemboli. Modestly increased D-dimer concentrations occur in other diseases such as neoplasia, liver disease, and IMHA. This could reflect subclinical TE disease or another clot activation mechanism, as these conditions are associated with a procoagulant state[7, 65]. Body cavity hemorrhage also causes a rise in D-dimers. Because this condition is associated with increased fibrin formation, elevated D-dimers may not indicate TE disease in these cases[6]. The specificity of D-dimer testing for pathologic thromboembolism is lower at lower D-dimer concentrations, but the high sensitivity at lower concentrations provides an important screening tool. D-dimer testing appears to be as specific for DIC as FDP measurement[6]. A number of assays have been developed to measure D-dimers in dogs; some are qualitative or semiquantitative (e.g. latex agglutination, immunochromatographic, and immunofiltration tests), others are more quantitative (e.g. immunoturbidity, enzymatic immunoassays)[66]. It is important to interpret D-dimer results in the context of other clinical and test findings. The applicability of D-dimer testing in cats is not yet clear. Assays for circulating AT III and proteins C and S are also available for dogs and cats. Deficiencies of these proteins are associated with increased risk of thrombosis[5, 30]. A number of methods are described to test for AT III activity. Sample submission instructions and normal reference values should be obtained from the laboratory performing the testing.

Arterial blood gas analysis is helpful when respiratory signs are severe or persistent (see Chapter 9, p. 114). Animals with pulmonary thromboemboli often have hypoxemia, hypocapnia, and an increased A-a gradient. Hypoxemia usually improves with supplemental O_2 because the mechanism is largely related to V/Q mismatch; however, massive embolization creates a large functional intrapulmonary shunt (venous admixture) and unresponsive hypoxemia. Progressively decreasing PaO_2 despite O_2 therapy suggests intrapulmonary shunting[54]. Cranial vena cava thrombosis with complete caval obstruction also leads to hypocapnia and hypoxemia. Respiratory alkalosis, from hyperventilation, and metabolic acidosis, possibly from poor tissue oxygenation induced by hypoxemia and low cardiac output, can occur. Partial improvement with O$_2$ therapy indicates some degree of V/Q mismatch, suggesting concurrent pulmonary thrombo-embolism.

DIAGNOSTIC IMAGING

Thoracic radiography is used to screen for cardiac abnormalities, especially in animals with systemic arterial TE disease, and for pulmonary changes in animals suspected to have pulmonary thromboemboli. Evidence for CHF or other pulmonary disease associated with thromboemboli (e.g. neoplasia, HWD,

or other infections) may also be found. Most cats with arterial TE disease have some degree of cardiomegaly, especially LA enlargement, when cardiomyopathy is underlying (see **46, 47**, p. 39, **432–437**, p. 302, **466, 467**, p. 313, and Chapter 21). A minority of affected cats have no radiographic evidence of cardiomegaly[15, 67]. Signs of CHF may or may not be present (e.g. dilated pulmonary veins, pulmonary edema, or pleural effusion [see **64–68**, p. 45]). Pulmonary TE disease produces variable radiographic findings (**218–223**). Pleural effusion, truncated lobar pulmonary arteries, alveolar infiltrates, hyperlucent lungs (suggesting reduced pulmonary blood flow), main

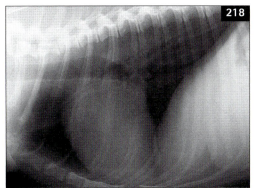
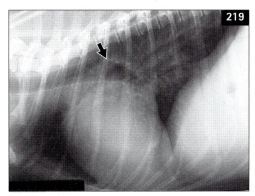
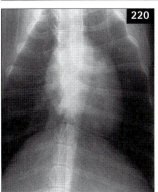
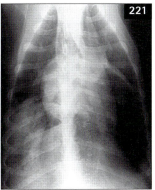
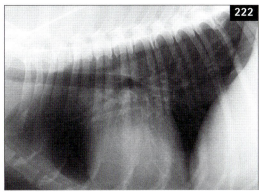
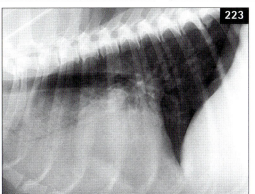

218–223 Radiographic changes caused by pulmonary thromboembolism (PTE). (**218**) Normal lateral view from the dog in 212 taken 12 days prior to PTE. (**219**) Radiograph from the dog in 218 after onset of acute dyspnea. Note increase in width of heart shadow (RV enlargement), prominent pulmonary artery (arrow), and dorsocaudal perivascular pulmonary infiltrates. (**220**) Normal DV radiograph from a 5-year-old Rottweiler at presentation for bloody diarrhea, anemia, and dehydration. (**221**) From the dog in 220 8 days later after acute onset of cough and respiratory distress. Skin staples are visible on the midline from abdominal surgery 1 week prior. Note pulmonary infiltrates localized near the right caudal pulmonary artery. (**222**) Lateral view from an 8-year-old Golden Retriever with severe hepatic disease, thrombocytopenia, and hypoproteinemia. (**223**) Radiograph from the dog in 222 5 days later, after respiratory signs and facial/neck swelling developed. Severe interstitial and alveolar infiltrates in the cranioventral lung and mild pleural effusion are seen. At postmortem examination, PTE in several medium sized arteries (but no evidence for bacterial pneumonia), malignant histiocytosis of the liver and spleen, membranous glomerulonephritis, and cranial caval and jugular vein thrombosis were found (see also **199**, p. 128).

pulmonary trunk enlargement, and, sometimes, lung atelectasis are described in dogs. But any radiographic pattern is possible[54, 68]. Cats with pulmonary thromboembolism can also develop pleural effusion, alveolar opacification, peribronchial and interstitial markings, or pulmonary vascular congestion similar to dogs[55, 56]. Radiographs are sometimes unremarkable, even with clinical signs of respiratory compromise[19].

A complete echocardiographic examination is important to define whether heart disease might be present and, if so, what type of heart disease. Thrombi within the left or right heart chambers and proximal great vessels can be readily seen with 2-D echocardiography (**224, 225**) (see also **454, 455**, p. 307, **464**, p. 312, and **549**, p. 345). Doppler modalities help define abnormal (or lack of) blood flow in affected regions. Most cats with arterial TE disease associated with cardiomyopathy have some degree of LA enlargement. An LA dimension of >20 mm (measured from the 2-D long-axis 4-chamber view) may increase the risk for TE disease[37, 67], although over half of aortic TE cases had a smaller LA size in one study[41]. The most common site for intracardiac thrombi is the left auricular appendage. Pulmonary TE disease that causes pulmonary hypertension variably produces RV enlargement and hypertrophy, interventricular septal

flattening, and high tricuspid regurgitation jet velocities (see Chapter 23 and **544–552**, pp. 345, 346). Sometimes, a clot is identified within the pulmonary artery or RA. Likewise, vena cava thrombosis may be visible ultrasonographically, especially when the clot extends into the RA. Portal vein thrombosis and thromboemboli in the aorta or other large peripheral vessels can also be documented on ultrasound examination (**225**). In animals with coronary TE disease, the echo examination may indicate reduced myocardial contractility with or without regional dysfunction. Areas of myocardial fibrosis secondary to chronic ischemia or infarction appear hyperechoic compared with the surrounding myocardium.

Angiography can document vascular occlusion when ultrasonography is inconclusive or unavailable, as well as show the extent of collateral circulation. The choice of selective or nonselective technique depends on patient size and the suspected location of the clot. Especially in cats, if echocardiography is unavailable, nonselective angiocardiography can help define the nature of underlying cardiac disease and determine the location and extent of the thromboembolus. Pulmonary angiography can identify major pulmonary flow obstructions (**226, 227**). Ventilation/perfusion scintigraphy may show unperfused lung regions.

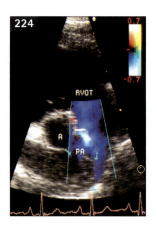

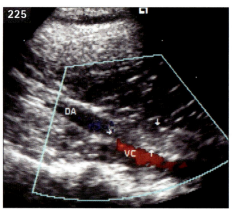

224, 225 (224) Echocardiography revealed a large PTE (arrows) in the main PA of an 8-year-old male mixed breed dog with a 2-week history of exercise intolerance and fainting. CF Doppler showed flow (coded blue) up to and around the edge of the mass. RV dilation and hypertrophy and small LV size were also evident. Severe renal amyloidosis, hypoproteinemia, and low AT III were identified. (225) Abdominal ultrasonography indicated a thromboembolus in the distal aorta of a cat with cardiomyopathy. CF Doppler showed flow (blue) in the descending aorta (DA) just proximal to the obstruction. Flow (red) is also seen in the adjacent vena cava (VC). (Courtesy Dr K Miles.)

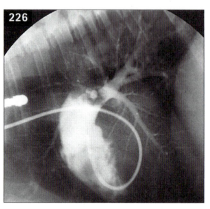

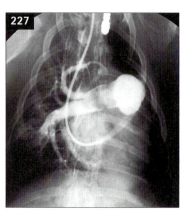

226, 227 Lateral (226) and DV (227) pulmonary angiograms from a 7-year-old female mixed breed dog with hypothyroidism, exercise intolerance, and postexercise cyanosis. A large thromboembolus (TE) obstructed flow into the left pulmonary artery (PA) and its branches. PAs serving the right cranial and ventral lung regions are perfused, but another TE obstructed flow to the right caudodorsal lung region. (Courtesy Dr E Riedesel.)

Nuclear scintigraphy can help evaluate perfusion in other obstructed regions as well[35, 69, 70]. CT and magnetic resonance angiography could also have applicability in delineating TE disease in animals.

GENERAL PRINCIPLES OF THERAPY FOR TE DISEASE

The goals of therapy are 1) to stabilize the patient by supportive treatment as indicated; 2) to prevent extension of the thrombus and additional TE events; and 3) to reduce the size of existing clots and restore perfusion. Management strategies used for TE disease are outlined in *Table 40*. Supportive care is given to improve and maintain adequate tissue perfusion, to minimize further endothelial damage and blood stasis, and to optimize organ function, as well as to allow time for collateral circulation development. Antiplatelet and anticoagulant therapies are used to reduce platelet aggregation and growth of existing thrombi. Although fibrinolytic therapy is used in some cases, dosage uncertainties, the need for intensive care, and the potential for serious complications limit its use. Correcting or managing underlying disease(s), as far as is possible, is also important.

Table 40 Management of thromboembolic disease.

1) Initial diagnostic tests:
   a) Complete physical examination and history.
   b) Hemogram, serum biochemical profile, urinalysis.
   c) Thoracic radiographs (rule out signs of CHF, other infiltrates, pleural effusion).
   d) Coagulation and D-dimer tests, if possible.

2) Initial management:
   a) Analgesia as needed (especially for systemic arterial thromboembolism).
   b) Morphine:
      ■ Dog: 0.5–2.0 mg/kg IM, SC q3–5h; 0.05–0.4 mg/kg IV q3–5h.
      ■ Cat: 0.05–0.2 mg/kg IM, SC q3–4h (dysphoria occurs in some cats).
   c) Oxymorphone or hydromorphone:
      ■ Dog: 0.05–0.2 mg/kg IM, IV, SC q2–4h.
      ■ Cat: 0.05–0.2 mg/kg IM, IV, SC q2–4h.
   d) Butorphanol:
      ■ Dog: 0.2–2.0 mg/kg IM, IV, SC q1–4h.
      ■ Cat: 0.2–1.0 mg/kg IM (cranial lumbar area), IV, SC q1–4h.
   e) Buprenorphine:
      ■ Dog: 0.005–0.02 mg/kg IM, IV, SC q6–8h.
      ■ Cat: 0.005–0.02 mg/kg IM, IV, SC q6–8h; can give PO for transmucosal absorption.

3) Supportive care:
   a) Supplemental O_2 if respiratory signs.
   b) IV fluid as indicated (and not in CHF).
   c) Monitor for and correct azotemia and electrolyte abnormalities.
   d) Manage CHF if present (see Chapters 16 and 21).
   e) External warming if persistent hypothermia after rehydration.
   f) Identify and manage underlying disease(s).
   g) Nutritional support if persistent anorexia.

4) Further diagnostic testing:
   a) Complete cardiac evaluation, including echocardiogram.
   b) Other tests as indicated (based on initial findings and cardiac exam) to rule out predisposing conditions (see *Table 38*, p. 148).

5) Prevent extension of existing clot and new TE events:
   a) Antiplatelet therapy:
      ■ Aspirin:
         • Dog: 0.5 mg/kg PO q12h.
         • Cat: 81 mg/cat PO 2–3 times a week; low-dose, 5 mg/cat q72h (see text).
      ■ Clopidogrel:
         • Cat: ?18.75 mg/cat PO q24h (dose not well established).
   b) Anticoagulant therapy:
      ■ Sodium heparin:
         • Dog: 200–250 IU/kg IV, followed by 200–300 IU/kg SC q6–8h for 2–4 days or as needed.
         • Cat: same.
      ■ Dalteparin sodium:
         • Dog: 100–150 U/kg SC q(12)–24h (see text).
         • Cat: 100 U/kg SC q(12)–24h (see text).
      ■ Enoxaparin:
         • Dog: same as cat?
         • Cat: 1 mg/kg SC q12–24h (see text).

6) Thrombolytic therapy (pursue only with caution, see text):
   a) Streptokinase:
      ■ Dog: 90,000 IU infused IV over 20–30 minutes, then at 45,000 IU/hour for 3 (or more) hours (see text).
      ■ Cat: same.
   b) rt-PA:
      ■ Dog: 1 mg/kg bolus IV q1h for 10 doses (see text).
      ■ Cat: 0.25–1 mg/kg/hour (up to a total of 1–10 mg/kg) IV (see text).

Fluid therapy is used to expand vascular volume, support blood pressure, and correct electrolyte and acid/base abnormalities depending on individual patient needs. However, for animals with heart disease, and especially CHF, fluid therapy is given only with great caution, if at all. Specific therapy for heart diseases, CHF, and arrhythmias is provided as indicated (see Chapters 16, 17, and other pertinent chapters). In patients with acute respiratory signs, it is important to determine if CHF is the cause or if pain or pulmonary thromboembolism is responsible. Diuretic or vasodilator therapy could worsen perfusion in animals without CHF.

Acute arterial embolization is particularly painful, so analgesic therapy is important in such cases, especially for the first 24–36 hours (*Table 40*, p. 157). Acepromazine is not recommended for animals with arterial thromboembolism, despite its alpha-adrenergic receptor-blocking effects. Improved collateral flow has not been documented, and hypotension or exacerbation of dynamic ventricular outflow obstruction, particularly in cats with hypertrophic obstructive cardiomyopathy, are potential adverse effects. Propranolol is also avoided in cats with cardiomyopathy and arterial thromboembolism. Propranolol's nonselective beta-blocking effect may contribute to peripheral vasoconstriction from unopposed alpha-receptors, and the drug has no antithrombotic effects at clinical doses.

Loosely bandaging the affected limb(s) to prevent self-mutilation may be needed in some animals with aortic TE disease. Hypothermia that persists after circulating volume is restored can be addressed with external warming. Renal function and serum electrolyte concentrations are monitored daily or more frequently if fibrinolytic therapy is used. Continuous ECG monitoring during the first several days can help the clinician detect acute hyperkalemia associated with reperfusion (see Chapter 4, p. 64). Nutritional support may become important if anorexia persists after the initial treatment period. Supplemental O_2 improves hypoxemia related to V/Q mismatch and alveolar hypoventilation. This is especially important with pulmonary TE events but may be helpful with other TE disease also.

ANTIPLATELET THERAPY

Aspirin (acetylsalicylic acid) is used commonly to block platelet activation and aggregation in patients with, or at risk for, TE disease. Aspirin irreversibly inhibits cyclo-oxygenase, which reduces prostaglandin and thromboxane A_2 synthesis and, therefore, subsequent platelet aggregation, serotonin release, and vasoconstriction. Because platelets cannot synthesize additional cyclo-oxygenase, this reduction of proco-agulant prostaglandins and thromboxane persists for the platelet's lifespan (7–10 days). Endothelial production of prostacyclin (also via the cyclo-

oxygenase pathway) is reduced by aspirin, but only transiently as endothelial cells synthesize additional cyclo-oxygenase. Aspirin's benefit may relate more to *in situ* thrombus formation; efficacy in acute arterial thromboembolism is unknown[35]. Adverse effects of aspirin tend to be mild and uncommon, but the optimal dose is unclear. Cats lack an enzyme (glucaronyl transferase) needed to metabolize aspirin, so less frequent dosing is required compared with dogs. In cats with experimental aortic thrombosis, 10–25 mg/kg (1.25 grains/cat) given PO once every (2–)3 days inhibited platelet aggregation and improved collateral circulation[27]. However, low-dose aspirin (5 mg/cat q72h) has also been used with fewer GI side-effects, although its efficacy in preventing TE events is unknown[41]. Aspirin therapy is started when the patient is able to take food and oral medications.

Other antiplatelet drugs are being studied. The thienopyridines inhibit ADP binding at platelet receptors and subsequent ADP-mediated platelet aggregation. Clopidogrel (18.75 mg/cat PO q24h) appears to have significant antiplatelet effects; dosing every other day may be possible[71]. The related drug ticlodipine caused a high rate of anorexia and vomiting at the effective antiplatelet dose in a preliminary study in cats[72]. Another group of antiplatelet agents block gp IIb/IIIa receptors, which interferes with binding of platelets and fibrinogen. A preliminary study showed that pretreatment with the gp IIb/IIIa receptor-blocker abciximab (0.25 mg/kg IV bolus, followed by 0.125 µg/kg/min CRI) plus aspirin was more effective than aspirin alone in reducing platelet aggregation and *in vivo* thrombosis in cats, although there was much intercat variability[73]. Clinical studies are needed to verify whether the drug is useful for acute TE disease management. A similar drug, eptifibatide, caused unpredictable CV collapse and death in an experimental cat study and is not recommended[74]. Other drugs have antiplatelet effects via calcium-blocking or phosphodiesterase-inhibiting mechanisms.

ANTICOAGULANT THERAPY

Heparin is indicated to limit extension of existing thrombi and prevent further TE episodes; it does not promote thrombolysis. Unfractionated heparin and a number of low-molecular-weight heparin (LMWH) products are available. Heparin's main anticoagulant effect is produced through AT III activation, which in turn inhibits factors IX, X, XI, and XII and thrombin[75]. Unfractionated heparin binds thrombin as well as AT III. Heparin also stimulates release of tissue factor inhibitor from vascular sites, which helps reduce (extrinsic) coagulation cascade activation. Optimal dosing protocols for animals are not known. Unfractionated heparin is usually given as an initial IV bolus followed by SC injections (*Table 40*, p. 157). Heparin is not given IM because of the risk for hemorrhage at the injection site. Heparin doses (from 75–500 U/kg) have been used with uncertain efficacy[41, 76]. Monitoring the patient's activated partial thromboplastin time (aPTT) has been recommended, although results may not accurately predict serum heparin concentrations[35]. Pretreatment coagulation testing is done for comparison, and the goal is to prolong the aPTT to 1.5–2.5 times baseline. Activated clotting time is not recommended to monitor heparin therapy. Hemorrhage is the major complication. Protamine sulfate can be used to counteract heparin-induced bleeding. Fresh frozen plasma may be needed to replenish AT III[76]. Heparin treatment is continued until the patient is stable and has been on antiplatelet therapy for a few days[35].

LMWH products are a diverse group of depolymerized heparins that vary in size, structure, and pharmacokinetics. Their smaller size prevents simultaneous binding to thrombin and AT III. LMWHs have more effect against factor Xa by catalyzing AT III inhibition of factor Xa. They have minimal ability to inhibit thrombin, so are less likely to cause bleeding. LMWHs have greater bioavailability and a longer half-life than unfractionated heparin when given SC, because of lesser binding to plasma proteins as well as endothelial cells and macrophages[75]. LMWHs do not markedly affect coagulation times, so monitoring aPTT is generally not necessary[76, 77]. The LMWH effect can be monitored indirectly by anti-Xa activity[77]. An anti-Xa activity level of 0.3–0.6 U/ml is considered sufficient in people. The most effective dosage for the various LMWHs is not clearly established in dogs and cats. Dalteparin sodium has been used (100–150 U/kg SC q[12-]24h), but some animals may need q8h dosing[35, 77, 78]. Enoxaparin has been used (1 mg/kg SC q12[-24]h).

FIBRINOLYTIC THERAPY
Drugs used to promote clot lysis include streptokinase and human recombinant tissue plasminogen activator (rt-PA). These agents increase conversion of plasminogen to plasmin to facilitate fibrinolysis. Veterinary experience with these agents is quite limited. Although they effectively break down clots, complications related to reperfusion injury and hemorrhage, high mortality rate, cost of therapy, intensive care required, and lack of clearly established dosing protocols have prevented their widespread use[19, 79, 80]. If used, this therapy is best instituted within 3–4 hours of vascular occlusion. An intensive care setting, including continuous serum potassium concentration (or ECG) monitoring to detect reperfusion-induced hyperkalemia, is recommended.

Streptokinase is a nonspecific plasminogen activator that promotes the breakdown of fibrin as well as fibrinogen. This leads to the degradation of fibrin within thrombi and clot lysis, but also potentially leads to systemic fibrinolysis, coagulopathy, and bleeding[81]. Streptokinase also degrades factors V and VIII, and prothrombin. Although its half-life is about 30 minutes, fibrinogen depletion continues for much longer[79]. Streptokinase has been used with variable success in a small number of dogs with arterial thromboembolism[79]. The reported protocol for dogs and cats is 90,000 IU of streptokinase infused IV over 20–30 minutes, then at a rate of 45,000 IU/hour for 3 hours (up to 8–12 in dogs)[39]. Dilution of 250,000 IU into 5 ml saline, then into 50 ml to yield 5,000 IU/ml for infusion with a syringe pump has been suggested for cats[35]. Adverse effects are minor in some cases and bleeding may respond to discontinuing streptokinase[81]; however, there is potential for serious hemorrhage and the mortality rate in clinical cases is high[39, 61, 81]. Acute hyperkalemia, secondary to thrombolysis and reperfusion injury, metabolic acidosis, bleeding, and other complications are thought to be responsible for causing death[61]. Streptokinase can increase platelet aggregability and induce platelet dysfunction. It is unclear if lower doses would be effective with fewer complications. Streptokinase combined with heparin therapy can increase the risk of hemorrhage, especially when coagulation times are increased. Streptokinase is potentially antigenic, as it is produced by beta-hemolytic streptococci. No survival benefit has been shown for streptokinase compared with 'conventional' (aspirin and heparin) treatment in cats[35].

rt-PA is a single-chain polypeptide serine protease with a higher specificity for fibrin within thrombi and a low affinity for circulating plasminogen. Although the risk of hemorrhage is less than with streptokinase, there is potential for serious bleeding as well as other side-effects. rt-PA is also potentially antigenic in animals because it is a human protein. Like streptokinase, rt-PA induces platelet dysfunction but not hyperaggregability. Experience with rt-PA is very limited and the optimal dosage is not known[79]. A dose of 0.25–1 mg/kg/hour up to a total of 1–10 mg/kg IV was used in a small number of cats; although signs of reperfusion occurred, there was a high mortality rate[82]. The cause of death in most cats was attributed to reperfusion (hyperkalemia, metabolic acidosis) and hemorrhage, although CHF and arrhythmias were also involved[82]. In dogs, rt-PA has been used as 1 mg/kg boluses IV q1h for 10 doses, with IV fluid, other supportive therapy, and close monitoring[80]. The half-life of t-PA is about 2–3 minutes in dogs, but effects persist longer because of binding to fibrin. The consequences of reperfusion injury present serious complications to thrombolytic therapy. The iron chelator deferoxamine mesylate has been used in an attempt to reduce oxidative damage from free radicals involving iron[80]. Allopurinol has also been used but with uncertain results[81].

OTHER CONSIDERATIONS

Surgical clot removal is generally not advised in cats. The surgical risk is high and significant neuromuscular ischemic injury is likely to have already occurred by the time of surgery. Clot removal using an embolectomy catheter has not been very effective in cats but might be more successful in dogs of larger size.

In general, the prognosis is poor in both dogs and cats with arterial TE disease. Historically, only a third of cats survive the initial episode; however, survival statistics improve when cats euthanized without therapy are excluded or when only cases from recent years are analyzed[15, 41, 61, 62]. Survival is better if only one limb is involved and/or if some motor function is preserved at presentation[15, 41, 61, 62]. Hypothermia and CHF at presentation are both associated with poor survival in cats[41, 61]. Rectal temperature at admission of 37.2°C (98.9°F) predicted a 50% probability of survival[41]. Other negative factors may include hyperphosphatemia, progressive hyperkalemia or azotemia, progressive limb injury (continued muscle contracture after 2–3 days, necrosis), severe LA enlargement, presence of intracardiac thrombi or spontaneous contrast ('swirling smoke') on echocardiogram, DIC, and history of thromboembolism.

Barring complications, limb function should begin to return within 1–2 weeks. Some cats become clinically normal within 1–2 months, although residual deficits may persist for a variable time. Tissue necrosis may require wound management and skin grafting. Permanent limb deformity develops in some cats (**228**) and amputation is occasionally necessary. Repeated events occur in at least a quarter of surviving cats[41]. Significant embolization of the kidneys, intestines, or other organs carries a grave prognosis.

TE DISEASE PROPHYLAXIS

Prophylactic therapy with an antiplatelet or anticoagulant drug is usually used in animals thought to be at increased risk for TE disease. These include cats with cardiomyopathy, especially those with marked LA enlargement, echo evidence for intracardiac spontaneous contrast or thrombus, or a previous TE event, and animals with sepsis, IMHA, severe pancreatitis, or other procoagulant conditions[19, 67, 79]. However, efficacy of TE disease prophylaxis is unknown and a strategy that consistently prevents thromboembolism is not yet identified. In cats, no strategy has shown clear advantage over others[35].

Drugs used for arterial TE disease prophylaxis include aspirin, warfarin (coumadin), and, more recently, LMWH. Clopidogrel may also prove useful (see above). As with the other agents, aspirin does not consistently prevent initial or recurrent TE events, but aspirin is often recommended because it is inexpensive, has little risk for serious hemorrhage, and requires less monitoring than warfarin. Adverse GI effects (e.g. vomiting, inappetence, ulceration, hematemesis) occur in some animals; a buffered formulation or aspirin-Maalox combination product may be helpful. Low-dose aspirin (5 mg/cat every 3rd day) has been advocated in cats[41]. Although adverse effects are unlikely with this dose, it is not known if antiplatelet effectiveness is compromised. Warfarin (see below) is associated with greater expense and a higher rate of fatal hemorrhage[15, 41, 61]. No survival benefit has been shown for warfarin compared with aspirin in cats[41]. In some reports, recurrent thromboembolism occurred in almost half of cats treated with warfarin[15, 61]. LMWH prophylaxis may be more efficacious, with less risk of hemorrhage, but more experience with this therapy is needed. Recurrent TE events occurred in 20% of cats in one study[77]. LMWH is expensive and must be given by daily SC injection, but many owners are motivated to do this. In cats without thrombocytopenia, aspirin can be used concurrently. Diltiazem at clinical doses does not appear to have significant platelet-inhibiting effects.

Warfarin inhibits the enzyme (vitamin K epoxide reductase) responsible for activating the vitamin-K dependent factors (II, VII, IX, and X), as well as proteins C and S. Initial warfarin treatment causes transient hypercoagulability because anticoagulant proteins have a shorter half-life than most procoagulant factors; therefore, heparin (e.g. 100 IU/kg SC q8h) is given for 2–4 days after warfarin is initiated. There is wide variability in dose response and potential for serious bleeding, even in cats that are monitored closely. Warfarin is highly protein bound; concurrent use of other protein-bound drugs or change in serum protein content can markedly

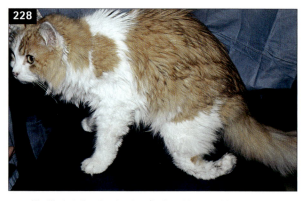

228 Hindlimb deformity developed after this cat with restrictive cardiomyopathy and AF survived an episode of caudal aortic thromboembolism. The cat was able to ambulate well, despite weight-bearing on the dorsal aspect of the left metatarsus.

alter the anticoagulant effect. Bleeding may be manifest as weakness, lethargy, or pallor rather than overt hemorrhage. A baseline coagulation profile and platelet count are obtained, and aspirin discontinued, before beginning treatment. The usual initial warfarin dose is 0.25–0.5 mg (total dose) PO q24(–48)h in cats; 0.1–0.2 mg/kg PO q24h in dogs. A loading dose of ~0.2 mg/kg for 2 days appears safe in dogs[83]. Uneven distribution of drug within the tablets is reported, so compounding rather than administering tablet fragments is recommended[35]. Drug administration and blood sampling times should be consistent.

The dose is adjusted either on the basis of PT or the international normalization ratio (INR)[67, 83]. The INR is a more precise method that has been recommended to avoid problems related to variation in commercial PT assays. The INR is calculated by dividing the animal's PT by the control PT and raising the quotient to the power of the international sensitivity index (ISI) of the thromboplastin used in the assay (i.e. INR = [animal PT/control PT]^{ISI}). The

ISI is provided with each batch of thromboplastin made. Extrapolation from human data suggests that an INR of 2–3 is as effective as higher values, with less chance for bleeding. Using a warfarin dose of 0.05–0.1 mg/kg/day in the dog achieves this INR in about 5–7 days. Heparin overlap until the INR is >2 is recommended. When using PT to monitor warfarin therapy, a goal of 1.25–1.5 (to 2) times pretreatment PT at 8–10 hours after dosing is advised; the animal is weaned off heparin when the INR is >1.25. The PT is evaluated several hours after dosing, daily initially, then at progressively increasing time intervals (e.g. twice a week, then once a week, then every month to 2 months) as long as the cat's condition appears stable.

If the PT or INR increases excessively, warfarin is discontinued and vitamin K_1 administered (1–2 mg/kg/day PO or SC) until the PT is normal and the PCV is stable. Transfusion with fresh frozen plasma, packed red blood cells, or whole fresh blood is sometimes necessary.

REFERENCES

1 Good LI, Manning AM (2003) Thromboembolic disease: physiology of hemostasis and pathophysiology of thrombosis. *Compend Contin Educ Pract Vet* **25**:650–658.

2 Turk JR (1998) Physiologic and pathophysiologic effects of endothelin: implications in cardiopulmonary disease. *J Am Vet Med Assoc* **212**:265–270.

3 Weiss DJ, Rashid J (1998) The sepsis-coagulant axis: a review. *J Vet Intern Med* **12**:317–324.

4 Boudreaux MK (1996) Platelets and coagulation. *Vet Clin North Am: Small Anim Pract* **26**:1065–1087.

5 Welles EG (1996) Antithrombotic and fibrinolytic factors. *Vet Clin North Am: Small Anim Pract* **26**:1111–1127.

6 Stokol T, Brooks MB, Erb HN *et al.* (2000) D-dimer concentrations in healthy dogs and dogs with disseminated intravascular coagulation. *Am J Vet Res* **61**:393–398.

7 Nelson OL, Andreasen C (2003) The utility of plasma D-dimer to identify thromboembolic disease in dogs. *J Vet Intern Med* **17**:830–834.

8 Howe LM, Booth HW (1999) Nitric oxide response in critically ill dogs. *J Vet Emerg Crit Care* **9**:195–202.

9 Williamson LH (1991) Antithrombin III: a natural anticoagulant. *Compend Contin Educ Pract Vet* **13**:100–109.

10 Van Winkle TJ, Hackner SG, Liu SM (1993) Clinical and pathological features of aortic thromboembolism in 36 dogs. *J Vet Emerg Crit Care* **3**:13–21.

11 Klein MK, Dow SW, Rosychuk RA (1989) Pulmonary thromboembolism associated with immune-mediated hemolytic anemia in dogs: ten cases (1982–1987). *J Am Vet Med Assoc* **195**:246–250.

12 Rawlings CA, Raynard JP, Lewis RE *et al.* (1993) Pulmonary thromboembolism and hypertension after thiacetarsemide vs melarsomine dihydrochloride treatment of *Dirofilaria immitis* infection in dogs. *Am J Vet Res* **54**:920–925.

13 Palmer KG, King LG, Van Winkle TJ (1998). Clinical manifestations and associated disease syndromes in dogs with cranial vena cava thrombosis: 17 cases (1989–1996) *J Am Vet Med Assoc* **213**:220–224.

14 Sottiaux J, Franck M (1998) Cranial vena cava thrombosis secondary to invasive mediastinal lymphosarcoma in a cat. *J Small Anim Pract* **39**:352–355.

15 Laste NJ, Harpster NK (1995) A retrospective study of 100 cases of feline distal aortic thromboembolism: 1977–1993. *J Am Anim Hosp Assoc* **31**:492–500.

16 Jaffe MH, Grooters AM, Partington BP *et al.* (1999) Extensive venous thrombosis and hindlimb edema associated with adrenocortical carcinoma in a dog. *J Am Anim Hosp Assoc* **35**:306–310.

17 Nichols R (1997) Complications and concurrent disease associated with canine hyperadrenocorticism. *Vet Clin North Am: Small Anim Pract* **27**:309–320.

18 Cook AK, Cowgill LD (1999) Clinical and pathological features of protein-losing glomerular disease in the dog: a review of 137 cases (1985–1992). *J Am Anim Hosp Assoc* **32**:313–332.

19 Good LI, Manning AM (2003) Thromboembolic disease: predis-positions and clinical management. *Compend Contin Educ Pract Vet* **25**:660–674.

20 Purvis D, Kirby R (1994) Systemic inflammatory response syndrome: septic shock. *Vet Clin North Am: Small Anim Pract* **24**:1225–1247.

21 Buchanan JW, Beardow AW, Sammarco CD (1997) Femoral artery occlusion in

Cavalier King Charles Spaniels. *J Am Vet Med Assoc* **211**:872–874.

22 De Laforcade AM, Freeman LM, Shaw SP *et al.* (2003) Hemostatic changes in dogs with naturally occurring sepsis. *J Vet Intern Med* **17**:674–679.

23 Olsen LH, Kristensen AT, Haggstrom J *et al.* (2001) Increased platelet aggregation response in Cavalier King Charles Spaniels with mitral valve prolapse. *J Vet Intern Med* **15**:209–216.

24 Thomas JS, Rodgers KS (1999) Platelet aggregation and adenosine triphosphate secretion dogs with untreated multicentric lymphoma. *J Vet Intern Med* **13**:319–322.

25 Welles EG, Boudreaux MK, Crager CS *et al.* (1994) Platelet function and antithrombin, plasminogen, and fibrinolytic activities in cats with heart disease. *Am J Vet Res* **55**:619–627.

26 Feldman BF, Thomason KJ, Jain NC (1988) Quantitative platelet disorders. *Vet Clin North Am: Small Anim Pract* **18**:35–49.

27 Fox PR, Petrie JP, Hohenhaus AE (2005) Peripheral vascular disease. In: *Textbook of Veterinary Internal Medicine*, 6th edn. SJ Ettinger, EC Feldman (eds). WB Saunders, Philadelphia, pp. 1145–1165.

28 Bateman SW, Mathews KA, Abrams-Ogg ACG *et al.* (1999) Diagnosis of disseminated intravascular coagulation in dogs admitted to an intensive care unit. *J Am Vet Med Assoc* **215**:798–804.

29 Bateman SW, Mathews KA, Abrams-Ogg ACG (1998) Disseminated intravascular coagulation in dogs: review of the literature. *J Vet Emerg Crit Care* **8**:29–45.

30 Green RA (1984) Clinical implications of antithrombin III deficiency in animal diseases. *Compend Contin Educ Pract Vet* **6**:537–545.

31 Carr AP, Panciera DL, Kidd L (2002) Prognostic factors for mortality and thromboembolism in canine immune-mediated hemolytic anemia: a retrospective study of 72 dogs. *J Vet Intern Med* **16**:504–509.

32 Driehuys S, Van Winkle TJ, Sammarco CD *et al.* (1998) Myocardial infarction in dogs and cats: 37 cases (1985–1994). *J Am Vet Med Assoc* **213**:1444–1448.

33 Burns MG, Kelly AB, Hornof WJ *et al.* (1981) Pulmonary artery thrombosis in three dogs with hyperadrenocorticism. *J Am Vet Med Assoc* **178**:388–393.

34 Liu SK (1970) Acquired cardiac lesions leading to congestive heart failure in the cat. *Am J Vet Res* **31**:2071–2088.

35 Smith SA, Tobias AH (2004) Feline arterial thromboembolism: an update. *Vet Clin North Am: Small Anim Pract* **34**:1245–1271.

36 Schober KE, Marz I (2003) Doppler echocardiographic assessment of left atrial appendage flow in cats with cardiomyopathy. Abstract. *J Vet Intern Med* **17**:739.

37 Rush JE, Freeman LM, Fenollosa NK *et al.* (2002) Population and survival characteristics of cats with hypertrophic cardiomyopathy: 260 cases (1990–1999). *J Am Vet Med Assoc* **20**:202–207.

38 Helenski CA, Ross JN (1987) Platelet aggregation in feline cardiomyopathy. *J Vet Intern Med* **1**:24–28.

39 Killingsworth CR, Eyster GE, Adams T *et al.* (1986) Streptokinase treatment of cats with experimentally induced aortic thrombosis. *Am J Vet Res* **47**:1351–1359.

40 McMichael MA, Freeman LM, Selhub FJ *et al.* (2000) Plasma homocysteine, B vitamins, and amino acid concentrations in cats with cardiomyopathy and arterial thromboembolism. *J Vet Intern Med* **14**:507–512.

41 Smith SA, Tobias AH, Jacob KA *et al.* (2003) Arterial thromboembolism in cats: acute crisis in 127 cases (1992–2001) and long-term management with low-dose aspirin in 24 cases. *J Vet Intern Med* **17**:73–83.

42 Boswood A, Lamb CR, White RN (2000) Aortic and iliac thrombosis in six dogs. *J Small Anim Pract* **41**:109–114.

43 Carter WO (1990) Aortic thromboembolism as a complication of gastric dilatation/volvulus in a dog. *J Am Vet Med Assoc* **196**:1829–1830.

44 Ware WA, Fenner WR (1988) Arterial thromboembolic disease in a dog with blastomycosis localized in a hilar lymph node. *J Am Vet Med Assoc* **193**:847–849.

45 Zandvliet MMJM, Stokhof AA, Boroffka S *et al.* (2005) Intermittent claudication in an Afghan hound due to aortic arteriosclerosis. *J Vet Intern Med* **19**:259–261.

46 Liu SK, Tilley LP, Tappe JP, *et al.* (1986) Clinical and pathologic findings in dogs with atherosclerosis: 21 cases (1970–1983). *J Am Vet Med Assoc* **189**:227–232.

47 Scott-Moncrieff JCR, Snyder PW, Glickman LT *et al.* (1992) Systemic necrotizing vasculitis in nine young Beagles. *J Am Vet Med Assoc* **201**:1553–1558.

48 Fox PR (1999) Feline cardiomyopathies: arterial thromboembolism. In: *Textbook of Canine and Feline Cardiology*, 2nd edn. PR Fox, D Sisson, NS Moise (eds). WB Saunders, Philadelphia, pp. 658–667.

49 Kidd L, Stepien RL, Amrheiw DP (2000) Clinical findings and coronary artery disease in dogs and cats with acute and subacute myocardial necrosis: 28 cases. *J Am Anim Hosp Assoc* **36**:199–208.

50 LaRue MJ, Murtaugh RJ (1990) Pulmonary thromboembolism in dogs: 47 cases (1986–987). *J Am Vet Med Assoc* **197**:68–1372.

51 Baines EA, Watson PJ, Stidworthy MF *et al.* (2001) Gross pulmonary thrombosis in a greyhound. *J Small Anim Pract* **42**:448–452.

52 Keyes ML, Rush JE, Knowles KE (1993) Pulmonary thromboembolism in dogs. *J Vet Emerg Crit Care* **3**:23–32.

53 Heseltine JC, Panciera DL, Saunders GK (2003) Systemic candidiasis in a dog. *J Am Vet Med Assoc* **223**:821–824.

54 Johnson LR, Lappin MR, Baker DC (1999) Pulmonary thrombo-embolism in 29 dogs:1985–1995. *J Vet Intern Med* **13**:338–345.

55 Schermerhorn TS, Pembleton-Corbett JR, Kornreich B (2004)

Pulmonary thromboembolism in cats. *J Vet Intern Med* 18:533–535.

56 Norris CR, Griffey SM, Samii VF (1999) Pulmonary thromboembolism in cats: 29 cases (1987–1997). *J Am Vet Med Assoc* 215:1650–1654.

57 Sottiaux J, Franck M (1999) Pulmonary embolism and cor pulmonale in a cat. *J Small Anim Pract* 40:88–91.

58 Van Winkle TJ, Bruce E (1993) Thrombosis of the portal vein in eleven dogs. *Vet Pathol* 30:28–35.

59 Lamb CR, Wrigley RH, Simpson KW *et al.* (1996) Ultrasonographic diagnosis of portal vein thrombosis in four dogs. *Vet Radiol Ultrasound* 37:121–129.

60 Diaz Espineira MM, Vink-Nooteboom M, Van den Ingh TSGAM *et al.* (1999) Thrombosis of the portal vein in a Miniature Schnauzer. *J Small Anim Pract* 40:540–543.

61 Moore KE, Morris N, Dhupa N *et al.* (2000) Retrospective study of streptokinase administration in 46 cats with arterial thromboembolism. *J Vet Emerg Crit Care* 10:245–257.

62 Schoeman JP (1999) Feline distal aortic thromboembolism: a review of 44 cases (1990–1998). *J Feline Med Surg* 1:221–231.

63 Feldman BF, Kirby R, Caldin M (2000) Recognition and treatment of disseminated intravascular coagulation. In: *Kirk's Current Veterinary Therapy XIII*. JD Bonagura (ed). WB Saunders, Philadelphia, pp. 190–194.

64 Otto CM, Rieser TM, Brooks MB, *et al.* (2000) Evidence of hypercoagulability in dogs with parvoviral enteritis. *J Am Vet Med Assoc* 217:1500–1504.

65 Scott-Moncrieff JC, Treadwell NG, McCullough SM *et al.* (2001) Hemostatic abnormalities in dogs with primary immune-mediated hemolytic anemia. *J Am Anim Hosp Assoc* 37:220–227.

66 Rossmeisl JH (2003) Current principles and applications of D-dimer analysis in small animal practice. *Vet Med* 98:224–234.

67 Harpster NK, Baty CJ (1995) Warfarin therapy of the cat at risk of thromboembolism. In: *Kirk's Current Veterinary Therapy XII*. JD Bonagura (ed). WB Saunders, Philadelphia, pp. 868–873.

68 Fluckiger MA, Gomez JA (1984) Radiographic findings in dogs with spontaneous pulmonary thrombosis or embolism. *Vet Radiol* 25:124–131.

69 Daniel GB, Wantschek L, Bright R *et al.* (1990) Diagnosis of aortic thromboembolism in two dogs with radionuclide angiography. *Vet Radiol* 31:182–185.

70 Pouchelon J-L, Chetboul V, Devauchelle P *et al.* (1997) Diagnosis of pulmonary thromboembolism in a cat using electrocardiography and pulmonary scintigraphy. *J Small Anim Pract* 38:306–310.

71 Hogan DF, Andrews DA, Green HW *et al.* (2004) Antiplatelet effects and pharmacodynamics of clopidogrel in cats. *J Am Vet Med Assoc* 225:1406–1411.

72 Hogan DF, Andrews DA, Talbott KK *et al.* (2004) Evaluation of antiplatelet effects of ticlopidine in cats. *Am J Vet Res* 65:327–332.

73 Bright JM, Dowers K, Powers BE (2003) Effects of the glycoprotein IIb/IIIa antagonist abciximab on thrombus formation and platelet function in cats with arterial injury. *Vet Ther* 4:35–46.

74 Bright JM, Dowers K, Hellyer P (2002) *In vitro* anti-aggregatory effects of the GP IIb/IIIa antagonist eptifibatide on feline platelets. Letter. *J Vet Intern Med* 16:v.

75 Weitz JI (1997) Low-molecular-weight heparins. *N Eng J Med* 337:688–698.

76 Mischke RH, Schuettert C, Grebe SI (2001) Anticoagulant effects of repeated subcutaneous injections of high doses of unfractionated heparin in healthy dogs. *Am J Vet Res* 62:1887–1891.

77 Smith CE, Rozanski EA, Freeman LM *et al.* (2004) Use of low molecular weight heparin in cats: 57 cases (1999–2003). *J Am Vet Med Assoc* 225:1237–1241.

78 Dunn M, Charland V, Thorneloe C (2004) The use of a low molecular weight heparin in 6 dogs. Abstract. *J Vet Intern Med* 18:389.

79 Thompson MF, Scott-Moncrieff JC, Hogan DF (2001) Thrombolytic therapy in dogs and cats. *J Vet Emerg Crit Care* 11:111–121.

80 Clare AC, Kraje BJ (1998) Use of recombinant tissue-plasminogen activator for aortic thrombolysis in a hypoproteinemic dog. *J Am Vet Med Assoc* 212:539–543.

81 Ramsey CC, Burney DP, Macintire DK *et al.* (1996) Use of streptokinase in four dogs with thrombosis. *J Am Vet Med Assoc* 209:780–785.

82 Pion PD, Kittleson MD (1989) Therapy for feline aortic thromboembolism. In: *Current Veterinary Therapy X*. RW Kirk (ed). WB Saunders, Philadelphia, pp. 295–301.

83 Monnet E, Morgan MR (2000) Effect of three loading doses of warfarin on the international normalized ratio for dogs. *Am J Vet Res* 61:48–50.

16
Management of Heart Failure

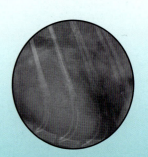

OVERVIEW

Heart failure is traditionally considered to occur when the heart either cannot provide blood flow adequate for metabolic demands or when it can do so only at elevated filling pressures. High cardiac filling pressure leads to the venous congestion and fluid accumulation that characterize congestive heart failure (CHF). CHF is a complex clinical syndrome rather than an etiologic diagnosis. It results from (over)expression of compensatory neurohormonal (NH) and other responses to an underlying cardiac injury or abnormality. Abnormal systolic (pumping) or diastolic (filling) function can lead to CHF.

While poor myocardial contractility often underlies CHF, chronic cardiac overload or injury from other causes can also initiate the cascade of NH and cardiac responses that ultimately produce circulatory congestion and further myocardial functional impairment. The development of CHF is described in three phases: 1) an initiating (and often undetected) cardiac injury or insult; 2) a phase of compensation, but with clinically silent progression; and 3) the onset of clinical CHF signs. For most veterinary patients, heart disease is identified only late in this process.

APPROACH TO HEART FAILURE MANAGEMENT

While some treatment principles are common to most causes of CHF, it is helpful to consider the functional abnormality(ies) present in an individual. The predominant or initiating pathophysiology usually involves either primary myocardial failure, volume (flow) overload, systolic pressure overload, or reduced ventricular compliance (impaired filling). Most causes of CHF can be grouped into one of these four categories. Nevertheless, the distinctions between them blur with disease progression, and patients with advanced heart failure develop features of several pathophysiologic categories.

Most current strategies for managing heart failure are aimed at modifying either the results of NH activation (e.g. Na$^+$ and water retention) or the activation process itself (e.g. ACE inhibition).

Emerging treatment strategies also focus on preventing or reversing pathologic cardiac remodeling and improving myocardial function. Whether a particular therapy increases survival as well as improves function and quality of life is a major impetus behind ongoing research. In general, current CHF therapy centers on controlling edema and effusions, improving cardiac output, reducing cardiac workload, supporting myocardial function, and managing concurrent arrhythmias or other complications. The approach to these goals varies somewhat with different diseases, most notably those that impair ventricular filling (see Chapters 21 and 22). So it is important to define the underlying cause of CHF and its associated pathophysiology, as well as any complicating factors. Besides arrhythmias, the latter often include azotemia, electrolyte abnormalities, and concurrent noncardiac disease.

Circulating concentrations of various neuro-hormones and other substances rise with CHF and/or cardiac damage. Assessment of plasma natriuretic peptides, cardiac troponins, and other substances has the potential to provide diagnostic and prognostic information, as well as to guide therapy. Exploration in this area is ongoing in both human and veterinary medicine. Measurement of specific cardiac and NH biomarkers will likely become an increasingly important clinical tool in dogs and cats.

PATHOPHYSIOLOGY OF HEART FAILURE

GENERAL PATHOPHYSIOLOGIC CATEGORIES

Primary myocardial failure is characterized by poor contractility (systolic dysfunction). The affected ventricle progressively dilates, and AV valve insufficiency usually develops as a consequence. Dilated cardiomyopathy (DCM) is the most common cause in animals (see Chapters 20 and 21). Long-standing tachyarrhythmias and some nutritional or metabolic deficiencies (see Chapters 20 and 21), as well as cardiac inflammation, infection, or infarction, also lead to myocardial failure.

Heart disease producing a ventricular volume overload usually involves a primary 'plumbing' problem (i.e. an incompetent valve or abnormal systemic-to-pulmonary shunt). A chronic high-output state (e.g. hyperthyroidism or anemia) can also underlie this. Cardiac pump function is often maintained near normal for a long time, but myocardial contractility eventually deteriorates. Chronic degenerative AV valve disease and, less often, mitral or aortic valve endocarditis in dogs (see Chapter 19), and some congenital malformations (see Chapter 18), are the usual causes of volume overload CHF.

Pressure overload occurs when the ventricle must generate greater than normal systolic pressure to eject blood. Common causes of ventricular pressure overload include stenosis of the pulmonic or (sub)aortic valve regions (see Chapter 18), pulmonary hypertension (see Chapters 23 and 24), and systemic hypertension (see Chapter 25). An excessive systolic pressure load stimulates concentric hypertrophy (see Chapter 1, p. 18) but also increases ventricular wall stiffness and can predispose to ischemia. Myocardial contractility eventually declines as well.

Impaired ventricular filling (diastolic dysfunction) results from hypertrophic and restrictive cardiomyopathies (see Chapters 21 and 20, p. 292) as well as pericardial diseases (see Chapter 22). Contractility is initially normal in most of these cases; however, elevated ventricular filling pressure leads to congestion behind the affected ventricle and may diminish cardiac output.

CARDIAC RESPONSES

The development of heart failure involves structural and functional changes in myocardial cells, vascular cells, and the extracellular matrix, as well as multiple systemic compensatory mechanisms. Progressive alterations in cardiac size and shape (remodeling) occur in response to mechanical, biochemical, and molecular signals that are induced by injury or stress[1, 2]. Valvular disease, genetic mutations, acute inflammation, ischemia, increased systolic pressure load, and other events can initiate this process. The triggering stimulus as well as the resulting cardiac hypertrophy and remodeling begin long before heart failure becomes manifest[1].

Ventricular remodeling can involve myocardial hypertrophy, cardiac cell loss or self-destruction (apoptosis), excessive interstitial matrix formation, and loss of normal collagen binding between individual myocytes[1, 2]. The latter (from the effects of myocardial collagenases or matrix metalloproteinases) promotes ventricular dilation and distortion from slippage of adjacent myocytes. Increased chamber size increases wall stress and myocardial O_2 demand. Stimuli for remodeling include mechanical forces (e.g. increased wall stress from volume or pressure overload), various neurohormones (e.g. AT II, NE,

aldosterone [ALD], and endothelin), and proinflammatory cytokines such as TNF, interleukins (ILs), and other factors[1, 3, 4]. Biochemical abnormalities of oxidative phosphorylation, high-energy phosphate metabolism, Ca^{++} fluxes, contractile proteins, protein synthesis, and catecholamine metabolism have also been identified in different heart failure models and in clinical patients.

Increased ventricular filling (preload) causes greater contraction force and stroke volume by the Frank–Starling mechanism (see Chapter 1 p. 17). This allows beat-to-beat adjustments, which balance RV and LV output and increase overall cardiac output when hemodynamic load rises. Causes of increased cardiac load include valvular insufficiency, arterial hypertension, and outflow obstruction. Although the Frank–Starling effect helps normalize cardiac output when pressure or volume load is increased, ventricular wall stress and O_2 consumption also rise. Wall stress is related directly to ventricular pressure and internal dimensions, and inversely to wall thickness (Laplace's law; Chapter 1, p. 18). Compensatory myocardial hypertrophy reduces wall stress and lessens the importance of the Frank–Starling mechanism in stable, chronic heart failure. The pattern of hypertrophy depends on the underlying cardiac disease: increased systolic pressure load stimulates 'concentric' hypertrophy, but volume loading promotes 'eccentric' hypertrophy and chamber dilation. Abnormal pressure and volume loads both impair cardiac performance over time. Volume loads are better tolerated because myocardial O_2 demand is not as severe; however, decompensation and myocardial failure eventually develop. In primary myocardial disease, loading conditions are initially normal. Intrinsic myocardial defect(s) lead to the hypertrophy and dilation observed, although secondary alterations in preload and afterload can contribute.

Myocyte hypertrophy and reactive fibrosis increase total cardiac mass and also ventricular stiffness. This promotes elevated filling pressures[1]. Hypertrophy predisposes to ischemia as the relative density of capillaries and mitochondria becomes reduced. Impaired relaxation and further fibrosis, ventricular stiffness, and diastolic dysfunction are consequences. Diastolic abnormalities result from delayed or incomplete (active) relaxation in early diastole, reduced passive compliance (see Chapter 1, p. 17), and external constraint caused by pericardial disease (see Chapter 22). Such diastolic function abnormalities can also contribute to systolic dysfunction. Clinical heart failure can be viewed as a state of decompensated hypertrophy, in which ventricular function progressively deteriorates as contractility and relaxation become more abnormal. Ventricular remodeling also promotes the development of arrhythmias.

NEUROHORMONAL MECHANISMS

Major NH changes in heart failure include increased sympathetic nervous tone, attenuated vagal tone, renin-angiotensin-aldosterone system (RAAS) activation, and release of antidiuretic hormone (ADH), also known as arginine vasopressin (AVP)[1, 5–10]. These NH systems work independently and together to increase vascular volume (by Na^+ and water retention and increased thirst) and vascular tone. Although these mechanisms support the circulation in the face of acute hypotension and hypovolemia, their chronic activation is maladaptive. Excessive volume retention causes edema and effusions. Systemic vasoconstriction increases cardiac workload and can reduce forward cardiac output and exacerbate valvular regurgitation. More importantly, these mechanisms accelerate cardiac function deterioration and pathologic remodeling. Increased production of endothelins and proinflammatory cytokines, as well as altered expression of vasodilatory and natriuretic factors, contribute to the complex interplay among these NH mechanisms and their consequences. The extent to which different NH mechanisms are activated varies with the severity and etiology of heart failure; however, in general, their intensity increases as failure worsens. NH activation is initially selective and regional; generalized activation is a late occurrence. Increased cardiac and renal sympathetic activity and natriuretic peptide release occurs initially with asymptomatic left ventricular dysfunction[2, 11]. This precedes congestive signs. While the initial stimulus for NH activation is unclear, it is thought that stimulation of low-pressure cardiac receptors, ventricular dilation, and early cardiac remodeling increase sympathetic afferent activity, which then initiates the NH activation process, rather than low cardiac output or effective circulating blood volume being the initial activator; however, reduced cardiac output and arterial baroreceptor unloading eventually lead to systemic NH activation and are late consequences of CHF[2]. Increased sympathetic (and decreased parasympathetic) tone increases heart rate, contractility, and relaxation rate, thereby raising cardiac output; however, chronic sympathetic stimulation has detrimental effects related to greater myocardial afterload stress and O_2 demand, cellular damage, myocardial remodeling and fibrosis, and enhanced potential for cardiac arrhythmias[1, 10, 12]. Diminished heart rate variability is another manifestation of high sympathetic tone. Norepinephrine (NE) promotes arrhythmias by increasing automaticity among other electro-physiologic effects[12]. NE, via beta$_1$-receptor activation, increases cyclic adenosine monophosphate (cAMP) production and intracellular Ca^{++} concentrations. Prolonged and excessive exposure can cause calcium overload and cell necrosis. NE can also stimulate

growth and increase oxidative stress which can promote apoptosis[11]. NE's peripheral vasoconstrictive effect as well as its renal effects to promote volume retention lead to increased ventricular size and pressure, which also raise myocardial O_2 demand. Increased NE release from sympathetic nerve terminals causes some NE spillover into the circulation. High circulating NE levels have been correlated with CHF severity and a worse prognosis[7, 10, 13, 14]. Chronic catecholamine exposure leads to reduced myocardial beta$_1$-receptor density (down-regulation), uncoupling of beta$_2$-receptors from G-regulatory protein complex, and other changes in cellular signaling that decrease myocardial sensitivity to changes in adrenergic tone[13–15]. Myocardial beta$_1$-receptor down-regulation may be a protective mechanism against the cardiotoxic and arrhyth-mogenic effects of catecholamines. But cardiac beta$_2$- and alpha$_1$-receptors are not down-regulated. These can also contribute to myocardial remodeling and arrhythmogenesis; cardiac beta$_3$-receptors may contribute to declining myocardial function by their negative inotropic effect[16].

The RAAS also has far-reaching effects. Renin is released from the renal juxtaglomerular apparatus in response to several stimuli, including renal beta$_1$-adrenergic stimulation, low perfusion pressure, and reduced Na^+ delivery to the macula densa of the distal renal tubule. Stringent dietary salt restriction and diuretic or vasodilator therapy also promote renin release[17]. Renin facilitates conversion of the precursor peptide AT (formed in the liver) to AT I. Angiotensin-converting enzyme (ACE), found in the lung and elsewhere, converts this inactive peptide into the active AT II[18, 19]. ACE also degrades certain vasodilator kinins, including bradykinin. Additionally, there are other pathways that generate AT II as well as the less potent peptide, AT III[10].

AT II is a potent vasoconstrictor that also causes Na^+ and water retention by a direct effect on the proximal tubule and by stimulating ALD release from the adrenal cortex[20]. The effects of AT II are mediated by AT1 receptors. Additional effects of AT II include increased thirst and salt appetite, enhanced neuronal NE synthesis and release, neuronal NE reuptake blockade, enhanced ADH/AVP release, and increased adrenal epinephrine secretion. Thus, inhibition of ACE can reduce NH activation as well as promote vasodilation and diuresis. Local AT II production also occurs in the heart, blood vessels, adrenal glands, and other tissues. This local activity affects cardiovascular structure and function by enhancing sympathetic effects and promoting tissue remodeling, including hypertrophy, inflammation, and fibrosis[10].

ALD secretion in CHF is stimulated by AT II, hyperkalemia, and chronically high plasma corticotrophin. Less important in increasing ALD release are circulating catecholamines, endothelins, and ADH/AVP[9, 10]. ALD promotes Na^+ and Cl^- reabsorption as well as K^+ and H^+ secretion in the renal collecting tubules; concurrent water reabsorption augments vascular volume[20]. Increased ALD can promote hypokalemia and hypomagnesemia. ALD also interferes with baroreceptor function in CHF. ALD is also produced locally in the cardiovascular system and mediates inflammation and fibrosis. Chronic ALD exposure has detrimental effects on ventricular function. It contributes to pathologic remodeling, inhibits myocardial NE uptake, and promotes myocardial fibrosis[10, 17]. Other ALD effects include vascular (e.g. coronary, renal) remodeling and fibrosis, and endothelial cell dysfunction. Reduced hepatic perfusion slows the clearance of ALD.

There is controversy as to whether the RAAS is activated systemically before overt CHF occurs[10, 21-23]. Plasma renin activity and ALD are not increased in all patients with CHF[19], and such increases can occur with mitral valve prolapse rather than MR *per se*[22, 24]. Furthermore, ACE inhibition may not prevent volume overload myocardial hypertrophy in dogs[25]; however, RAAS activation has been shown in animals with CHF caused by DCM, especially after diuretic therapy[6, 8, 26, 27].

ADH/AVP is another endogenous vasoconstrictor that also increases free water reabsorption in the distal nephron. Provasopressin, which is synthesized by neurons in the hypothalamus, is converted to ADH/AVP within transport vesicles. These become secretory granules in nerve endings within the posterior pituitary. V1A receptors in the vasculature and heart mediate the vasoconstrictive and inotropic effects of ADH/AVP. V2 receptors in the kidney mediate water reabsorption[10]. Although increased plasma osmolality or low blood volume are the normal stimuli for ADH/AVP release, reduced effective circulating volume and other nonosmotic stimuli (e.g. AT II and sympathetic stimulation) cause its continued production in CHF. Excessive ADH/AVP contributes to dilutional hyponatremia in some animals with severe CHF. ADH/AVP structure is highly conserved among people, dogs, and cats.

Normal feedback regulation of the sympathetic nervous and hormonal systems depends on arterial and atrial baroreceptor function, but baroreceptor responsiveness becomes attenuated in chronic heart failure. This contributes to sustained sympathetic and hormonal activation and reduced inhibitory vagal effects. Baroreceptor dysfunction can improve, with reversal of heart failure, increased myocardial contractility, decreased cardiac loading conditions, or inhibition of AT II, which directly attenuates baroreceptor sensitivity. Digoxin has a positive effect on baroreceptor sensitivity.

Endothelin (ET)-1 is one of several ETs produced by the vascular endothelium. The normal function of these vasoconstrictor peptides is to maintain vascular tone in opposition to endothelial-derived vasodilators (nitric oxide [NO] and prostacyclin). ET-1 is produced in a series of steps leading to conversion from an inactive precursor (proendothelin or 'big' endothelin) to the active ET-1 via endothelin-converting enzyme. ET production is stimulated by hypoxia and vascular mechanical factors, but also by AT II, ADH/AVP, NE, bradykinin, and cytokines, including TNF and IL-1[10]. ET-1 acts on two receptors, ET_A and ET_B. ET_A mediates smooth muscle vasoconstriction, increased myocardial contractility, ALD secretion, and renin suppression. Circulating ET (and pro-ET) are increased in dogs, cats, and people with CHF as well as pulmonary hypertension[10, 28, 29]. Chronically increased ET-1 promotes vascular smooth muscle and myocardial hypertrophy and so contributes to remodeling[10]. ET-1 is highly conserved across species.

Cytokines are endogenous peptides that act as autocrine and paracrine mediators. They are also involved in modulating cardiovascular structure and function. Increased circulating levels are seen in CHF and their overexpression contributes to heart failure progression. Chronic increases in sympathetic activity, AT II, and ALD stimulate further cytokine production, although the initiating stimulus is unknown[30]. TNF is a proinflammatory cytokine that additionally has negative inotropic effects and contributes to remodeling, hypertrophy, and apoptosis. TNF is produced by the heart, macrophages, and other tissues in response to stress. While this is initially an adaptive and protective response after ischemia and hemodynamic overload, the response becomes maladaptive over time. Exuberant production in the heart spills over and can cause secondary circulatory immune stimulating effects. Proinflammatory cytokines stimulate production of large amounts of NO by increased inducible-NO synthetase (NOS) expression. This has negative inotropic and cytotoxic effects on the myocardium[30, 31].

Endogenous mechanisms, which oppose the vasoconstrictor neurohormones, are also invoked with cardiac dysfunction. These include the natriuretic peptides, NO, which is important in the physiologic regulation of vascular tone, and vasodilator prostaglandins; however, the influence of the vasoconstrictor mechanisms becomes predominant as heart failure progresses, despite increased activation of vasodilator mechanisms. Natriuretic peptides synthesized in the heart play an important physiologic role in regulating blood volume and pressure. Atrial natriuretic peptide (ANP) and, to a minor degree, brain natriuretic peptide (BNP) are produced by atrial myocytes as preprohormones. Mechanical stretch of the atrial wall stimulates their release. With myocardial dysfunction the cardiac ventricles become the main source of BNP[10, 32]. Other natriuretic peptides have been identified as well. Natriuretic peptides promote diuresis, natriuresis, and peripheral vasodilation. They antagonize the effects of the RAAS, but can also alter vascular permeability and inhibit smooth muscle cell growth[33]. Natriuretic peptides are degraded by neutral endopeptidases. Circulating concentrations of ANP and BNP increase in patients with heart failure. Their elevation has been correlated with pulmonary capillary wedge pressure and heart failure severity in dogs as well as in people [11, 33–35].

NO (also known as endothelium-derived relaxing factor) is an important functional antagonist of ET and AT II. It is expressed in vascular endothelium and in the myocardium. Endothelial release of NO (via endothelial-NOS) is impaired in CHF. Concurrently, myocardial NO release is enhanced because of increased inducible-NOS expression. The consequences of this are reduced vasodilatory capacity, negative inotropic and chronotropic effects, and myocyte damage[36, 37].

Vasodilatory prostaglandins are produced to a much greater degree in the renal glomerular afferent (compared with the efferent) arterioles. By this means, they attenuate AT II's vasoconstrictive effects on afferent (but not efferent) arterioles. The use of prostaglandin synthesis inhibitors in severe heart failure could increase afferent arteriolar resistance and thereby reduce glomerular filtration and renal blood flow, as well as enhance Na^+ retention[20]; however, the clinical significance of this in dogs and cats is not known. Adrenomedullin is another peptide with natriuretic and vasodilating effects. Increased release occurs with inflammation and other stimuli. Elevated circulating levels have been observed in people with CHF[10, 36].

RENAL RESPONSES

The balance (or imbalance) between vasoconstrictive /volume retentive stimuli and vasodilatory/natriuretic factors is reflected by the kidney. Renal efferent glomerular arteriolar constriction, mediated by sympathetic stimulation and AT II, helps maintain glomerular filtration when cardiac output and renal blood flow are reduced. The higher oncotic and lower hydrostatic pressures that develop in the peritubular capillaries enhance fluid and Na^+ reabsorption. AT II also promotes renal cortical blood flow redistribution toward the juxtomedullary regions, where longer loops of Henle penetrate more deeply into the hypertonic medullary region. This promotes greater Na^+ and water reabsorption[20]. AT II-induced ALD release stimulates further Na^+ and water retention. Afferent arteriolar vasodilation, mediated by intrarenal vasodilator prostaglandins and natriuretic peptides, can partially offset the

effects of strong efferent vasoconstriction[1]. However, progressive reduction in renal blood flow leads to renal insufficiency. Diuretic use can magnify azotemia and electrolyte loss, further reducing circulating volume and cardiac output, and exacerbating NH activation[1].

EXERCISE CAPACITY

Reduced exercise capacity as well as skeletal muscle atrophy occur with heart failure[38, 39]. Poor diastolic filling, inadequate forward cardiac output, and impaired pulmonary function from edema or pleural effusion can certainly interfere with exercise ability; however, abnormal peripheral vasodilatory responses also contribute to inadequate skeletal muscle perfusion and fatigue during exercise. Altered skeletal muscle metabolism secondary to chronic physical deconditioning may contribute to fatigue[38, 39]. High sympathetic tone, AT II (both circulating and locally produced), and ADH/AVP can contribute to impaired skeletal muscle vasodilatory capacity in chronic heart failure. Increased vascular wall Na^+ content and interstitial fluid pressure cause vascular stiffening and compression; however, impaired endothelium-dependent relaxation, increased ET levels, and vascular wall remodeling induced by the growth factor effects of various NH vasoconstrictors are also implicated. Normal physiologic production of endothelial-dependent NO (mediated by endothelial-NOS) is down-regulated in CHF. This contributes to endothelial dysfunction and reduced responsiveness in exercise[31]. Treatment with an ACE inhibitor, with or without spironolactone, may improve endothelial vasomotor function and exercise capacity. Pulmonary endothelial function is improved by ACE inhibitors in dogs with CHF[40].

CLINICAL MANIFESTATIONS OF CONGESTIVE HEART FAILURE

PRESENTING SIGNS

The clinical signs of CHF result largely from chronic NH activation (*Table 41*). Excessive volume retention and elevated ventricular filling pressure cause congestion ('backward' failure), manifested as edema and body cavity effusions (see Chapter 2 and *Table 1*, p. 26). Pulmonary venous congestion and edema are characteristic of left-sided CHF. Signs typical for right-sided CHF commonly occur with biventricular failure as well as pure right heart disease. Additional information can be found in Chapters 8–12, which focus on clinical problems that can arise from CHF, as well as other diseases.

Low cardiac output ('forward' failure) can cause such signs as weakness, prerenal azotemia, and syncope (see *Table 1*, p. 26 and Chapter 15). Profoundly

Table 41 Typical presentation for common causes of chronic heart failure.

Left-sided CHF signs*	Either left- or right-sided CHF signs	Right-sided CHF signs
Myocardial failure		
Drug toxicities (e.g. doxorubicin)	Idiopathic DCM	
Myocardial ischemia/infarction	Infective myocarditis	
Volume-flow overload		
Mitral endocardiosis	Chronic anemia	Tricuspid endocardiosis
Mitral/aortic endocarditis	Thyrotoxicosis	Tricuspid endocarditis
Ventricular septal defect		Tricuspid dysplasia
Patent ductus arteriosus		
Mitral dysplasia		
Pressure overload		
(Sub)aortic stenosis		Pulmonic stenosis
Systemic hypertension		Pulmonary hypertension
		Heartworm disease
Restriction to ventricular filling		
Hypertrophic cardiomyopathy		Cardiac tamponade
Restrictive cardiomyopathy		Constrictive pericardial disease

*See *Table 1*, p. 26 for clinical signs characteristic of left-sided and right-sided congestion as well as low cardiac output.

impaired cardiac pumping ability leads to cardiogenic shock; severe DCM is the most common cause in veterinary patients. Other causes besides severe myocardial dysfunction include acute valve disruption with massive regurgitation, sustained and severe brady- or tachyarrhythmias, overdose of hypotensive or negative inotropic drug, especially with preexisting cardiac disease, and intracardiac flow obstruction (e.g. heartworm caval syndrome or intracardiac tumor). Extracardiac causes of blood flow obstruction (e.g. cardiac tamponade, pulmonary hypertension, or massive pulmonary embolism) can also severely reduce cardiac output. Acute myocardial infarction is a rare cause of cardiogenic shock in animals. Signs of cardiogenic shock relate to low cardiac output, arterial hypotension, and the compensatory mechanisms activated to increase vascular volume and pressure. Evidence of the animal's underlying disease (e.g. murmur, gallop sound, arrhythmia, muffled sounds) as well as congestive signs are also likely.

DIAGNOSIS

Identification of the underlying etiology leading to CHF, as well as any complicating factors, is important in the individual animal. The diagnostic process involves the cardiovascular examination (see Chapter 2) as well as additional graphical testing (see Chapters 3–5) to explore the basis for any clinical problems (see Chapters 6–15). Other chapters, or chapter, related to the suspected underlying disease provide additional information useful in diagnosis and management.

Routine clinical laboratory test results are often nonspecific, but they can reveal evidence of low cardiac output (e.g. prerenal azotemia), systemic congestion (e.g. mild liver enzyme elevation), or concurrent noncardiac disease. Prerenal azotemia, mild electrolyte abnormalities, and, sometimes, mild anemia occur more commonly with DCM. Dilutional hyponatremia and hypoproteinemia can develop with chronic heart failure; when marked or progressive these are negative prognostic signs. Animals with severe myocardial failure occasionally present with hyperkalemia, hyponatremia, and azotemia that mimics hypoadrenocorticism. Primary renal disease and the effects of drug therapy often contribute to biochemical abnormalities. Nonspecific markers of cardiac injury, such as CK, aspartate dehydrogenase, lactate dehydrogenase, and myoglobin, become elevated after severe myocardial necrosis, but they also increase with liver or skeletal muscle injury and other conditions[41]. The more cardiac-specific isoenzyme of CK (CK-MB) is found mainly in the myocardial cytosol; synthesis increases after cardiac injury. Nevertheless, CK-MB is relatively nonspecific in that it is also produced by skeletal muscle and other tissues. Furthermore, CK-MB is not well-conserved among species and human assays are not recommended[36].

CARDIAC BIOMARKERS

More specific biochemical markers of cardiac injury are being evaluated for their potential to provide diagnostic and prognostic information. Circulating concentrations of cardiac troponin (cTn) proteins I (cTnI) and T (cTnT) provide a specific indicator of myocardial cell injury[36]. The troponin proteins (I, T, and C) are attached to the thin filaments of the contractile apparatus; cTnI inhibits binding of Ca^{++} to cTnC (and thus actin–myosin interaction) during diastole. Serum levels of cTnI and cTnT are normally very low. Cardiac membrane damage and cell necrosis cause cTn release into the circulation[36, 41–47]. The pattern of release depends on the type and severity of myocyte injury[36]. With acute injury, the degree of myocardial damage is associated with serum cTn elevation, but in chronic heart disease this association is less clear[36]. Minimal cTn elevation may also occur after strenuous exercise or noncardiac disease[36]. After myocyte damage, serum cTn increases within 4 hours; this peaks within 12–24 hours, then declines over 1–3 weeks[41]. Increased cTn concentrations have been found with myocardial inflammation, trauma, CHF, hypertrophic cardiomyopathy (HCM), and also gastric dilatation/volvulus[41, 44, 45, 47–50]. cTn elevation with CHF and HCM is consistent with a process of continued myocardial remodeling, not just acute damage from myocardial infarction. cTnI appears to be more specific than cTnT[41, 51, 52]. In a recent study the highest concentrations of cTnI were found in dogs with CHF. Variable elevation was seen with different cardiac diseases, but in the absence of CHF there was overlap with control dogs[41]. Human assays for cTnI and cTnT can be used in dogs and cats; however, nonstandardized methodology among various cTnI assays results in variable cut-off values for normal[36, 53, 54]. Furthermore, cTn values that indicate clinically relevant myocardial disease or damage in animals are unclear.

Other biomarkers that may become useful in assessing the presence and possibly prognosis of CHF in individuals include the natriuretic peptides ANP and, especially in cats, BNP[11, 21, 26, 33–35, 55–57]. Circulating natriuretic peptide levels rise when vascular volume is increased, renal clearance is decreased, and production is stimulated (e.g. with ventricular strain and hypertrophy, hypoxia, or tachycardia). The natriuretic peptides could serve more as functional markers of cardiac disease, rather than of specific pathology; however, at present, standardization among different commercial assays and methodologies, and universal reference values, are lacking. The N-terminal fragments (NT-proANP and NT-proBNP) of the natriuretic peptide precursor molecules remain in circulation longer and reach higher plasma levels than the active hormone molecules[10, 36]. ANP and NT-proANP amino acid sequences are highly conserved among people, dogs, and cats, so human assays can be used[10, 36]; however, although canine and feline BNP are similar to each other, differences from people preclude the use of most human BNP assays[10]. Circulating BNP levels respond more slowly and fluctuate less than ANP[36].

Plasma BNP and NT-proBNP are considered sensitive and specific markers for chronic left ventricular dysfunction in people, and high concentrations are negatively correlated with prognosis. BNP as well as NT-proANP seem to be elevated in cats with hypertrophic cardiomyopathy[10]. The potential utility of plasma natriuretic peptides in dogs with cardiac disease is unclear, but plasma NT-proANP concentration may be a more useful marker than BNP in this species[6, 10, 33–35, 55].

Other biomarkers are being explored. Because the ET system is activated in dogs and cats with CHF, as well as pulmonary hypertension, assays for plasma ET-like immunoreactivity may have future usefulness[28, 36]. TNF may also be a useful marker of cardiac disease progression, but it is not cardiac specific.

CLASSIFICATION OF HEART FAILURE

The clinical severity of heart failure is sometimes described according to a modified New York Heart Association (NYHA) classification scheme or the International Small Animal Cardiac Health Council (ISACHC) criteria (*Table 42*)[30]. These systems group patients into functional categories based on clinical observations rather than underlying cardiac disease or myocardial function. Such classification can be helpful conceptually and for categorizing study patients. However, identifying underlying etiology and pathophysiology as well as CHF severity is also important for individual therapy. Newer guidelines for clinical staging of heart failure (based on the American Heart Association and American College of Cardiology [AHA/ACC] system) are also being applied to veterinary patients and these describe progression through four stages over time. This staging system emphasizes the importance of early diagnosis and evidence-based management of heart dysfunction. It also deemphasizes the term 'congestive' heart failure because volume overload is not consistently present at all stages, although the fluid status of the patient is highly important.

MANAGEMENT OF ACUTE DECOMPENSATED CONGESTIVE HEART FAILURE

Severe cardiogenic pulmonary edema requires urgent therapy (*Table 43*). Some patients also have body cavity effusion or poor cardiac output that must be addressed. Thoracocentesis is indicated for moderate to large volume pleural effusion to improve ventilation. Large volume ascites that impairs ventilation should also be partially drained. Curtailing the patient's physical activity helps reduce total O_2 consumption. When transported, the animal should be placed on a cart or carried. Unnecessary

Table 42 Heart failure severity classification schemes.

Modified AHA/ACC heart failure staging system

A Patient 'at risk' for the development of heart failure, but without apparent structural abnormality of the heart.

B Structural cardiac abnormality present, but no clinical signs of heart failure.

C Structural cardiac abnormality with past or present clinical heart failure signs.

D Persistent or end-stage heart failure signs, refractory to standard therapy.

Modified New York Heart Association functional classification

I Heart disease is present, but no evidence of heart failure or exercise intolerance; cardiomegaly is minimal to absent.

II Signs of heart disease with evidence of exercise intolerance; radiographic cardiomegaly is present.

III Signs of heart failure with normal activity or at night (e.g. cough, orthopnea); radiographic signs of significant cardiomegaly and pulmonary edema or pleural/abdominal effusion.

IV Severe heart failure with clinical signs at rest or with minimal activity; marked radiographic signs of CHF and cardiomegaly.

International Small Animal Cardiac Health Council functional classification

I Asymptomatic patient.

   Ia Signs of heart disease without cardiomegaly.

   Ib Signs of heart disease and evidence of compensation (cardiomegaly).

II Mild to moderate heart failure. Clinical signs of failure evident at rest or with mild exercise, and adversely affect quality of life.

III Advanced heart failure. Clinical signs of CHF are immediately obvious.

   IIIa Home care is possible.

   IIIb Hospitalization recommended (cardiogenic shock, life-threatening edema, large pleural effusion, refractory ascites).

AHA/ACC = American Heart Association and American College of Cardiology

---

Table 43 Management of acute decompensated congestive heart failure.

1) Avoid stress!

2) Provide cage rest.

3) Enhance oxygenation:

   a) Check airway patency.

   b) Give supplemental O_2 (avoid >50% for >24 hours).

   c) If frothing is evident, suction airways.

   d) Intubate and mechanically ventilate if needed.

   e) Perform thoracocentesis if pleural effusion suspected.

4) Remove alveolar fluid:

   a) Initiate diuresis:

     ■ Furosemide (dogs: 2–5 [–8] mg/kg IV or IM q1–4h until respiratory rate decreases, then 1–4 mg/kg q6–12h, or 0.6–1 mg/kg/hour CRI see p. 172; cats: 1–2 (–4) mg/kg IV or IM q1–4h until respiratory rate decreases, then q6–12h).

   b) Redistribute blood volume:

     ■ Vasodilators (sodium nitroprusside: 0.5–1 mcg/kg/minute (initial) CRI in D5W, titrate upward as needed to 5–15 mcg/kg/minute, monitor arterial pressure (see text); or 2% nitroglycerin ointment (+/- with hydralazine): dogs: 1/2–1 1/2 inch cutaneously q6h; cats: 1/4–1/2 inch cutaneously q6h.

     ■ ± morphine (dogs only, see below).

     ■ ± phlebotomy (6–10 ml/kg).

5) Reduce bronchoconstriction:

   a) Aminophylline (dogs: 4–8 mg/kg slow IV, IM, SC or 6–10 mg/kg PO q6–8h; cats: 4–8 mg/kg IM, SC, PO q8–12h) or similar drug.

6) Mild sedation to reduce anxiety:

   a) Butorphanol (dogs: 0.2–0.3 mg/kg IM; cats: 0.2–0.25 mg/kg IM); or   (continued over)

Table 43 (*continued*)

b) Morphine (dogs: 0.025–0.1 mg/kg IV boluses q2–3min to effect, or 0.1–0.5 mg/kg single IM or SC dose).

c) Acepromazine (cats: 0.05–0.2 mg/kg SC; or 0.05–0.1 mg/kg IM with butorphanol).

d) Diazepam (cats: 2–5 mg IV; dogs: 5–10 mg IV).

7) Reduce afterload:

a) Hydralazine: dogs: initial 0.5–1.0 mg/kg PO, repeat in 2–3 hours (until systolic arterial pressure is 90–110 mm Hg), then q12h (see text) (avoid nitroprusside); or

b) Enalapril (0.5 mg/kg PO q12–24h) or other ACE inhibitor (avoid nitroprusside); or

c) Amlodipine (dogs: 0.1–0.3 mg/kg PO q12–24h; see text).

8) Increase contractility (if myocardial failure present):

a) Dobutamine* (1–10 mcg/kg/minute CRI; start low), or dopamine** (dogs: 1–10 mcg/kg/min CRI; cats: 1–5 mcg/kg/min CRI; start low).

b) Amrinone (1–3 mg/kg IV; 10–100 mcg/kg/minute CRI).

c) Milrinone (50 mcg/kg IV over 10 minutes initially; 0.375–0.75 mcg/kg/minute CRI [human dose]).

d) Digoxin (see *Table 44* for PO maintenance dosage; loading dose [see text for indications]: PO - 1 or 2 doses at twice calculated maintenance; dog IV: 0.01–0.02 mg/kg – give 1/4 of this total dose in slow boluses over 2–4 hours to effect; cat IV: 0.005 mg/kg – give 1/2 of total, then 1–2 hours later give 1/4 dose bolus(es), if needed).

9) Monitor and manage abnormalities as possible:

a) Respiratory rate, heart rate and rhythm, arterial blood pressure, body weight, urine output, hydration, attitude, serum biochemistry and blood gas analyses, and pulmonary capillary wedge pressure (if available).

10) Diastolic dysfunction (e.g. cats with hypertrophic cardiomyopathy):

a) General recommendations, O_2 therapy, and furosemide as above.

b) +/- Nitroglycerin and mild sedation.

c) Consider IV esmolol (200–500 mcg/kg IV over 1 minute, followed by 25–200 mcg/kg CRI) or diltiazem (0.15–0.25 mg/kg over 2–3 minutes IV).

* Dilution of 250 mg dobutamine into 500 ml of fluid yields 500 mcg/ml; infusion at 0.6 ml/kg/hour provides 5 mcg dobutamine/kg/minute (also see *Table 49*, p. 201 for CRI rate calculation).

** Dopamine is diluted in saline solution, 5% dextrose in water, or lactated Ringer's solution. 40 mg of dopamine into 500 ml of fluid provides 80 mcg/ml; infusion at 0.75 ml/kg/hour provides 1 mcg dopamine/kg/minute (also see *Table 49*, p. 201 for CRI rate calculation).

handling and use of oral medications should be avoided when possible to reduce patient stress. Environmental stressors including excessive heat, humidity, or noise should also be avoided.

OXYGEN

Supplemental O_2 can be provided by face mask or improvised O_2 hood, nasal or nasopharyngeal catheter, oxygen cage, or endotracheal tube. Whatever the means, patient struggling should be avoided. If an oxygen cage with temperature and humidity controls is available, a setting of 18.3°C (65°F) is recommended for normothermic animals; an O_2 flow of 6–10 l/minute is usually adequate[58, 59]. Although 50–100% O_2 may be needed initially, this is reduced to 40% or less within a few hours to avoid lung injury[59]. With a nasal or nasopharyngeal tube, humidified O_2 at a rate of 50–100 ml/kg/minute is suggested. Extreme cases of pulmonary edema with respiratory failure may respond to endotracheal or tracheotomy tube placement and mechanical ventilation. Frothy edema fluid in the airways requires immediate suctioning. Positive end-expiratory pressure ventilation helps clear small airways and expand alveoli; however, positive airway pressure can adversely affect hemodynamics, and continuous monitoring is essential. Further information on assisted ventilation can be found elsewhere[60–63].

DIURETIC THERAPY

Strategies used to control cardiogenic pulmonary edema include circulating volume reduction and blood redistribution. Furosemide is used IV for rapid diuresis; this also provides a mild venodilating effect[64, 65]. The actions of IV furosemide begin within 5 minutes, peak by 30 minutes, and last about 2 hours. An aggressive initial dosage or cumulative doses administered at frequent intervals may be needed. Administration by constant rate infusion (CRI) may provide greater diuresis than bolus injections[66]. The veterinary formulation (50 mg/ml) can be diluted to 10 mg/ml in 5% dextrose in water (D5W), 0.9% NaCl, lactated Ringer's solution (LRS), or sterile water[67]. Alternatively, it can be diluted to 5 mg/ml in D5W or sterile water. The aggressiveness of continued furosemide therapy is guided by the patient's respiratory rate, among other parameters (see p. 175). Once diuresis has begun and respiration improves, the dosage is reduced to prevent excessive volume contraction and electrolyte depletion.

VASODILATOR THERAPY

Vasodilator drugs reduce pulmonary edema by increasing systemic venous capacitance, lowering pulmonary venous pressure, and/or reducing systemic arterial resistance. Although ACE inhibitors have greater advantage for long-term treatment, more immediate afterload reduction is desired for acute CHF **not** caused by diastolic dysfunction or ventricular outflow obstruction. Sodium nitroprusside causes potent arteriolar and venous dilation through direct action on vascular smooth muscle. Blood pressure must be closely monitored. The dose is titrated to maintain mean arterial pressure >70 mm Hg (ideally about 80 mm Hg; or systolic blood pressure of 90–110 mm Hg). Nitroprusside by CRI is usually continued for 12–24 hours. Tolerance develops rapidly, so dosage adjustments are usually needed. Profound hypotension is the major adverse effect. Cyanide toxicity can result from excessive or prolonged use (e.g. over 48 hours). Nitroprusside should not be infused with other drugs and it should be protected from light.

Hydralazine, with or without nitroglycerin, is an alternative to nitroprusside infusion. Hydralazine is a pure arteriolar dilator that is useful for refractory pulmonary edema caused by MR (and sometimes DCM) because it reduces the regurgitant fraction and lowers LA pressure. An initial PO dose (*Table 44*, p. 174) can be repeated every 2–3 hours until systolic blood pressure is 90–110 mm Hg or clinical improvement is obvious. If blood pressure cannot be monitored, an initial dose (1 mg/kg) is repeated once in 2–4 hours if sufficient clinical improvement has not occurred. Concurrent application of 2% nitroglycerin ointment may provide a complementary venodilating effect. Another choice for vasodilation is an ACE inhibitor or amlodipine, with or without nitroglycerin ointment, although the onset of action is slower and immediate effects are less pronounced (see p. 178). Arteriolar vasodilators are generally not used in animals with LV outflow obstruction (e.g. hypertrophic obstructive cardiomyopathy) because they can exacerbate the obstruction.

Nitroglycerin, and other orally or transcutaneously administered nitrates, act mainly on venous smooth muscle to increase venous capacitance and reduce cardiac filling pressure. Nitroglycerin has been shown to produce splanchnic vasodilation in experimental dogs[68, 69]. The major indication for nitroglycerin is acute cardiogenic pulmonary edema. Nitroglycerin ointment (2%) is usually applied to the skin of the groin, axillary area, or ear pinna, although the efficacy of this in CHF is unclear. An application paper or glove is used to avoid skin contact by the person applying the drug. Self-adhesive, sustained-release nitrate preparations may be useful, but they have not been well evaluated in small animals. Transdermal nitrate patches (5 mg) applied for 12 hours/day have been used with anecdotal success in large dogs.

OTHER ACUTE THERAPY

Bronchodilator therapy may benefit some dogs with severe, acute pulmonary edema and bronchoconstriction. Aminophylline (slowly IV or IM) also has transient diuretic properties and a mild positive inotropic effect. The oral route can be used when respiration improves; GI absorption is rapid. Long-term bronchodilator administration is not recommended. Adverse effects include increased sympathomimetic activity and arrhythmias.

Mild sedation can reduce patient anxiety. Morphine or butorphanol can be used in dogs; acepromazine with butorphanol is effective in cats. Morphine's other beneficial effects include slower, deeper respiration and blood redistribution via splanchnic vasodilation[70]; however, morphine can induce vomiting, which could trigger cardiac arrest. Morphine can raise intracranial pressure and so is contraindicated in dogs with neurogenic pulmonary edema. Morphine is not used in cats.

INOTROPIC SUPPORT

Positive inotropic therapy is indicated for animals with poor myocardial contractility or marked hypotension. Oral therapy with digoxin or pimobendan, where available, is begun as soon as practical for patients needing chronic support (*Table 44*, p. 174, and pp. 178 and 181). Acute (1–3 day) inotropic support with an IV sympathomimetic (catecholamine) or phosphodiesterase (PDE) inhibitor agent can help support arterial pressure, forward cardiac output, and organ perfusion when myocardial failure or hypotension is severe. Catecholamines augment contractility by a cAMP-mediated increase in intracellular Ca^{++}; however, they can provoke arrhythmias as well as increase pulmonary and systemic vascular resistance, potentially exacerbating interstitial fluid accumulation. Their short half-life and extensive hepatic metabolism necessitate constant IV infusion. Dobutamine (a synthetic analog of dopamine) is preferred over dopamine because of its lesser effect on heart rate and afterload. Dobutamine stimulates $beta_1$-receptors, but has only weak action on $beta_2$- and alpha-receptors. Lower doses increase contractility with minimal effects on heart rate and blood pressure. A low initial infusion rate can be gradually increased over hours to achieve greater inotropic effect and

Table 44 Drugs for long-term congestive heart failure management.

Drug	Dog	Cat
Diuretics		
Furosemide	1–3 mg/kg PO q8–24h (long term); use smallest effective dose	1–2 mg/kg PO q8–12h; use smallest effective dose
Spironolactone	0.5–1 mg/kg PO q(12–)24h	0.5–1 mg/kg PO q(12–)24h
Chlorothiazide	20–40 mg/kg PO q12h	20–40 mg/kg PO q12h
Hydrochlorothiazide	2–4 mg/kg PO q12h	1–2 mg/kg PO q12h
ACE inhibitors		
Enalapril	0.5 mg/kg PO q24(–12)h	0.25–0.5 mg/kg PO q24(–12)h
Benazepril	0.25–0.5 mg/kg PO q(12–)24h	0.25–0.5 mg/kg PO q(12–)24h
Captopril	0.5–2.0 mg/kg PO q8–12h (low initial dose)	0.5–1.25 mg/kg PO q12–24h
Lisinopril	0.25–0.5 mg/kg PO q(12–)24h	0.25–0.5 mg/kg PO q24h
Fosinopril	0.25–0.5 mg/kg PO q24h	—
Ramipril	0.125–0.25 mg/kg PO q24h	—
Imidapril	0.25 mg/kg PO q24h	—
Other vasodilators		
Hydralazine	0.5–2 mg/kg PO q12h (to 1 mg/kg initial)	2.5 (up to 10) mg/cat PO q12h
Amlodipine	0.05 (initial) to 0.3(–0.5) mg/kg PO q(12–)24h	0.3125–0.625 mg/cat PO q24(–12)h
Prazosin	Medium dogs: 1 mg PO q8–12h; large dogs: 2 mg PO q8h	—
Nitroglycerin 2% ointment	1/2–1 1/2 inch cutaneously q4–6h	1/4–1/2 inch cutaneously q4–6h
Isosorbide dinitrate	0.5–2 mg/kg PO q(8–)12h	—
Isosorbide mononitrate	0.25–2 mg/kg PO q12h	—
Positive inotropic agents		
Digoxin	PO: dogs <22 kg, 0.005–0.008 mg/kg q12h; dogs >22 kg, 0.22 mg/m^2 or 0.003–0.005 mg/kg q12h. Decrease by 10% for elixir. Maximum: 0.5 mg/day or 0.375 mg/day for Doberman Pinchers.	0.007 mg/kg (or 1/4 of 0.125 mg tab) PO q48h
Digitoxin	0.02–0.03 mg/kg PO q8h (small dogs) to q12h (large dogs)	Do not use in cats
Pimobendan	0.1–0.3 mg/kg PO q12h, start low; give at least 1 hour before feeding	?1.25 mg/cat PO q12h
Drugs for diastolic dysfunction		
Diltiazem	0.5–2 mg/kg PO q8h	1.5–2.5 mg/kg or 7.5–10 mg/cat PO q8h; sustained release: Dilacor XR, 30 mg/cat (1/2 internal [60 mg] tablet from the 240 mg capsule size) q24(–12)h; or Cardizem CD, 10 mg/kg q24h, (must be compounded)
Atenolol	0.2–1 mg/kg PO q12–24h	6.25–12.5 mg/cat PO q(12–)24h

maintain systolic arterial pressure between 90 and 120 mm Hg. Heart rate, rhythm, and blood pressure should be closely monitored. Although less arrhythmogenic than other catecholamines, higher infusion rates can precipitate supraventricular and ventricular arrhythmias. Adverse effects are more likely in cats; these include seizures at relatively low doses. Dopamine at low doses (<2–5 mcg/kg/minute) also stimulates vasodilator dopaminergic receptors in some regional circulations. Low to moderate doses enhance contractility and cardiac output, but high doses (10–15 mcg/kg/minute) cause peripheral vasoconstriction and increase heart rate, O_2 consumption, and the risk of ventricular arrhythmias.

Bipyridine PDE inhibitors such as amrinone and milrinone increase intracellular Ca^{++} by inhibiting PDE III, an intracellular enzyme that degrades cAMP. These drugs also cause vasodilation as increased cAMP promotes vascular smooth muscle relaxation. High doses can cause hypotension, tachycardia, and GI signs. These drugs may exacerbate ventricular arrhythmias[71]. Amrinone is sometimes used as an initial slow IV bolus followed by CRI; half the original bolus dose can be repeated after 20–30 minutes. Milrinone has a much greater potency than amrinone, but there is little veterinary experience with the IV form. Oral milrinone (0.5–1 mg/kg), used in clinical trials in dogs with myocardial failure, produced clinical, hemodynamic, and echocardiographic improvement[72, 73]. A PDE inhibitor can be used concurrently with digoxin and a catecholamine. Digoxin is generally not used IV, except for some supraventricular tachyarrhythmias when other acute therapy is unavailable or ineffective. Acidosis and hypoxemia associated with severe pulmonary edema can increase myocardial sensitivity to digitalis-induced arrhythmias. If digoxin is used IV, it must be given slowly (over at least 15 minutes), as rapid injection causes peripheral vasoconstriction. The calculated dose is usually divided, and boluses of one-fourth the dose are given slowly over several hours.

If arrhythmias develop during IV inotropic therapy, the infusion rate is reduced or the drug is discontinued. In animals with atrial fibrillation, catecholamine infusion is likely to increase the ventricular response rate by enhancing AV conduction. If dobutamine or dopamine is deemed necessary for such a case, rapid PO or cautious IV diltiazem will help reduce the heart rate. Digoxin, either PO (loading) or cautiously IV, is an alternative.

HEART FAILURE FROM DIASTOLIC DYSFUNCTION

For cats (or dogs) with acute CHF from diastolic dysfunction (e.g. HCM), diuretic and O_2 therapy are given as outlined above. Topical nitroglycerin is also used for acute pulmonary edema. Moderate to large pleural effusion should be drained. Once severe dyspnea has abated, diltiazem or a beta$_1$-blocker (e.g. atenolol) is often instituted to control heart rate and increase filling time. Alternatively, IV esmolol or diltiazem can be used acutely. Propranolol or other nonselective beta-blockers are generally avoided with fulminant pulmonary edema because beta$_2$-blockade could induce bronchoconstriction; however, the use of a beta-blocker or diltiazem for long-term management of cats with CHF has been called into question, as benefit appears lacking in an ongoing clinical trial. Arteriolar vasodilators can be detrimental in animals with dynamic LV outflow obstruction, because afterload reduction provokes greater systolic obstruction (see Chapter 21); however, ACE inhibitors at a standard dose do not appear to worsen the LV outflow gradient.

MONITORING AND FOLLOW-UP

Frequent patient assessment is important to monitor therapeutic effectiveness as well as to avoid hypotension or severe azotemia from excessive diuresis. Mild azotemia is to be expected. Hypokalemia and metabolic alkalosis can occur with aggressive diuresis. Serum biochemical testing every 24–48 hours is advised until the patient is eating and drinking well. Maintaining serum potassium concentration within the mid- to high-normal range is especially important for animals with arrhythmias (see below). Arterial blood pressure can be monitored directly or indirectly. Indirect measures of organ perfusion, such as CRT, mucous membrane color, urine output, toe-web temperature, and mentation, can also be useful. Body weight should be monitored, especially with aggressive diuretic therapy. CVP does not adequately reflect left heart filling pressures or, when right heart function is poor, circulating blood volume status. CVP is likely to be misleading if used to guide diuretic or fluid therapy in such patients. Although pulmonary capillary wedge pressure can reliably guide therapy, the placement and care of an indwelling pulmonary artery catheter requires meticulous attention to asepsis and close monitoring. Pulse oximetry is a helpful noninvasive means of monitoring oxygen saturation. Supplemental O_2 should be given if the hemaglobin saturation is <90%; mechanical ventilation is indicated if the hemaglobin saturation is <80% despite O_2 therapy. Arterial sampling for blood gas analysis is more accurate, but is stressful for the patient. Resolution of radiographic evidence for pulmonary edema usually lags behind clinical improvement by a day or two.

Once diuresis has begun and respiratory signs begin to abate, water is offered by mouth. Fluid administration, either SC or IV, is generally not advised in patients with fulminant CHF. In most cases, gradual rehydration by free choice (low sodium) water intake is preferred even after aggressive diuretic therapy. However, there are some patients that need fluid therapy, including those with persistent anorexia, renal failure, moderate/severe hypokalemia, hypotension, digoxin toxicity, or other serious systemic disease[74]. Some animals require high cardiac filling pressure to maintain cardiac output, especially those with myocardial failure or markedly reduced ventricular compliance (e.g. from HCM or pericardial disease). The preload reduction achieved by diuresis and vasodilation in such cases can cause inadequate cardiac output and hypotension. When fluid therapy is necessary, D5W or a reduced sodium fluid (e.g. 0.45% NaCl with 2.5% dextrose) with added KCl is administered at a conservative rate (e.g. 15–30 ml/kg/day IV). Alternatively, 0.45% NaCl with 2.5% dextrose or LRS can be administered SC. A maintenance rate for potassium supplementation is 0.05–0.1 mEq/kg/hour (or, more conservatively, 0.5–2.0 mEq/kg/day). For animals with potassium deficiency, increased supplementation is suggested: for mild K+ deficiency, 0.15–0.2 mEq/kg/hour; for moderate deficiency, 0.25–0.3 mEq/kg/hour; and for severe deficiency, 0.4–0.5 mEq/kg/hour. Serum K+ measurement after 4–6 hours is advised with supplementation for moderate to severe deficiency. Some patients develop hyponatremia and worsened fluid retention with low sodium IV solutions and require a more balanced crystalloid solution[74]. In decompensated CHF, the smallest fluid volume possible is used to deliver a drug by CRI. Careful monitoring and continued diuretic use is important to avoid recurrent pulmonary edema. Other supportive therapies for CHF and any underlying disease(s) depend on individual patient needs. Parenteral fluid administration is tapered as the animal is able to resume oral food and water intake.

MANAGEMENT OF CHRONIC HEART FAILURE

While the treatment focus for fulminant pulmonary edema is on rapid diuresis, the evolving perspective for chronic heart failure management is based on reducing maladaptive NH activity, myocardial remodeling, and progressive cardiac dysfunction[1]. Diuretics are used as needed to control signs of congestion, but the current focus is on neurohormone blockers to prevent heart failure progression. In people, chronic therapy with ACE inhibitors, certain beta-blockers, and the ALD receptor antagonist spironolactone have improved clinical status and survival. Conversely, potent positive inotropic agents (milrinone and others) have decreased long-term survival. Likewise, drugs that simply reduce afterload (pure arteriolar vasodilators) have not improved long-term survival[1]. Future strategies may involve drugs that block cytokines, antagonize ETs, and enhance

natriuretic peptide actions, as well as other strategies to block the effects of NH activation.

A summary of long-term heart failure management strategies is presented (see **229** and the chapters on specific diseases for additional information). Long-term therapy is tailored to the individual patient's needs. Dosage adjustments, addition or substitution of drugs, and lifestyle or diet modifications become necessary as heart disease progresses. Support of cardiac function with pimobendan or digoxin is often indicated in dogs. Cardiac arrhythmias requiring specific antiarrhythmic therapy develop commonly (see Chapter 17). Moderate and large volume pleural effusion and large volume ascites are drained to aid ventilation. Likewise, pericardial effusion that compromises cardiac filling must be drained (see Chapter 22).

DIURETICS
Furosemide

Furosemide (frusomide) is used most commonly to control edema and effusion. Although aggressive diuretic therapy is indicated for fulminant pulmonary edema, the lowest effective doses given at consistent time intervals are used for chronic CHF therapy. Furosemide, or other diuretic, alone is not recommended as the sole treatment for chronic heart failure, because it can exacerbate NH activation and reduce renal function[75]. Furosemide therapy increases RAAS activation; while other therapy (e.g. ACE inhibitors) can mitigate this, ALD release can occur despite ACE inhibition (see p. 178). Experimentally, furosemide is associated with faster development of LV dysfunction, increased ALD levels, and altered Ca++ handling[17].

Furosemide, like other 'loop' diuretics, inhibits active Cl-, K+, and Na+ cotransport in the ascending limb of the loop of Henle, thereby promoting excretion of these electrolytes. Ca++ and Mg++ are also lost in the urine. Furosemide may also promote salt loss by increasing total renal blood flow and by preferentially enhancing renal cortical flow. The effects of oral furosemide begin in 1 hour, peak at 1–2 hours, and last about 6 hours. Long-term furosemide dosage depends on the patient's clinical situation and is guided by respiratory pattern, hydration, body weight, exercise tolerance, renal function, and serum electrolyte concentrations. Hypokalemia and alkalosis are uncommon adverse effects, especially in animals without anorexia or vomiting. Cautious potassium supplementation may be used for documented hypokalemia, but hyperkalemia can develop, especially with concurrent ACE inhibitor and/or spironolactone therapy, or if renal disease is present. Furosemide with a low salt diet can reduce serum Cl- as well as K+, Mg++, and Na+[75, 76].

A diuretic acting at a different segment of the nephron (e.g. spironolactone or a thiazide) is

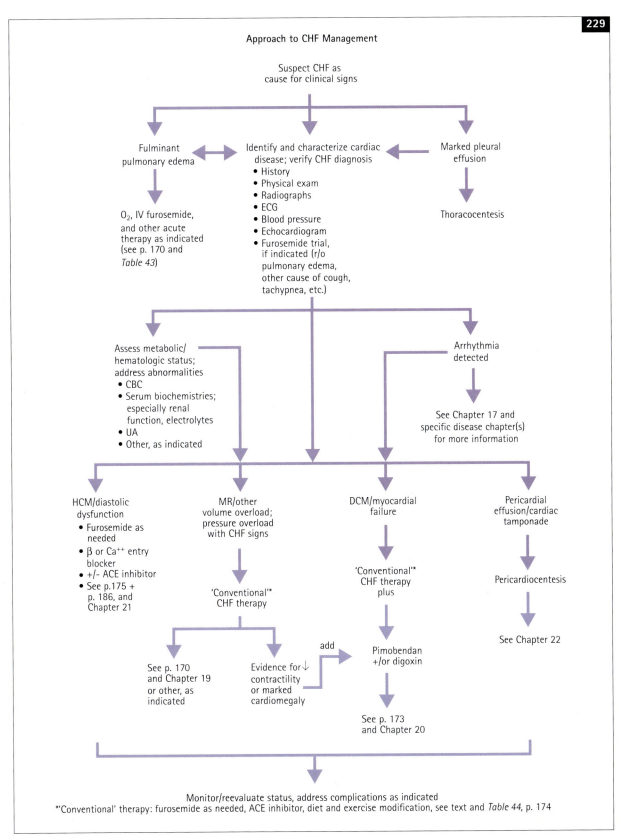

229 Approach to the patient with suspected CHF.

sometimes combined with furosemide for refractory CHF therapy. Multiple diuretic therapy can promote excessive volume contraction and RAAS activation, as well as cause or exacerbate azotemia and electrolyte imbalances. Therefore, the indications for use should be clearly established and the lowest effective doses administered.

Spironolactone

Spironolactone is a potassium-sparing agent. It is thought to be a useful adjunct for chronic refractory CHF when furosemide and an ACE inhibitor, with or without digoxin, does not control congestive signs. As a competitive antagonist of ALD, spironolactone promotes Na+ loss and K+ retention in the distal renal tubule. It is more effective when circulating ALD concentration is high; however, it appears to lack diuretic effect in normal dogs at standard doses[77]. Spironolactone's onset of action is slow and peak effect occurs in 2–3 days. Potassium-sparing diuretics are contraindicated in patients with hyperkalemia and must be used cautiously in those receiving an ACE inhibitor or potassium supplements. Adverse effects relate to excess K+ retention and GI disturbances. Spironolactone may decrease the clearance of digoxin.

ALD release can occur despite ACE inhibitor use. This phenomenon of 'aldosterone escape' can involve reduced hepatic clearance, increased release stimulated by K+ elevation or Na+ depletion, and local tissue ALD production[17]. Therefore, in addition to ACE inhibitors, furosemide, and digoxin, spironolactone is gaining favor for chronic CHF therapy. Spironolactone's anti-ALD effects are also known to mitigate ALD-induced cardiovascular remodeling and fibrosis in people and experimental animals. It also improves survival in people with moderate to severe CHF[9, 78, 79]. Whether similar survival benefit occurs clinically in dogs and cats is not known, but it is important to monitor for hyperkalemia and azotemia when using an ACE inhibitor and potassium-sparing diuretic, because serious hyperkalemia can develop[80, 81].

Thiazide diuretics

Thiazide diuretics reduce Na+ and Cl- absorption and increase Ca++ absorption in the distal convoluted tubule. This causes mild to moderate diuresis and excretion of Na+, Cl-, K+, and Mg++. The thiazides reduce renal blood flow and therefore must not be given to animals with azotemia. Adverse effects are uncommon in nonazotemic animals, but hypokalemia, other electrolyte disturbance, and dehydration can occur with anorexia or excessive use. They are relatively contraindicated with hyponatremia because they impair free-water clearance. Thiazides can cause hyperglycemia in

diabetic or prediabetic animals by inhibiting conversion of proinsulin to insulin. Chlorothiazide produces diuresis within 1 hour, with a peak effect in 4 hours and duration of 6–12 hours. Hydrochlorothiazide's effects begin within 2 hours, peak at 4 hours, and last 12 hours.

ANGIOTENSIN–CONVERTING ENZYME INHIBITORS

ACE inhibitors are indicated for chronic CHF of most causes, especially DCM and chronic valvular insufficiency. Their main benefits arise from opposing the effects of NH activation and potentially reducing abnormal cardiovascular remodeling[1]. Because of their multiple effects in moderating excess NH responses, ACE inhibitors have advantages over hydralazine and other arteriolar dilators. ACE inhibitors have only modest diuretic and vasodilatory effects. These arise as decreased AT II levels permit some arteriolar and venous dilation and reduce Na+ and water retention, via decreased circulating ALD. The vasodilating effects of ACE inhibitors may be partially due to vasodilator kinins normally degraded by ACE. Inhibition of ACE present in the vasculature may produce a local vasodilating effect, even in the absence of high circulating renin levels. Local ACE inhibition is also thought to be beneficial by modulating vascular smooth muscle and myocardial remodeling. Sustained clinical improvement and lowered mortality rates have occurred when an ACE inhibitor is added to diuretic and digoxin therapy in people. Similar benefits seem to occur in dogs with heart failure from myocardial disease or volume overload, as well as in cats with diastolic dysfunction[82–84]. ACE inhibitors reduce ventricular arrhythmias and the sudden death rate in people (and probably animals) with heart failure; this is probably because AT II-induced enhancement of NE and epinephrine release is inhibited. ACE inhibitors may attenuate progressive LV dilation and secondary MR in dogs with DCM, as well as improve clinical status and survival in DCM and chronic MR, and possibly other causes of heart failure as well[85]. ACE inhibitors may delay the onset of clinical heart failure in patients with myocardial dysfunction. Reduced heart rate, cardiac filling pressure, peripheral vascular resistance, as well as improved cardiac output, have been variably reported. The secondary inhibition of ALD presumably helps reduce edema and also direct adverse cardiac effects. However, in asymptomatic dogs with chronic MR, ACE inhibitor use does not appear to delay significantly the onset of CHF signs[18, 86, 87]. There are conflicting reports as to whether ACE inhibitors prevent ventricular remodeling and dilation in canine heart disease[19, 25].

Several ACE inhibitors are available. Most, except captopril and lisinopril, are prodrugs that are converted in the liver to their active form; severe liver dysfunction will interfere with this conversion. ACE inhibitors commonly used in animals include enalapril, benazepril, and, previously, captopril.

Enalapril
Enalapril has been used in several clinical studies[18, 82, 83, 85, 87]. It is hydrolyzed in the liver to its most active form, enalaprilat. Enalapril is well-absorbed orally; bioavailability is not decreased by food. Peak ACE inhibiting activity occurs within 4–6 hours in dogs[88]. Duration of action is 12–14 hours; effects are minimal by 24 hours at the recommended once daily dose. Dogs with more advanced CHF may respond better when dosed every 12 hours. Maximal activity in cats occurs within 2–4 hours after an oral dose; some ACE inhibition (50% of control) persists for 2–3 days. Enalapril and its active metabolite are excreted in the urine. Enalapril does not cause significant adverse effects on renal function in dogs with advanced MR[89]; however, renal failure and severe CHF prolong its elimination, so reduced dosage or benazepril are used in such patients[90]. Injectable enalaprilat is available, but there is little veterinary experience with it.

Benazepril
Benazepril, like enalapril, is well-tolerated in CHF and improves exercise tolerance, clinical status, and survival[91, 92]. Benazepril is metabolized to its active form (benazeprilat) in the liver. Only about 40% is absorbed when administered orally, but feeding does not affect absorption. Peak ACE inhibition occurs within 2 hours of PO administration in dogs and cats[88, 93]. Complete ACE inhibition occurs in cats at doses of 0.25–0.5 mg/kg, with maintenance of >90% inhibition at 24 hours[94]. Repeated dosing moderately increases drug plasma concentrations. Benazepril is eliminated equally in urine and bile in dogs, an advantage for animals with renal disease[86, 94]. In cats, about 85% is excreted in the feces and only 15% in the urine. Benazepril may also slow renal function deterioration and partially mitigate hypertension in cats with renal disease[95].

Captopril
Captopril was the first ACE inhibitor used clinically. In contrast to other ACE inhibitors, captopril contains a sulfhydryl group. This may confer a beneficial free-radical scavenging effect, although the clinical significance of this is unclear. Captopril appears less effective in reducing ACE activity than other ACEIs in normal dogs[88]. Captopril is well-absorbed orally (75% bioavailable), but food decreases bioavailability by 30–40%. Hemodynamic effects appear within 1 hour, peak in 1–2 hours, and last <4 hours in dogs. Captopril is excreted in the urine.

Lisinopril
Lisinopril is a lysine analog of enalaprilat with direct ACE inhibiting effects. It is 25–50% bioavailable; absorption is not affected by feeding. Time to peak effect is 6–8 hours. Once daily lisinopril administration appears to be effective.

Fosinopril
Fosinopril is structurally different from other ACE inhibitors in that it contains a phosphinic acid radical (rather than sulfhydryl or carboxyl). It may be retained longer in myocytes. Fosinopril is converted to its active form (fosinoprilat) in the GI mucosa and liver. Elimination occurs equally by the kidney and liver. Its duration of action is >24 hours in people. Fosinopril may falsely lower serum digoxin measurements by radioimmunoassay (RIA) tests.

Other ACE inhibitors
Other ACE inhibitors that have been used in animals include **ramipril, quinipril,** and **imidapril**[88, 96]. Imidapril has comparable efficacy to enalapril and is available in liquid form, although other ACE inhibitors can be compounded into suspension[96].

Adverse effects of ACE inhibitors
Adverse effects of ACE inhibitors include hypotension, GI upset, azotemia, acute renal failure, and hyperkalemia (especially when used with a potassium-sparing diuretic or potassium supplement). AT II is important in mediating renal efferent arteriolar constriction, which maintains glomerular filtration when renal blood flow decreases. As long as cardiac output and renal perfusion improve with therapy, renal function is usually maintained. Poor glomerular filtration is more likely to occur with excessive diuresis or vasodilation, volume depletion, and severe myocardial dysfunction. Azotemia is addressed by first decreasing the diuretic dosage. If necessary, the ACE inhibitor dose is reduced, or discontinued. Occasionally, cautious fluid therapy is needed (see p. 175). Hypotension can usually be avoided with low initial doses. Other adverse effects reported in people include rash, pruritus, impaired taste, proteinuria, cough, and neutropenia. The mechanism of ACE inhibitor-induced cough is unclear, but may involve inhibition of endogenous bradykinin degradation or possibly increased NO generation. NO has an inflammatory effect on bronchial epithelial cells[97]. Aspirin does not appear to reduce the beneficial effects of ACE inhibition in CHF, but it is unclear if other nonsteroidal antiinflammatory drugs do[98].

DIGITALIS GLYCOSIDES
Digoxin
Digoxin has mild positive inotropic as well as antiarrhythmic effects. Probably more importantly, it

modulates baroreceptor function to alter autonomic tone favorably in CHF. By improving baroreceptor sensitivity, digoxin can blunt sympathetic activation. Indications for digoxin include reduced myocardial contractility and supraventricular tachyarrhythmias (see Chapter 17 p. 202). Digoxin is often added to diuretic and ACE inhibitor therapy in advanced MR and other chronic volume overload conditions. Digoxin improves clinical status in people with CHF; it has a neutral effect on long-term mortality[99]. Digoxin is usually contraindicated for HCM, especially where there is ventricular outflow obstruction. It is not indicated for treating pericardial disease. Digoxin alone is only moderately effective in slowing the ventricular response rate to atrial fibrillation (see Chapter 17). Digoxin is relatively contraindicated in the presence of sinus or AV node disease or serious ventricular arrhythmias.

Digoxin, as is the case with other digitalis glycosides, increases the Ca^{++} available for contraction by inhibiting myocardial membrane Na/K-ATPase pump activity. The drug binds competitively to the extracellular K^+ site. Subsequent intracellular Na^+ accumulation promotes increased Ca^{++} entry via the transmembrane Na^+/Ca^{++} exchange mechanism. Digoxin does not increase cAMP. Digoxin's antiarrhythmic effects stem primarily from increased parasympathetic tone to the sinus and AV nodes and atrial tissue. AV conduction time and refractory period are also directly prolonged to some degree. These effects cause a slowed sinus rate, reduced ventricular response to atrial fibrillation, and suppression of atrial premature depolarizations. Although enhanced vagal tone might help suppress some ventricular arrhythmias, the potential arrhythmogenic effects of digoxin should be considered in animals with CHF.

Digoxin is well-absorbed orally: ~60% for the tablet form and 75% for the elixir; there is minimal hepatic metabolism. The presence of food, kaolin–pectin compounds, antacids, and malabsorption syndromes decreases bioavailability; about 27% of the drug in serum is protein-bound. Therapeutic serum concentrations occur in dogs within 2–4 1/2 days with q12h dosing (half-life in dogs is ~23–39 hours). Cats have more variable pharmacokinetics and the half-life ranges widely (~25 to over 78 hours)[100–102]. The alcohol-based digoxin elixir is poorly palatable in cats and yields ~50% higher serum concentrations than the tablet form. Steady state concentrations are achieved in about 10 days with q48h dosing in cats with CHF. Digoxin is eliminated primarily by glomerular filtration and renal secretion in dogs; renal and hepatic elimination are equally important in cats[100]. Serum digoxin concentration (and risk of toxicity) increases with renal dysfunction, but the degree of azotemia is not well-correlated with serum digoxin concentration

in dogs. Lower doses and monitoring of serum digoxin concentration are recommended for animals with renal disease. Digitoxin, if available, is an alternative to digoxin in dogs with renal failure; digitoxin should not be used in cats.

Digoxin therapy is usually begun with the PO maintenance dose. If a faster increase in serum concentration is urgent, digoxin can be given at twice the PO maintenance dose for 1–2 doses. An alternative is cautious IV administration (see p. 175). However, for supraventricular tachycardia, other therapy is usually more effective (see Chapter 17, p. 202). Other IV positive inotropic agents (see p. 173) are safer and more effective than digoxin for immediate support of myocardial contractility.

The correlation between digoxin dose and serum concentration in dogs with heart failure is quite weak[103]. Because digoxin has poor lipid solubility, the dose should be based on the animal's estimated lean body weight; this is especially important in obese animals. The risk of toxicity at usual doses is increased in animals with reduced muscle mass or cachexia, because much of the drug is bound to skeletal muscle. Conservative dosing and measurement of serum concentration help to prevent toxicity. In some dogs, toxicity seems to develop at relatively low dosages; a total maximum daily dose of 0.25–0.375 mg/day is used for Doberman Pinschers, and a total of 0.5 mg or less for other large and giant breed dogs.

Measurement of serum digoxin concentration is recommended at 7–10 days after therapy is initiated or the dosage changed. Samples are drawn 8–10 hours after the previous dose. The therapeutic serum concentration range is (0.5 or) 1–2 ng/ml. Serum concentrations in the low to mid therapeutic range are desired. A greater risk for sudden death was found in people with serum digoxin concentrations toward the higher end of normal[99]. If serum concentration is below the therapeutic range, the dose can be increased by 25% and serum concentration measured the following week. If serum levels cannot be measured and toxicity is suspected, the drug is discontinued for 1–2 days and then reinstituted at half of the original dose.

Digitoxin

Digitoxin is another digitalis glycoside. It may be available in some areas, but is now almost never used. Its indication was for dogs with CHF and renal dysfunction, because it is cleared mainly by the liver. Digitoxin is well-absorbed orally, highly (90%) protein-bound in serum, and lipid soluble. Its half-life in dogs is 8–12 hours, but in cats it is extremely long (>100 hours); therefore it is not used in cats. Serum digitoxin concentration is measured 6–8 hours post dose; the therapeutic range is 15–35 ng/ml. Quinidine does not increase serum concentrations of digitoxin.

Digitalis toxicity

Digitalis toxicity is more likely with renal dysfunction, hypokalemia, and concurrent use of certain drugs. Renal function and serum electrolyte concentrations should be monitored during digoxin therapy. Quinidine increases serum digoxin concentration by reducing renal clearance and competing for Na/K binding sites in skeletal muscle. Verapamil and amiodarone also increase serum digoxin concentration; other drugs that may do so include diltiazem, prazosin, and spironolactone. Hypokalemia promotes myocardial toxicity by leaving more membrane Na/K-ATPase binding sites available; conversely, hyperkalemia displaces digitalis from those binding sites. Hypercalcemia and hypernatremia potentiate both the inotropic and toxic effects of the drug. Hyperthyroidism and hypoxia may potentiate the toxic myocardial effects of the drug.

Toxicity causes GI, myocardial, or sometimes CNS signs[104, 105]. GI toxicity can develop before signs of myocardial toxicity and sometimes occurs with digoxin concentrations in the therapeutic range. Signs include anorexia, depression, vomiting, borborygmus, and diarrhea. Direct effects of digitalis on chemoreceptors in the brainstem are responsible for some GI effects. CNS signs can include depression and disorientation. Because these are also manifestations of hypotension or arrhythmias from underlying disease, digoxin serum concentration should be verified.

Myocardial toxicity causes many cardiac rhythm disturbances, including ventricular tachyarrhythmias, supraventricular premature complexes and tachycardia, sinus arrest, Mobitz type I 2nd degree AV block, and junctional rhythms. Myocardial toxicity can occur before any other signs and can lead to collapse and death, especially in animals with myocardial failure. Therefore, using the criteria of PR interval prolongation on ECG or signs of GI toxicity to guide progressive dosing of digoxin is not advised. Loading doses are generally avoided in cases with myocardial failure because digitalis can aggravate cellular calcium overloading and electrical instability. Digitalis can provoke spontaneous automaticity in myocardial cells by inducing late afterdepolarizations; cellular stretch, Ca^{++} overloading, and hypokalemia enhance this effect. Toxic concentrations further enhance automaticity by increasing cardiac sympathetic tone. The parasympathetic effects of slowed conduction and altered refractory period also facilitate reentrant arrhythmias. Digoxin should be used at low doses or withheld until the arrhythmia is controlled in patients with serious preexisting ventricular arrhythmias. In animals receiving digoxin, toxicity should be suspected if tachyarrhythmias appear, especially with evidence of impaired conduction.

Treatment for digitalis toxicity depends on the manifestations. GI signs usually respond to drug withdrawal and correction of fluid or electrolyte disturbances. Abnormal AV conduction should resolve after drug withdrawal, although anticholinergic therapy may be needed. Digitalis-induced ventricular tachyarrhythmias are treated with lidocaine (see Chapter 17, p. 208). This agent reduces sympathetic tone and suppresses reentry and late afterdepolarizations, with little effect on sinus rate or AV node conduction. Phenytoin (diphenylhydantoin) is the drug of second choice in dogs. It has effects similar to lidocaine (see Chapter 17, p. 213). Also helpful is IV potassium supplementation if the serum potassium concentration is <4 mEq/l. Magnesium supplementation may also be effective in suppressing arrhythmias (see Chapter 17, p. 208). Cautious fluid therapy is indicated to correct dehydration and maximize renal function. Sometimes, a beta-blocker helps control ventricular tachyarrhythmias, but beta-blockers should not be used with AV conduction block. Quinidine is not used. The steroid-binding resin cholestyramine, given PO, is useful only very soon after accidental digoxin overdose, because enterohepatic circulation of this drug is minimal. A preparation of digoxin-specific antigen–binding fragments (digoxin-immune Fab) derived from ovine antidigoxin antibodies has occasionally been used for digoxin and digitoxin overdose[104]. The Fab binds with antigenic determinants on the digoxin molecule, preventing and reversing the pharmacologic and toxic effects of digoxin. The Fab–digoxin complex is subsequently excreted by the kidney. Each 38 mg vial will bind about 0.6 mg digoxin. For acute oral ingestion, the dose (1 vial for every milligram of digoxin consumed) is based on total digoxin intake. After prolonged overdose (i.e. steady state concentration), the following modified formula[105], taking the volume of distribution of digoxin in the dog into account, is used: number of vials needed = body load of digoxin (mg)/0.6. The body load of digoxin = (serum digoxin concentration [ng/ml]/1,000) x 14 liters/kg x body weight in kg.

PIMOBENDAN

Pimobendan is known as an 'inodilator', because it increases contractility while also causing systemic and pulmonary vasodilation. This leads to improved cardiac pump function. This drug is a benzimidazole derivative PDE III inhibitor. As such it slows cAMP breakdown and enhances adrenergic effects on Ca^{++} fluxes and myocardial contractility. Pimobendan also has a calcium sensitizing effect on the contractile proteins, which increases contractility without greater myocardial O_2 consumption[71, 106]. The drug may have other beneficial effects by modulating NH and proinflammatory cytokine activation[106, 108]. Reports conflict about pimobendan's effect on heart rate. Concurrent calcium channel- or beta-blocker therapy may diminish the drug's positive inotropic effect[106].

Peak plasma levels occur within an hour of PO dosing. Bioavailability is about 60% in dogs, but this decreases in the presence of food. Pimobendan is highly protein-bound. Elimination is mainly via hepatic metabolism and biliary excretion; there is an active metabolite[106].

Many dogs appear to experience marked clinical improvement when this agent is added to conventional CHF therapy (e.g. furosemide, an ACE inhibitor, and digoxin). Controlled clinical trials are ongoing in dogs with heart failure from DCM as well as chronic MR. Pimobendan appears to improve clinical status and increase survival time in DCM and chronic mitral valve disease[107-110]. Pimobendan does not appear to increase the frequency of ventricular arrhythmias and sudden death, as has occurred with other PDE inhibitors. Nevertheless, a trend toward increased overall mortality was seen in one large human trial despite improvement in clinical status with pimobendan[106]. There are limited anecdotal reports of pimobendan use in cats with systolic dysfunction. Pimobendan is available in many countries. It is not yet marketed in the US, but it can be legally imported on an individual case, compassionate use basis.

OTHER VASODILATORS

Arteriolar dilators reduce systemic vascular resistance and LV afterload, thereby enhancing forward cardiac output. They also diminish regurgitant flow in animals with MR, which reduces LA pressure and pulmonary congestion. LA size may decrease somewhat as well. Arterial vasodilators have the potential to cause hypotension, especially in animals with a low cardiac reserve and those already receiving ACE inhibitor and diuretic therapy. Low initial doses are used, with up-titration to effect. Venodilators relax systemic veins, which increases venous capacitance and reduces cardiac filling pressure (preload) and pulmonary congestion.

Hydralazine

Hydralazine is a pure arteriolar dilator that directly relaxes smooth muscle. It can improve cardiac output, congestion, and exercise tolerance. It can also precipitate marked hypotension and reflex tachycardia; the dosage should be reduced if this occurs. Hydralazine can further increase NH activation, which makes it less desirable than ACE inhibitors for long-term use[19]. A common indication for hydralazine is severe acute CHF from MR (see p. 173). Long term, hydralazine is sometimes used with a nitrate for dogs that do not tolerate ACE inhibitors. Hydralazine or amlodipine (see below) is also used as adjunct therapy for dogs with refractory heart failure; a very low starting dose is used. If the initial dose is well-tolerated, the next dose is increased to a low maintenance level. Ideally, blood pressure measurement over several hours should follow each incremental dose; pressures <70–80

mm Hg mean, or <90–100 mm Hg systolic, should be avoided. Clinical evaluation also helps guide dose titration; increasing tachycardia, weakened pulses, lethargy, and poor peripheral perfusion can signal hypotension. Jugular venous PO_2 can indicate directional changes in cardiac output; venous PO_2 >30 mm Hg is desirable[111]. Reduction in concurrent diuretic dosage may be advisable. Hydralazine has a faster onset of action than amlodipine. Its effect peaks within 3 hours and lasts up to 12 hours. Administration with food decreases bioavailability by >60%. First-pass hepatic metabolism is extensive; however, bioavailability in dogs increases over time via saturation of this mechanism. Besides hypotension, GI upset is an adverse effect.

Amlodipine

Amlodipine is a dihydropyridine L-type calcium channel-blocker. Its major effect is peripheral vasodilation, which offsets any negative inotropic effect[112, 113]. It has little effect on AV conduction. Amlodipine is used to treat hypertension in cats and, sometimes, dogs (see Chapter 25), but it is also used as adjunctive therapy for refractory CHF, combined with an ACE inhibitor, furosemide, and digoxin. Amlodipine could be used with a nitrate for dogs that cannot tolerate ACE inhibitors. When added to conventional CHF therapy in people, it does not increase morbidity or mortality, and possibly improves survival with nonischemic DCM. Other calcium channel-blockers have increased morbidity and mortality[114]. Amlodipine has good PO bioavailability and a long duration of action (at least 24 hours in dogs). Plasma concentration peaks in 3–8 hours; half-life is about 30 hours. Plasma concentrations increase with long-term therapy. Maximal effect develops over 4–7 days after therapy is begun in dogs. The drug is metabolized in the liver, so caution is warranted in animals with impaired liver function. Excretion is through the urine and feces. Because of the delay in achieving maximum effect, low initial doses and weekly blood pressure monitoring during slow up-titration are recommended.

Prazosin

Prazosin is a selective alpha$_1$-adrenergic receptor-blocker that promotes arteriolar and venous dilation. It is not often used for chronic CHF management because drug tolerance can develop over time and the capsule dose size is inconvenient in small animals.

Nitrates

Nitrates act as venodilators. They are metabolized in vascular smooth muscle to produce NO, which indirectly mediates vasodilation. Nitroglycerin ointment or isosorbide dinitrate[115] are used occasionally in chronic CHF management, either combined with standard therapy for refractory CHF or with hydralazine or amlodipine in animals that cannot tolerate ACE inhibitors.

Nitrates effect blood redistribution in people, but there are few studies involving dogs, especially using the oral route for CHF management. There is extensive first-pass hepatic metabolism, and the efficacy of oral nitrates is questionable. PO isosorbide mononitrate did not cause a demonstrable shift in blood volume to the splanchnic circulation in one study[110]. Although hypotension might occur from excessive or inappropriate use of nitrates, this is not a common clinical problem. Large doses, frequent application or long-acting formulations are most likely to be associated with drug tolerance. Whether intermittent treatment (with drug-free intervals) would prevent nitrate tolerance from developing in dogs and cats is unknown.

DIETARY CONSIDERATIONS

Heart failure can impair renal ability to excrete excessive Na^+ and water. Dietary Na^+ restriction has long been recommended to reduce fluid accumulation and necessary drug therapy; Cl^- restriction also appears important. However, stringent dietary salt restriction can increase RAAS activation[23, 75]. Nevertheless, a low salt diet appears to improve heart size and end-systolic volume index in dogs with CHF from chronic MR, without apparent change in NH activation[116].

There is controversy about whether a reduced sodium diet should be fed before clinical CHF develops; however, it seems prudent at least to avoid a high-salt diet (and table scraps or treats). When clinical CHF develops, moderate salt restriction is advised; this represents a sodium intake of about 30 mg/kg/day (about 0.06% sodium for canned food or 210–240 mg/100 g of dry food). Diets designed for geriatric animals or animals with renal disease usually provide this amount. Further sodium restriction (~13 mg/kg/day) found in some cardiac diets (about 0.025% sodium for canned food or 90–100 mg/100 g of dry food) may be useful in advanced CHF. Severe sodium restriction (e.g. 7 mg/kg/day) is not recommended because this can exacerbate NH activation and contribute to hyponatremia[23, 116, 117]. A home-made reduced-salt diet can be fed and may be more palatable, but providing a well balanced nutrient content can be challenging. Some drinking water contains considerable amounts of sodium; nonsoftened water or distilled water can be used in these areas.

Poor appetite is common with CHF; caloric intake is likely to be suboptimal, especially in dogs with DCM[118]. When appetite is poor, helpful strategies include warming the food to enhance its flavor, adding small amounts of palatable 'people' foods (e.g. nonsalted meats or low-sodium soup or gravy), using a salt substitute (KCl) or garlic powder, hand feeding, and providing small quantities of food several times a day. If a dietary change is indicated, gradually mixing an increasing proportion of the new food with the old over several days improves its acceptance. Malaise, increased respiratory effort, and adverse effects of medication all contribute to poor appetite. Concurrently, greater caloric intake may be needed due to increased cardiopulmonary energy consumption or stress. Poor splanchnic perfusion, bowel and pancreatic edema, and secondary intestinal lymphangiectasia can reduce nutrient absorption and promote protein loss.

Cardiac cachexia

Cardiac cachexia is the syndrome of muscle wasting as well as fat loss that can accompany chronic CHF. Weakness and fatigue occur when lean body mass is lost. Cardiac mass also declines with cachexia. In people, cardiac cachexia is also associated with reduced immune function and it is a predictor of poor survival[118]. Multiple factors are involved in the pathogenesis of cardiac cachexia, including the proinflammatory cytokines TNF and IL-1[118, 119]. These substances suppress appetite and increase catabolism. Dietary supplementation with fish oils, which are high in n-3 fatty acids (eicosapentaenoic [EPA] and docosahexaenoic [DHA] acids) can reduce cytokine production[118]. They may also improve endothelial function and confer other beneficial effects. Reduced cachexia and circulating IL-1 concentrations occur in dogs with DCM given ~27 mg/kg/day EPA and 18 mg/kg/day DHA[118]. The latter correlated with survival in these dogs, although there was no effect of fish oil on overall mortality[118]. Whether higher EPA and DHA doses would provide added benefit is not known; 30–40 mg/kg/day EPA and 20–25 mg/kg/day DHA orally have been recommended[74].

Supplementation of specific nutrients

Specific nutrient supplementation is important in some cases.

Taurine

Taurine is considered an essential amino acid for cats, although not for dogs[120]. Prolonged deficiency causes myocardial failure as well as other abnormalities (e.g. feline DCM, see Chapter 21, p. 312)[121]. Increased supplementation of commercial cat foods dramatically reduced the prevalence of taurine-responsive DCM in cats; however, taurine levels should be measured in cats diagnosed with DCM, as the diet of some could still be deficient. Taurine-deficient cats are given 250–500 mg taurine q12h.

Some dogs with DCM appear deficient in taurine and/or L-carnitine (see Chapter 20, p. 290)[120, 122–124]. Taurine deficiency DCM is seen mainly in American Cocker Spaniels, some Golden Retrievers, and other 'atypical' breeds. Dogs fed protein-restricted diets can become taurine deficient and some develop evidence of DCM[125, 126]. Taurine supplementation for dogs <25 kg is 500–1,000 mg q8h; for dogs 25–40 kg the dose is 1–2 g q8–12h[120]. Although not all taurine-deficient American Cocker Spaniels need both taurine and L-carnitine, most appear to[120, 123, 127].

L-carnitine

L-carnitine deficiency has been identified in several Boxers and Doberman Pinschers with DCM. However, the prevalence of carnitine-deficiency DCM in dogs of these breeds is thought to be low, and the number responsive to L-carnitine supplementation even lower. L-carnitine plays an essential role in transporting fatty acids into mitochondria for use in ATP generation. Oral L-carnitine supplementation for dogs <25 kg is 1 g q8h; for dogs 25–40 kg the dose is 2 g q8h. (About 1/2 teaspoonful of pure L-carnitine powder is the equivalent of 1 g.) Both taurine and L-carnitine can be mixed with food for easier administration. However, the minimum effective dose, especially of L-carnitine, is not known, and it may vary with the type of deficiency, if deficiency is present at all. L-carnitine has also been recommended at 50–100 mg/kg q8–12h for systemic deficiency, or 200 mg/kg q8h for myopathic deficiency[120]. When it is not known whether carnitine deficiency exists and the client wishes to try supplementation, the higher dosage is recommended for at least 4 months. The dog is then reassessed by echocardiography for evidence of functional improvement. High L-carnitine doses can cause diarrhea.

Other supplements

The role of antioxidant and other dietary supplements is unclear. There is evidence of oxidative stress in patients with myocardial failure, and free-radical damage probably plays a role in the pathogenesis of myocardial dysfunction[128, 129]. TNF and other cytokines that increase in circulation during heart failure can promote oxidative stress. Vitamin C supplementation appears to have a beneficial effect on endothelial function, cardiac morbidity, and mortality in people[130–132], although its role and that of other antioxidant vitamin supplementation in CHF is still unclear, especially in dogs and cats. There is controversy as to whether coenzyme Q_{10} provides measurable benefit. Coenzyme Q_{10} is synthesized in the body and is present in meat-based diets. Its purported benefit in CHF relates to support of ATP synthesis when energy status is depleted, and possibly to oxidative stress reduction. Some human CHF trials with coenzyme Q_{10} suggest functional improvement, while others do not[133]. Neither its efficacy in veterinary patients, nor optimal dose or formulation (if efficacious), are known.

EXERCISE

Exercise restriction is recommended in the face of decompensated CHF; strenuous exercise can provoke dyspnea and potentially serious cardiac arrhythmias. However, in chronic heart failure, skeletal muscle alterations occur that contribute to fatigue and dyspnea. Physical training can improve cardiopulmonary function and quality of life in patients with chronic heart failure[39]. This is partly mediated by improved vascular endothelial function and enhanced flow-dependent vasodilation. It is difficult to know how much exercise is beneficial in an individual. In general, regular (not sporadic) mild to moderate activity is encouraged, as long as signs of excessive respiratory effort do not develop. Strenuous bursts of activity should be avoided.

BETA-BLOCKERS IN CHRONIC HEART FAILURE

The traditional use of beta-blockers in dogs and cats with CHF is for arrhythmia management (e.g. atrial fibrillation and some ventricular tachyarrhythmias; see Chapter 17). The negative inotropic effect of these agents must be taken into account, especially in animals with marked systolic dysfunction. Apart from arrhythmia control, their use in patients with myocardial failure seemed counterintuitive historically, but it is now well known that in people with myocardial failure, long-term (>4 month) therapy with certain beta-blockers improves cardiac function, reverses pathologic ventricular remodeling, and reduces mortality[1, 134]. Protection from the toxic effects of endogenous catecholamines improves myocardial function with time, which overcomes the negative inotropic effect of adrenergic blockade[12]. Not all beta-blockers are effective in this regard. The 3rd generation beta-blocker carvedilol, and some 2nd generation agents (metoprolol, bisoprolol), have produced a survival benefit in people. Carvedilol appears most effective in human clinical trials; it also improves clinical status and survival in people with severe heart failure[135]. The possibility that carvedilol, or metoprolol, might play a similar beneficial role in dogs, especially those with DCM, is appealing, but the clinical efficacy of this drug in dogs, and cats, is presently not known.

Carvedilol

Carvedilol blocks $beta_1$-, $beta_2$-, and $alpha_1$-adrenergic receptors, has antioxidant effects, and decreases ET release[136]. Carvedilol also has some Ca^{++} blocking properties and it lacks intrinsic sympathomimetic activity. Carvedilol, and to a lesser extent metoprolol, was shown to reduce circulating proinflammatory cytokine levels in people with DCM[137]. The attenuation or reversal of pathologic myocardial remodeling seen with carvedilol in heart failure may be related partly to reduced oxygen free radicals, which contribute to myocardial dysfunction and cell death[13]. Carvedilol's combined beta-blockade reduces cardiac adrenergic activity without up-regulating beta-receptors; metoprolol does not[13]. The alpha$_1$-blocking effect of carvedilol offsets its beta$_1$-blocking effect on contractility. In healthy dogs, low doses of carvedilol cause minimal hemodynamic effect[136, 138]. Doses of 0.2–0.4 mg/kg in experimental MR lowered blood pressure and heart rate within 3 hours without changing other hemodynamic parameters; values returned to baseline by 24 hours[139]. Decreased systemic vascular resistance with IV carvedilol was observed in dogs[140]. In people, the optimal plasma concentration is 100 ng/ml; IV infusion to a cumulative dose of 0.15–0.31 mg/kg achieved that plasma level in dogs[136]. Oral doses of 1.5 mg/kg in healthy dogs produce a wide range of peak plasma concentrations, from well below to almost 2.5 times the human optimal level[141, 142]. Dogs in heart failure may not tolerate this dose and caution is urged. Peak plasma concentration correlates with the degree of attenuation in heart rate response to isoproterenol challenge[142]. Carvedilol is eliminated mainly through hepatic metabolism; the terminal half-life in dogs is <1–2 hours (i.e. shorter than in people) and the drug is highly protein-bound[136]. A substantial nonselective beta-blocking effect lasts for 12 hours, with minimal effect on resting heart rate and blood pressure in normal dogs; some residual effect persists for up to 24 hours[139, 141, 142]. An active metabolite is probably responsible[139, 141]. These findings suggest q12h dosing is adequate.

Metoprolol

Metoprolol has been used in dogs with chronic MR and DCM. The drug seems well-tolerated, but its long-term effect on myocardial function and survival has not been reported[143]. In an experimental dog model of ischemic DCM, 3 months of metoprolol treatment prevented progressive left ventricular dilation, remodeling, and dysfunction[144, 145]. Atenolol, another 2nd generation beta-blocker, also produced beneficial effects on myocardial function in dogs with iatrogenic MR[146]. Heart rate reduction (from atenolol) was thought to have a positive effect on myocardial energetics.

General considerations when using beta-blockers in CHF

Caution is warranted when using a beta-blocker in CHF. Some patients experience clinical deterioration, including hypotension, bradycardia, and worsening failure, before any long-term benefit is seen. The risk of CHF decompensation is mitigated by delaying beta-blocker therapy until the patient is clinically stabilized, and using low initial doses and slow drug up-titration. Considering the short survival time for most dogs with overt CHF from DCM, many may not live long enough to realize significant myocardial functional improvement; however, beta-blocker initiation during the clinically occult stage would appear rational.

Carvedilol, or metoprolol, could be considered for dogs with occult DCM, dogs with stable compensated CHF (e.g. no evidence of congestion for at least a week or more) caused by DCM, or dogs with chronic MR that have evidence for myocardial dysfunction and compensated CHF. A very low initial dose is used, along with conventional CHF therapy as indicated. Beta-blocker up-titration is done slowly. The dosage is increased every 1–2 weeks, if possible, over a 2-month period, to a target dose or as tolerated. Anecdotal experience with carvedilol suggests an initial dose of 0.05–0.1 mg/kg q24h, with an eventual target of 0.2–0.3 mg/kg q12h (or higher) if tolerated. An initial metoprolol dose might be 0.1–0.2 mg/kg/day, with an eventual target of 1 mg/kg if tolerated[13]. Frequent monitoring is important, especially during up-titration; bradycardia, hypotension, and CHF decompensation are potential adverse effects; dosage reduction, at least temporarily, or increased diuretic dose are recommended to counteract this in people[147]. An interesting consideration could be the use of pimobendan for inotropic support during beta-blocker titration. Results of veterinary clinical studies are needed before definitive guidelines can be established.

POSSIBLE FUTURE THERAPY

Because there are alternative pathways besides ACE for AT II production, blockade of AT II receptors presents another possible therapeutic strategy. AT II receptor-blockers act at AT II-subtype 1 receptors, which mediate AT II's cardiovascular effects. These receptors occur mainly in vascular smooth muscle, kidney, heart, and adrenal gland tissue. AT II receptor-blockers, used in place of or in combination with an ACE inhibitor, appear to have beneficial effects in people with CHF. Their use in dogs and cats has not been well studied.

Blockade of other NH pathways activated in CHF may provide new treatment strategies in the future, although initial experience with some approaches has been disappointing. These include inhibitors of neutral endopeptidase (an enzyme that inactivates natriuretic peptides, angiotensins, and bradykinins), vasopeptidase (which inhibits both neutral endopeptidase and ACE), and ET. The possible role of pentoxifylline for CHF therapy is not known. Improved clinical signs and ventricular function were seen in people when pentoxifylline was added to digoxin, ACE inhibitor, and carvedilol therapy for idiopathic DCM[148, 149]. Pentoxifylline is a methylxanthine drug with immunologic and hematologic properties, and less potent chronotropic and inotropic effects than theophylline. It reportedly reduces inflammatory mediators, including TNF and IL-1, and stimulates collagenase[150]. Another approach that seems effective as adjunctive therapy in people with severe CHF is recombinant human BNP (nesiritide) given SC (~10 mcg/kg q12h)[151]. Veterinary experience with this is lacking. Cardiac resynchronization therapy, using artificial biventricular pacing, has improved systolic function, clinical status, and survival in people with abnormal intraventricular conduction and myocardial failure. Applicability of this therapy in dogs has not been explored. Stem cell transplantation is another emerging modality for human heart failure that may have future applicability in veterinary patients.

LONG-TERM MANAGEMENT OF DIASTOLIC DYSFUNCTION

Following management for acute CHF, if needed, furosemide PO is used at the lowest effective dose. A common starting dose for cats is 6.25 mg q12h, with adjustment up or down as indicated. After other long-term therapy has begun, some animals can be weaned off, or reduced to a very low dose, of furosemide, at least for a time. A beta-blocker or calcium channel-blocker has been the traditional therapy for diastolic dysfunction (e.g. HCM), although controversy now exists. ACE inhibitor therapy is probably beneficial (see also Chapter 21)[152, 153]. Spironolactone can be added, especially for cats with recurrent pleural effusion.

Calcium channel-blockers as a group can cause coronary and systemic vasodilation, enhance myocardial relaxation, and reduce cardiac contractility. Some of these agents have antiarrhythmic effects by their action on the slow inward Ca^{++} current (see Chapter 17, p. 217). calcium channel-blockers are thought to exert their beneficial effects in HCM by modestly reducing heart rate and contractility, which reduces myocardial O_2 demand. Diltiazem may have a positive effect on myocardial relaxation. Although verapamil has a greater negative inotropic effect than diltiazem, which is advantageous for reducing ventricular outflow obstruction, it is not recommended because of its variable bioavailability and risk of toxicity in cats[154]. Calcium channel-blockers with primarily vasodilatory effects (e.g. amlodipine, nifedipine) can provoke reflex tachycardia and worsen a systolic outflow gradient; therefore, they are not used for HCM.

Beta-blockers are thought to have a greater ability to reduce heart rate and dynamic LV outflow obstruction compared with diltiazem. Beta-blockers are also indicated to control tachyarrhythmias in cats.

By inhibiting catecholamine-induced myocyte damage, they may reduce myocardial fibrosis; however, beta-blockers can potentially slow active relaxation. Atenolol (see Chapter 17, p. 214) is the beta-blocker used most commonly.

PATIENT MONITORING AND FOLLOW-UP EVALUATION

Periodic reevaluation is important in animals with heart failure (*Table 45*). Disease progression and complications often occur. Medications and dosage schedules should be reviewed with the owner at each visit. Problems with giving the drug, including compliance in dosing as prescribed, or adverse effects should be ascertained. The animal's diet, appetite, and activity levels, and any concerns are also discussed. Client education is crucial to successful long-term heart failure management. Early identification of complications is more likely when the owner has a good understanding of their pet's underlying disease, CHF signs, and the purpose and potential adverse effects of each medication. Home monitoring of the animal's resting/sleeping respiratory rate is helpful. Most animals normally breathe at ≤30 breaths/minute when resting in the home environment. Because pulmonary edema increases lung stiffness, it induces faster, more shallow respirations; a persistent increase in resting respiratory rate can be an early sign of CHF decompensation. Likewise, a persistent increase in resting heart rate occurs with the heightened sympathetic tone of CHF.

A thorough physical examination, with emphasis on the cardiovascular system (see Chapter 2), is important at each evaluation. Depending on the patient's status, other tests might include a resting ECG or ambulatory monitoring (see Chapter 4), thoracic radiographs (see Chapter 3), CBC and serum biochemical tests, an echocardiogram (see Chapter 5), serum digoxin concentration, or others. Serum electrolyte and creatinine (or urea nitrogen) concentrations are monitored frequently. Electrolyte imbalances (especially hypokalemia or hyperkalemia, hypomagnesemia, and sometimes hyponatremia) can occur with the use of diuretics, ACE inhibitors, and salt restriction[155]. Prolonged anorexia can contribute to hypokalemia; however, potassium supplements are not used without documented hypokalemia, especially when an ACE inhibitor and spironolactone are prescribed. Serum magnesium concentration does not accurately reflect total body stores; however, supplementation may help animals that develop ventricular arrhythmias while receiving furosemide and digoxin.

Many factors can exacerbate the signs of CHF, including physical exertion, infection, anemia, fluid administration, high-salt diet or dietary indiscretion,

Table 45 Reevaluation of the chronic heart failure patient.

1) Review recent history:

   a) Attitude and activity level.

   b) Appetite and water intake.

   ■ Verify diet being eaten.

2) Respiratory (+/- heart) rate when resting/sleeping at home.

3) Any coughing? (see Chapter 8):

   a) How often and when does it occur?

   b) Dry/honking or moist sound?

4) Any episodes of respiratory difficulty? (see Chapter 9).

5) Verify all medications (prescription and nonprescription):

   a) Drug name.

   b) Tablet size/liquid concentration.

   c) Dosage and frequency.

5) Any concerns about possible adverse drug effects?

6) Any problems with medication administration?

7) Have all doses been given as prescribed?

   a) Are any refills needed?

8) Physical examination:

   a) Thorough general examination.

   b) Careful cardiovascular examination (see Chapters 2, 6, and 10–12).

   c) Note heart rate and rhythm (see Chapter 13).

   d) Note respiratory rate and effort.

   e) Note changes since last examination:

   ■ Heart sounds/murmurs.

   ■ Heart rhythm.

   ■ Pulmonary sounds.

   ■ Body weight/condition.

   ■ Any abnormal fluid accumulation?

9) Laboratory and other testing:

   a) Blood pressure.

   b) Check renal function, Na^+, and K^+ at minimum.

   c) Complete biochemistry panel, hemogram, and urinalysis periodically or if other concerns.

   d) Thoracic radiographs if suspect pulmonary edema (e.g. increased home resting respiratory rate, pulmonary crackles, new or worsened cough) or other concerns based on history/physical examination (see Chapter 3).

   e) ECG if an arrhythmia is suspected, an unexpectedly low or high heart rate is auscultated, or to document heart rate with atrial fibrillation (see Chapter 4).

   f) Ambulatory ECG monitoring if indicated (e.g. to identify occult arrhythmias or assess efficacy of antiarrhythmic therapy).

   g) Serum digoxin concentration, indicated especially if therapy recently begun, dosage changed, or any signs suspicious for toxicity (see p. 181).

   h) Echocardiogram periodically, to assess myocardial function and evidence for disease progression (see Chapter 5).

   i) Heartworm testing and prophylaxis as indicated in endemic areas.

   j) Other tests as indicated.

erratic administration of medication, inappropriate medication dosage for the level of disease, development of cardiac arrhythmias, environmental stress, development or worsening of concurrent extracardiac disease (e.g. systemic hypertension, hyperadrenocorticism, hypo- or hyperthyroidism, renal failure, neoplasia, pneumonia, pulmonary hypertension, anemia), and progression of underlying heart disease. Repeated episodes of decompensated CHF are relatively common in patients with chronic progressive heart failure.

APPROACH TO REFRACTORY CONGESTIVE HEART FAILURE

Chronic CHF that is difficult to control with initial furosemide and ACE inhibitor doses is usually handled by either intensifying the dosage of either or both drugs, adding digoxin (if not previously used), or adding pimobendan or other ancillary therapy. Administering furosemide SC can improve diuretic effectiveness in patients with splanchnic congestion and poor oral absorption. As dosages approach maximum recommended levels, another diuretic or vasodilator can be added as needed. Spironolactone is recommended first because of its ALD antagonist action and the possibility of aldosterone escape. While the use of spironolactone earlier in the course of therapy may be advantageous in dogs and cats with CHF, documentation of improved cardiac function and survival is awaited.

Further therapeutic intensification for dogs with CHF from chronic MR or DCM is also achieved by adding a low dose of another vasodilator (e.g. amlodipine or hydralazine) to further reduce afterload. Blood pressure should be monitored in these cases. Arteriolar vasodilation is not recommended for cats with hypertrophic cardiomyopathy or dogs with fixed ventricular outflow obstruction (e.g. subaortic stenosis). Some animals benefit from the addition of a thiazide diuretic or nitrate as failure becomes more refractory.

REFERENCES

1 Francis GS (2005) Pathophysiology of chronic heart failure. *Am J Med* 110:37S–46S.
2 Davila DF, Nunez TJ, Odreman R *et al.* (2005) Mechanisms of neurohormonal activation in chronic congestive heart failure: pathophysiology and therapeutic implications. *Int J Cardiol* 101:343–346.
3 Turk JR (1998) Physiologic and pathophysiologic effects of endothelin: implications in cardiopulmonary disease. *J Am Vet Med Assoc* 212:265–270.
4 Meurs KM, Fox PR, Miller MW *et al.* (2002) Plasma concentrations of tumor necrosis factor–alpha in cats with congestive heart failure. *Am J Vet Res* 63:640–642.
5 Tidholm A, Haggstrom J, Hansson K (2005) Vasopressin, cortisol, and catecholamine concentrations in dogs with dilated cardiomyopathy. *Am J Vet Res* 66:1709–1717.
6 Tidholm A, Haggstrom J, Hansson K (2001) Effects of dilated cardiomyopathy on the renin-angiotensin-aldosterone system, atrial natriuretic peptide activity, and thyroid hormone concentrations in dogs. *Am J Vet Res* 62:961–967.
7 Ware WA, Lund DD, Subieta AR *et al.* (1990) Sympathetic activation in dogs with congestive heart failure caused by chronic mitral valve disease and dilated cardiomyopathy. *J Am Vet Med Assoc* 197:1475–1481.
8 Knowlen GG, Kittleson MD, Nachreiner RF *et al.* (1983) Comparison of plasma aldosterone concentration among clinical status groups of dogs with chronic heart failure. *J Am Vet Med Assoc* 183:991–996.
9 Weber KT (2001) Aldosterone in congestive heart failure. *N Engl J Med* 345:1689–1697.
10 Sisson DD (2004) Neuroendocrine evaluation of cardiac disease. *Vet Clin North Am: Small Anim Pract* 34:1105–1126.
11 Chetboul V, Tessier-Vetzel D, Escriou C *et al.* (2004) Diagnostic potential of natriuretic peptides in occult phase of Golden Retriever muscular dystrophy cardiomyopathy. *J Vet Intern Med* 18:845–850.
12 Packer M (2001) Current role of beta-adrenergic blockers in the management of chronic heart failure. *Am J Med* 110:81S–94S.
13 Abbott JA (2004) Beta-blockade in the management of systolic dysfunction. *Vet Clin North Am: Small Anim Pract* 34:1157–1170.
14 Re G, Bergamasco L, Badino P *et al.* (1999) Canine dilated cardiomyopathy: lymphocyte and cardiac alpha(1)- and beta-adrenoreceptor concentrations in normal and affected Great Danes. *Vet J* 158:1475–1481.
15 Borgarelli M, Badino P, Bergamasco L *et al.* (1999) Lymphocyte beta-adrenoreceptor down-regulation in Great Danes with occult dilated cardiomyopathy (DCM) and with DCM and heart failure. *Vet J* 158:128–134.
16 Cheng HJ, Zhang ZS, Onishi K *et al.* (2001) Upregulation of functional beta(3)-adrenergic receptor in the failing canine myocardium. *Circ Res* 89:599–606.
17 McCurley JM, Hanlon SU, Wei SK *et al.* (2004) Furosemide and the progression of left ventricular dysfunction in experimental heart failure. *J Am Coll Cardiol* 44:1301–1307.
18 Kvart C, Haggsrom J, Pedersen HD *et al.* (2002) Efficacy of enalapril for prevention of congestive heart failure in dogs with myxomatous valve disease and asymptomatic mitral

regurgitation. *J Vet Intern Med* **16**:80–88.

19 Haggstrom J, Hansson K, Karlberg BE *et al.* (1996) Effects of long-term treatment with enalapril or hydralazine on the renin-angiotensin-aldosterone system and fluid balance in dogs with naturally acquired mitral valve regurgitation. *Am J Vet Res* **57**:1645–1652.

20 Itkin RJ (1994) Effects of the renin-angiotensin system on the kidneys. *Compend Cont Educ Small Anim Pract* **16**:753–764.

21 Haggstrom J, Hansson K, Kvart C *et al.* (1997) Effects of naturally acquired decompensated mitral valve regurgitation on the renin-angiotensin-aldosterone system and atrial natriuretic peptide concentration in dogs. *Am J Vet Res* **58**:77–82.

22 Pedersen HD, Koch J, Poulsen K *et al.* (1995) Activation of the renin-angiotensin system in dogs with asymptomatic and mildly symptomatic mitral valvular insufficiency. *J Vet Intern Med* **9**:328–331.

23 Pedersen HD (1996) Effects of mild mitral valve insufficiency, sodium intake, and place of blood sampling on renin-angiotensin system in dogs. *Acta Vet Scand* **37**:109–118.

24 Pedersen HD, Olsen LH, Mow T *et al.* (1999) Neuroendocrine changes in Dachshunds with mitral valve prolapse examined under different study conditions. *Res Vet Sci* **66**:11–17.

25 Dell'italia L, Balcells E, Meng Q *et al.* (1997) Volume-overload cardiac hypertrophy is unaffected by ACE inhibitor treatment in dogs. *Am J Physiol* **273**:H961–H970.

26 Sisson DD, Oyama MA, Solter PF (2003) Plasma levels of ANP, BNP, epinephrine, norepinephrine, serum aldosterone, and plasma renin activity in healthy cats and cats with myocardial disease. Abstract. *J Vet Intern Med* **17**:438.

27 Koch J, Pedersen HD, Jensen AL *et al.* (1995) Activation of the renin-angiotensin system in dogs with asymptomatic and symptomatic dilated cardiomyopathy. *Res Vet Sci* **59**:172–175.

28 Prosek R, Sisson D, Oyama M *et al.* (2004) Plasma endothelin-1 immunoreactivity in normal dogs and dogs with acquired heart disease. *J Vet Intern Med* **18**:840–844.

29 Prosek R, Sisson D, Oyama M *et al.* (2004) Measurements of plasma endothelin immunoreactivity in healthy cats and cats with cardiomyopathy. *J Vet Intern Med* **18**:826–830.

30 deMorais HA, Schwartz DS (2005) Pathophysiology of heart failure. In: *Textbook of Veterinary Internal Medicine*, 6th edn. SJ Ettinger, EC Feldman (eds). WB Saunders, Philadelphia, pp. 914–940.

31 deLaforcade AM, Freeman LM, Rush JE (2003) Serum nitrate and nitrite in dogs with spontaneous cardiac disease. *J Vet Intern Med* **17**:315–318.

32 Turk JR (2000) Physiologic and pathophysiologic effects of natriuretic peptides and their implication in cardiopulmonary disease. *J Am Vet Med Assoc* **216**:1970–1976.

33 MacDonald KA, Kittleson MD, Munro C *et al.* (2003) Brain natriuretic peptide concentration in dogs with heart disease and congestive heart failure. *J Vet Intern Med* **17**: 172–177.

34 Haggstrom J, Hansson K, Kvart C *et al.* (2000) Relationship between different natriuretic peptides and severity of naturally acquired mitral regurgitation in dogs with chronic myxomatous valve disease. *J Vet Cardiol* **2**:7–16.

35 Asano K, Masuda K, Okumura M *et al.* (1999) Plasma atrial and brain naturietic peptide levels in dogs with congestive heart failure. *J Vet Med Sci* **61**:523–529.

36 Schober KE (2005) Biochemical markers of cardiovascular disease. In: *Textbook of Veterinary Internal Medicine*, 6th edn. SJ Ettinger, EC Feldman WB Saunders, (eds). Philadelphia, pp. 940–948.

37 Pedersen HD, Schuett T, Sondergaard R *et al.* (2003) Decreased plasma concentration of nitric oxide metabolites in dogs with untreated mitral regurgitation. *J Vet Intern Med* **17**:8–184.

38 Boddy KN, Roche BM, Schwartz DS *et al.* (2004) Evaluation of the six-minute walk test in dogs. *Am J Vet Res* **65**:331–313.

39 Hornig B, Maier V, Drexler H (1996) Physical training improves endothelial function in patients with chronic heart failure. *Circulation* **93**:210–214.

40 Straeter-Knowlen IM, Dell'Italia LJ, Dai J *et al.* (1999) ACE inhibitors in HF restore canine pulmonary endothelial function and ANGII vasoconstriction. *American Physiology Soc* **277**:H1924–H1930.

41 Spratt DP, Mellanby RJ, Drury N *et al.* (2005) Cardiac troponin I: evaluation of a biomarker for the diagnosis of heart disease in the dog. *J Small Anim Pract* **46**:139–145.

42 Sleeper MM, Clifford CA, Laster LL (2001) Cardiac troponin I in the normal dog and cat. *J Vet Intern Med* **15**:501–503.

43 De Francesco TC, Atkins CE, Keene BW *et al.* (2002) Prospective clinical evaluation of serum cardiac troponin I in dogs admitted to a veterinary teaching hospital. *J Vet Intern Med* **16**:553–555.

44 Herndon WE, Kittleson MD, Sanderson K *et al.* (2002) Cardiac troponin I in feline hypertrophic cardiomyopathy. *J Vet Intern Med* **16**:558–564.

45 Lobetti R, Dvir E, Pearson J (2002) Cardiac troponins in canine babesiosis. *J Vet Intern Med* **16**:63–68.

46 Pelander L, Haggstrom J, Jones B(2002) Troponin I: a possible marker of myocardial cell damage in the dog? *Eur J Compan Anim Pract* **12**:66–71.

47 Schober KE, Cornand C, Kirbach B *et al.* (2002) Serum cardiac troponin I and cardiac troponin T concentrations in dogs with gastric dilatation-volvulus. *J Am Vet Med Assoc* **221**:381–388.

48 Schober KE, Kirbach B, Oechtung G (1999) Noninvasive assessment of myocardial cell injury in dogs with suspected cardiac contusion. *J Vet Cardiol* **1**:17–25.

49 Connolly DJ, Cannata J, Boswood A et al. (2003) Cardiac troponin I in cats with hypertrophic cardiomyopathy. *J Fel Med Surg* 5:209–216.

50 Oyama MA, Sisson DD (2004) Cardiac troponin I concentration in dogs with cardiac disease. *J Vet Intern Med* 18:831–839.

51 Oyama MA, Solter PF (2004) Validation of an immunoassay for measurement of canine cardiac troponin-I. *J Vet Cardiol* 6, 17–24.

52 Shaw SP, Rozanski EA, Rush JE (2004) Cardiac troponins I and T in dogs with pericardial effusion. *J Vet Intern Med* 18:322–324.

53 Adin DB, Milner RJ, Berger KD et al. (2005) Cardiac troponin I concentrations in normal dogs and cats using a bedside analyzer. *J Vet Cardiol* 7:27–32.

54 Oyama MA, Solter PF (2004) Validation of an immunoassay for measurement of canine cardiac troponin I. *J Vet Cardiol* 7:17–24.

55 Haggstrom J, Hansson K, Karlberg BE et al. (1994) Plasma concentration of atrial natriuretic peptide in relation to severity of mitral regurgitation in Cavalier King Charles Spaniels. *Am J Vet Res* 55:698–703.

56 Sisson D (2001) The diagnostic potential of natriuretic peptides in heart failure. *J Vet Cardiol* 2:5–6.

57 Boswood A, Attree A, Page K (2003) Clinical validation of a pro-ANP 31-67 fragment ELISA in the diagnosis of heart failure in the dog. *J Small Anim Pract* 44:104–108.

58 Crowe DT (2003) Supplemental oxygen therapy in critically ill or injured patients. *Vet Med* 98:935–953.

59 Tseng LW, Drobatz KJ (2004) Oxygen supplementation and humidification. In: *Textbook of Respiratory Disease in Dogs and Cats*. LG King (ed.) Elsevier Saunders, St. Louis, pp. 205–213.

60 Clare M, Hopper K (2005) Mechanical ventilation: indications, goals and prognosis. *Compend Cont Educ Pract Vet* 27:195–207.

61 Lee JA, Drobatz KJ (2004) Respiratory distress and cyanosis in dogs. In: *Textbook of Respiratory Disease in Dogs and Cats*. LG King (ed.) Elsevier Saunders, St. Louis, pp. 1–12.

62 Clare M, Hopper K (2005) Mechanical ventilation: ventilator settings, patient management, and nursing care. *Compend Cont Educ Pract Vet* 27:256–268.

63 Haskins SC, King LG (2004) Positive pressure ventilation. In: *Textbook of Respiratory Disease in Dogs and Cats*. LG King (ed.) Elsevier Saunders, St. Louis, pp. 217–229.

64 Silke B (1993) Central hemodynamic effects of diuretic therapy in chronic heart failure. *Cardiovasc Drugs Ther* 7(**Suppl 1**):45–53.

65 Pickkers P, Dormans TPJ, Russel FGM et al. (1997) Direct vascular effects of furosemide in humans. *Circulation* 96:1847–1852.

66 Adin DB, Taylor AW, Hill RC et al. (2003) Intermittent bolus injection versus continuous infusion of furosemide in normal adult greyhound dogs. *J Vet Intern Med* 17:632–636.

67 Adin DB, Hill RC, Scott KC (2003) Short-term compatibility of furosemide with crystalloid solutions. *J Vet Intern Med* 17:724–726.

68 Parameswaran N, Hamlin RL, Nakayama T et al. (1999) Increased splenic capacity in response to transdermal application of nitroglycerine in the dog. *J Vet Intern Med* 13:44–46.

69 Wang SY, Manyari DE, Scott-Douglas N et al. (1995) Splanchnic venous pressure-volume relation during experimental acute ischemic heart failure: differential effects of hydralazine, enalaprilat, and nitroglycerine. *Circulation* 91:1205–1212.

70 Green JF, Jackman AP, Parsons G (1978) The effects of morphine on the mechanical properties of the systemic circulation in the dog. *Circ Res* 42:474–478.

71 Perrone SV, Kaplinsky EJ (2005) Calcium sensitizer agents: a new class of inotropic agents in the treatment of decompensated heart failure. *Int J Cardiol* 103:248–255.

72 Keister DM, Kittleson MD, Bonagura JD et al. (1990) Milrinone: a clinical trial in 29 dogs with moderate-to-severe congestive heart failure. *J Vet Intern Med* 4:79–86.

73 Kittleson MD, Johnson LE, Pion PD (1987) The acute hemodynamic effects of milrinone in dogs with severe idiopathic myocardial failure. *J Vet Intern Med* 1:121–127.

74 Bonagura JB, Lehmkuhl LB, de Morais HA (2006) Fluid and diuretic therapy in heart failure. In *Fluid, Electrolyte, and Acid-Base Disorders in Small Animal Practice*, 3rd edn. SP DiBartola (ed). Elsevier Saunders, St Louis, pp. 490–518.

75 Lovern CS, Swecker WS, Lee JC et al (2001) Additive effects of a sodium chloride restricted diet and furosemide administration in healthy dogs. *Am J Vet Res* 62:1793–1796.

76 Cobb M, Michell AR (1992) Electrolyte concentrations in dogs receiving diuretic therapy for cardiac failure. *J Small Anim Pract* 33:526–529.

77 Riordan L, Estrada A (2005) Diuretic efficacy of oral spironolactone when used in conjunction with furosemide in healthy adult greyhounds. Abstract. *J Vet Intern Med* 19:451.

78 Pitt B, Zannad F, Remme WJ et al. (1999) The effect of spironolactone on morbidity and mortality in patients with severe heart failure. Randomized Aldactone Evaluation Study Investigators. *N Engl J Med* 341:709–717.

79 Tsutamoto T, Wada A, Maeda K et al. (2001) Effect of spironolactone on plasma brain natriuretic peptide and left ventricular remodeling in patients with congestive heart failure. *J Am Coll Cardiol* 37:1228–1233.

80 Svensson M, Gustafsson F, Galatius S et al. (2004) How prevalent is hyperkalemia and renal dysfunction during treatment with spironolactone in patients with congestive heart failure? *J Card Fail* 10:297–303.

81 Juurlink DN, Mamdani MM, Lee DS et al. (2004) Rates of hyperkalemia after publication of the Randomized Aldactone Evaluation Study. *N Engl J Med* 351:526–528.

82 COVE Study Group (1995) Controlled clinical evaluation of

enalapril in dogs with heart failure: results of the Cooperative Veterinary Study Group. *J Vet Intern Med* 9:243–252.

83 IMPROVE Study Group (1995) Acute and short-term hemodynamic, echocardiographic, and clinical effects of enalapril maleate in dogs with naturally acquired heart failure: results of the Invasive Multicenter Prospective Veterinary Evaluation of Enalapril study. *J Vet Intern Med* 9:234–242.

84 Hamlin RL, Benitz AM, Ericsson GF *et al.* (1996) Effects of enalapril on exercise tolerance and longevity in dogs with heart failure produced by iatrogenic mitral regurgitation. *J Vet Intern Med* 10:85–87.

85 Ettinger SJ, Benitz AM, Ericsson GF *et al.* (1998) Effects of enalapril maleate on survival of dogs with naturally acquired heart failure. *J Am Vet Med Assoc* 213:1573–1577.

86 Kitagawa H, Wakamiya H, Kitoh K *et al.* (1997) Efficacy of monotherapy with benazepril, an angiotensin converting enzyme inhibitor, in dogs with naturally acquired chronic mitral insufficiency. *J Vet Med Sci* 59:513–520.

87 Atkins CE (2002) Enalapril monotherapy in asymptomatic mitral regurgitation, results of Vetproof. In: *Proceedings of the 20th ACVIM Forum*, Nashville, pp. 75–76.

88 Hamlin RL, Nakayama T (1998) Comparison of some pharmacokinetic parameters of 5 angiotensin-converting enzyme inhibitors in normal Beagles. *J Vet Intern Med* 12:93–95.

89 Atkins CE, Brown WA, Coats JR *et al.* (2002) Effects of long-term administration of enalapril on clinical indicators of renal function in dogs with compensated mitral regurgitation. *J Am Vet Med Assoc* 221:654–658.

90 Lefebvre HP, Laroute V, Concordet D *et al.* (1999) Effects of renal impairment on the disposition of orally administered enalapril, benazepril and their active metabolites. *J Vet Intern Med* 13:21–27.

91 Pouchelon JL, King J, Martignoni L *et al.* (2004) Long-term tolerability of benazepril in dogs with congestive heart failure. *J Vet Cardiol* 6:7–13.

92 BENCH study group (1999) The effect of benazepril on survival times and clinical signs of dogs with congestive heart failure: results of a multicenter, prospective, randomized, double-blinded, placebo-controlled, long-term clinical trial. *J Vet Cardiol* 1:7–18.

93 King JN, Mauron C, Kaiser G (1995) Pharmacokinetics of the active metabolite of benazepril, benazeprilat, and inhibition of plasma angiotensin-converting enzyme activity after single and repeated administration to dogs. *Am J Vet Res* 56:1620–1628.

94 King JN, Humbert-Droz E, Maurer M (1996) Pharmacokinetics of benazepril and inhibition of plasma ACE activity in cats. Abstract. *J Vet Intern Med* 10, 63.

95 Brown SA, Brown CA, Jacobs G *et al.* (2001) Effects of the angiotensin-converting enzyme inhibitor benazepril in cats with induced renal insufficiency. *Am J Vet Res* 62:375–383.

96 Amberger C, Chetboul V, Bomassi E *et al.* (2004) Comparison of the effects of imidapril and enalapril in a prospective, multicentric randomized trial in dogs with naturally acquired heart failure. *J Vet Cardiol* 6:9–16.

97 Lee SC, Park SW, Kim DK *et al.* (2001) Iron supplementation inhibits cough associated with ACE inhibitors. *Hypertension* 38:166–170.

98 Teo KK, Yusuf S, Pfeffer M *et al.* (2002) Effects of long-term treatment with angiotensin-converting enzyme inhibitors in the presence or absence of aspirin: a systematic review. *Lancet* 360:1037–1043.

99 Hood WB, Dans AL, Guyatt GH *et al.* (20040 Digitalis for treatment of congestive heart failure in patients in sinus rhythm: a systematic review and meta-analysis. *J Card Fail* 10:155–164.

100 Bolton GR, Powell W (1982) Plasma kinetics of digoxin in the cat. *Am J Vet Res* 43,1994–1999.

101 Erichsen DF, Harris SG, Upson DW (1980) Therapeutic and toxic plasma concentrations of digoxin in the cat. *Am J Vet Res* 41:2049–2058.

102 Atkins CE, Snyder PS, Keene BW *et al.* (1989) Effects of compensated heart failure on digoxin pharmacokinetics in cats. *J Am Vet Med Assoc* 195:945–950.

103 Bonagura JD, Ware WA (1986) Atrial fibrillation in the dog: clinical findings in 81 cases. *J Am Anim Hosp Assoc* 22:111–120.

104 Ward DM, Forrester SD, DeFrancesco TC *et al.* (1999) Treatment of severe chronic digoxin toxicosis in a dog with cardiac disease, using ovine digoxin-specific immunoglobulin G Fab fragments. *J Am Vet Med Assoc* 215:1808–1812.

105 Senior DF, Feist EH, Stuart LB *et al.* (1991) Treatment of acute digoxin toxicosis with digoxin immune Fab (ovine). *J Vet Intern Med* 5:302–303.

106 Luis Fuentes V (2004) Use of pimobendan in the management of heart failure. *Vet Clin North Am: Small Anim Pract* 34:1145–1155.

107 O'Grady MR, Minors SL, O'Sullivan LM *et al.* (2003) Evaluation of the efficacy of pimobendan to reduce mortality and morbidity in Doberman Pinschers with congestive heart failure due to dilated cardiomyopathy. Abstract. *J Vet Intern Med* 17, 410.

108 Lombard CW, Jöns O, Bussadori CM (2006) Clinical effeciency of pimobendan versus benazepril for the treatment of acquired atrioventricular valvular disease in dogs. *J Am Anim Hosp Assoc* 42:249–261.

109 Smith PJ, French AT, Van Israël N *et al.* (2005) Efficacy and safety of pimobendan in canine heart failure caused by myxomatous mitral valve disease. *J Small Anim Pract* 46:121–130.

110 Luis Fuentes V, Corcoran B, French A *et al.* (2002) A double-blind, randomized, placebo-controlled study of pimobendan in dogs with cardiomyopathy. *J Vet Intern Med* 16:255–261.

111 Kittleson MD, EysterGE, Olivier NB *et al.* (1983) Oral hydralzaine for chronic mitral regurgitation in the dog. *J Am Vet Med Assoc* 182:1205–1209.

112 Arnold RM (2001) Amlodipine. *Compend Cont Educ Pract Vet* 23:558–559.

113 Tissier R, Perrot S, Enriquez B (2005) Amlodipine: one of the main anti-hypertensive drugs in veterinary therapeutics. *J Vet Cardiol* 7:53–58.

114 Packer M, O'Connor CM, Ghali JK *et al.* (1996) Effect of amlodipine on morbidity and mortality in severe chronic heart failure. *N Engl J Med* 335:1107–1114.

115 Adin DB, Kittleson MD, Hornof WJ *et al.* (2001) Efficacy of a single oral dose of isosorbide 5-mononitrate in normal dogs and in dogs with congestive heart failure. *J Vet Intern Med* 15:105–111.

116 Rush JE, Freeman LM, Brown DJ *et al.* (2000) Clinical, echocardiographic, and neurohormonal effects of a sodium-restricted diet in dogs with heart failure. *J Vet Intern Med* 14:512–520.

117 Pedersen H, Koch J, Jensen A *et al.* (1994) Some effects of a low sodium diet high in potassium on the renin-angiotensin system and plasma electrolyte concentrations in normal dogs. *Act Vet Scand* 35:133–140.

118 Freeman LM, Rush JE, Kehayias JJ *et al.* (1998) Nutritional alterations and the effect of fish oil supplementation in dogs with heart failure. *J Vet Intern Med* 12:440–448.

119 Freeman LM, Rush JE, Brown DJ *et al.* (1994) Elevated concentrations of tumor necrosis factor in dogs with congestive heart failure. *J Vet Intern Med* 8:146.

120 Pion PD, Sanderson SL, Kittelson MD (1998) The effectiveness of taurine and levo-carnitine in dogs with heart disease. *Vet Clin North Am: Small Anim Pract* 28:1495–1514.

121 Pion PD, Kittleson MD, Rogers QR *et al.* (1987) Myocardial failure in cats associated with low plasma taurine: a reversible cardiomyopathy. *Science* 237:764–768.

122 Kramer GA, Kittleson MD, Fox PR *et al.* (1995) Plasma taurine concentrations in normal dogs and in dogs with heart disease. *J Vet Intern Med* 9:253–258.

123 Kittleson MD, Keene B, Pion PD *et al.* (1997) Results of the multicenter spaniel trial (MUST): taurine- and carnitine-responsive dilated cardiomyopathy in American Cocker Spaniels with decreased plasma taurine concentration. *J Vet Intern Med* 11:204–211.

124 Keene BW, Panciera DP, Atkins CE *et al.* (1991) Myocardial L-carnitine deficiency in a family of dogs with dilated cardiomyopathy. *J Am Vet Med Assoc* 201:647–650.

125 Sanderson SL, Gross KL, Ogburn PH *et al.* (2001) Effects of dietary fat and L-carnitine on plasma and whole blood taurine concentrations and cardiac function in healthy dogs fed protein-restricted diets. *Am J Vet Res* 62:1616–1623.

126 Freeman LM, Michel KE, Brown DJ *et al.* (19960 Idiopathic dilated cardiomyopathy in Dalmations: nine cases (1990–1995). *J Am Vet Med Assoc* 209:1592–1596.

127 Gavaghan BJ, Kittleson MD (1997) Dilated cardiomyopathy in an American Cocker Spaniel with taurine deficiency. *Aust Vet J* 75:862–868.

128 Freeman LM, Rush KE, Milbury PE *et al.* (2005) Antioxidant status and biomarkers of oxidative stress in dogs with congestive heart failure. *J Vet Intern Med* 19:537–541.

129 Freeman LM, Brown DJ, Rush JE (1999) Assessment of degree of oxidative stress and antioxidant concentration in dogs with idiopathic dilated cardiomyopathy. *J Am Vet Med Assoc* 215:644–646.

130 Shite J, Qin F, Mao W *et al.* (2001) Antioxidant vitamins attenuate oxidative stress and cardiac dysfunction in tachycardia-induced cardiomyopathy. *J Am Coll Cardiol* 38:1734–1740.

131 Richartz BM, Werner GS, Ferrari M *et al.* (2001) Reversibility of coronary endothelial vasomotor dysfunction in idiopathic dilated cardiomyopathy: acute effects of vitamin C. *Am J Cardiol* 88:1001–1005.

132 Hoffman RL, Hugel J, Mallat B *et al.* (2001) Vitamin C inhibits endothelial cell apoptosis in congestive heart failure. *Circulation* 104:2182–2187.

133 Tran MT, Mitchell TM, Kennedy DT *et al.* (2001) Role of coenzyme Q10 in chronic heart failure, angina, and hypertension. *Pharmacotherapy* 21:707–806.

134 Ko DT, Hebert PR, Coffey CS *et al.* (2004) Adverse effects of beta-blocker therapy for patients with heart failure: a quantitative overview of randomized trials. *Arch Intern Med* 164:1389–1394.

135 Fowler MB (2004) Carvedilol prospective randomized cumulative survival (COPERNICUS) trial: carvedilol in severe heart failure. *Am J Cardiol* 93:35–39.

136 Sawangkoon S, Miyamoto M, Nakayama T *et al.* (2000) Acute cardiovascular effects and pharmacokinetics of carvedilol in healthy dogs. *Am J Vet Res* 61:57–60.

137 Cinquegrana G, D'Aniello L, Landi M *et al.* (2005) Effects of different degrees of sympathetic antagonism on cytokine network in patients with ischemic dilated cardiomyopathy. *J Card Fail* 11:213–219.

138 Abbott JA, Broadstone RV, Ward DL *et al.* (2005) Hemodynamic effects of orally administered carvedilol in healthy conscious dogs. *Am J Vet Res* 66:637–641.

139 Uechi M, Sasaki T, Ueno K *et al.* (2002) Cardiovascular and renal effects of carvedilol in dogs with heart failure. *J Vet Med Sci* 64:469–475.

140 Strein K, Sponer G, Muller-Beckmann B *et al.* (1987) Pharmacological profile of carvedilol, a compound with beta-blocking and vasodilating properties. *J Cardiovasc Pharmacol* 10(suppl11):S33–41.

141 Arsenault WG, Boothe DM, Gordon SG *et al.* (2005) Pharmacokinetics of carvedilol after intravenous and oral administration in conscious healthy dogs. *Am J Vet Res* **66**:2172–2176.

142 Gordon SG, Arsenault WG, Longnecker M *et al.* (2006) Pharmacodynamics of carvedilol in conscious, healthy dogs. *J Vet Intern Med* **20**:297–304.

143 Rush JE, Freeman LM, Hiler C *et al.* (2002) Use of metoprolol in dogs with acquired cardiac disease. *J Vet Cardiol* **4**:23–28.

144 Sabbah HN, Shimoyama H, Kono T *et al.* (1994) Effects of long-term monotherapy with enalapril, metoprolol, and digoxin on the progression of left ventricular dysfunction and dilation in dogs with reduced ejection fraction. *Circulation* **89**:2852–2859.

145 Morita H, Suzuki G, Mishima T *et al.* (2002) Effects of long-term monotherapy with metoprolol CR/XL on the progression of left ventricular dysfunction and remodeling in dogs with chronic heart failure. *Cardiovasc Drugs Ther* **16**:443–449.

146 Nemoto S, Hamawaki M, DeFreitas G *et al.* (2002) Differential aspects of the angiotensin-converting enzyme inhibitor lisinopril versus beta-receptor blocker atenolol on hemodynamics and left ventricular contractile function in experimental mitral regurgitation. *J Am Coll Cardiol* **40**:149–154.

147 Packer M, Coats AJ, Fowler MB *et al.* (2001) Effects of carvedilol on survival in severe chronic heart failure. *N Engl J Med* **344**:1651–1658.

148 Skudicky D, Bergemann A, Sliwa K *et al.* (2001) Beneficial effects of pentoxifylline in patients with idiopathic dilated cardiomyopathy treated with angiotensin-converting enzyme inhibitors and carvedilol: results of a randomized study. *Circulation* **103**:1083–1088.

149 Strickland KN (2003) Pentoxifylline as an adjunctive therapy for congestive heart failure. In: *Proceedings of the 21st ACVIM Forum*, Charlotte, pp. 105–106.

150 Rees CA, Boothe DM, Boeckh A *et al.* (2003) Dosing regimen and hematologic effects of pentoxifylline and its active metabolites in normal dogs. *Vet Ther* **4**:188–196.

151 Chen HH, Redfield MM, Nordstrom LJ *et al.* (2004) Subcutaneous administration of the cardiac hormone BNP in symptomatic human heart failure. *J Card Fail* **10**:115–119.

152 Sisson DD, Oyama MA, Solter PF (2003) Plasma levels of ANP, BNP, epinephrine, norepinephrine, serum aldosterone, and plasma renin activity in healthy cats and cats with myocardial disease. Abstract. *J Vet Intern Med* **17**:438–439.

153 Oyama MA, Gidlewski J, Sisson DD (2003) Effect of ACE inhibition on dynamic left ventricular obstruction in cats with hypertrophic obstructive cardiomyopathy. Abstract. *J Vet Intern Med* **17**, 372.

154 Bright JM, Golden AL, Gompf RE *et al.* (1991) Evaluation of the calcium channel blocking agents diltiazem and verapamil for treatment of feline hypertrophic cardiomyopathy. *J Vet Intern Med* **5**:272–282.

155 Roudebush P, Allen TA, Kuehn NF *et al.* (1994) The effect of combined therapy with captopril, furosemide, and a sodium-restricted diet on serum electrolyte levels and renal function in normal dogs and dogs with congestive heart failure. *J Vet Intern Med* **8**:337–342.

17
Management of Arrhythmias

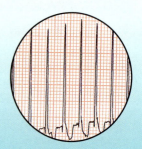

OVERVIEW

Cardiac arrhythmias can present a number of challenges for the clinician. Some arrhythmias clearly produce serious hemodynamic compromise that can be fatal, but some cause no clinically evident problems. Other arrhythmias may portend increased risk for sudden arrhythmic death. In addition to identifying the presence and type of arrhythmia, the clinician is faced with the issues of whether antiarrhythmic drug therapy is warranted, which drug would be most effective, and whether the benefits of therapy outweigh potential risks. The cardiac rhythm is ultimately determined by a complex interplay of factors. Some of these factors can be modified by means other than antiarrhythmic drugs in a way that reduces the occurrence or severity of the arrhythmia.

The issue of whether to use antiarrhythmic drug therapy for arrhythmias that cause no clinical signs is controversial and influenced by individual circumstances. Based on human medicine experience, there is much less advocacy for antiarrhythmic drug use in animals with asymptomatic ventricular ectopy, especially when ventricular function is normal[1–3]. Whether this conservative approach is also justified in animals with disease known to be associated with sudden death is not clear; however, there is agreement that arrhythmias that cause acute clinical signs should be treated. Furthermore, aggressive management of persistent tachycardias, especially those of supraventricular origin, is prompted by their negative long-term myocardial consequences[4, 5].

When antiarrhythmic drug therapy is chosen, it is helpful to define specific treatment goals for the patient, (e.g. to stabilize hemodynamic parameters). While ideal goals might be to restore sinus rhythm, correct underlying disease, and prevent further arrhythmias and sudden death, they may not be realistic. Likewise, suppression of all abnormal beats is not a realistic goal. Successful therapy usually means sufficient reduction in frequency (e.g. by ≥70–80%) or repetitive rate of ectopic beats to restore normal hemodynamic status and eliminate clinical

signs. It is important to recognize that even apparently complete arrhythmia suppression does not remove the risk of lethal arrhythmia and sudden cardiac death.

PATHOPHYSIOLOGY

Sinus rhythms, as well as abnormal rhythms, are influenced greatly by the autonomic nervous system. Many extracardiac conditions as well as cardiac diseases affect prevailing autonomic tone (see *Table 10*, p. 52). Sinus arrhythmia, with its recurring fluctuations in rate and P wave morphology (see Chapter 4, p. 51), is a normal rhythm variation in dogs over a month old[6]. It often becomes very prominent in dogs with respiratory disease. Sinus arrhythmia usually changes to a regular sinus rhythm at rates above 150 beats/minute, as sympathetic influence increases and vagal tone is withdrawn[6]. In cats, sinus arrhythmia in the clinic setting is rare and may indicate pathology, but resting cats normally do manifest some degree of sinus arrhythmia at home[7, 8].

ARRHYTHMOGENESIS

The development of abnormal cardiac arrhythmias depends on several factors (see Chapter 13). Overt or subclinical changes in cardiac structure or function can alter cell electrophysiologic characteristics in ways that predispose to arrhythmia formation (i.e. that create a substrate for arrhythmia development); for example, an increasing heterogeneity of repolarization and conduction velocity that develops across the ventricular wall from endocardium to epicardium in cardiomyopathy, enhances the propensity for ventricular arrhythmias[9]. These structural or functional changes can occur during cardiac remodeling with heart disease and failure (see Chapter 16), or can result from genetic or environmental factors. They can involve myocyte hypertrophy, abnormal ion channel structure or function, tissue inflammation or fibrosis, and other changes. Despite such underlying abnormalities, an arrhythmia may not occur unless provoked by some triggering event; for example, abrupt change in cardiac cycle length (heart rate) or a premature stimulus can trigger sustained arrhythmia when the underlying conditions are favorable[10]. Ca++ overloading of myocardial cells promotes spontaneous Ca++ release from the sarcoplasmic reticulum, delayed afterdepolarizations, and triggered electrical activity[11]. Additional modulating factors can further influence whether an arrhythmia occurs or is sustained. These factors include changes in cardiac adrenergic or vagal tone, circulating catecholamine concentrations, electrolyte disturbances, and ischemia[12–14]; for example, increased adrenergic activity associated with anger-like behavior can precipitate lethal arrhythmias[15, 16]. Such factors also influence the response to antiarrhythmic drugs.

Electrophysiologic mechanisms

The electrophysiologic mechanisms that underlie cardiac arrhythmias involve either abnormal impulse formation (automaticity or excitability), abnormal impulse conduction, or a combination of both abnormal excitation and conduction (see Chapter 13). The sympathetic nervous system can potentiate arrhythmias caused by increased automaticity, triggered activity, and reentry[17, 18]. Increased excitability is appropriate in the case of sinus tachycardia from increased sympathetic tone or subsidiary pacemaker activation after sinus arrest; however, abnormal automaticity can underlie atrial, junctional, and ventricular extrasystoles and tachycardias[4, 6]. Examples include automatic atrial tachycardia, ventricular parasystole (caused by a protected automatic ventricular focus), and some ventricular tachycardias. Decreased excitability can ultimately cause bradycardia or asystole (arrest).

Conduction delay or 'block' can occur within the SA or AV nodes, major ventricular conduction pathways (bundle branches), or within small areas of myocardium. Not all conduction blocks cause bradycardia. The phenomenon of reentry (see Chapter 13, p. 132) can promote rapid sustained tachycardias via a small anatomic or functional circuit (microreentry) or via a larger circuit (macroreentry). The latter includes AV node reciprocating tachycardias in animals with a functional AV node bypass tract (see Chapter 4, p. 53). Atrial and ventricular fibrillation are other arrhythmias driven by reentry. Multiple reentrant circuits are more likely to develop when there is greater variation (dispersion) of refractoriness across the myocardium.

Abnormalities of both impulse formation and conduction underlie the sick sinus syndrome (SSS) as well as preexcitation syndromes. With preexcitation, the accessory conduction pathway, bypassing the AV node, allows part of the ventricle to be activated early during sinus rhythm, and also allows rapid reentrant tachycardias to be sustained. The SSS, or bradycardia–tachycardia syndrome (see Chapter 13, p. 134), involves abnormal SA node activation, (leading to sinus bradycardia and arrest); delays in AV node conduction (causing 1st degree and 2nd degree heart block); and variable disturbances in excitability (provoking junctional or atrial tachyarrhythmias and, sometimes, ventricular ectopy). The mechanism underlying an arrhythmia is not always clear, especially based on surface ECG morphology. Nevertheless, the ECG sometimes can provide clues as to arrhythmia mechanism.

HEMODYNAMIC AND CARDIAC CONSEQUENCES

The hemodynamic effects of an arrhythmia depend on a number of factors. These include whether underlying disease is present and its effect on cardiac function, the ventricular activation rate, the duration of the arrhythmia, the temporal relation between atrial and ventricular activation, the sequence or coordination of ventricular activation, drug therapy, and the animal's activity level[6]. Arrhythmias that compromise cardiac output and coronary perfusion promote hypotension, myocardial ischemia, impaired pump function, and, sometimes, sudden death. These arrhythmias tend to be either very rapid (e.g. sustained ventricular or supraventricular tachycardias) or very slow (e.g. advanced AV block with a slow or unstable ventricular escape rhythm).

Cardiac output depends on heart rate and the factors that influence stroke volume (CO = HR x SV). Within a physiologic range, as HR increases so does cardiac output; however, excessively fast ventricular rates reduce cardiac output, because diastole becomes too abbreviated for adequate ventricular filling. Conversely, when HR is very low, cardiac output can fall below that needed for the animal's activity level if further increase in SV cannot be achieved. Inadequate cardiac output can cause systemic hypotension. Consequently, coronary perfusion pressure (aortic pressure minus RA pressure) also decreases. Rapid tachycardias especially can promote myocardial ischemia because they reduce coronary perfusion pressure and markedly abbreviate diastole (when most coronary blood flow occurs). Rapid ventricular tachycardia (VT) can quickly degenerate into ventricular fibrillation (VF). Supraventricular tachycardia (SVT) could promote secondary ventricular arrhythmias related to poor myocardial perfusion, ischemia, and increased sympathetic stimulation.

Loss of sequential atrial and ventricular contraction (e.g. with AF) negatively affects ventricular end-diastolic volume and can lower cardiac output. Although this may be unimportant at rest, atrial contraction can contribute up to 30% of total ventricular filling at high HRs. During exercise or with heart failure, the detrimental effect on cardiac output can be marked. Ventricular tachyarrhythmias are likely to have greater negative impact on cardiac output at any given HR because of incoordinated LV and RV contraction. Major bundle branch blocks also cause dyssynchronous ventricular contraction that could reduce cardiac output depending on HR and myocardial function.

Chronic tachycardia of either supraventricular or ventricular origin can cause myocardial failure (see Chapter 20, p. 292)[5, 19]. Persistently rapid ventricular rates (e.g. 180–200 beats/minute) will cause myocardial failure within a few weeks. The cardiac enlargement, myocardial structural and functional changes, and NH activation that occur mimic spontaneous cardiomyopathy[5]. Tachycardia-induced cardiomyopathy is reversible if HR is controlled within a few weeks of onset.

GENERAL ARRHYTHMIA MANAGEMENT CONSIDERATIONS

PATIENT ASSESSMENT

All aspects of the patient's clinical situation should be considered when evaluating an arrhythmia's significance (*Table 46*); this includes signalment, medical history, physical examination findings, and all other available data (see Chapter 13). When cardiac output is inadequate for the level of activity, the animal is likely to exhibit weakness, lethargy, syncope, or pre-syncope (see Chapter 14). The arrhythmia's immediate effects on cardiac function can be estimated by the presence or absence of such

clinical signs and the quality of perfusion during the arrhythmia (e.g. pulse quality, mentation, blood pressure). Another consequence of arrhythmias can be the onset or exacerbation of CHF. The arrhythmias of greatest concern are those that cause marked hemodynamic compromise and those that occur in animals with a clinical condition known to be associated with sudden death.

Various arrhythmias occur without causing hemodynamic impairment or clinical signs, especially in animals with normal heart size and function. These can include isolated premature beats, accelerated idioventricular rhythm, brief episodes of paroxysmal tachycardia, and intermittent AV block (see Chapters 4 and 13). Healthy animals, especially of older age, are known to have occasional ventricular premature complexes (VPCs)[7, 20, 21]. Accelerated idioventricular rhythm (at about 60–100 beats/minute in the dog) appear commonly after thoracic trauma (see Chapter 20, p. 295).

Some clinical conditions are associated with frequent VPCs as well as more complex ventricular tachyarrhythmias and higher risk of sudden cardiac death. Most of these involve marked structural heart disease, but some do not. Sometimes, a lethal arrhythmia (e.g. VF) is triggered without a prior sustained arrhythmia and its clinical manifestations. Cardiomyopathy in dogs (see Chapter 20) is associated with sudden death, especially in Doberman Pinschers and Boxers, although myocardial function is preserved in many Boxers[22–26]. There is some evidence that signal-averaged electrocardiography, where

Table 46 Approach to the patient with an arrhythmia.

1) Identify and define the arrhythmia (see *Table 34*, p. 131, *Table 36*, p. 135, and **202**, p. 136):
   a) An extended recording period may be necessary (ambulatory or prolonged in-hospital monitoring).
2) Evaluate the whole patient:
   a) Include history, physical findings, biochemical tests (especially electrolytes), cardiac and respiratory function, acid/base status, other tests as indicated. Correct what can be corrected.
3) Decide whether to use antiarrhythmic drug therapy (see text):
   a) Consider case context and clinical signs.
   b) Consider benfits/risks of therapeutic choice.
4) Define goals of antiarrhythmic drug therpay, if used.
5) Initiate therpay and determine drug effectiveness:
   a) Adjust dose and/or try alternate agent(s) as necessary (see text).
6) Monitor and follow up:
   a) Assess arrhythmia control (continuous ECG monitoring for acute cases; consider repeated Holter studies for chronic cases).
   b) Manage underlying disease/abnormalities.
   c) Watch for adverse drug effects and other complications.

available, could identify individual animals at greater risk for sudden cardiac death[27, 28]. Ventricular tachyarrhythmias in people with impaired myocardial function are associated with greater risk of sudden death[29], but overall prognosis does not seem to be significantly affected by how well-tolerated these ventricular tachyarrhythmias are hemodynamically[30]. Similar information is not yet available in animals. Cardiac diseases associated with marked ventricular hypertrophy, and greater likelihood for ischemia, are also associated with sudden death. Severe subaortic stenosis (see Chapter 18, p. 229) and hypertrophic cardiomyopathy (see Chapters 20, p. 292 and 21, p. 300) are examples. Familial ventricular arrhythmias, affecting young dogs in some lines of German Shepherd Dogs, can cause sudden arrhythmic death. Although gross structural lesions are lacking in these dogs, abnormalities of cardiac sympathetic innervation and repolarization have been demonstrated[31–34].

RHYTHM DIAGNOSIS

Accurate ECG interpretation is important for defining the origin, timing, and severity of the rhythm disturbance (see Chapter 4) and to guide treatment decisions; however, cardiac arrhythmias can vary tremendously in frequency and severity over time. Potentially critical arrhythmias can easily be missed on a routine ECG. Holter or other ambulatory monitoring allows the clinician to better assess arrhythmia frequency and severity as well as treatment efficacy (see Chapter 4, p. 66 and Chapter 14, p. 142)[12, 35].

The identification of arrhythmias recorded on ECG begins with a cursory, left-to-right visual scan of the entire tracing. Normal P-QRS-T waveforms are identified, HR determined, and an orientation to the overall rhythm gained. Some ECG artifacts may resemble rhythm disturbances, so critical evaluation is warranted to avoid misinterpretation. Ectopic (abnormal) complexes are identified and classified, insofar as possible, as to their origin (supraventricular or ventricular) and timing (premature or escape).

Clues to the underlying mechanism (e.g. automatic focus or reentry) may also be evident. More information on the general approach to ECG interpretation can be found in Chapter 4, followed by descriptions of common rhythm disturbances. *Table 34* (p. 131) provides additional guidelines for ECG interpretation. *Table 36* (p. 135) lists differential diagnoses for irregular and regular cardiac rhythms.

Rapid, narrow-QRS tachycardias can be caused by sinus tachycardia, sustained automatic atrial tachycardia, AV node reciprocating (or other reentry) tachycardia, or even a 'high' ventricular tachyarrhythmia. Differentiation can be challenging, especially because P waves may not be seen well, or at all, if buried in preceding QRS or T waveforms. A vagal maneuver (see p. 202) can help define the arrhythmia. It is important to differentiate sinus tachycardia from other tachyarrhythmias. Ectopic rhythms with a ventricular rate over 250/minute usually require immediate IV antiarrhythmic drug therapy.

Wide QRS tachycardias also can present a diagnostic challenge. If the rhythm is fairly regular, a ventricular origin (i.e. VT) is most likely. But SVT with aberrant ventricular conduction must also be considered, especially if there is no response to initial ventricular antiarrhythmic drug therapy. Irregular, wide QRS tachycardias without visible P waves are usually AF with concurrent ventricular aberrancy (**230**).

DECISION TO TREAT

Standards for choosing and continuing antiarrhythmic therapy are not clearly defined for most situations. There are few controlled veterinary clinical studies on efficacy and outcomes of various antiarrhythmic strategies. Many questions remain regarding which patients should receive antiarrhythmic drug therapy and which strategies are most effective in suppressing arrhythmias as well as in preventing sudden death. Isolated supraventricular and VPCs generally lack hemodynamic importance and do not require specific drug therapy. There is general agreement that antiarrhythmic drug therapy is indicated when rhythm

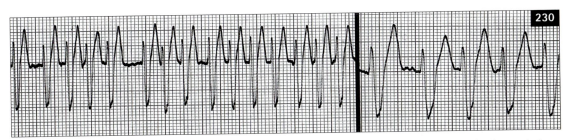

230 ECG from a female German Shepherd Dog with dilated cardiomyopathy. This wide QRS tachycardia could be mistaken for ventricular tachycardia, but note the irregularity and absence of P waves typical for AF. Aberrant ventricular conduction (right bundle branch block) caused the wide, negative QRS configuration. Lead aVF, 25 mm/sec (left), and 50 mm/sec (right).

disturbances cause clinical signs or hemodynamic instability, or when the risk of a lethal arrhythmia is high. Control of persistent tachycardia is warranted based not only on immediate hemodynamic effects but also on the longer-term risk of tachycardia-induced cardiomyopathy. The use of antiarrhythmic therapy in an asymptomatic animal that has complex ventricular arrhythmias as well as a disease associated with increased risk of sudden death may appear compelling; however, it is not clear whether, or which, antiarrhythmic therapy prolongs survival. Drugs that suppress extrasystoles may or may not have antifibrillatory activity, and sudden cardiac death can occur from asystole or electrical–mechanical dissociation as well as VF.

Symptomatic ventricular arrhythmias and syncope predict increased risk for sudden death in people with heart failure, but asymptomatic ventricular arrhythmias do not[29]. Some antiarrhythmic agents can actually increase mortality via their proarrhythmic effects[29]. The only antiarrhythmic agents shown to reduce arrhythmia mortality in people with severe LV dysfunction are beta-blockers and amiodarone[29]. Some drugs used for heart failure are more effective in reducing sudden death than antiarrhythmic drugs *per se* (e.g. beta-blockers, ACE inhibitors, AT receptor-blockers, statins, aldosterone receptor-blockers, n-3 polyunsaturated fatty acids, aspirin)[29, 36, 37]. There is evidence that ACE inhibitors and AT receptor-blockers may protect from AT II-induced atrial structural and electrical remodeling associated with AF in patients with heart disease[38]. Some people with heart failure benefit from cardiac resynchronization therapy (biventricular pacing) to improve ventricular coordination as well as cardioverter/defibrillator (ICD) implantation[29]. Whether these therapies have application in veterinary medicine remains to be seen; there are a number of technical and practical issues of concern. An interventional therapy used commonly in animals is artificial pacing for symptomatic bradyarrhythmias (see p. 219). Intracardiac electrical mapping and catheter ablation procedures have been successful in abolishing tachyarrhythmias in some animals[39].

When deciding whether to use antiarrhythmic drug therapy, the animal's clinical status (see above), underlying disease(s), and current medications, as well as the potential benefits/risks of specific drugs are considered. Treatment for concurrent cardiac or extracardiac disease can markedly reduce some arrhythmias; therefore, abnormalities that can be corrected should be. Conditions commonly associated with various arrhythmias are shown in *Table 35* (p. 133). Hypokalemia and hypomagnesemia predispose to ventricular arrhythmias by affecting cell electrophysiologic properties, and can reduce the effectiveness of many antiarrhythmic drugs[12, 40–42].

Predictors of hypomagnesemia in hospitalized animals include decreases in serum albumin, K^+, total CO_2, and urea nitrogen, as well as the presence of cardiovascular disease[41]. Some patients with a total body Mg^{++} deficit can have a normal serum magnesium level[41].

The decision to use an antiarrhythmic drug also includes consideration of treatment goals for the individual patient. An obvious immediate goal is to restore hemodynamic stability. Conversion to sinus rhythm and correcting underlying cause(s) may or may not be achievable goals. It is generally not realistic to expect total suppression of all premature ectopic activity. Successful therapy usually means reducing the frequency (e.g. by ≥70–80%) or repetitive rate of ectopic beats sufficiently to restore normal hemodynamics and eliminate clinical signs; however, even apparently complete conversion to sinus rhythm does not assure protection from sudden death. Antiarrhythmic agents with greater antifibrillatory activity (e.g. class III drugs) are thought to provide increased protection, but such agents do not prevent other lethal arrhythmias such as asystole. It is important that the owner also understand what antiarrhythmic therapy can and cannot do, especially over the long term.

Potential antiarrhythmic drug adverse effects must be considered and weighed against the desired benefits. Besides their expense, these drugs have multiple adverse effects that can include provoking new arrhythmias (proarrhythmia)[12, 22]. Proarrhythmic effects may be more pronounced in patients with myocardial dysfunction, CHF, hypokalemia, or hypomagnesemia[12]. In all cases, careful monitoring of the patient as well as the ECG is warranted to determine drug effectiveness. Dosage adjustments as well as alternate antiarrhythmic agents may be needed. It is important to watch for adverse drug effects and other complications, especially with chronic therapy. Initially, effective therapy sometimes loses efficacy over time. Repeated Holter monitoring can be helpful for assessing arrhythmia control over time.

ANTIARRHYTHMIC DRUG CLASSIFICATION

Antiarrhythmic drugs can serve to slow a tachycardia's rate, terminate a reentrant arrhythmia, or prevent abnormal impulse formation or conduction[6]. These effects can occur through modulation of tissue electrophysiologic properties and/or autonomic nervous system effects. The traditional (Vaughan Williams) drug classification system consists of four classes based on the drug's predominant cardiac electrophysiologic effects (*Table 47*). Shortcomings of this classification system relate to the exclusion of some drugs with antiarrhythmic effects (e.g. digoxin), the multiple-class effects of several drugs, dissimilarity among some drugs within the same class, and the focus on electrophysiologic blocking mechanisms rather than ion channels and/or receptor activation. Another classification scheme, the Sicilian Gambit, was proposed to categorize antiarrhythmic drugs by their actions on underlying arrhythmia mechanisms, with emphasis on how they affect ion currents, membrane pumps, and receptors[43–45]; however, this has not markedly facilitated clinical arrhythmic management.

Vaughan Williams class I agents have membrane-stabilizing effects that tend to slow conduction as well as decrease automaticity and excitability. The 'traditional' ventricular antiarrhythmic drugs belong to this class. Class II consists of beta-adrenergic antagonists, which act by inhibiting catecholamine effects on the heart. Class III drugs prolong the effective refractory period of cardiac action potentials without decreasing conduction velocity. The class III

agents may be most effective in suppressing reentrant arrhythmias or in preventing VF. Class IV contains calcium-entry blocking drugs. These are most useful for supraventricular tachyarrhythmias; ventricular arrhythmias are usually unresponsive to them. Additional information on specific agents can be found below. Suggested drug dosages are listed in *Table 48* (p. 200); methods for CRI dosage are described in *Table 49* (p. 201).

Other drugs are also useful in managing arrhythmias. These include digoxin, anticholinergic agents, and other drugs not typically considered to have antiarrhythmic effects. Modification of various modulating factors important in arrhythmogenesis may prevent some arrhythmias; for example, catecholamines, free radicals, AT II, cytokines, and

Table 47 Classification of antiarrhythmic drugs.

Class	Drug	Mechanism and ECG effects
I		Decrease fast inward Na^+ current; membrane-stabilizing effects (slowed conduction, decreased excitability and automaticity)
IA	Quinidine Procainamide Disopyramide	Moderately slows conduction, increases action potential duration; can prolong QRS complex and Q-T interval
IB	Lidocaine Mexiletine Tocainide Phenytoin	Little change in conductivity, decreases action potential duration; QRS complex and Q-T interval unchanged
IC	Flecainide Encainide Propafenone	Markedly slows conduction without change in action potential duration
II	Propranolol Atenolol Esmolol Metoprolol Carvedilol, others	Beta-adrenergic blockade, reduces effects of sympathetic stimulation (no direct myocardial effects at clinical doses)
III	Sotalol Amiodarone Bretylium Ibutilide Dofetilide, others	Selectively prolongs action potential duration and refractory period; antiadrenergic effects; Q-T interval prolonged
IV	Verapamil Diltiazem	Decreases slow inward Ca^{++} current (greatest effect on SA and AV nodes)
Other agents with antiarrhythmic effects include:	Digoxin	Antiarrhythmic action results mainly from indirect autonomic effects, especially increased vagal tone
	Atropine and other anticholinergic agents	Oppose vagal effects on SA and AV nodes

Table 48 Dosages of antiarrhythmic drugs.

Agent	Dosage
Class I	
Lidocaine	Dog: initial boluses of 2 mg/kg slowly IV, up to 8 mg/kg; or rapid IV infusion at 0.8 mg/kg/minute; if effective, then 25–80 mcg/kg/minute CRI; can also be used intratracheally for CPR
	Cat: initial bolus of 0.25–0.5 (or 1.0) mg/kg slowly IV; can repeat boluses of 0.15–0.25 mg/kg, up to total of 4 mg/kg; if effective, 10–40 mcg/kg/minute CRI
Procainamide	Dog: 6–10 (up to 20) mg/kg IV over 5–10 minutes; 10–50 mcg/kg/minute CRI; 6–20 (up to 30) mg/kg IM q4–6h; 10–25 mg/kg PO q6h (sustained release: q6–8h)
	Cat: 1.0–2.0 mg/kg slowly IV; 10–20 mcg/kg/minute CRI; 7.5–20 mg/kg IM or PO q(6–)8h
Quinidine	Dog: 6–20 mg/kg IM q6h (loading dose, 14–20 mg/kg); 6–16 mg/kg PO q6h; sustained action preparations, 8–20 mg/kg PO q8h
	Cat: 6–16 mg/kg IM or PO q8h
Tocainide	Dog: 10–20 (–25) mg/kg PO q8h
	Cat: *
Mexiletine	Dog: 4–10 mg/kg PO q8h
	Cat: *
Phenytoin	Dog: 10 mg/kg slowly IV; 30–50 mg/kg PO q8h
	Cat: do not use
Propafenone	Dog: (?) 3–4 mg/kg PO q8h
	Cat: *
Flecainide	Dog: (?) 1–5 mg/kg PO q8–12h
	Cat: *
Class II	
Atenolol	Dog: 0.2–1.0 mg/kg PO q12–24h
	Cat: 6.25–12.5 mg/cat PO q(12–)24h
Propranolol	Dog: 0.02 mg/kg initial bolus slowly IV (up to maximum of 0.1 mg/kg); initial dose, 0.1–0.2 mg/kg PO q8h, up to 1 mg/kg q8h
	Cat: Same IV instructions; 2.5 up to 10 mg/cat PO q8–12h
Esmolol	Dog: 0.1–0.5 mg/kg IV over 1 minute (loading dose), followed by infusion of 0.025–0.2 mg/kg/minute
	Cat: same
Metoprolol	Dog: initial dose, 0.2 mg/kg PO q8h, up to 1 mg/kg q8(–12)h
	Cat: *
Class III	
Sotalol	Dog: 1–3.5 (–5) mg/kg PO q12h
	Cat: 10–20 mg/cat PO q12 h (or 2–4 mg/kg PO q12h)
Amiodarone	Dog: 10 mg/kg PO q12h for 7 days, then 8 mg/kg PO q24h (lower as well as higher doses have been used); 3(–5) mg/kg slowly (over 10–20 minutes) IV (can repeat but do not exceed 10 mg/kg in 1 hour)
	Cat: *
Bretylium	Dog: 2–6 mg/kg IV; can repeat in 1–2 hours (people)
	Cat: *
Class IV	
Diltiazem	Dog: Oral maintenance: initial dose 0.5 mg/kg (up to 2+ mg/kg) PO q8h; acute IV for supraventricular tachycardia: 0.15–0.25 mg/kg over 2–3 minutes IV, can repeat every 15 minutes until conversion or maximum 0.75 mg/kg; CRI: 5–15 mg/kg/hr; PO loading dose: 0.5 mg/kg PO followed by 0.25 mg/kg PO q1h to a total of 1.5(–2.0) mg/kg or conversion
	Cat: Same?; for HCM: 1.5–2.5 mg/kg (or 7.5–10 mg/cat) PO q8h; sustained-release preparations: Cardizem-CD, 10 mg/kg/day (45 mg/cat is about 105 mg of Cardizem-CD or the amount that fits into the small end of a No. 4 gelatin capsule); Diltiazem (Dilacor) XR, 30 mg/cat/day (one half of a

Table 48 (Continued)

	60 mg controlled-release tablet within the 240 mg gelatin capsule), can increase to 60 mg/day in some cats if necessary
Verapamil	Dog: initial dose, 0.02–0.05 mg/kg slowly IV, can repeat q5min up to a total of 0.15(–0.2) mg/kg; 0.5–2 mg/kg PO q8h
	Cat: initial dose, 0.025 mg/kg slowly IV, can repeat every 5 minutes up to a total of 0.15(–0.2) mg/kg; 0.5–1 mg/kg PO q8h
Anticholinergic	
Atropine	Dog: 0.02–0.04 mg/kg IV, IM, SC; can also be given intratracheally for CPR; 0.04 mg/kg PO q6–8h
	Cat: same
Glycopyrrolate	Dog: 0.005–0.01 mg/kg IV or IM; 0.01–0.02 mg/kg SC
	Cat: same
Propantheline	Dog: 3.73–7.5 mg PO q8–12h
	Cat: *
Hyoscyamine	Dog: 0.003–0.006 mg/kg PO q8h
	Cat: *
Sympathomimetic	
Isoproterenol	Dog: 0.045–0.09 mcg/kg/minute CRI
	Cat: same
Terbutaline	Dog: 2.5–5 mg/dog PO q8–12h
	Cat: 1.25 mg/cat PO q12h
Other agents	
Digoxin	See *Tables 43* and *44*, pp. 171 and 174
Adenosine	Dog: up to 12 mg as rapid IV bolus
	Cat: *
Edrophonium	Dog: 0.05 to 0.1 mg/kg IV (have atropine and endotracheal tube available)
	Cat: same?
Phenylephrine	Dog: 0.004 to 0.01 mg/kg IV
	Cat: same?

CRI = constant rate infusion; CPR = cardiopulmonary resuscitation; * = effective dosage not known.

Table 49 Formulas for constant rate infusion.

1) Method 1 (Allows for 'fine-tuning' fluid as well as drug administration rate)
   a) Determine desired drug infusion rate: mcg/kg/minute x kg body weight = mcg/minute (A).
   b) Determine desired fluid infusion rate: ml/hour ÷ 60 = ml/minute (B).
   c) (A) ÷ (B) = mcg/minute ÷ ml/minute = mcg drug/ml of fluid.
   d) Convert from mcg to mg of drug needed (1 mcg = 0.001 mg).
   e) mg drug/ml fluid x ml of fluid in bag (or bottle or burette) = mg of drug to add to fluid bag.
2) Method 2 (for total dose over a 6-hour period, must also calculate fluid volume and administration rate)
   a) Total dose in mg to infuse over a 6-hour period = body weight (kg) x dose (mcg/kg/minute) x 0.36.
3) Method 3
   a) Drug dose (mcg/kg/minute) x body weight (kg) = mg drug to add to 250 ml fluid to administer at drip rate of 15 ml/hour.
4) Method 4 (for lidocaine) (faster but less helpful if fluid rate is important or fine drug-dosage adjustments are needed)
   a) For CRI of 44 mcg/kg/minute of lidocaine, add 25 ml of 2% lidocaine to 250 ml of D5W.
   b) Infuse at 0.25 ml/25 lb of body weight/minute.

nitric oxide are involved in the cardiac remodeling process that underlies various heart diseases (see Chapter 16) and that can also promote arrhythmias. Control of these factors may reduce arrhythmias. ACE inhibitors and fish oil (η–3 polyunsaturated fatty acids) have antiarrhythmic effects in some people and presumably animals as well[46]. There is evidence that statin drugs may play a role in arrhythmia prevention by virtue of their antioxidant and antiinflammatory properties[47]. The increased survival in human heart failure patients receiving ACE inhibitors, spironolactone, and some beta-blockers supports this approach.

MANAGEMENT OF SUPRAVENTRICULAR TACHYARRHYTHMIAS

Occasional premature beats do not require antiarrhythmic therapy. Predisposing factors should be minimized as far as possible (see *Table 35*, p. 133). For frequent atrial premature contractions or paroxysmal SVT, digoxin (see *Table 44*, p. 174) is the initial PO drug of choice in dogs with heart failure and in cats with DCM. A beta-blocker or the calcium channel-blocker diltiazem can be added if the arrhythmia is not sufficiently controlled with digoxin (along with an ACE inhibitor and furosemide for heart failure). For cats with HCM or hyperthyroidism, a beta-blocker such as atenolol or propranolol is used, although diltiazem could be an alternative. Recurrent supraventricular tachyarrhythmias that are refractory to these drugs may respond to amiodarone, sotalol, procainamide, quinidine, or a class IC agent.

ACUTE THERAPY FOR SUSTAINED OR FREQUENT PAROXYSMS OF SUPRAVENTRICULAR TACHYCARDIA

Rapid SVT (including automatic atrial tachycardia) is often associated with underlying heart disease as well as marked hemodynamic compromise. Various mechanisms cause SVTs. These include reentry involving an accessory pathway or the AV node and ectopic automatic foci within atrial or junctional tissue[10, 12, 48]. The underlying mechanism can affect response to treatment.

A **vagal maneuver** is tried initially for sustained SVT (**231**). This can help the clinician differentiate between tachycardias caused by an ectopic automatic focus, those dependent on a reentrant circuit involving the AV node, or excessively rapid sinus node activation. Increasing vagal tone should temporarily slow the rate of sinus tachycardia and allow normal P waves to be seen, although some atrial tachycardias also slow. Reentrant tachycardias involving the AV node are sometimes abruptly terminated by a vagal maneuver, as an increase in AV refractoriness blocks further conduction around the reentry circuit. The

vagal maneuver may transiently slow or intermittently block AV conduction to expose abnormal atrial P' waves from an automatic ectopic atrial focus.

Vagal maneuvers are performed by massaging the carotid sinus region (with gentle continuous pressure over the carotid sinuses, just caudodorsal to the larynx), or by applying firm bilateral ocular pressure, over closed eyelids, for 15–20 seconds. The latter technique is contraindicated in animals with ocular disease. Although a vagal maneuver is often ineffective at first, it can be repeated after antiarrhythmic drug administration if the rhythm disturbance persists. An IV drug that increases vagal or decreases sympathetic tone can potentiate the vagal maneuver in cases where it was initially unsuccessful. These agents include propranolol, esmolol, edrophonium chloride, and phenylephrine; morphine sulfate (0.2 mg/kg IM) has also been suggested. IV fluids are administered concurrently to maintain blood pressure and enhance endogenous vagal tone; however, patients with known or suspected heart failure should receive a small volume slowly, if at all. Further cardiac diagnostic tests are indicated once conversion is achieved or the ventricular rate falls below 200 beats/minute.

When SVT persists, a calcium channel-blocker is usually administered next. Diltiazem (IV or PO loading) is preferred. Although verapamil (IV) is also effective, it is not recommended for dogs with myocardial dysfunction or heart failure because of its greater negative inotropic effect. A beta-blocker given slowly IV (e.g. propranolol or esmolol) is an alternative therapy, but its negative inotropic effect is also of concern in animals dependent on high underlying sympathetic tone. Lidocaine (IV) can be effective in some cases of SVT caused by an accessory pathway or ectopic atrial focus, although it is most often used for wide QRS tachyarrhythmias[49]. IV digoxin is another alternative, but it is generally less effective than calcium channel-blockers. Digoxin's onset of action is slower and, while it increases vagal tone, IV administration can also increase central sympathetic output[12, 50]. The combination of a calcium channel- and beta-blocker can be considered in animals with refractory SVT and reasonably normal myocardial function and blood pressure, but the second agent should be dosed cautiously to avoid hypotension.

If calcium channel- or beta-blocker or lidocaine therapy does not control persistent SVT, IV procainamide may be helpful[4, 51]. Again, caution is advised for patients in heart failure. Refractory SVT (AV node independent) may respond to sotalol or amiodarone[12]. Adenosine has abolished SVT in people by slowing AV conduction, but it is rarely effective in dogs[4, 12]; moreover, it has an extremely short duration of effect, requires rapid central IV injection, and is expensive. Other drugs that might be useful for refractory SVT include the alpha$_1$

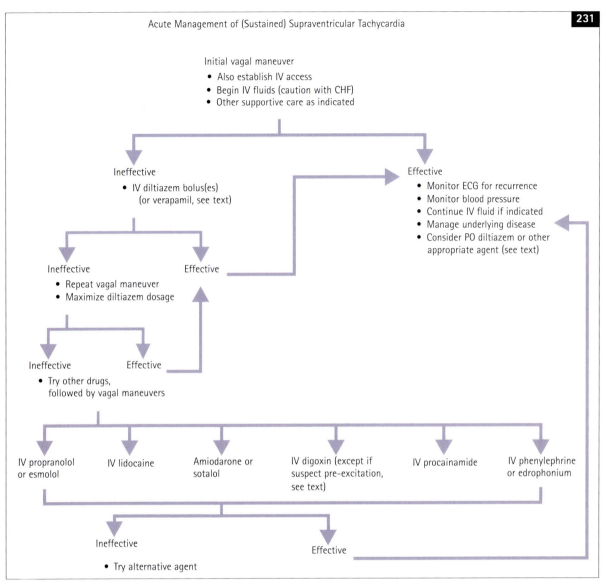

231 Approach to the acute management of rapid supraventricular tachycardia.
* See text (p. 202) for additional information and for long-term management of supraventricular tachyarrhythmias. CHF = congestive heart failure

agonist phenylephrine, which reflexly increases vagal tone, or the anticholinesterase edrophonium chloride[12]. Some class IC agents, as well as synchronized direct current (DC) cardioversion, have also been used successfully in people and could be considered[12, 52].

Once the rhythm is controlled, PO maintenance digoxin and/or diltiazem or a beta-blocker are used most often for long-term therapy. Amiodarone or sotalol are alternative agents in cases refractory to conventional drugs. Procainamide, quinidine, or a class IC drug have also been used.

Catheter ablation therapy is effective for certain persistent tachyarrhythmias. Those cases where a point lesion or small linear burn would disrupt the arrhythmia, and where patient size is sufficient to accommodate the mapping catheters, are most likely to benefit[39]. Although of limited availability, this technique is a therapeutic alternative for dogs with nonresponsive tachycardias and tachycardia-induced CHF.

ORTHODROMIC AV RECIPROCATING TACHYCARDIA (PREEXCITATION SYNDROMES)

Reentrant SVT involving an accessory pathway (bypass tract) and the AV node occurs in cats and dogs with ventricular preexcitation. This arrhythmia develops when a ventricular impulse is conducted backwards through the accessory pathway into the atrium, then travels down the AV node in the normal (orthodromic) direction to reenter the ventricles. This macroreentry circuit can perpetuate itself and cause rapid tachycardia with attendant clinical signs[4, 53]. The QRS complexes are usually narrow unless an intraventricular conduction abnormalitiy (such as a major bundle branch block) causes aberrancy.

AV reciprocating tachycardia may respond to a vagal maneuver if AV conduction slows enough to break the reentry cycle there. Drugs that slow conduction or prolong the refractory period of the bypass tract, AV node, or both tissues also interrupt the tachycardia. When vagal maneuvers fail to interrupt the tachycardia, IV diltiazem or verapamil can be tried, although they are not used in the setting of preexisting AF (see p. 205). Another alternative is procainamide or lidocaine, administered slowly IV. Vagal maneuvers can be repeated after these drugs are given. Procainamide (and quinidine) lengthen the refractory period of the accessory pathway and may prevent AV reciprocating tachycardia. High-dose procainamide, with or without a beta-blocker or diltiazem, has been successful in preventing the recurrence of tachycardia in some cases. If these approaches are unsuccessful, an IV beta-blocker or amiodarone can be effective, but amiodarone may be a better agent to use. Class III and class IC antiarrhythmic agents are also used in people with ventricular preexcitation. Digoxin slows AV conduction, but it can decrease the refractory period of the accessory pathway; therefore, it is avoided with preexcitation syndromes. Intracardiac electrophysiologic mapping with radiofrequency catheter ablation of the accessory pathway(s) has been successful in abolishing refractory supraventricular tachycardia associated with preexcitation in dogs[5].

ATRIAL TACHYCARDIA (AUTOMATIC FOCUS)

Acute therapy for automatic atrial tachycardia is as outlined above for sustained SVTs in general. If the arrhythmia is suppressed, therapy is continued PO; however, this rhythm can be unrelenting (232, 233). If the ectopic focus cannot be suppressed, the goal of therapy becomes ventricular rate control. This is accomplished by slowing AV conduction and increasing refractoriness so that fewer atrial impulses reach the ventricles. Combinations of diltiazem or a beta-blocker, and digoxin, sotalol, or amiodarone can be effective. The patient with persistent automatic atrial tachycardia could be a candidate for intracardiac electrophysiologic mapping and catheter ablation, if available. Alternatively, another strategy to control heart rate could be AV node ablation, with permanent pacemaker implantation.

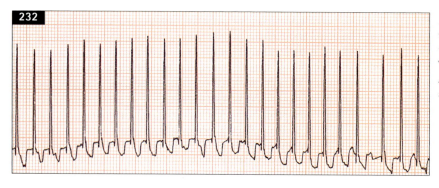

232 Sustained atrial tachycardia in a 9-month-old female Jack Russell Terrier with cardiomegaly and myocardial failure. Ventricular rate is about 280/minute, 2:1 AV conduction of P' waves (except briefly at right of strip).

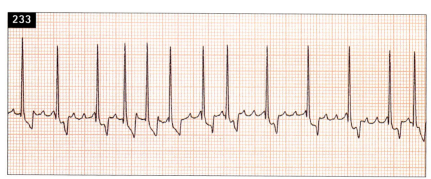

233 ECG from the dog in **232** showing persistent atrial tachycardia (atrial rate ~460/minute) with variable AV block (ventricular rate ~140/minute) on therapy with digoxin, diltiazem, enalapril, and sotalol. Signs of congestion had resolved and the dog was normally active. Amiodarone was later substituted for sotalol and partially suppressed the tachycardia. Lead II, 25 mm/sec, 1 cm = 1 mV.

ATRIAL FIBRILLATION

AF is a common arrhythmia in the dog, although it rarely occurs in puppies under a year old[54–57]. Most dogs and all cats with AF have significant underlying cardiac disease, with marked atrial enlargement[56, 58, 59]. A certain 'critical mass' of atrial tissue is needed to sustain AF. The prevalence is greater in large and giant breed dogs[54, 60, 61]. Up to 21% of all Irish Wolfhounds, and virtually every one with heart failure, are estimated to have AF[62, 63]. AF is almost always persistent and only occasionally paroxysmal[64]. Even if pharmacologic or electrical cardioversion to sinus rhythm is successful, AF usually recurs within a short time because of pathologic changes in atrial tissue.

Because permanent conversion to sinus rhythm is unlikely with significant underlying disease, the usual goals of therapy are to slow AV conduction and to manage underlying disease. The ventricular response rate to AF and, therefore, HR depends on the prevailing level of sympathetic tone and the conduction velocity and recovery rate of the AV node. HR control provides similar survival benefit (and fewer adverse effects) than conversion to sinus rhythm in human AF, with a trend toward lower mortality in the rate control group[29, 65, 66]. A slower HR allows more time for ventricular filling and lessens the relative importance of atrial contraction (which is lacking in AF).

In-hospital HRs less than 150 beats/minute in dogs (or 180 beats/minute in cats) are desirable. Ideal target HR probably depends on animal size and underlying disease; ~130–145 beats/minute is reported for 20–25 kg dogs[67–69]. The animal's HR at home will be less than this; HRs of 70–120 beats/minute in dogs and 80–140 beats/minute in cats are probably acceptable. An ECG recording is recommended to document the ventricular rate. HR estimation by auscultation or palpation can be quite inaccurate, depending on the skill of examiner[70]. Femoral pulses should not be used to assess HR when AF is present because of frequent pulse deficit.

If rapid HR reduction is indicated, IV diltiazem is recommended because it has less negative inotropic effect than verapamil and propranolol. IV diltiazem can improve ventricular performance by reducing HR, increasing filling time, and lowering myocardial O_2 requirement[56]. In experimental dogs with induced AF, IV diltiazem doses from 0.4–0.9 mg/kg produced plasma concentrations between 68–117 ng/ml and HRs closest to baseline sinus rhythm[68]. Although cautious use of IV esmolol is an alternative, IV digoxin is usually avoided. When dobutamine or dopamine infusion is needed to support myocardial function (see *Table 43*, p.171), IV diltiazem or (cautiously) IV digoxin could be used, but a beta-blocker should be avoided.

Long-term oral therapy usually includes digoxin in dogs and in cats with DCM. If the HR exceeds 200–220 beats/minute at rest, twice the eventual PO maintenance dosage can be given for 1 (to 2) days. Digoxin by itself does not adequately slow the HR in many animals. The increase in sympathetic tone that occurs with exercise, excitement, or CHF often overrides the vagal effect of digoxin on the AV node[56, 71]. Either a beta-blocker or diltiazem can be added to further slow AV conduction. Because of their potential myocardial depressive effects, low initial doses are used and titrated upward to effect. PO diltiazem at 5 mg/kg in experimental dogs with acute AF produced therapeutic blood levels (32–100 ng/ml) 3 hours post dose and hemodynamic values similar to baseline sinus rhythm[69]; however, animals with heart disease may not tolerate such high doses. On occasion, a dog will revert to sinus rhythm with diltiazem. Simultaneous use of diltiazem and a beta-blocker is not recommended in patients with heart failure because of the risk for hypotension and reduced contractility[72]. Amiodarone can be added if additional rate control is needed. For cats with HCM and AF, diltiazem or a beta-blocker is used without digoxin.

If preexcitation is also present in a patient with AF, AV nodal blocking drugs (i.e. calcium channel-blockers, digoxin, and, possibly, beta-blockers) should not be used because they can paradoxically increase the ventricular response rate[52]. Amiodarone is recommended in these cases[52]. Sotalol or procainamide can also be used.

AF can occur transiently in medium to large sized dogs without structural heart disease, usually in association with anesthesia, hypothyroidism, rapid removal of large volume pericardial effusion, GI disease, or volume infusion-induced atrial distension[57]. Changes in autonomic balance can provoke the onset and maintenance of AF[73]. AF sometimes occurs spontaneously in overtly normal giant breed dogs, especially Irish Wolfhounds. This is known as 'lone AF'. Males are affected more often than females[56, 61]. It is possible that some of these cases represent a familial AF, as is known to occur in people[74]. It is unclear if affected dogs are destined to eventually develop DCM[56, 75]. Likewise, it is not known if those with persistently slow HR response to AF have comparable survival times to dogs that convert to sinus rhythm. Dogs that do not convert to sinus rhythm can be given digoxin or diltiazem for rate control, or monitored periodically without therapy if the ventricular rate appears consistently low; however, excessively high HRs still can occur with exercise and excitement.

Acute AF without signs of heart disease or failure may convert to sinus rhythm, either spontaneously or with drug treatment or electrical cardioversion. Conversion is more likely with AF of recent onset and normal atrial size. Pharmacologic cardioversion is sometimes achieved with quinidine, but this is only used where there is no or only mild underlying disease. Doses of 5–20 mg/kg PO q2–6h are recommended. Side-effects can be serious, including torsades de pointes (TdP) (related to QT prolongation), weakness, ataxia, and seizures[76]. Quinidine's vagolytic effect can increase the ventricular response rate initially. Simultaneous use of diltiazem or a beta-blocker might be useful[56]. Alternatively, high dose diltiazem alone (PO for 3 days) has sometimes been effective. The drug is discontinued after sinus rhythm is achieved. In people with recent onset AF, ibutilide seems most effective (0.01 mg/kg IV over 10 minutes to a maximum of 1 mg/kg)[52, 77, 78]. However, caution is warranted; in experimental pacing-induced cardiomyopathy in dogs, ibutilide caused increased dispersion of ventricular repolarization and episodes of TdP[79]. Other drugs that have successfully converted AF in people include amiodarone, propafenone, flecainide, and dofetilide[52, 80]. Amiodarone, propafenone, and sotalol have had anecdotal success in some dogs[56]. Acute onset AF associated with high vagal tone may convert with IV lidocaine[81]. Magnesium supplementation is useful in some people with AF and rapid ventricular rate[52].

Electrical cardioversion has been of limited success in animals; most revert to AF after a variable time period. DC cardioversion (low-energy shock) is synchronized with endogenous electrical activity (R wave) to avoid stimulation during the cardiac vulnerable period and precipitation of VF. Biphasic current delivery followed by amiodarone therapy may be more effective and safer than older methods of cardioversion[82]. DC cardioversion can be done after a loading dose of a class III (ibutilide, amiodarone, sotalol) or IC (propafenone, flecainide) agent. Greater success is reported in people with prior drug loading[56]. Multiple complicating factors related to the animal as well as equipment can potentially prevent successful DC cardioversion[56]. Other treatments for AF used in people include catheter interventional and surgical techniques. Their applicability in clinical veterinary patients has not been described.

MANAGEMENT OF VENTRICULAR TACHYARRHYTHMIAS

Occasional VPCs in an otherwise asymptomatic animal do not cause hemodynamic disturbance and generally are not treated. Based on 24-hour Holter studies, occasional VPCs (<25 or so/day) are seen in normal dogs and cats, especially older animals[7, 21, 83]. Even moderately frequent VPCs may not require antiarrhythmic drug treatment if underlying heart function is normal. Accelerated idioventricular rhythm (see Chapter 4, p. 56) and ventricular parasystole tend to be well-tolerated and benign rhythms. Parasystole is an unusual arrhythmia caused by an accelerated automatic ventricular focus that is electrically protected (entrance block) from depolarization by sinus (or other) impulses[84]. Specific antiarrhythmic therapy is usually unnecessary, unless the ventricular rate increases or the animal shows hemodynamic compromise. If underlying disease is identified, therapy is directed at that disease.

Previous guidelines for instituting ventricular antiarrhythmic therapy were based on VPC frequency, prematurity, and variability of the QRS configuration of the arrhythmia. Characteristics thought to imply increased electrical instability include rapid paroxysmal or sustained ventricular tachycardia (e.g. at rates > 150 beats/minute), multiform (polymorphic) VPCs, or close coupling of the VPCs to preceding complexes (R-on-T phenomenon), but it is not clear if the frequency or morphologic complexity predict greater risk of sudden death[1–3]. The animal's underlying disease and whether the arrhythmia causes signs of hypotension or inadequate CO are probably more important in the decision to treat. Animals thought to be hemodynamically unstable or to have disease associated with sudden cardiac death are treated earlier and more aggressively.

General goals for managing ventricular tachyarrhythmias are to optimize CO by controlling HR and rhythm, and to avoid adverse effects of antiarrhythmic therapy. VT can degenerate into increasingly unstable rhythms. But reducing the number of VT episodes or VPCs with antiarrhythmic drugs does not necessarily prevent sudden cardiac death.

ACUTE THERAPY FOR SUSTAINED OR FREQUENT PAROXYSMS OF VENTRICULAR TACHYCARDIA

Rapid paroxysmal or sustained VT is treated aggressively because marked hypotension can result. IV lidocaine is usually the first-choice antiarrhythmic agent in dogs. It can suppress arrhythmias from multiple underlying mechanisms and has minimal adverse hemodynamic effects. Because the effect from IV boluses lasts about 10–15 minutes, CRI is warranted if the drug is effective. Small supplemental IV boluses can be given with the CRI to maintain therapeutic concentrations until steady state is achieved. IV infusions can be continued for several days, if needed. If lidocaine is ineffective after maximal recommended doses, several other approaches can be used (234). Procainamide (given IV, IM, or PO) or quinidine (given IM or PO) has often been used (234).

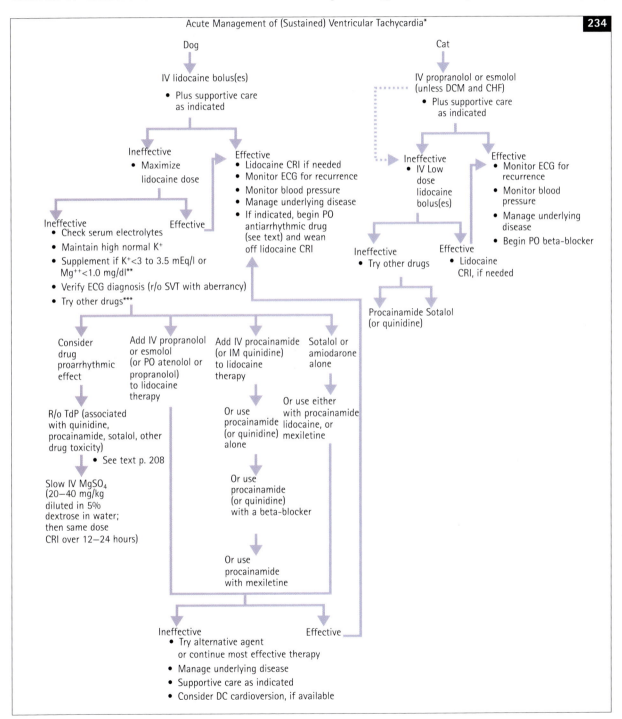

234 Approach to the acute management of sustained ventricular tachycardia.

* See text for additional information, and for long-term management of ventricular tachyarrhythmias.

** KCl infusion rate: if serum K^+ is <3 mmol/l (<3 mEq/l), use 0.5 mEq/kg/hour; if serum K^+ is between 3.0 and 3.5 mmol/l (3.0 and 3.5 mEq/l), use 0.25 mEq/kg/hour. $MgSO_4$ or $MgCl$ infusion rate: if serum Mg^{++} is 0.41 mmol/l (<1 mg/dl), use 0.75–1.0 mEq/kg/day.

*** Use IV phenytoin for refractory ventricular tachycardia caused by digoxin toxicity.

Quinidine is not given IV because of its hypotensive effects. It is also avoided in animals receiving digoxin or with prolonged QT intervals. Effects of a single IM or PO loading dose of either drug should occur within 2 hours. If this is effective, maintenance doses can be given every 4–6 hours IM or PO. If ineffective, the dose can be increased or another antiarrhythmic agent chosen. Another strategy is to add a beta-blocker to lidocaine or procainamide. Other approaches that are more effective in some cases include using mexiletine, sotalol, or amiodarone. IV amiodarone is now recommended as the first line treatment for regular wide QRS tachycardia in people[52]. Veterinary experience with this drug is growing but still limited. IV amiodarone effectively suppresses VT in some dogs[22, 85], but hypotension can occur. Very slow injection of conservative doses and blood pressure monitoring are recommended.

DC cardioversion can be attempted for refractory VT if the equipment is available. ECG synchronization and anesthesia or sedation are required. High-energy, nonsynchronized shock (defibrillation) can be used for rapid polymorphic VT or flutter degenerating into VF.

Cats with serious ventricular tachyarrhythmias are usually given a beta-blocker first. Alternatively, low doses of lidocaine can be used; however, cats are quite sensitive to lidocaine's neurotoxic effects. Procainamide, quinidine, and sotalol have also been used in cats.

Digoxin is not used for treating ventricular tachyarrhythmias specifically, although it is often indicated for concurrent heart failure or supraventricular arrhythmias. Digoxin can predispose to arrhythmia development. In animals with preexisting ventricular tachyarrhythmias, the use of another antiarrhythmic drug before or with digoxin therapy may be necessary.

Digoxin toxicity-induced ventricular tachyarrhythmias

Digoxin-induced ventricular tachyarrhythmias are treated first with IV lidocaine. If these are refractory to lidocaine, phenytoin is used (in dogs only) slowly IV to avoid hypotension (see p. 213) Phenytoin is used PO occasionally to treat or prevent digitalis-induced ventricular arrhythmias. IV potassium supplementation is also given for digitalis toxicity if the serum potassium concentration is <4 mmol/l (<4 mEq/l). Magnesium supplementation can help suppress arrhythmias as well. MgSO₄ has been used at 25–40 mg/kg slow IV bolus, followed by infusion of the same dose over 12–24 hours.

Torsades de pointes

TdP is a form of polymorphic VT associated with underlying QT prolongation[86, 87]. TdP is typically preceded by a period of slow HR with prolonged QT intervals (e.g. >0.25 seconds in dogs); its onset is triggered by a VPC during the ventricular repolarization period (R on T). TdP is characterized by a rapid VT of continuously changing amplitude and polarity (as if its axis is 'rotating around a point'). It usually occurs as a brief paroxysm, but can degenerate into VF. Anything that causes QT interval prolongation (with increased dispersion of refractoriness) can predispose to TdP, including hypokalemia, hypocalcemia, antiarrhythmic drug toxicity, especially class IA agents, and congenital long QT syndromes. When TdP is suspected, all antiarrhythmic, and other, drugs that can prolong the QT interval should be discontinued and electrolyte imbalances corrected. Slow IV injection of MgSO₄ (20–40 mg/kg, diluted in 5% dextrose in water) may suppress the arrhythmia[87]. As MgSO₄ contains 8.13 mEq magnesium/gram, a similar magnesium dose is provided by calculating 0.15–0.3 mEq/kg. Isoproterenol or ventricular pacing can also be effective for TdP[52], but isoproterenol infusion can provoke VF if TdP is not present. Polymorphic VT that is not associated with prolonged QT intervals may respond to amiodarone[52].

Ventricular fibrillation

VF (see Chapter 4, p. 56 and 98, p. 57) is usually preceded by VT or flutter. It quickly causes circulatory collapse. Severe disease usually underlies this lethal arrhythmia (including myocardial anoxia or ischemia, trauma, severe electrolyte imbalance, shock). After verifying pulselessness/unconsciousness (and ruling out ECG artifact), immediate cardiopulmonary resuscitation and electrical defibrillation (high-energy unsynchronized shock) are indicated. Other treatments are only rarely effective (e.g. precordial thump, KCl and CaCl₂, class III agents)[6].

Follow-up monitoring

Close ECG monitoring and further diagnostic testing should follow initial therapy for ventricular tachyarrhythmias. Total suppression of VPCs is not expected. Consideration of the animal's clinical status and underlying disease, how well the drug has suppressed the arrhythmia, and the drug dosage used influence the decision whether to continue or discontinue current treatment or to use a different drug. Clinical status and results of diagnostic testing also guide decisions about long-term PO therapy.

LONG-TERM ORAL THERAPY FOR VENTRICULAR TACHYARRHYTHMIAS

Animals treated successfully for acute ventricular tachyarrhythmias are usually continued PO on the same (or similar) agent that was most effective parenterally. Any concurrent or underlying abnormalities should also be addressed as possible.

Patients with underlying heart disease and arrhythmias can benefit from the use of beta-blockers and ACE inhibitors, as well as other appropriate therapies[30].

Historically, class I antiarrhythmic drugs, sometimes in combination with a beta-blocker, were used most often for long-term therapy. These agents may effectively suppress ventricular arrhythmias, but there is concern that they do not reduce the risk of sudden death[12, 76, 88]. Sustained release procainamide has suppressed ventricular ectopia in some cases, but there are concerns about long-term efficacy, lack of protection from sudden death, and adverse effects including GI disturbances, lethargy, and proarrhythmia. Quinidine is a less desirable agent because of its frequent adverse effects, and its interference with digoxin pharmacokinetics[73]. Mexiletine (similar to lidocaine) has been effective against ventricular tachyarrhythmias, with fewer adverse effects than tocainide[89]. Uncontrolled observations in dogs suggest it may be more effective than procainamide or quinidine[12, 90]. The combination of mexiletine with quinidine may be effective against arrhythmias refractory to each agent alone[90]. The class III agents appear to have greater antifibrillatory effects than the class I drugs. In people, use of the traditional class I drugs has been largely replaced by class III agents, especially amiodarone, or invasive techniques such as catheter ablation or implantable cardioverter defibrillators[30, 35].

A beta-blocker can help prevent both ventricular and supraventricular tachyarrhythmias that are provoked by sympathetic stimulation or catecholamines. Beta-blockers have protected people and experimental dogs with myocardial ischemia or infarction against VF[83]. Beta-blockers alone have not been very effective in suppressing ventricular tachyarrhythmias in Doberman Pinschers with cardiomyopathy[22]; however, they are often used in combination with a class I agent (e.g. procainamide or mexiletine). Beta-blockers must be used cautiously in animals with myocardial failure because of their potential negative inotropic effect[22].

A significant decrease in the number of VPCs and arrhythmia severity was seen in Boxers with arrhythmogenic RV cardiomyopathy using mexiletine combined with atenolol and with sotalol alone, but not with procainamide or atenolol alone[91]; however, there was no difference in the occurrence of syncope. This study did not determine if there was any survival benefit, although anecdotally, sotalol seems to reduce the occurrence of sudden death[86]. Antiarrhythmic therapy may possibly prolong survival in Doberman Pinschers with cardiomyopathy and VT[92]. Some dogs with DCM have experienced worsening myocardial function while on sotalol[22]. Amiodarone is an effective alternative antiarrhythmic, although there are concerns about its prolonged half-life and an array of potential adverse effects (see p. 216); however, amiodarone may have lesser proarrhythmic effects and confer greater antifibrillatory protection than other agents.

In summary, drugs currently used for the long-term management of ventricular tachyarrhythmias in dogs include sustained-release procainamide or mexiletine (or possibly tocainide); sustained-release procainamide or mexiletine combined with atenolol or propranolol; sotalol; or amiodarone. The latter three options are favored because they are thought to provide a greater antifibrillatory effect.

Animals on long-term antiarrhythmic therapy, for any rhythm disturbance, should be reevaluated frequently. Besides determining treatment effectiveness, it is important to screen for adverse drug effects and disease progression. Pretreatment and post-treatment 24- to 48-hour ambulatory ECG recordings showing at least a 70–80% reduction in arrhythmia frequency provide the best indicator of antiarrhythmic drug efficacy. Intermittent ECG recordings cannot truly differentiate between drug effect, or lack thereof, and the often marked variability in arrhythmia frequency that occurs spontaneously, but in-hospital ECG recordings are often used in an attempt to monitor arrhythmias. Also, clients can be shown how to use a stethoscope or palpate the chest wall to count the number of 'skipped' beats/minute at home; this may yield an approximation of the frequency of arrhythmic events, either single or paroxysms. Likewise, the presence or frequency of clinical signs caused by the arrhythmia can be a rough guide to treatment efficacy. The decision to continue or discontinue successful antiarrhythmic therapy is also based on consideration of the clinical situation and underlying cardiac disease.

MANAGEMENT OF BRADYARRHYTHMIAS

Abnormally slow rhythms occur with excessive vagal tone, certain drugs, hyperkalemia, and pathology within the heart (see *Table 36*, p. 135 and Chapter 4). When the bradycardia is drug induced, the agent is discontinued or its dosage reduced; additional therapy is used if indicated (e.g. reversal of anesthesia, calcium salts for calcium channel-blocker overdose, dopamine or atropine for beta-blocker toxicity). Underlying disease is addressed as possible.

Sinus bradycardia or AV conduction block associated with clinical signs, such as weakness, exercise intolerance, syncope, or worsening cardiac disease, may respond to anticholinergic, or adrenergic, therapy (235). An atropine response test can reveal the extent to which excessive vagal tone underlies the bradycardia and, thus, whether an oral anticholinergic agent might be useful. If medical therapy does not improve symptomatic bradycardia, temporary or permanent artificial pacing is indicated (see p. 219).

ATROPINE RESPONSE TEST

The atropine response test is used to determine the degree of vagal influence on sinus and AV nodal function. Atropine increases HR and improves AV block in vagally-mediated bradycardia. It has little to no effect on bradyarrhythmias caused by intrinsic disease of the sinus or AV node. Response to atropine challenge is most consistent with IV administration of 0.04 mg/kg[93, 94]. An ECG is recorded within 5–10 minutes after atropine injection. If the HR has not increased by at least 150%, the ECG is repeated 15 (to 20) minutes after the atropine injection; sometimes, an initial vagomimetic effect on the AV node lasts longer than 5 minutes (see p. 218). The normal sinus node response is a rate increase to 150–160 beats/minute (or >135 beats/minute).

A positive response may not predict response to oral anticholinergic therapy.

SICK SINUS SYNDROME

SSS (or bradycardia–tachycardia syndrome) is described further in Chapter 13, p. 134. Oral therapy with an anticholinergic agent, methylxanthine bronchodilator, or terbutaline temporarily helps some animals. Response to oral anticholinergic agents is not necessarily correlated with positive response to IV atropine challenge[95], but PO therapy often is, or over time becomes, unrewarding. Drugs used to accelerate the sinus rate can also exacerbate tachyarrhythmias and so are relatively contraindicated. Conversely, drugs that suppress supraventricular tachyarrhythmias can magnify the bradycardia. Digoxin is relatively contraindicated for this reason[6]. SSS that causes frequent or severe clinical signs is best managed by permanent artificial pacing. Dogs that remain symptomatic because of supraventricular tachyarrhythmias are treated with an appropriate antiarrhythmic drug after successful pacemaker implantation.

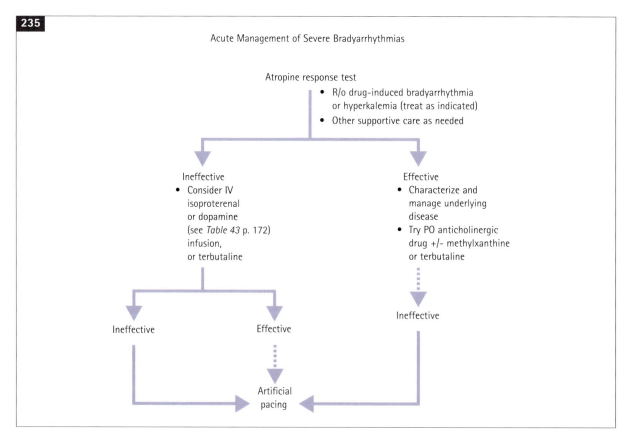

235

Acute Management of Severe Bradyarrhythmias

Atropine response test
- R/o drug-induced bradyarrhythmia or hyperkalemia (treat as indicated)
- Other supportive care as needed

Ineffective
- Consider IV isoproterenal or dopamine (see *Table 43* p. 172) infusion, or terbutaline

Effective
- Characterize and manage underlying disease
- Try PO anticholinergic drug +/- methylxanthine or terbutaline

Ineffective   Effective

Ineffective

Artificial pacing

235 Approach to the acute management of severe bradyarrhythmias.

ATRIAL STANDSTILL

An apparent lack of atrial electrical and mechanical activity ('silent atrium') can occur in animals with hyperkalemia (see Chapter 4, p. 64). It is important to exclude hyperkalemia as a cause for flat or absent P waves and relatively slow HR. When serum potassium concentration is normalized, sinus P waves become evident.

Medical treatment for persistent atrial standstill (see Chapter 13, p. 135) is rarely rewarding, but an anticholinergic drug or infusion of dopamine or isoproterenol sometimes accelerates the escape rhythm temporarily. Terbutaline PO may also have some beneficial effect. If ventricular tachyarrhythmias are provoked, the drug is discontinued or used at a lower dose. Ventricular antiarrhythmic drugs are contraindicated because they can suppress the escape focus as well as the tachyarrhythmia. Permanent pacemaker implantation is the treatment of choice, although long-term prognosis is poor in dogs with concurrent ventricular myocardial dysfunction.

AV CONDUCTION BLOCK

AV conduction disturbances vary in cause and severity (see Chapter 4, p. 58). 1st degree and 2nd degree AV blocks with occasional nonconducted P waves cause no clinical signs and need no treatment. However, a search for the underlying cause (e.g. high vagal tone or drug therapy that slows AV conduction) and appropriate disease management are indicated. Whether AV block causes clinical signs is related to the overall ventricular rate as well as the underlying cardiac function. High-grade or advanced 2nd degree and 3rd degree AV blocks are more likely to cause signs of low cardiac output; however, some dogs are fairly asymptomatic, as are most cats with persistent 3rd degree AV block. Cats usually have a ventricular escape rhythm rate of 90–120 beats/minute. Cats with syncope from AV block are likely to have intermittent 3rd degree AV block, with delayed ventricular escape rhythm activation[6, 96]. Most advanced forms of AV block are associated with underlying structural disease (e.g. endocarditis/myocarditis, cardiomyopathy, endocardiosis, fibrosis, trauma), although this may not be detectable antemortem. Occasional cases have functional AV block (e.g. digoxin toxicity, alpha$_2$-agonist anesthetics, hyperkalemia).

Atropine challenge and oral anticholinergic therapy are often ineffective for high-grade 2nd degree and complete AV block, so artificial pacing is usually indicated. An emergency infusion of dopamine (see *Table 43*, p. 172) or isoproterenol may increase the ventricular escape rate in these animals, but such therapy can provoke ventricular tachyarrhythmias. Isoproterenol PO is usually ineffective. Some cats with complete AV block survive for years without artificial pacing, even with underlying cardiac disease or heart failure at presentation[97].

OVERVIEW OF ANTIARRHYTHMIC DRUGS

CLASS I ANTIARRHYTHMIC DRUGS

These agents block membrane Na$^+$ channels and depress the action potential upstroke (phase 0). This slows conduction velocity and can interrupt reentrant rhythms[40]. The class I drugs are subclassified according to other electrophysiologic characteristics (*Table 47*, p. 199) that influence their efficacy against particular arrhythmias. The electrophysiologic effects of class I drugs are extremely dependent on extracellular potassium concentration; hypokalemia may render these drugs ineffective, whereas hyperkalemia intensifies their depressant effects on cardiac membranes. All these agents are contraindicated in animals with complete heart block and should be used only cautiously in animals with sinus bradycardia, SSS, and 1st or 2nd degree AV block.

Lidocaine

Lidocaine HCl is usually the IV ventricular antiarrhythmic agent of first choice in dogs. Lidocaine has little effect on sinus rate, AV conduction rate, and refractoriness. It is generally ineffective against supraventricular arrhythmias. Lidocaine suppresses automaticity in normal Purkinje fibers and diseased myocardium, slows conduction, and reduces the dispersion of refractoriness. Its effects are greater on diseased and hypoxic cardiac cells and at faster stimulation rates[12]. Lidocaine produces little or no depression of contractility when given slowly IV at therapeutic doses[40]. Toxic concentrations can cause hypotension.

Lidocaine is rapidly metabolized in the liver; some metabolites are active. It is not effective PO because of almost complete first-pass hepatic elimination. Lidocaine is administered as slow IV boluses followed by CRI. Antiarrhythmic effects after an IV bolus occur within 2 minutes and abate within 10–20 minutes[12]. CRI without a loading dose produces steady-state concentrations in 4–6 hours. The half-life is <1 hour in the dog. Therapeutic plasma concentrations are thought to be 1.5–6 mcg/ml in dogs. Lidocaine's half-life is about 1.7 hours in awake cats, but only 1 hour in cats anesthetized with isoflurane[98]. The anesthetized cats reached higher initial serum concentrations; other pharmacokinetic properties of lidocaine and an active metabolite are also affected by isoflurane[98]. Only lidocaine without epinephrine should be used for antiarrhythmic therapy. IM administration could be considered if IV access is not possible, but IV is much preferred.

The toxic effects of lidocaine most often relate to the CNS. They include agitation, disorientation, mental depression, ataxia, muscle twitches, nystagmus, and generalized seizures. The latter may require diazepam (0.25–0.5 mg/kg IV) or a short-acting barbiturate. Nausea can also occur. Toxicity signs usually dissipate shortly after the drug is discontinued; a lower infusion rate can then be reinstituted. Worsening of arrhythmia (proarrhythmia) occurs occasionally, as with any drug having cardiac electrophysiologic effects. Cats are particularly sensitive to lidocaine's toxic effects; bradycardia and respiratory arrest can occur, along with seizures. There are anecdotal reports of respiratory depression and arrest after administration of lidocaine to unconscious dogs and cats. Hepatic disease can delay elimination. Propranolol, cimetidine, chloramphenicol, halothane, and other drugs that decrease liver blood flow slow lidocaine's metabolism and predispose to toxicity. Heart failure also can reduce hepatic blood flow.

Procainamide

Procainamide HCl is similar to quinidine in its electrophysiologic effects, but it causes fewer GI side-effects, less QT prolongation, less hypotension, and no interaction with digoxin[99]. Procainamide prolongs the effective refractory period and slows conduction in the accessory pathway of dogs with orthodromic AV reciprocating tachycardia[51]. Procainamide has both direct and indirect (vagolytic) effects. It is indicated for ventricular (and sometimes supraventricular) tachyarrhythmias, but is less effective than quinidine for atrial tachyarrhythmias. Procainamide should be used only cautiously in hypotensive animals.

Procainamide is well-absorbed orally in the dog (food may delay absorption), but its half-life is only 2.5–4 hours. The sustained-release preparation has a slightly longer half-life of 3–6 hours but may be poorly absorbed. The drug undergoes hepatic metabolism and renal excretion. The metabolite N-acetylprocainamide is not present to any significant degree in dogs and cats. The PO or IM administration of procainamide does not cause marked hemodynamic effects, but rapid IV injection can produce hypotension and cardiac depression, although to a much lesser degree than quinidine. Time to peak plasma concentration is similar for both the IM and PO routes. Procainamide CRI is useful for arrhythmias responsive to an IV bolus. Steady state concentration occurs in 12–22 hours. Therapeutic plasma concentrations are thought to be 4–12 mcg/ml. Serum concentration can be measured 4–5 hours after an oral procainamide dose (or 8 hours after a sustained release preparation). Procainamide is often used with a beta-blocker or another class I agent (e.g. lidocaine) for refractory arrhythmias.

Procainamide's toxic effects are similar but usually milder than those of quinidine (see below). GI upset and QRS or QT interval prolongation can occur. Procainamide can increase the ventricular response rate to AF (vagolytic effect) if used without digoxin or a beta- or calcium channel-blocker. More serious toxic effects include hypotension, depressed AV conduction, sometimes causing 2nd or 3rd degree AV block, and proarrhythmia. The latter can cause syncope or VF. IV fluids, catecholamines, or Ca^{++}-containing solutions can be used to treat hypotension. GI signs associated with PO therapy may respond to a dosage reduction. High-dose PO procainamide in people has been associated with a reversible lupus-like syndrome characterized by neutropenia, fever, depression, and hepatomegaly, but this has not been documented in dogs. Long-term use can cause brown discoloration of the haircoat in black Doberman Pinschers.

Quinidine

Quinidine is useful for ventricular and, occasionally, supraventricular tachyarrhythmias. It may convert recent onset AF to sinus rhythm in dogs with normal ventricular function. Quinidine must be used with caution in animals with heart failure or hyperkalemia. Quinidine characteristically depresses automaticity and conduction velocity and prolongs effective refractory period. Corresponding dose-dependent ECG changes (e.g. prolonged PR, QRS, and QT intervals) result from direct electrophysiologic and vagolytic effects; however, at low doses the drug's vagolytic effects can offset its direct effects and increase the sinus rate or the ventricular response rate to AF. Hypokalemia reduces quinidine's antiarrhythmic effectiveness, as with other class I agents.

The drug is well absorbed PO, but has fallen out of favor for long-term oral therapy. Quinidine undergoes extensive hepatic metabolism. Its half-life is about 6 hours in dogs and 2 hours in cats. It is highly protein-bound; severe hypoalbuminemia can predispose to toxicity. Cimetidine can also predispose to toxicity by slowing the drug's elimination. Quinidine can precipitate digoxin toxicity, when used simultaneously, by displacing digoxin from skeletal muscle-binding sites and decreasing its renal clearance. Anticonvulsants and other drugs that induce hepatic microsomal enzymes can speed quinidine's metabolism. Quinidine is not given IV because of its propensity to cause vasodilation, cardiac depression, and hypotension. The PO and IM routes do not usually cause adverse hemodynamic effects but close monitoring is warranted, especially in animals with cardiac disease. Therapeutic blood concentration is thought to be 2.5–5 mcg/ml. Slow-release sulfate (83% active drug), gluconate (62% active drug), and polygalacturonate (80% active drug) salts of quinidine prolong the drug's absorption and elimination. The sulfate salt is more rapidly absorbed than the gluconate. A peak effect is usually achieved 1–2 hours after PO administration.

Quinidine toxicity extends from the drug's electrophysiologic and hemodynamic effects. Manifestations include marked QT prolongation, right bundle branch block, QRS widening >25% of pretreatment value, various conduction blocks, and ventricular tachyarrhythmias. Marked QT prolongation implies increased temporal dispersion of myocardial refractoriness, which predisposes to TdP and VF. Transient episodes of these serious arrhythmias are known to cause syncope in people taking quinidine. Quinidine's negative inotropic and vasodilatory effects (and subsequent hypotension) can lead to lethargy, weakness, and CHF. Cardiotoxicity and hypotension are partially reversed by sodium bicarbonate (1 mEq/kg IV), which temporarily reduces serum K^+ concentration and enhances quinidine's binding to albumin. GI signs (nausea, vomiting, and diarrhea) are common with PO quinidine. Thrombocytopenia (reversible after drug cessation) can occur in people and possibly in dogs and cats.

Mexiletine
Mexiletine HCl is similar to lidocaine in its electrophysiologic, hemodynamic, toxic, and antiarrhythmic properties. It is used for ventricular tachyarrhythmias in dogs. The combination of a beta-blocker (or procainamide or quinidine) with mexiletine may be more effective and cause fewer adverse effects than mexiletine alone[90, 91]. The drug is well-absorbed PO (<10% first-pass elimination), but antacids, cimetidine, and narcotic analgesics reportedly slow its absorption in people. Mexiletine undergoes hepatic metabolism, influenced by liver blood flow, and renal excretion, which is slower if the urine is alkaline. Hepatic microsomal enzyme inducers may accelerate its clearance. The half-life in dogs is about 4.5–7 hours. Approximately 70% of the drug is protein-bound. Therapeutic serum concentration is thought to be 0.5–2.0 mcg/ml (as in people). The effects of this drug in cats are not known. Adverse effects have included vomiting, anorexia, tremor, ataxia, disorientation, sinus bradycardia, and thrombocytopenia[6, 90]. Administration with food can reduce GI side-effects[12]. Overall, mexiletine appears to produce fewer adverse effects than tocainide[89].

Tocainide
Tocainide HCl is another effective lidocaine congener. It is not often used long term because of frequent side-effects. Tocainide is well absorbed PO, without extensive first-pass metabolism. The plasma concentration peaks about 2 hours after administration in dogs. Effective serum concentrations are maintained for 6–8 hours after three doses. A 'loading' dose is achieved using two doses 2 hours apart, and a third dose 6 hours later, but this is not recommended for dogs concurrently receiving lidocaine. The PO dose does not appear closely correlated with plasma concentration in dogs. Effective plasma concentrations in dogs are reportedly 6 mcg/ml 8 hours after administration (trough) and 10 mcg/ml 2 hours after administration (peak). Concentrations >12 mcg/ml can cause neurotoxicity[89]. Toxicity signs sometimes also occur at 'therapeutic' plasma concentrations. The drug is eliminated by both renal and hepatic routes. The process is not significantly influenced by liver blood flow. GI adverse effects (anorexia and vomiting) seem to be common; occasional neurotoxic signs such as ataxia, disorientation, and twitching can occur. Long-term (>3 months) tocainide use has been associated with serious ocular and renal toxicity in some dogs[89].

Phenytoin
Phenytoin sodium has electrophysiologic effects similar to those of lidocaine. It also has some Ca^{++} channel inhibitory and CNS effects that may contribute to its effectiveness against digitalis-induced arrhythmias. Phenytoin is currently used only in dogs to treat digitalis-induced ventricular tachyarrhythmias that are not responsive to lidocaine. Contraindications to its use are the same as those for lidocaine. Rapid IV injection is avoided because the propylene glycol vehicle can depress myocardial contractility and cause vasodilation, hypotension, respiratory arrest, and exacerbation of arrhythmias. Slow IV infusion and PO administration do not cause relevant hemodynamic disturbance; however, phenytoin's oral bioavailability is poor in dogs. The half-life is only about 3 hours in the dog. Hepatic metabolism occurs and is accelerated by hepatic microsomal enzyme stimulation. Coadministration of cimetidine, chloramphenicol, and other drugs that inhibit microsomal enzyme activity increases phenytoin's serum concentration. Manifestations of phenytoin toxicity include bradycardia, AV block, ventricular tachycardia, and cardiac arrest as well as central nervous system signs (depression, nystagmus, disorientation, and ataxia). The drug is not used in cats; the half-life is very long (>40 hours) in this species and toxicity can occur even at low doses.

Other class I agents
Disopyramide is similar to quinidine and procainamide, but it is not used clinically because of a very short half-life (<2 hours) as well as marked cardiodepressive effects in the dog. **Flecainide** and

propafenone are class IC agents. They slow cardiac conduction velocity markedly but have little effect on sinus rate or refractoriness. High doses depress automaticity in the sinus node and specialized conducting tissues. Vasodilation and myocardial depression can cause severe hypotension after IV injection, especially in animals with underlying cardiac disease. Proarrhythmia is a serious potential adverse effect of these class IC agents. Bradycardia, intraventricular conduction disturbance, and consistent, although transient, hypotension, as well as nausea, vomiting, and anorexia, have occurred in dogs. Flecainide, and **encainide**, have been associated with increased mortality in people[29]; therefore, these agents are used only rarely, with caution, and for life-threatening ventricular arrhythmias refractory to other therapy.

CLASS II ANTIARRHYTHMIC DRUGS: BETA–ADRENERGIC BLOCKERS

Beta-blockers act by inhibiting catecholamine effects. These drugs slow HR, reduce myocardial oxygen demand, and increase AV conduction time and refractoriness[100–102]. They are unlikely to affect repolarization. The antiarrhythmic effect of beta-blockers relates to beta$_1$-receptor blockade rather than direct electrophysiologic effects. Beta$_1$-receptors, located primarily in the myocardium, mediate increases in contractility, HR, AV conduction velocity, and automaticity in specialized fibers. Beta$_2$-receptors in extracardiac regions mediate bronchodilation and vasodilation, as well as renin and insulin release. There are also some beta$_2$-receptors in the heart. In patients with heart failure and beta$_1$-receptor downregulation, the increased relative responsiveness to beta$_2$ stimulation affects diastolic Ca^{++} fluxes, which may magnify the risk for VF in these cases[103]. 'Nonselective' beta-blockers inhibit catecholamine binding to both beta$_1$- and beta$_2$-receptors. Other beta-blockers are more selective and antagonize primarily one or the other receptor subtype. First generation beta-blockers (e.g. propranolol) have nonselective beta-blocking effects. Second generation agents (e.g. atenolol, metoprolol, esmolol) are relatively beta$_1$ selective. Third generation beta-blockers (e.g. carvedilol) affect both beta$_1$ and beta$_2$-receptors, but also antagonize alpha$_1$-receptors and have other effects. A few beta-blockers have some degree of intrinsic sympathomimetic activity.

Beta-receptor blockers are used in animals with HCM (see Chapter 21), congenital (see Chapter 18) and acquired ventricular outflow obstruction, systemic hypertension (see Chapter 25), hyperthyroid heart disease, supraventricular or ventricular tachyarrhythmias, especially those provoked by increased sympathetic tone, and other diseases or toxicities associated with excessive sympathetic

stimulation. A beta-blocker is often used in conjunction with digoxin to slow the ventricular response rate to AF. Beta-blockers are also considered the first line antiarrhythmic agent in cats for both supraventricular and ventricular tachyarrhythmias. In dogs, the combination of a beta-blocker with a class I agent often produces better ventricular tachyarrhythmia suppression than either agent alone[91]. Beta-blockers enhance the depression of AV conduction produced by digitalis, class I antiarrhythmic drugs, and calcium channel-blockers. Long-term therapy with certain beta-blockers improves cardiac function and prolongs survival in people, and possibly animals, with stable heart failure (see Chapter 16, p. 184).

Because the effects of beta-blockers depend on the level of sympathetic activation, individual patient response is quite variable. Initial doses should be low and titrated upward as needed, according to the animal's response. These drugs must be used cautiously in animals with severe myocardial disease, which may be dependent on increased sympathetic drive to maintain cardiac output, because marked depression of cardiac contractility, conduction, or HR could result. Prior institution of inotropic support is advised in these cases. Beta-blockers are generally contraindicated in animals with sinus bradycardia, SSS, high-grade AV block, or severe CHF. The simultaneous use of a beta-blocker and a calcium channel-blocker is generally not recommended because marked decrease in HR and myocardial contractility can result; however, selected cases may benefit from the cautious use of both agents. Because of possible beta-receptor upregulation (increased number or affinity of receptors) during long-term beta-blockade, abrupt discontinuation of therapy could result in serious cardiac arrhythmias[12]. Nonselective beta-blockers may increase peripheral vascular resistance, because of unopposed alpha effects, and promote bronchoconstriction by beta$_2$ antagonism. Other adverse effects of beta-blockers can include lethargy, fatigue, anorexia, vomiting, diarrhea, hypotension, onset or recurrence of CHF, sinus bradycardia, and AV block. Beta-blockers can also mask early signs of acute hypoglycemia in diabetics (e.g. tachycardia and blood pressure changes), and reduce insulin release in response to hyperglycemia[102].

Propanolol

Propranolol HCl is the prototypical nonselective beta-blocker, but it is now used less often than atenolol. Propranolol is avoided with pulmonary edema because of the potential for bronchoconstriction from beta$_2$-receptor antagonism. A beta$_1$-selective agent can be used instead. Propranolol's beta$_2$-receptor blocking effects also make it relatively contraindicated in patients with asthma or chronic small airway disease.

Propranolol has a relatively low oral bioavailability because of extensive first-pass hepatic metabolism, but long-term use and higher doses saturate hepatic enzymes and increase bioavailability. Propranolol decreases hepatic blood flow and so prolongs its own elimination and that of other drugs dependent on liver blood flow for their metabolism (e.g. lidocaine). Feeding delays PO absorption and increases drug clearance by increasing hepatic blood flow. The half-life of propranolol in the dog is only about 1.5 hours (0.5–4.2 hours in cats), but active metabolites exist. Peak plasma concentration is higher in hyperthyroid cats[104]. IV propranolol is used mainly for refractory ventricular tachycardia, in conjunction with a class I drug, and for acute management of atrial or junctional tachycardia.

Propranolol toxicity is usually related to excessive beta-blockade. Some animals cannot tolerate even small doses. Bradycardia, heart failure, hypotension, bronchospasm, and hypoglycemia can occur. Infusion of a catecholamine (e.g. dopamine or dobutamine) mitigates these effects. Propranolol and other lipophilic beta-blockers can cause depressed attitude and disorientation because of CNS effects.

Atenolol
Atenolol is a selective beta$_1$-blocker used commonly in dogs and cats to slow sinus rate and AV conduction, and to suppress ventricular premature depolarizations. The half-life of atenolol is slightly over 3 hours in dogs and about 3.5 hours in cats. Oral bioavailability in both species is 90%. Atenolol is excreted in the urine; renal impairment delays clearance. Its beta-blocking effects are evident for 12 hours, but are gone by 24 hours in normal cats[105]. This hydrophilic drug does not readily cross the blood–brain barrier, so adverse CNS effects are unlikely; However, weakness or exacerbation of heart failure can be observed, as with other beta-blockers.

Metoprolol
Metoprolol tartrate is another longer acting beta$_1$-selective agent that has been used in dogs with DCM and chronic valvular disease. It is well absorbed PO, but bioavailability is reduced by a large first-pass effect. There is minimal protein-binding. The drug is metabolized in the liver and excreted in the urine. Half-life is 1.6 hours in dogs, and 1.3 hours in cats. Experimental heart failure studies in dogs show efficacy of the sustained release formulation, and suggest possible improvement in ejection fraction over time[106].

Esmolol
Esmolol HCl is an ultra-short acting agent with beta$_1$-receptor selectivity. It's half-life is less than 10 minutes[107]. It is rapidly metabolized by blood esterases. Steady state occurs in 5 minutes with, or 30 minutes without, a loading dose. Effects dissipate within 10–20 minutes of discontinuing infusion. Although expensive, this drug has been used for acute treatment of tachyarrhythmias and feline hypertrophic obstructive cardiomyopathy.

Other beta-blocking drugs
Other beta-blocking drugs are available. Their basic effects are similar, although their relative selectivity for beta$_1$-receptors as well as their pharmacologic characteristics vary. Certain beta-blockers, particularly carvedilol and also metoprolol, were shown to improve cardiac function and survival in people with heart failure. (see Chapter 16, p. 184). Nonselective (1st generation) agents and some later generation agents do not appear to confer these survival benefits. Those with intrinsic sympathomimetic activity appear to have deleterious effects.

CLASS III ANTIARRHYTHMIC DRUGS
These agents prolong action potential duration and effective refractory period without decreasing conduction velocity. They act mainly by inhibiting the repolarizing potassium channel I$_K$ (delayed rectifier). The effects of some drugs in this class (e.g. amiodarone) are greater at higher HRs ('use-dependence'), although others exhibit reverse use-dependence (e.g. sotalol)[108]. They are useful for refractory ventricular arrhythmias, especially those caused by reentry. These drugs can have antifibrillatory effects on atrial and ventricular tissues[76]. Currently available agents share some characteristics of other antiarrhythmic drug classes in addition to their class III effects.

Sotalol
Sotalol HCl is a nonselective beta-blocker with class III effects at higher doses. Beta-blocking effects, from the l-isomer, occur at lower doses and are about 30% of propranolol's potency[109]. These are important to sotalol's antiarrhythmic effectivness. d-Sotalol alone has no beta-blocking effect; it prolongs repolarization, but nonuniformity probably explains the increased mortality in human clinical trials with this isomer. The racemic mixture is used clinically. Sotalol prolongs the refractory period by selectively blocking the rapid component of K$^+$ channels responsible for repolarization (delayed rectifier current). Bioavailability of sotalol is high with negligible first-pass effect, but absorption is reduced with food. The half-life is about 5 hours in dogs. It is eliminated unchanged by the kidneys; renal dysfunction prolongs elimination. Sotalol's beta-blocking effects last longer than its plasma half-life. The drug has minimal hemodynamic effects,

although it can cause hypotension. Slowed sinus rate and 1st degree heart block can occur. Sotalol can be proarrhythmic (as can all antiarrhythmic agents). Dogs require much higher doses than people to manifest the class III effects. Doses that are used clinically in dogs probably produce primarily beta-blocking effects[110]; however, the high rate of proarrhythmia, especially TdP, of concern in people taking sotalol has not been reported clinically in dogs. Experimentally, in hypokalemic dogs, coadministration of mexiletine reduced this proarrhythmia potential[111]. Sotalol has also been used in cats with severe ventricular tachyarrhythmias.

Some dogs with DCM experience worsened myocardial function on sotalol[22], but sotalol has less negative inotropic effect than propranolol. Its ability to prolong action potential duration can confer a mild positive inotropic effect related to increased intracellular Ca^{++}, but this may not be realized at doses used in dogs[112]. Other adverse effects of sotalol can include hypotension, depression, nausea, vomiting, diarrhea, and bradycardia[40]. There are a few anecdotal reports of aggression that resolved after sotalol was discontinued.

Amiodarone

Amiodarone HCl is considered a 'broad-spectrum' antiarrhythmic drug. It prolongs the action potential duration and effective refractory period in both atrial and ventricular tissues. It also shares properties with all three other antiarrhythmic drug classes. Amiodarone is an iodinated compound that has effects on Na^+, K^+, and Ca^{++} channels, and has noncompetitive alpha$_1$- and beta-blocking properties[52]. Its beta-blocking effects occur soon after administration, but maximal class III effects, and prolongation of the action potential and QT interval, are not achieved for weeks with long-term administration. The Ca^{++} channel-blocking effects may inhibit triggered arrhythmias by reducing afterdepolarizations. Therapeutic doses slow the sinus rate, decrease AV conduction velocity, and minimally depress myocardial contractility and blood pressure. Indications for amiodarone include refractory tachyarrhythmias of both atrial and ventricular origin, especially reentrant arrhythmias using an accessory pathway. IV amiodarone has been used in people with AT, VT, and during cardiopulmonary resuscitation from recurrent VT and fibrillation. Amiodarone is effective without causing increased mortality in people, unlike several other antiarrhythmic agents[113].

Veterinary experience with amiodarone is growing, although still limited. The drug has been used PO more often than IV. Experimentally, boluses of 3–5 mg/kg IV suppressed ventricular arrhythmias

of various causes in dogs[85]; however, IV use can cause hypotension and bradycardia. Conservative dosing with slow injection over 10–20 minutes is recommended. The drug is also given by CRI in people; 10–15 mg/kg/day has been used in children[114]. Human CRI dosage schedules account for the known adsorption of amiodarone to polyvinyl chloride; the drug can also leach out plasticizers from IV tubing. Veterinary CRI recommendations have not been established. Amiodarone's pharmacokinetics are complex, with a delayed onset of action, prolonged time to steady state, concentration in myocardial and other tissues (especially fat), and accumulation of an active metabolite (desethylamiodarone) with long-term PO use. The drug is metabolized in the liver. The half-life in dogs after a single PO dose is about 7.5 hours, but increases to 3.2 days with long-term use. Therapeutic serum concentration is thought to be 1–2.5 mcg/ml. Amiodarone can be compounded into an oral suspension for easier dosing.

Amiodarone has uniform effects on repolarization throughout the ventricles. Experimentally in dogs, long-term amiodarone treatment moderately prolongs action potential duration and QT interval without affecting dispersion of repolarization, protects from TdP in dogs with long QT intervals, and suppresses Purkinje fiber automaticity[115–117]. The long-term electrophysiologic effects of amiodarone are somewhat different from its acute effects[118]. PO loading doses (25 mg/kg q12h) of amiodarone in normal dogs lowered HR and prolonged PR and QT intervals, but maintenance doses (of 30 mg/kg/day) caused no ECG or echo changes of significance in normal dogs[119]. Steady state was reached only after 11 weeks of treatment[119]. Adverse effects may increase at this dose; lower doses are generally used clinically[22]. IV amiodarone administered to normal dogs did not decrease myocardial contractility (dP/dtmax) until cumulative doses of 12.5 and 15 mg/kg were reached (given in 2.5 mg/kg increments q15min)[120]. However, the potential for more profound cardiac depression and hypotension with IV amiodarone is of concern in dogs with myocardial disease[120, 121]. Amiodarone use is not described in cats.

Many potential side-effects occur with long-term use, including depressed appetite, GI upset, pneumonitis leading to pulmonary fibrosis, hepatopathy, thyroid dysfunction, positive Coombs test, thrombocytopenia, and neutropenia[122–124]. Some of these resolve with drug discontinuation or dosage reduction. There are anecdotal reports in dogs of occasional hypersensitivity reactions, with acute angioedema formation, or of tremors. Other adverse effects noted with long-term use in people include corneal microdeposits, photosensitivity, bluish skin discoloration, and peripheral neuropathy; however, amiodarone may have a lesser proarrhythmic effect than other agents and reduce the risk of sudden death[22, 120, 125]. Amiodarone can increase serum concentrations of digoxin, diltiazem, and, possibly, procainamide and quinidine[126].

Bretylium tosylate

Bretylium tosylate prolongs action potential duration and effective refractory period in ventricular muscle and Purkinje fibers, and also increases the VF threshold. Bretylium initially causes norepinephrine release from sympathetic nerve terminals, before inhibiting its further release. Concurrently, the drug transiently increases then decreases sinus rate, AV conduction velocity, vascular resistance, and arterial blood pressure. Bretylium is eliminated through the kidneys; renal disease reduces drug clearance. Bretylium's half-life in dogs is about 10.4 hours. Extremely poor oral absorption limits its use to the IM or IV routes. Tissue concentrations rise slowly to peak in 1.5–6 hours after administration and are more closely related to the antifibrillatory effects of the drug than plasma concentrations. Bretylium is not often used. It is potentially indicated for life-threatening ventricular arrhythmias that are nonresponsive to other therapy or for animals at risk for VF, although its antifibrillatory effects may be delayed 4–6 hours after administration. Adverse effects of bretylium after rapid IV injection include ataxia, nausea, and vomiting. Aggravation of arrhythmias and tachycardia (early) can occur. It is contraindicated with extreme bradycardia or hypotension.

Other Class III agents

Ibutilide fumarate is used for converting recent onset AF in people, but there is little veterinary experience with it. Ibutilide has caused TdP in dogs with experimental cardiomyopathy[79]. **Dofetilide** is another drug that selectively blocks the rapid component of the repolarizing K^+ current. It also is used in people to convert AF and maintain sinus rhythm. Efficacy for this appears comparable to other Class III drugs; it does not exacerbate left ventricular dysfunction.

CLASS IV ANTIARRHYTHMIC DRUGS: CALCIUM CHANNEL–BLOCKERS

This diverse group of drugs reduces cellular Ca^{++} influx by blocking transmembrane L-type Ca^{++} channels[127]. Calcium channel-blockers as a group can cause coronary and systemic vasodilation, as well as diminished myocardial contractility with enhanced relaxation, but various agents differ in these effects. Some calcium channel-blockers (i.e. the nondihydropyridines: diltiazem and verapamil) have antiarrhythmic effects, especially on tissues dependent on the slow inward Ca^{++} current, particularly the sinus and AV nodes. They slow the sinus rate, increase AV nodal refractory period, and can interrupt some arrhythmias caused by abnormal automaticity, triggered mechanisms, and reentry. These agents are most effective against SVTs, although they might suppress ventricular arrhythmias dependent on abnormal Ca^{++} fluxes. Calcium channel-blockers are also used to manage HCM, myocardial ischemia, and hypertension.

Low initial doses are used and increased as needed to effect or to maximal recommended dose. Side-effects of these agents can include reduced contractility, vasodilation, hypotension, depression, anorexia, lethargy, bradycardia, and AV block. Contraindications to calcium channel-blocker use include sinus bradycardia, AV block, SSS, digoxin toxicity, and myocardial failure (for agents with pronounced negative inotropic effect). They are usually not prescribed with a beta-blocker, but if so, only with caution. An overdose or exaggerated response to a calcium channel-blocker is treated with supportive care; atropine (*Table 48*, p. 200) for bradycardia or AV blocks; dopamine or dobutamine (see *Table 43*, p. 171) and furosemide (see *Table 44*, p. 174) for heart failure; and dopamine or IV calcium salts for hypotension.

Diltiazem

Diltiazem HCl is a benzothiazepine calcium channel-blocker that slows AV conduction and causes potent coronary and mild peripheral vasodilation. It is usually preferred over verapamil because it has less negative inotropic effect and does not interfere with digoxin elimination[4, 12, 127]. Diltiazem is indicated for supraventricular tachyarrhythmias. Its channel-blocking effect in the AV node is greater at faster rates (use-dependence)[68]. Diltiazem can be used as a CRI after IV bolus injection[12]. It is often combined with digoxin to further slow the ventricular response rate to AF in dogs. Diltiazem is the calcium channel-blocker recommended in cats with HCM (see Chapter 21, p. 300).

Diltiazem's bioavailability is only about 43% in dogs because of extensive first-pass effect[127]. Effects peak within 2 hours after PO dosing and last at least 6 hours in dogs. The half-life in dogs is just over 2 hours, but is longer with long-term PO use because of its enterohepatic circulation. The half-life in cats is about 2–3 hours; plasma concentrations peak within 30–90 minutes and effects last for 8 hours[128, 129]. The therapeutic range is 50–300 mg/ml. Bioavailability of conventional diltiazem is greater in cats than in dogs. Diltiazem is metabolized in the liver; active metabolites exist. Drugs that inhibit hepatic enzyme systems (e.g. cimetidine) reduce diltiazem's metabolism. A sustained-release preparation (Cardizem CD capsules) (10 mg/kg daily in cats) produces plasma concentrations that peak in 6 hours and remain in the therapeutic range for 24 hours[129]. A dose of 45 mg/cat is about 105 mg of Cardizem CD, or the amount that fits into the small end of a No. 4 gelatin capsule. Diltiazem XR is another sustained-release preparation. The 240 mg capsules contain four tablets of 60 mg each. However, much variability in pharmacokinetics exists among individual cats; higher doses are more likely to be associated with anorexia and other GI signs[130].

Adverse effects are uncommon at therapeutic doses, but anorexia, nausea, bradycardia, and, rarely, other GI, cardiac, or neurologic effects may occur. Cats sporadically develop liver enzyme elevation with anorexia. Anecdotally, some cats become aggressive or show other personality change when treated with diltiazem. Sustained-release diltiazem may have less efficacy in preventing sinus tachycardia compared with atenolol. Adverse effects may also be more frequent, including anorexia, vomiting, lethargy, and evidence of hepatopathy in cats[6].

Verapamil

Verapamil HCl, a phenylalkylamine, has the most potent cardiac effects of the clinically used calcium channel-blockers. It causes dose-related slowing of the sinus rate and AV conduction. The drug prolongs nodal tissue refractoriness and thus is effective in abolishing reentrant SVT and slowing the ventricular response rate to AF. Verapamil's half-life in dogs is about 2.5 hours. It is poorly absorbed and undergoes first-pass hepatic metabolism, resulting in low PO bioavailability. The pharmacokinetics in cats are similar to dogs.

Verapamil has important negative inotropic and some vasodilatory effects that can precipitate hypotension, heart failure, and even death in animals with underlying myocardial disease. Verapamil is avoided in animals with heart failure. For SVTs in animals without heart failure, a low initial dose is given slowly IV. This can be repeated at 5(or more)–minute intervals if no adverse effects have occurred and the arrhythmia persists. Blood pressure should be monitored. The drug is contraindicated with CHF, SSS, AV conduction disturbance, and digitalis toxicity. The concurrent use of verapamil and a beta-blocker can cause a sudden decrease in sinus rate or complete AV block. Toxic effects of verapamil include sinus bradycardia, AV block, hypotension, reduced myocardial contractility, and cardiogenic shock. The negative inotropic effects of verapamil may be reversed with IV calcium salts, sympathomimetic drugs, or amrinone (see *Table 43*, p. 171). Atropine may mitigate bradycardia or AV block precipitated by verapamil. Verapamil reduces the renal clearance of digoxin.

Other calcium channel-blockers

Other calcium channel-blockers are available. Most (i.e. the dihydropyridines) are used as antihypertensives. **Amlodipine** besylate is recommended as the first line antihypertensive agent in cats and it is also used in some hypertensive dogs (see Chapter 25 p. 379). It is also used for chronic refractory heart failure in dogs (see Chapter 16, p. 182).

ANTICHOLINERGIC DRUGS

Atropine sulfate and **glycopyrrolate** are anticholinergic agents. They increase sinus rate and AV conduction when excessive vagal tone is present. Parenteral atropine or glycopyrrolate is indicated for bradycardia or AV block induced by anesthesia, CNS lesions, and certain other diseases or toxicities. Atropine is a competitive muscarinic receptor antagonist that is used to determine underlying vagal influence in animals with AV block or sinus bradycardia/arrest (see p. 210). Atropine's effect peaks within 5 minutes after IV administration. It is metabolized in the liver and excreted in the urine. Parenteral atropine can transiently exacerbate vagally-mediated AV block when the atrial rate increases faster than AV conduction can respond. IV administration (0.02 mg/kg) causes the fastest and most consistent onset and resolution of the exacerbated block, as well as the most rapid postbradycardia HRs, compared with the IM and SC routes. Experimental evaluation of HR variability after different atropine doses indicated that 0.04 mg/kg completely abolished parasympathetic tone, but 0.02 mg/kg did not[94]. In animals with organic AV nodal disease, AV block may remain unchanged or worsen after anticholinergic injection. Glycopyrrolate has longer duration of action than atropine, without centrally-mediated effects.

Bradyarrhythmias responsive to parenteral atropine or glycopyrrolate sometimes also respond to oral anticholinergic agents, at least for a time; however, animals with persistent bradyarrhythmias usually require permanent pacemaker implantation to effectively control HR and clinical signs. **Propantheline bromide** and **hyoscyamine sulfate** are used commonly, but other oral anticholinergic agents are also available. PO absorption of propantheline is variable; individual dosage is adjusted to effect. Food may decrease the drug's absorption. Vagolytic drugs may aggravate paroxysmal supraventricular tachyarrhythmias (as in SSS). Other adverse effects of anticholinergic therapy include vomiting, dry mouth, constipation, keratoconjunctivitis sicca, increased intraocular pressure, and drying of respiratory secretions.

SYMPATHOMIMETIC DRUGS

Isoproterenol

Isoproterenol HCl is a beta-receptor agonist that has been used to treat TdP as well as symptomatic AV block and bradycardia refractory to atropine, although artificial pacing is safer and more effective. Because of its affinity for $beta_2$-receptors, it can cause hypotension and it is not used for treating either heart failure or cardiac arrest. Isoproterenol can be arrhythmogenic, like other catecholamines. The lowest effective dose is used and the animal monitored closely for arrhythmias. Administration PO is not effective because of marked first-pass hepatic metabolism.

Terbutaline

PO terbutaline sulfate, a $beta_2$-receptor agonist, may have a mild stimulatory effect on HR.

Methylxanthine bronchodilators

The methylxanthine bronchodilators aminophylline and theophylline can increase HR in some dogs with SSS when used at higher doses.

OTHER DRUGS

Edrophonium

Edrophonium chloride is a short-acting anti-cholinesterase with nicotinic and muscarinic effects. The drug is used primarily for diagnosing myasthenia gravis, but its effect of slowing AV conduction can help diagnose and terminate some cases of acute SVT. Edrophonium's effect begins within 1 minute and lasts up to 10 minutes after IV injection. Adverse effects are primarily cholinergic and include GI (vomiting, diarrhea, salivation), respiratory (bronchospasm, respiratory paralysis, edema), cardiovascular (bradycardia, hypotension, cardiac arrest), and muscular (twitching, weakness) signs. Atropine and supportive care are used if necessary.

Phenylephrine

Phenylephrine HCl is an alpha-adrenergic agonist that increases blood pressure by causing peripheral vasoconstriction. A baroreflex-mediated increase in vagal tone slows AV conduction and is thought to underlie its effects on SVT. Phenylephrine's pressor effect begins rapidly after IV injection and persists for up to 20 minutes. The drug is contraindicated in patients with hypertension or VT. Extravasation can cause ischemic necrosis of surrounding tissue.

Adenosine

Adenosine is an endogenous purine nucleoside that briefly opens K^+ channels and indirectly slows Ca^{++} current, with greatest effect on SA and AV nodes. By transiently depressing AV node activity it can terminate reentrant SVTs in people, but the drug has been largely ineffective for this in dogs. Adenosine must be administered rapidly IV, preferably into a central vein. It is degraded within seconds by enzyme systems in the vascular endothelium and blood cells. Doses of 6–12 mg are used in people, but body weight-adjusted doses over twice this have been unsuccessful in dogs[4].

OVERVIEW OF PACING THERAPY

Permanent artificial pacing therapy is indicated for bradyarrhythmias (such as SSS, AV block, and atrial standstill) that are unresponsive to medical management[131–137]. Pacemaker implantation is performed at many larger veterinary centers. Factors that limit the use of this therapy include the availability of pulse generators and pacing leads, the expense involved with the procedure, and advanced age or concurrent disease in some patients. Pacemakers obtained for veterinary use are human devices that either have an expired shelf-life or have been previously used and explanted.

A thorough workup is indicated before pacemaker implantation. Some underlying conditions (e.g. myocardial dysfunction, endocarditis) are associated with a poor prognosis, even after pacing. Temporary transvenous pacing is sometimes used for 1–2 days to assess the animal's response to a normal HR before permanent pacemaker surgery is performed. Animals with CHF complicated by bradyarrhythmia can improve with pacing, although their prognosis is less favorable (60% 1 year mortality) than those animals without heart failure (25% 1 year mortality)[131]. Some animals do well for several years with artificial pacing.

The transvenous approach is currently used most commonly (236, 237)[131–133, 137]. Both unipolar and bipolar lead wires are available; the pulse generator used must be compatible with the lead type. Before implantation it is important to verify the pulse generator's programmed parameters, battery status, and its compatibility with the available lead. The pacing lead must be consistent with the approach planned (transvenous or epicardial) as well as be of adequate length for the animal's size. Transvenous pacemaker implantation usually involves inserting the lead wire through the right jugular vein, fixing the electrode tip in the endocardium of the RV apex, and placing the pulse generator subcutaneously in the dorsolateral cervical region; however, other methods may be better in individual cases. Placement of an epicardial electrode via the transdiaphragmatic approach may be necessary occasionally[138–140]. The epicardial approach is probably better for cats requiring artificial pacing. Cats implanted with a transvenous pacing electrode often subsequently develop chylothorax[6, 96]. Prolonged survival without artificial pacing is possible in cats with 3rd degree AV block[97]. A temporary transvenous pacing lead is generally inserted (or at least must be immediately available) prior to permanent lead placement and fixation[132]. An alternative, where available, is transthoracic temporary pacing[141]. There are several reports detailing pacing methods, outcomes, and complications in animals[131–145]. These should be consulted for additional information, especially by clinicians planning to implant a pacemaker.

Identification of pacemaker functional mode is provided by a three (or more) letter code[133, 147]. The first letter refers to the chamber that is paced and the second to the chamber where endogenous electrical activity is sensed. The third letter describes the response to sensed activity (Table 50). The VVI mode has been used most often in animals, although the DDD mode is preferred in people. Current pacemakers have multiple programmable features, including rate responsiveness to patient activity.

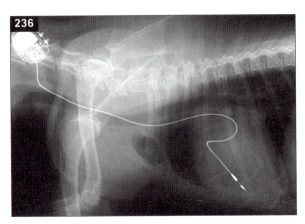

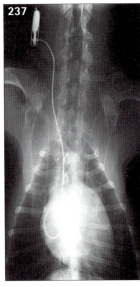

236, 237 Lateral (236) and DV (237) radiographs from a 6-year-old female Labrador Retriever with 3rd degree AV block after implantation of a permanent transvenous pacemaker.

Table 50 Pacemaker nomenclature.

NBG* Code			
I	II	III	IV
Chamber paced	Chamber sensed	Response to sensing	Programmability, rate modulation
0 = none	0 = none	0 = none	0 = none
A = atrium	A = atrium	T = triggered	P = simple programmable
V = ventricle	V = ventricle	I = inhibited	M = multiprogrammable
D = dual (A and V)	D = dual (A and V)	D = dual (T and I)	R = rate modulation

* The North American Society of Pacing and Electrophysiology and the British Pacing and Electrophysiology Group.[147]

Single chamber (ventricular) pacing has been employed almost exclusively in dogs and cats. Dual chamber (atrial and ventricular) pacing may be an option for some cases, but dual lead systems are more challenging to implant and program. Nevertheless, dual chamber pacing provides the hemodynamic benefit of synchronized atrial then ventricular contraction. Newer single lead systems that allow both atrial sensing and sequential ventricular (VDD) pacing may make physiologic pacing more practical for animals with AV block, although not yet for those with sinus node dysfunction[148, 149]. Single chamber ventricular pacing is also associated with dyssynchronous RV and LV activation. Although this is not a clinical issue for most paced animals, it could contribute to the development or progression of ventricular dysfunction. Experimental biventricular pacing improves LV performance[150]. The potential role for biventricular pacing (cardiac re-synchronization therapy) in animals with myocardial failure is not known. It is a beneficial strategy in people.

Complications associated with pacing therapy are common[131–136, 139, 145]. The major complications of lead malfunction, lead dislodgement, generator failure (or battery depletion), and cardiac arrest are more prevalent[131]. Lead dislodgement appears to be particularly common in large breed dogs[144]. Major complications can also include infection, associated with either the lead wire or pulse generator, RV perforation, VT, profound bradycardia, chylothorax, and others[96, 131, 144–146]. Minor complications include seroma formation at the generator site, muscle twitch, minor ventricular or atrial arrhythmias, and mild hemorrhage, among others[131, 133, 139].

The potential role of pacing therapy to interrupt tachyarrhythmias or provide defibrillation shocks with ICD devices is currently undefined. Aside from device availability and advanced programming requirements and other technical issues, there is a propensity for T-wave (as well as R-wave) oversensing. This causes inaccurate rhythm assessment by the device and can trigger inappropriate (and painful) defibrillation shocks to the animal.

REFERENCES

1 Knight DH (2000) Reason must supersede dogma in the management of ventricular arrhythmias. In: *Kirk's Current Veterinary Therapy XIII*. JD Bonagura (ed). WB Saunders, Philadelphia, pp. 730–733.

2 Myerburg RJ, Mitrani R, Interian A Jr *et al.* (1998) Interpretation of outcomes of antiarrhythmic clinical trials. *Circulation* 97:1514–1521.

3 Marinchak RA, Rials SJ, Filart RA *et al.* (1997) Top ten fallacies of nonsustained ventricular tachycardia. *Pacing Clin Electrophysiol* 20:2825–2847.

4 Wright KN (2000) Assessment and treatment of supraventricular tachyarrhythmias. In: *Kirk's Current Veterinary Therapy XIII*. JD Bonagura (ed). WB Saunders, Philadelphia, pp. 726–729.

5 Wright KN, Mehdirad AA, Giacobbe P *et al.* (1999) Radiofrequency catheter ablation of atrioventricular accessory pathways in 3 dogs with subsequent resolution of tachycardia-induced cardiomyopathy. *J Vet Intern Med* 13:361–371.

6 Cote E, Ettinger SJ (2005) Electrocardiography and cardiac arrhythmias. In: *Textbook of Veterinary Internal Medicine*, 6th edn. SJ Ettinger, EC Feldman (eds). Elsevier Saunders, St Louis, pp. 1040–1076.

7 Ware WA (1999) Twenty-four-hour ambulatory electrocardiography in normal cats. *J Vet Intern Med* 13:175–180.

8 Rishniw M, Bruskiewicz K (1996) ECG of the month. Respiratory sinus arrhythmia and wandering pacemaker in a cat. *J Am Vet Med Assoc* 208:1811–1812.

9 Akar FG, Spragg DD, Tunin RS *et al.* (2004) Mechanisms underlying conduction slowing and arrhythmogenesis in nonischemic dilated cardiomyopathy. *Circ Res* 95:717–725.

10 Dangman KH (1999) Electrophysiologic mechanisms for arrhythmias. In: *Textbook of Canine and Feline Cardiology*, 2nd edn. PR Fox, D Sisson, NS Moise (eds). WB Saunders, Philadelphia, pp. 291–305.

11 Katra RP, Laurita KR (2005) Cellular mechanism of calcium-mediated triggered activity in the heart. *Circ Res* 96:535–542.

12 Moise NS (1999) Diagnosis and management of canine arrhythmias. In: *Textbook of Canine and Feline Cardiology*, 2nd edn. PR Fox, D Sisson, NS Moise (eds). WB Saunders, Philadelphia, pp. 331–385.

13 Coumel P, Leenhardt A (1991) Mental activity, adrenergic modulation, and cardiac arrhythmias in patients with heart disease. *Circulation* 83(suppl II): II58–II70.

14 Schwartz PJ, Priori SG (2000) Autonomic modulation of cardiac arrhythmias. In: *Cardiac Electrophysiology: From Cell To Bedside*, 3rd edn. DP Zipes, J Jalife (eds). WB Saunders, Philadelphia, pp. 300–314.

15 Kovach JA, Nearing BD, Verrier RL (2001) Anger-like behavioral state potentiates myocardial ischemia-induced T-wave alternans in canines. *J Am Coll Cardiol* 37:1719–1725.

16 Pinson DM (1997) Myocardial necrosis and sudden death after an episode of aggressive behavior in a dog. *J Am Vet Med Assoc* 211:1371–1372.

17 Steinberg SF, Robinson RB, Rosen MR (2000) Molecular and cellular

bases of β-adrenergic modulation of cardiac rhythm. In: *Cardiac Electrophysiology: From Cell To Bedside*, 3rd edn. DP Zipes, J Jalife (eds). WB Saunders, Philadelphia, pp. 283–294.

18 Tatewaki T, Inagaki M, Kawada T *et al.* (2003) Biphasic response of action potential duration to sudden sympathetic stimulation in anesthetized cats. *Circ J* **67**:876–880.

19 Zupen I, Rakovec P, Budihna N *et al.* (1996) Tachycardia-induced cardiomyopathy in dogs: relation between chronic supraventricular and chronic ventricular tachycardia. *Int J Cardiol* **56**:75–81.

20 Hall LW, Dunn JK, Delaney M *et al.* (1991) Ambulatory electrocardiography in dogs. *Vet Rec* **129**:213–216.

21 Ulloa HM, Houston BJ, Altrogge DM (1995) Arrhythmia prevalence during ambulatory electrocardiographic monitoring of Beagles. *Am J Vet Res* **56**:275–281.

22 Calvert CA, Meurs KM (2000) CVT update: Doberman Pinscher occult cardiomyopathy. In: *Kirk's Current Veterinary Therapy XIII*. JD Bonagura (ed). WB Saunders, Philadelphia, pp. 756–760.

23 Moise NS (2000) CVT Update: ventricular arrhythmias. In: *Kirk's Current Veterinary Therapy XIII*. JD Bonagura (ed). WB Saunders, Philadelphia, pp. 733–737.

24 Calvert CA, Hall G, Jacobs G *et al.* (1997) Clinical and pathological findings in Doberman Pinschers with occult cardiomyopathy that died suddenly or developed congestive heart failure: 54 cases (1984–1991). *J Am Vet Med Assoc* **210**:505–511.

25 Harpster NK (1983) Boxer cardiomyopathy. In: *Current Veterinary Therapy VIII*. RW Kirk RW (ed). WB Saunders, Philadelphia, pp. 329–337.

26 Meurs KM (2003) Familial arrhythmic cardiomyopathy of Boxers (ARVC). In: *Proceedings of the 21st Annual ACVIM Forum*, Charlotte.

27 Spier AW, Meurs KM (2004) Use of signal-averaged electrocardiography in the evaluation of arrhythmogenic right ventricular cardiomyopathy in Boxers. *J Am Vet Med Assoc* **225**:1050–1055.

28 Calvert CA, Jacobs GJ, Kraus M (1998) Possible ventricular late potentials in Doberman Pinschers with occult cardiomyopathy. *J Am Vet Med Assoc* **213**:235–239.

29 Wellens HJJ (2004) Cardiac arrhythmias: the quest for a cure. *J Am Coll Cardiol* **44**:1155–1163.

30 Pinski SL, Yoa Q, Epstein AE *et al.* (2000) Determinants of outcome in patients with sustained ventricular tachyarrhythmias: the antiarrhythmics versus implantable defibrillators (AVID) study registry. *Am Heart J* **139**:804–813.

31 Moise NS, Gilmour RF, Riccio ML *et al.* (1997) Diagnosis of inherited ventricular tachycardia in German shepherd dogs. *J Am Vet Med Assoc* **210**:403–410.

32 Merot J, Probst V, Debailleul M *et al.* (2000) Electropharmacological characterization of cardiac repolarization in German shepherd dogs with an inherited syndrome of sudden death: abnormal response to potassium channel blockers. *J Am Coll Cardiol* **36**:939–947.

33 Moise NS, Riccio ML, Flahive WJ *et al.* (1997) Age dependence of the development of ventricular arrhythmias in a canine model of sudden cardiac death. *Cardiovasc Res* **34**:483–492.

34 Dae MW, Lee RJ, Ursell PC *et al.* (1997) Heterogeneous sympathetic innervation in German shepherd dogs with inherited ventricular arrhythmias and sudden death. *Circulation* **96**:1337–1342.

35 Raeder EA, Hohnloser SH, Graboys TB *et al.* (1988) Spontaneous variability and circadian distribution of ectopic activity in patients with malignant ventricular arrhythmia. *J Am Coll Cardiol* **12**:656–661.

36 Linseman JV, Bristow MR (2003) Drug therapy and heart failure prevention. *Circulation* **107**:1234–1236.

37 Leaf A, Kang JX, Xioa YF *et al.* (1999) The antiarrhythmic and anticonvulsant effects of dietary N-3 fatty acids. *J Membr Biol* **172**:1–11.

38 Ehrlich JR, Hohnloser SH, Nattel S (2006) Role of angiotensin system and effects of its inhibition in atrial fibrillation: clinical and experimental evidence. *Eur Heart J* **25**(5):512–518.

39 Wright KN (2004) Interventional catheterization for tachyarrhythmias. *Vet Clin North Am: Small Anim Pract* **34**:1171–1185.

40 Muir WW, Sams RA, Moise NS (1999) Pharmacology and pharmacokinetics of antiarrhythmic drugs. In: *Textbook of Canine and Feline Cardiology*. 2nd edn. PR Fox, D Sisson, NS Moise (eds). WB Saunders, Philadelphia, pp. 307–330.

41 Khanna C, Lund EM, Raffe M *et al.* (1998) Hypomagnesemia in 188 dogs: a hospital population-based prevalence study. *J Vet Intern Med* **12**:304–309.

42 Nakayama T, Nakayama H, Miyamoto M *et al.* (1999) Hemodynamic and electrocardiographi effects of magnesium sulfate in healthy dogs. *J Vet Intern Med* **13**:485–490.

43 Zipes DP (1997) Management of specific arrhythmias: pharmacological, electrical, and surgical techniques. In: *Heart Disease*, 5th edn. E Braunwald (ed). WB Saunders, Philadelphia, pp. 593–639.

44 Sicilian Gambit members (2001) New approaches to antiarrhythmic therapy: Part I. *Circulation* **104**:2865–2873.

45 Sicilian Gambit members (2001) New approaches to antiarrhythmic therapy: Part II. *Circulation* **104**:2990–2994.

46 Lee KW, Lip GY (2003) The role of omega-3 fatty acids in the secondary prevention of cardiovascular disease. *Quarterly J Med* **96**:465–480.

47 Shiroshita-Takeshita A, Schram G, Lavoie J *et al.* (2004) Effect of simvastatin and antioxidant vitamins on atrial fibrillation promotion by atrial-tachycardia remodeling in dogs. *Circulation* **110**:2313–2319.

48 Ganz LI, Friedman PL (1995) Supraventricular tachycardia. *N Engl J Med* **332**:162–173.

49 Stafford Johnson M, Martin M, Smith P (2006) Cardioversion of supraventricular tachycardia using lidocaine in five dogs. *J Vet Intern Med* **20**:272–276.

50 Sarter BH, Marchlinski FE (1992) Redefining the role of digoxin in the treatment of atrial fibrillation. *Am J Cardiol* **69**:71G–78G.

51 Atkins CE, Kanter R, Wright K *et al.* (1995) Orthodromic reciprocating tachycardia and heart failure in a dog with a concealed posteroseptal accessory pathway. *J Vet Intern Med* **9**:43–49.

52 American Heart Association Guidelines (2005) Management of symptomatic bradycardia and tachycardia. *Circulation* **112**:IV67–IV77.

53 Santilli RA, Bussadori C (2000) Orthodromic incessant reciprocating atrioventricular tachycardia in a dog. *J Vet Cardiol* **2**:23–27.

54 Bonagura JD, Ware WA (1986) Atrial fibrillation in the dog: clinical findings in 81 cases. *J Am Anim Hosp Assoc* **22**:110–120.

55 Brownlie SE (1991) An electrocardiographic survey of cardiac rhythm in Irish Wolfhounds. *Vet Rec* **129**:470–471.

56 Gelzer ARM, Kraus MS (2004) Management of atrial fibrillation. *Vet Clin North Am: Small Anim Pract* **34**:1127–1144.

57 Patterson DF, Detweiler DK, Hubben K *et al.* (1961) Spontaneous abnormal cardiac arrhythmias and conduction disturbances in the dog: a clinical and pathologic study of 3,000 dogs. *Am J Vet Res* **22**:355–369.

58 Cote E, Harpster NK, Laste NJ *et al.* (2004) Atrial fibrillation in cats: 50 cases (1979–2002). *J Am Vet Med Assoc* **225**:256–260.

59 Brundel BJJM, Melnyk P, Rivard L *et al.* (2005) The pathology of atrial fibrillation in dogs. *J Vet Cardiol* **7**:121–129.

60 Buchanan JW (1965) Spontaneous arrhythmias and conduction disturbances in domestic animals. *Ann NY Acad Sci* **127(I)**:224–238.

61 Menaut P, Belanger MC, Beauchamp G *et al.* (2005) Atrial fibrillation in dogs with and without structural or functional cardiac disease: a retrospective study of 109 cases. *J Vet Cardiol* **7**:75–83.

62 Vollmar AC (2000) The prevalence of cardiomyopathy in the Irish Wolfhound: a clinical study of 500 dogs. *J Am Anim Hosp Assoc* **36**:125–132.

63 Brownlie SE, Cobb MA (1999) Observations on the development of congestive heart failure in Irish Wolfhounds with dilated cardiomyopathy. *J Small Anim Pract* **40**:371–377.

64 Bolton GR, Ettinger SJ (1971) Paroxysmal atrial fibrillation in the dog. *J Am Vet Med Assoc* **158**:64–76.

65 Wyse DG *et al.* for the AFFIRM investigators (2002) A comparison of rate control and rhythm control in patients with atrial fibrillation. *New Engl J Med* **347**:1825–1833.

66 Saxonhouse SJ, Curtis AB (2003) Risks and benefits of rate control versus maintenance of sinus rhythm. *Am J Cardiol* **91(6A)**:27D–32D.

67 Hamlin RL (1995) What is the best heart rate for a dog in atrial fibrillation? In: *Proceedings of the 13th Annual ACVIM Forum*, Lake Buena Vista, pp. 325–326.

68 Miyamoto M, Nishijima Y, Nakayama T *et al.* (2000) Cardiovascular effects of intravenous diltiazem in dogs with iatrogenic atrial fibrillation. *J Vet Intern Med* **14**:445–451.

69 Miyamoto M, Nishijima Y, Nakayama T *et al.* (2001) Acute cardiovascular effects of diltiazem in anesthetized dogs with induced atrial fibrillation. *J Vet Intern Med* **15**:559–563.

70 Glaus TM, Hassig M, Keene BW (2003) Accuracy of heart rate obtained by auscultation in atrial fibrillation. *J Am Anim Hosp Assoc* **39**:237–239.

71 Boriani G, Biffi M, Branzi A *et al.* (1998) Pharmacological treatment of atrial fibrillation: a review on prevention of recurrences and control of ventricular response. *Arch Gerontol Geriatr* **27**:127–139.

72 Hamann SR, McAllister RG Jr (1994) Cardiodepressant actions of combined diltiazem and propranolol in dogs. *J Cardiovasc Pharmacol* **23**:31–36.

73 Sharifov OF, Fedorov VV, Beloshapko GG *et al.* (2004) Roles of adrenergic and cholinergic stimulation in spontaneous atrial fibrillation in dogs. *J Am Coll Cardiol* **43**:483–490.

74 Darbar D, Herron KJ, Ballew JD *et al.* (2003) Familial atrial fibrillation is a genetically heterogenous disorder. *J Am Coll Cardiol* **41**:2185–2192.

75 Guglielmini C, Chetboul V, Pietra M *et al.* (2000) Influence of left atrial enlargement and body weight on the development of atrial fibrillation: retrospective study on 205 dogs. *Vet J* **160**:235–241.

76 Kittleson MD (1998) Diagnosis and treatment of arrhythmias (dysrhythmias). In: *Small Animal Cardiovascular Medicine*. MD Kittleson, RD Kienle (eds). Mosby, St. Louis, pp. 449–494.

77 Volgman AS, Carberry PA, Stambler B *et al.* (1998) Conversion efficacy and safety of intravenous ibutilide compared with intravenous procainamide in patients with atrial flutter or fibrillation. *J Am Coll Cardiol* **31**:1414–1419.

78 Stambler BS, Wood MA, Ellenbogen KA *et al.* (1996) Efficacy and safety of repeated intravenous doses of ibutilide for rapid conversion of atrial flutter or fibrillation. *Circulation* **94**:1613–1621.

79 Hsieh MH, Chen YJ, Lee SH *et al.* (2000) Proarrhythmic effects of ibutilide in a canine model of pacing induced cardiomyopathy. *Pacing Clin Electrophysiol* **23**:149–156.

80 McNamara RL, Tamariz LJ, Segal JB *et al.* (2003) Management of atrial fibrillation: review of the evidence for the role of pharmacologic therapy, electrical cardioversion, and echocardiography. *Ann Intern Med* **139**:1018–1033.

81 Moise NS, Pariaut R, Gelzer ARM *et al.* (2005) Cardioversion with lidocaine of vagally associated atrial

fibrillation in two dogs. *J Vet Cardiol* 7:143–148.

82 Bright JM, Martin JM, Mama K (2005) A retrospective evaluation of transthoracic biphasic electrical cardioversion for atrial fibrillation in dogs. *J Vet Cardiol* 7:85–96.

83 Meurs KM, Spier AW, Wright NA *et al.* (2001) Use of ambulatory electrocardiography for detection of ventricular premature complexes in healthy dogs. *J Am Vet Med Assoc* 218:1291–1292.

84 de Madron E, Quagliariello RM (1991) Ventricular parasystole in a dog and a cat. *J Am Vet Med Assoc* 198:286–290.

85 Awaji T, Wu ZJ, Hashimoto K (1995) Acute antiarrhythmic effects of intravenously administered amiodarone on canine ventricular arrhythmias. *J Cardiovasc Pharmacol* 26:869–878.

86 Moise NS, Antzelevitch C, Shimizu W (1999) As Americans, we should get this right. Letter. *Circulation* 100:1462.

87 Baty CJ, Sweet DC, Keene BW (1994) Torsades de pointes-like polymorphic ventricular tachycardia in a dog. *J Vet Intern Med* 8: 439–442.

88 Poole JE, Bardy GH (2000) Sudden cardiac death. In: *Cardiac Electrophysiology: From Cell To Bedside*, 3rd edn. DP Zipes, J Jalife (eds). WB Saunders, Philadelphia, pp. 615–639.

89 Calvert CA, Pickus CW, Jacobs GJ (1996) Efficacy and toxicity of tocainide for the treatment of ventricular tachyarrhythmias in Doberman Pinschers with occult cardiomyopathy. *J Vet Intern Med* 10:235–240.

90 Lunney J, Ettinger SJ (1991) Mexiletine administration for management of ventricular arrhythmia in 22 dogs. *J Am Anim Hosp Assoc* 27:597–600.

91 Meurs KM, Spier AW, Wright NA *et al.* (2002) Comparison of the effects of four antiarrhythmic treatments for familial ventricular arrhythmias in Boxers. *J Am Vet Med Assoc* 221:522–527.

92 Calvert CA, Brown J (2004) Influence of antiarrhythmia therapy on survival times of 19 clinically healthy Doberman Pinschers with dilated cardiomyopathy that experienced syncope, ventricular tachycardia, and sudden death (1985–1998). *J Am Anim Hosp Assoc* 40:24–28.

93 Rishniw M, Tobias AH, Slinker BK (1996) Characterization of chronotropic and dysrhythmogenic effects of atropine in dogs with bradycardia. *Am J Vet Res* 57:337–341.

94 Rishniw M, Kittleson MD, Jaffe RS *et al.* (1999) Characterization of parasympatholytic chronotropic responses following intravenous administration of atropine to clinically normal dogs. *Am J Vet Res* 60:1000–1003.

95 Moneva-Jordan A, Corcoran BM, French A *et al.* (2001) Sick sinus syndrome in nine West Highland White Terriers. *Vet Rec* 148:142–147.

96 Ferasin L, van de Stad M, Rudorf H *et al.* (2002) Syncope associated with paroxysmal atrioventricular block and atrial standstill in a cat. *J Small Anim Pract* 43:124–128.

97 Kellum HB, Stepien RL (2006) Third degree atrioventricular block in 21 cats (1997–2004). *J Vet Intern Med* 20:97–103.

98 Thomasy SM. Pypendop BH, Ilkiw JE *et al.* (2005) Pharmacokinetics of lidocaine and its active metabolite, monoethylglycinexylidide, after intravenous administration of lidocaine to awake and isoflurane-anesthetized cats. *Am J Vet Res* 66:1162–1166.

99 Marcus FI, Opie LH (1995) Antiarrhythnmic agents. In: *Drugs for the Heart*. LH Opie (ed.) WB Saunders, Philadelphia, p. 207

100 Bristow MR (2000) Beta-adrenergic receptor blockade in chronic heart failure. *Circulation* 101:558–569.

101 Capomolla S, Febo O, Gnemmi M *et al.* (2000) Beta-blockade therapy in chronic heart failure: diastolic function and mitral regurgitation improvement by carvedilol. *Am Heart J* 139:596–608.

102 Singh BN, Sarma JSM (2000) Beta-blockers and calcium channel blockers as antiarrhythmic drugs. In *Cardiac Electrophysiology: From Cell To Bedside*, 3rd edn. DP Zipes, J Jalife (eds). WB Saunders, Philadelphia, pp. 903–921.

103 Altschuld RA, Billman GE (2000) Beta(2)-adrenoceptors and ventricular fibrillation. *Pharmacol Ther* 88:1–14.

104 Jacobs G, Whittem T, Sams R *et al.* (1997) Pharmacokinetics of propranolol in healthy cats during euthyroid and hyperthyroid states. *Am J Vet Res* 58:398–403.

105 Quinones M, Dyer DC, Ware WA (1996) Pharmacokinetics of atenolol in clinically normal cats. *Am J Vet Res* 57:1050–1053.

106 Morita H, Suzuki G, Mishima T *et al.* (2002) Effects of long-term monotherapy with metoprolol CR/XL on the progression of left ventricular dysfunction and remodeling in dogs with chronic heart failure. *Cardiovasc Drugs Ther* 16:443–449.

107 Frishman WH (1988) β-adrenergic blockers. *Med Clin North Am* 72:37–81.

108 Nattel S (2002) Class III drugs: amiodarone, bretylium, ibutilide, and sotalol. In: *Cardiac Electrophysiology: From Cell To Bedside*, 3rd edn. DP Zipes, J Jalife (eds). WB Saunders, Philadelphia, pp. 921–932.

109 Anderson JL (1995) Sotalol, bretylium, and other class 3 antiarrhythmics. In: *Cardiac Arrhythmia: Mechanisms, Diagnosis, and Management.* PJ Podrid, PR Kowey (eds). Williams and Wilkins, Baltimore, p. 450.

110 Gomoll AW, Lekich RF, Bartek MJ *et al.* (1990) Comparability of the electrophysiologic responses and plasma and myocardial tissue concentrations of sotalol and its d stereoisomer in the dog. *J Cardiovasc Pharmacol* 16:204–211.

111 Chezalviel-Guilbert F, Davy JM, Poirier JM *et al.* (1995) Mexiletine antagonizes the effects of sotalol on

QT interval duration and its proarrhythmic effects in a canine model of torsade de pointes. *J Am Coll Cardiol* **26**:787–792.

112 Seidler RW, Mueller K, Nakayama T *et al.* (1999) Influence of sotalol on the time constant of isovolumic left ventricular relaxation in anesthetized dogs. *Am J Vet Res* **60**:717–721.

113 Cappato R (1999) Secondary prevention of sudden death: the Dutch Study, the antiarrhythmics versus implantable defibrillator trial, the Cardiac Arrest Study Hamburg, and the Canadian Implantable Defibrillator Study. *Am J Cardiol* **83**:68D–73D.

114 Perry JC, Fenrich AL, Hulse JE *et al.* (1996) Pediatric use of intravenous amiodarone: efficacy and safety in critically ill patients from a multicenter protocol. *J Am Coll Cardiol* **27**:1246–1250.

115 Merot J, Charpentier F, Poirier JM *et al.* (1999) Effects of chronic treatment by amiodarone on transmural heterogeneity of canine ventricular repolarization *in vivo*: interactions with acute sotalol. *Cardiovasc Res* **44**:303–314.

116 van Opstal JM, Schoenmakers M, Verduyn SC *et al.* (2001) Chronic amiodarone evokes no torsades de pointes arrhythmias despite QT lengthening in an animal model of acquired long-QT syndrome. *Circulation* **104**:2722–2727.

117 Bicer S, Nakayama H, Nakayama T *et al.* (2001) Effects of chronic, oral amiodarone on left ventricular pressure, electrocardiograms, and action potentials from myocardium in vivo and from Purkinje fibers *in vitro*. *Vet Ther* **2**:325–333.

118 Huang J, Skinner JL, Rogers JM *et al.* (2002) The effects of acute and chronic amiodarone on activation patterns and defibrillation threshold during ventricular fibrillation in dogs. *J Am Coll Cardiol* **40**:375–383.

119 Bicer S, Nakayama T, Hamlin RL (2002) Effects of chronic oral amiodarone on left ventricular function, ECGs, serum chemistries, and exercise tolerance in healthy dogs. *J Vet Intern Med* **16**:247–254.

120 Bicer S, Schwartz DS, Nakayama T *et al.* (2000) Hemodynamic and electrocardiographic effects of graded doses of amiodarone in healthy dogs anesthetized with morphine/alpha chloralose. *J Vet Intern Med* **14**:90–95.

121 Ware WA, Muir WW, Swanson C (1991) Effects of amiodarone on myocardial performance in normal canine hearts and canine hearts with infarcts. *Am J Vet Res* **52**:891–897.

122 Jacobs G, Calvert CA, Kraus M (2000) Hepatopathy in 4 dogs treated with amiodarone. *J Vet Intern Med* **14**:96–99.

123 Calvert CA, Sammarco C, Pickus C (2000) Positive Coombs test results in two dogs treated with amiodarone. *J Am Vet Med Assoc* **216**:1933–1936.

124 Kraus MS, Ridge LG, Gelzer ARM *et al.* (2005) Toxicity in Doberman Pinscher dogs with ventricular arrhythmias treated with amiodarone. Abstract. *J Vet Intern Med* **19**:406.

125 Sicouri S, Moro S, Litovsky S *et al.* (1997) Chronic amiodarone reduces transmural dispersion of repolarization in the canine heart. *J Cardiovasc Electrophysiol* **8**:1269–1279.

126 Mason JW (1993) A comparison of electrophysiologic testing with Holter monitoring to predict antiarrhythmic drug efficacy for ventricular tachyarrhythmias. *N Engl J Med* **329**:445–451.

127 Cooke KL, Snyder PS (1998) Calcium channel blockers in veterinary medicine. *J Vet Intern Med* **12**:123–131.

128 Chapman E, Bullock NR, Swift S (2000) Pharmacokinetics of diltiazem hydrochloride and its efficacy in the treatment of feline hypertrophic cardiomyopathy. Abstract. *J Small Anim Pract* **41**:391.

129 Johnson LM, Atkins CE, Keene BW *et al.* (1996) Pharmacokinetic and pharmacodynamic properties of conventional and CD-formulated diltiazem in cats. *J Vet Intern Med* **10**:316–320.

130 Wall M, Calvert CA, Sanderson SL *et al.* (2005) Evaluation of extended-release diltiazem once daily in cats with hypertrophic cardiomyopathy. *J Am Anim Hosp Assoc* **41**:98–103.

131 Oyama MA, Sisson DD, Lehmkuhl LB 2001) Practices and outcome of artificial cardiac pacing in 154 dogs. *J Vet Intern Med* **15**:229–239.

132 Côté E, Laste NJ (2000) Transvenous cardiac pacing. *Clin Tech Small Anim Pract* **15**:165–176, (erratum: *Clin Tech Small Anim Pract* **15**, 260).

133 Moise NS (1999) Pacemaker therapy. In *Textbook of Canine and Feline Cardiology*, 2nd edn. PR Fox, D Sisson, NS Moise (eds). WB Saunders, Philadelphia, pp. 400–426.

134 Sisson D, Thomas WP, Woodfield J *et al.* (1991) Permanent transvenous pacemaker implantation in forty dogs. *J Vet Intern Med* **5**:322–331.

135 Darke PGG, McAreavey D, Been M (1989) Transvenous cardiac pacing in 19 dogs and one cat. *J Small Anim Pract* **30**:491–499.

136 Francois L, Chetboul V, Nicolle A *et al.* (2004) Pacemaker implantation in dogs: results of the last 30 years. *Schweiz Arch Tierheilkd* **146**:335–344.

138 Fox PR, Matthiesen DT, Purse D *et al.* (1986) Ventral abdominal, transdiaphragmatic approach for implantation of cardiac pacemakers in the dog. *J Am Vet Med Assoc* **189**:1303–1308.

139 Bonagura JD, Helphrey ML, Muir WW (1983) Complications associated with permanent pacemaker implantation in the dog. *J Am Vet Med Assoc* **182**:149–155.

140 Buchanan JW (2003) The first pacemaker in a dog: a historical note. *J Vet Intern Med* **17**:713–714.

141 DeFrancesco TC, Hansen BD, Atkins CE *et al.* (2003) Noninvasive transthoracic

temporary cardiac pacing in dogs. *J Vet Intern Med* **17**:663–667.

142 Stamoulis ME, Bond BR, Fox PR (1992) Permanent pacemaker implantation for treatment of symptomatic bradycardia in two cats. *Vet Emerg Crit Care* **2**:67–72.

143 Forterre S, Nürnberg J-H, Skrodzki M *et al.* (2001) Transvenous demand pacemaker treatment for intermittent complete heart block in a cat. *J Vet Cardiol* **3**:21–26.

144 Flanders JA, Moise NS, Gelzer AR *et al.* (1999) Introduction of an endocardial pacing lead through the costocervical vein in six dogs. *J Am Vet Med Assoc* **215**:46–48.

145 Snyder PS, Atkins CE, Sato T (1991) Syncope in three dogs with cardiac pacemakers. *J Am Anim Hosp Assoc* **27**:611–616.

146 Zimmerman SA, Bright JM (2004) Secure pacemaker fixation critical for prevention of Twiddler's syndrome. *J Vet Cardiol* **6**:40–44.

147 Hayes DL, Zipes DP (2001) Cardiac pacemakers and cardioverter defibrillators. In: *Heart Disease: A Textbook of Cardiovascular Medicine*, 6th edn. E Braunwald, DP Zipes, P Libby (eds). WB Saunders, Philadelphia, pp. 775–814.

148 Bulmer BJ, Oyama MA, Lamont LA *et al.* (2002) Implantation of a single-lead atrioventricular synchronous (VDD) pacemaker in a dog with naturally occurring 3rd degree atrioventricular block. *J Vet Intern Med* **16**:197–200.

149 Bulmer BJ, Sisson DD, Oyama MA *et al.* (2006) Physiologic VDD versus nonphysiologic VVI pacing in canine 3rd degree atrioventricular block. *J Vet Intern Med* **20**:257–271.

150 Frias PA, Corvera JS, Schmarkey L *et al.* (2003) Evaluation of myocardial performance with conventional single-site ventricular pacing and biventricular pacing in a canine model of atrioventricular block. *J Cardiovasc Electrophysiol* **14**:996–1000.

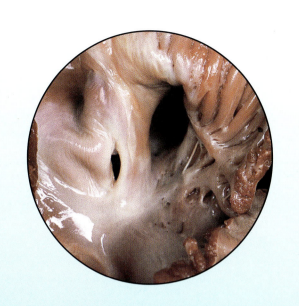

Section 3

Cardiovascular Diseases

18
Congenital Cardiovascular Diseases

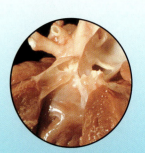

OVERVIEW

Congenital cardiac malformations most often involve either a valve (or valve region) or an abnormal communication between the systemic and pulmonary circulations; valve malformations can cause insufficiency, stenosis, or both. Other cardiac defects occur sporadically. Multiple anomalies sometimes occur in the same patient. Certain breed predispositions are recognized (*Table 51*)[1, 2]. Most congenital cardiac defects cause an audible murmur (see Chapter 6), but some do not. Murmur intensity (loudness) as well as clinical signs commonly relate to the defect's severity, although other factors can modify this. Some serious anomalies have no associated murmur. 'Innocent' murmurs are also relatively common in young animals[1]. Innocent murmurs are usually soft, systolic ejection-type murmurs heard best at the left heart base; their intensity may vary with heart rate or body position. Innocent murmurs diminish with time and generally disappear by about 4 months of age. Murmurs associated with congenital disease usually persist and some get louder as the animal grows (e.g. subaortic stenosis). Careful evaluation at full maturity is especially important in animals that might be used for breeding. Radiographic and ECG findings can be useful, but echocardiography with Doppler provides greater diagnostic accuracy[3].

Malformations that cause ventricular outflow obstruction can occur at the semilunar valve, just below the valve (subvalvular), or in the proximal great vessel (supravalvular). In the left heart, stenosis below the aortic valve (subaortic) is most common. Malformations of the pulmonary valve itself occur most commonly in dogs and cats; subvalvular (infundibular) narrowing from muscular hypertrophy is a frequent accompaniment. Stenotic lesions impose a systolic pressure overload on the affected ventricle. Downstream from the stenosis, measured pressure is normal but turbulence from the high velocity blood flow jet distends

Table 51 Breed predispositions for congenital heart disease.	
Defect	**Breed**
SAS	Newfoundland, Golden Retriever, Rottweiler, Boxer, German Shepherd Dog, English Bulldog, Great Dane, German Shorthaired Pointer, Bouvier des Flandres, Samoyed
PS	English Bulldog (males > females), Mastiff, Samoyed, Miniature Schnauzer, West Highland White Terrier, Cocker Spaniel, Beagle, Airedale Terrier, Boykin Spaniel, Chihuahua, Scottish Terrier, Boxer, Fox Terrier(?)
PDA	Maltese, Pomeranian, Shetland Sheepdog, English Springer Spaniel, Keeshond, Bichon Frise, Toy and Miniature Poodles, Yorkshire Terrier, Collie, Cocker Spaniel, German Shepherd Dog; Chihuahua, Kerry Blue Terrier, Labrador Retriever, Newfoundland; females > males
VSD	English Bulldog, English Springer Spaniel, Keeshond; cats
ASD	Samoyed, Doberman Pinscher, Boxer
Mdys	Bull Terrier, German Shepherd Dog, Great Dane, Golden Retriever, Newfoundland, Mastiff, Rottweiler(?); cats (males > females)
Tdys	Labrador Retriever, German Shepherd Dog, Boxer, Weimaraner, Great Dane, Old English Sheepdog, Golden Retriever; other large breeds; (males > females?)
T of F	Keeshond, English Bulldog
PRAA	German Shepherd Dog, Great Dane, Irish Setter

the proximal great vessel (poststenotic dilation) and causes the murmur (see Chapter 1, p. 21). The magnitude of systolic pressure difference (gradient) across the stenotic area is related to the severity of obstruction, as well as ventricular contractility and flow volume. Concentric hypertrophy is the ventricle's response to systolic pressure overload (see Chapter 1, p. 18), but some dilation of the affected ventricle can also occur. Secondary AV valve regurgitation and impaired diastolic filling (from increased ventricular stiffness) can develop. High ventricular diastolic and atrial pressures lead to congestive signs. Cardiac arrhythmias can also contribute to the development of congestive failure. The combination of outflow obstruction, paroxysmal tachyarrhythmias, and/or inappropriate bradycardia secondary to ventricular baroreceptor stimulation can result in exercise intolerance, syncope, and sudden death. These low-output signs are most often associated with severe outflow tract obstruction[1, 4].

Abnormal systemic-to-pulmonary shunts occur across atrial or ventricular septal defects (ASDs, VSDs) or, more commonly, through a patent ductus arteriosus (PDA). These shunts cause a volume overload on the left (PDA, VSD) or right (ASD) heart and pulmonary overcirculation as long as pulmonary vascular resistance is relatively normal. If right heart pressures increase as a result of pulmonary hypertension or concurrent pulmonic stenosis (PS), shunt flow may equilibrate or reverse (i.e. become right-to-left). The amount of blood flow across a shunt is related to the size of the defect and the pressure gradient across it. Left-to-right shunts cause total blood volume and cardiac output to increase in response to the partial diversion of blood away from the systemic circulation. Malformations that cause valvular insufficiency also cause volume overload to the affected side of the heart.

Cardiac malformations that allow unoxygenated blood to reach the systemic circulation cause hypoxemia. Visible cyanosis occurs with 50 g/l (5 g/dl) or more of desaturated hemoglobin. Chronic arterial hypoxemia stimulates erythropoiesis and polycythemia in an attempt to increase oxygen carrying capacity[1, 5]; however, blood viscosity and resistance to flow also rise along with the PCV. Severe polycythemia (e.g. PCV >0.65 l/l [>65%]) can cause microvascular sludging and poor tissue oxygenation, intravascular thrombosis, hemorrhage, stroke, and cardiac arrhythmias. Right-to-left shunts can allow a venous embolus to cross to the systemic circulation. Some collateral blood flow to the lungs can develop from the bronchial arteries of the systemic circulation. These small tortuous vessels may increase the radiographic opacity of the central lung fields.

Physical exertion exacerbates right-to-left shunting and cyanosis because peripheral vascular resistance decreases with greater skeletal muscle blood flow. Despite the pressure overload on the right heart, congestive failure is rare because the shunt acts as a 'pop-off' valve. The most common anomalies that cause cyanosis in dogs and cats are tetralogy of Fallot (T of F) and pulmonary arterial hypertension with shunt reversal from a large PDA, VSD, or ASD. Other complex anomalies, such as transposition of the great vessels or truncus arteriosus, occur rarely[1].

PDA and subaortic stenosis (SAS) have each been identified in different surveys as the most common congenital cardiovascular anomaly in the dog[1, 2, 6–8]. PS is also quite common. Persistent right aortic arch (PRAA) (a vascular ring anomaly), VSD, malformations (dysplasia) of the AV valves, ASD, and T of F occur less frequently but are not rare. The most common malformations in cats involve defects of the atrial or ventricular septum, which may occur together as an AV septal (endocardial cushion) defect, AV valve dysplasias, PDA, and endocardial fibroelastosis (mainly in Burmese and Siamese cats)[1, 9]. An endocardial cushion defect (common AV canal) consists of all or some of the following: a high VSD, a low ASD, and malformations of one or both AV valves. Congenital malformations are more prevalent in male than female cats.

SUBAORTIC STENOSIS

PATHOPHYSIOLOGY

Subvalvular narrowing caused by a fibrous or fibromuscular ring is the usual cause in dogs (238). The spectrum of SAS severity, described in Newfoundlands[10], varies widely and ranges from subtle,

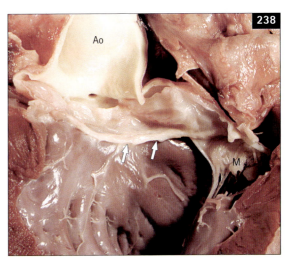

238 A band of fibrous tissue (arrows) extends around the LV outflow tract and involves the anterior mitral leaflet in this postmortem specimen from a dog with SAS. Ao = aortic root; M = anterior mitral leaflet.

subclinical fibrous tissue ridges to a complete fibrous ring around the LV outflow tract causing severe obstruction. Some cases have an elongated, tunnel-like obstruction. Malformation of the mitral valve apparatus may coexist. Outflow tract narrowing and dynamic obstruction with or without a discrete subvalvular ridge have also been noted in Golden Retrievers[11] and may be important in other dogs as well. The obstructive lesion of SAS develops during the first few months of life, and there may be no audible murmur at an early age[1]. In some dogs, no murmur is detected until 1–2 years of age and the obstruction may continue to worsen beyond that age[12, 13]. Exercise or excitement generally increases the murmur's intensity. These factors, and the common occurance of physiologic murmurs in some dogs, make definitive diagnosis of mild cases and genetic counseling to breeders problematic[14, 15].

The stenosis severity determines the degree of LV pressure overload and resulting concentric hypertrophy. Coronary perfusion is easily compromised in animals with severe SAS. Intramural coronary arteries are commonly narrowed[16]. High systolic LV wall tension with coronary narrowing can cause systolic flow reversal in small coronary arteries. Furthermore, myocardial capillary density may become inadequate as hypertrophy progresses. These factors contribute to the development of myocardial ischemia and fibrosis. Clinical sequelae can include arrhythmias, syncope, left-sided heart failure, and sudden death[4, 17]. Because of related malformations or secondary changes, aortic or mitral valve regurgitation also adds an LV volume overload in many animals. SAS predisposes to aortic valve endocarditis because of jet lesion injury to the underside of the valve leaflets (see Chapter 19, p. 272 and **402, 403**, p. 276)[4, 18].

CLINICAL FEATURES

SAS is more common in larger breeds of dog (*Table 51*, p. 229). SAS is thought to be inherited as an autosomal dominant trait with modifying genes that influence its phenotypic expression[14]. SAS also occurs in cats; supravalvular lesions have been reported in this species as well[1]. Historical signs of fatigue, exertional weakness, syncope, or sudden death occur in about a third of dogs with SAS[1, 4]. Dyspnea is the most commonly reported sign in cats with SAS[19]. With severe outflow obstruction, either tachyarrhythmias or abrupt reflex bradycardia and hypotension from activation of ventricular mechanoreceptors can cause low-output signs. Left-sided CHF can develop, usually in conjunction with concurrent mitral or aortic regurgitation, other cardiac malformations, or acquired endocarditis.

Characteristic physical findings with moderate to severe stenosis include weak and late-rising femoral pulses (*pulsus parvus et tardus*), a precordial thrill low on the left heart base, and the absence of a jugular pulse. There may be evidence of pulmonary edema or arrhythmias. A harsh systolic ejection murmur is heard at or below the aortic valve area on the left hemithorax (see **173, 174**, p.94). This murmur radiates equally or more loudly to the right heart base because of the course of the aortic arch. Often the murmur is also heard over the carotid arteries, and it may radiate to the calvarium in severe cases. In mild cases a soft, poorly radiating ejection murmur at the left and, sometimes, the right heart base may be the only abnormality noted. Aortic regurgitation may produce a diastolic murmur at the left base or it may be inaudible.

DIAGNOSIS

Radiographic abnormalities (*Table 52*) may be subtle, especially with mild SAS. The LV can look normal or enlarged. A prominent cranial waist in the cardiac silhouette on lateral projection and cranial mediastinal widening are manifestations of poststenotic dilation in the ascending aorta (**239–244**).

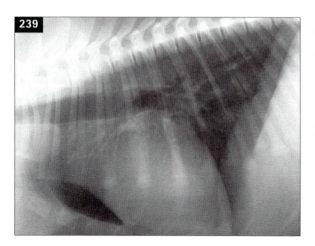
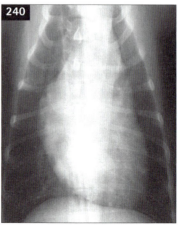

(**239, 240**) Radiographs from a 4-month-old female Golden Retriever with severe SAS (Doppler gradient 225 mm Hg) show LV enlargement and a very wide cranial cardiac waist on the lateral view (**239**).

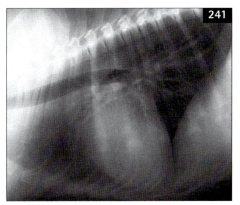

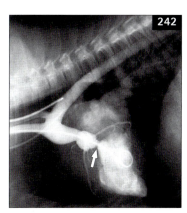

241–242 Dorsocranial cardiac widening is less prominent in other cases, although left heart enlargement is seen. (241) Lateral view from a 5-month-old male German Shepherd Dog (catheter gradient 130 mm Hg). (242) LV angiocardiogram from the dog in 241; fairly discrete subaortic narrowing (arrow), LV hypertrophy with stout left coronary arteries, LA enlargement, and modest ascending aortic dilation are seen.

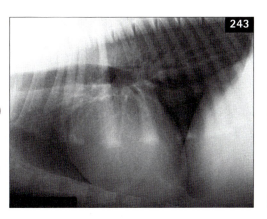

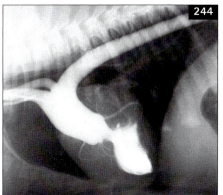

243, 244 (243) Lateral view from a 4-month-old male Rottweiler (catheter gradient 55 mm Hg). (244) LV angiocardiogram from the dog in 243 shows a tunnel-like stenosis with marked poststenotic aortic dilation that extends into the brachycephalic trunk.

Table 52 Characteristic radiographic findings with selected congenital heart defects.

Defect	Heart	Pulmonary vessels	Other
SAS	± LAE, LVE	Normal	Wide cranial cardiac waist (dilated ascending aorta)
PS	RAE, RVE; reverse D	Normal to undercirculated	Pulmonary trunk bulge
PDA	LAE, LVE; left auricular bulge; ± increased cardiac width	Overcirculated	Bulge(s) in descending aorta + pulmonary trunk; ± pulmonary edema
VSD	LAE, LVE; ± RVE	Overcirculated	± Pulmonary edema; ± pulmonary trunk bulge (large shunts)
ASD	RAE, RVE	± Overcirculated	± Pulmonary trunk bulge
Mdys	LAE, LVE	± Venous hypertension	± Pulmonary edema
Tdys	RAE, RVE; ± globoid shape	Normal	Caudal cava dilation; ± pleural effusion, ascites, hepatomegaly
T of F	RVE, RAE; reverse D	Undercirculated; ± prominent bronchial vessels	Normal to small pulmonary trunk; ± cranial aortic bulge on lateral view
PRAA	Normal	Normal	Focal leftward and ventral tracheal deviation ± narrowing cranial to heart; wide cranial mediastinum; megaesophagus; (± aspiration pneumonia)

LAE = left atrial enlargement; LVE = left ventricular enlargement; RAE = right atrial enlargement; RVE = right ventricular enlargement.

The ECG is often normal, although there can be evidence of LV hypertrophy (left axis deviation; **245**) or enlargement (tall complexes). ST segment depression resulting from myocardial ischemia or changes secondary to hypertrophy may be present in leads II and aVF (see **112**, p. 62). Exercise can induce further ischemic ST-segment changes. Ventricular tachyarrhythmias are common.

The extent of LV hypertrophy and subaortic narrowing are seen with echocardiography (**246–250**). A discrete subaortic tissue ridge is evident in many animals with moderate to severe disease (**248**). Premature closure of the aortic valve, systolic anterior motion (SAM) of the anterior mitral leaflet, and increased LV subendocardial echogenicity (probably from fibrosis) are common in animals with severe

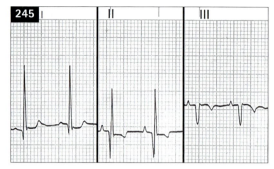

245 ECG from a 1-year-old female Mastiff with SAS shows sinus rhythm with a left axis deviation. Leads as marked; 25 mm/sec.

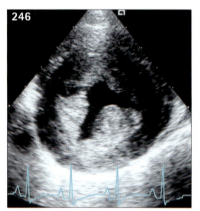 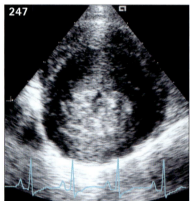 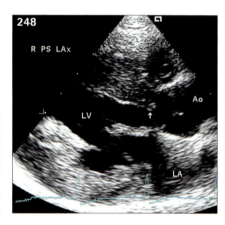

1 cm = 1 mV.

246–248 Right parasternal short-axis echocardiograms at end-diastole (**246**) and in systole (**247**) from the puppy in **239** and **240** show marked LV hypertrophy with increased echogenicity of papillary muscles and inner LV wall. In systole the LV lumen is almost obliterated. (**248**) The subaortic ridge (arrow) is prominent in a 4-month-old female German Shepherd Dog with severe SAS; one aortic leaflet is seen in closed position

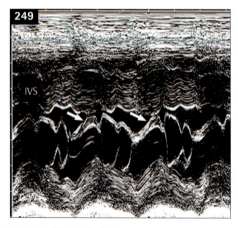 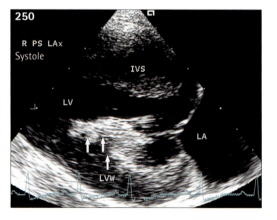

in this right parasternal long-axis view.

249, 250 Images from the puppy in **239** and **240**. (**249**) M-mode echocardiogram; SAM of the mitral valve (arrows) indicates dynamic as well as fixed LV outflow obstruction in this case. Note the thick LVW and IVS; cm marks along left edge. (**250**) Marked hyperechogenicity (arrows) of this hypertrophied papillary muscle and surrounding myocardium suggests chronic ischemia with fibrosis. IVS = interventricular septum; LA = left obstruction. Dilation of the ascending aorta, aortic valve thickening, and LA enlargement with hypertrophy may also be seen. Normal or equivocal M-mode and 2-D findings may be noted in mildly affected animals.

Systolic flow acceleration originating below the aortic valve and turbulence extending into the aorta, as well as high peak systolic outflow velocity, can be identified using Doppler echocardiography (251–253). Aortic or mitral regurgitation is also shown by color-flow and spectral Doppler studies (252). The severity of the stenosis is estimated using spectral Doppler. Doppler-estimated systolic pressure gradients in unanesthetized animals are usually 40–50% higher than those recorded during cardiac catheterization under general anesthesia[20]. Peak estimated gradients of more than 100 mmHg are associated with severe stenosis[21]. The LV outflow tract should be interrogated from more than one position to achieve the best possible alignment with blood flow. The subcostal (subxiphoid) position usually yields the highest velocity signals[17], although in some animals the left apical position is better. With optimal beam alignment, aortic root velocities of 1.7 m/sec or less are normal in unsedated dogs; velocities exceeding 2–2.25 m/sec are considered abnormal[1, 14, 22]. Peak velocities between these values may indicate the presence of mild SAS, especially if other supportive evidence exists, such as disturbed flow in the outflow tract or ascending aorta and aortic regurgitation. This is mainly of concern when selecting animals for breeding. However, velocities in this 'equivocal' range (1.8–2.25 m/sec) may occur from breed-related differences in LV outflow tract anatomy or response to sympatheic stimulation[23–25]. Use of the estimated pressure gradient to assess SAS severity is also limited by the dependence of this gradient on blood flow. Increased sympathetic activation and other causes of high cardiac output (e.g. excitement, fever, PDA) will increase outflow velocities, while myocardial failure, cardiodepressant drugs, and other causes of reduced stroke volume will decrease recorded velocities. Calculations related to LV outflow tract effective orifice area have been proposed as a way to address this concern[14, 26, 27]. Cardiac catheterization and angiocardiography (242 and 244 [p. 231], 254) are

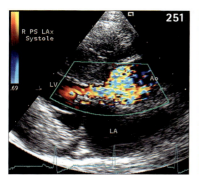 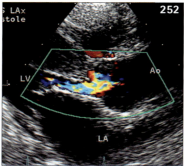 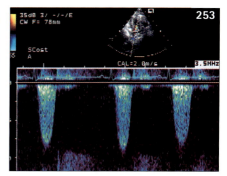

251–253 (251) Systolic turbulence originating in the narrowed LV outflow tract is evident in this right parasternal long-axis color flow Doppler image from a German Shepherd Dog puppy with severe SAS. (252) Diastolic frame from the same case shows moderate aortic regurgitation. (253) CW Doppler recorded from the subcostal position in a Golden Retriever indicates maximal LV outflow velocity of 7.5 m/sec, consistent with an instantaneous pressure gradient of about 225 mm Hg. An aortic insufficiency signal is seen above baseline and aliased faintly at the bottom of this spectral image. Ao = aorta; LA = left atrium; LV = left ventricle.

254 ECG (top) and pressure (bottom) recordings obtained during cardiac catheterization of a 2-year-old female German Shorthaired Pointer with SAS. The catheter tip was in the ascending aorta at the left side of the trace (pressure range indicated in mm Hg). As the catheter was pushed just past the aortic valve, LV diastolic and normal systolic pressures are seen (arrow) because the catheter tip was above the stenosis; continued insertion past the subvalvular obstruction reveals LV systolic pressure of well over 200 mm Hg (arrowhead).
255 Postmortem specimen opened through the RV outflow tract into

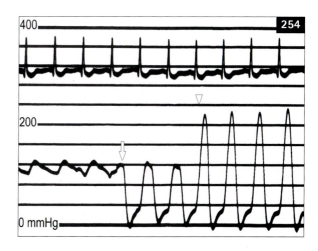

used infrequently now except in conjunction with balloon dilation of the stenotic area.

MANAGEMENT

Various techniques have been used to reduce outflow obstruction in dogs with severe SAS[28, 29]. Cardiopulmonary bypass and open-heart surgery are necessary to reach the lesion directly[30, 31]. Although surgical resection of the stenotic region can significantly reduce the LV systolic pressure gradient and possibly improve exercise ability, in one study, no improvement in long-term survival was found compared with dogs not undergoing the procedure[32]. Transcatheter balloon dilation of the stenotic area has reduced the measured gradient in some dogs, but partial restenosis may develop with time. Some improvement in signs has been noted, but no survival benefit has been documented with this procedure when compared with treatment with atenolol[33–35].

Beta-adrenergic blockers have been advocated to reduce myocardial oxygen demand and minimize the frequency and severity of arrhythmias. Animals with severe stenosis, marked ST-segment depression, frequent ventricular ectopy, or a history of syncope may be more likely to benefit from this therapy. Whether beta-blockers prolong survival is unclear. Exercise should be restricted in animals with moderate to severe SAS. Prophylactic antibiotic therapy is indicated prior to procedures with the potential to cause bacteremia (e.g. dentistry).

The prognosis with severe stenosis (catheterization pressure gradient >80 mmHg or Doppler gradient >100–125 mmHg) is guarded. More than 50% of severely affected dogs die suddenly before the age of 3 years[4]. The overall prevalence of sudden death in dogs with SAS appears to be just over 20%. Infective endocarditis and CHF may be more likely to develop later[4]. Atrial and ventricular arrhythmias and worsened MR are complicating factors. Dogs with mild stenosis (e.g. catheterization gradient <35 mmHg or Doppler gradient <60–70 mmHg) are more likely to be asymptomatic and live longer.

PULMONIC STENOSIS

PATHOPHYSIOLOGY

Valve dysplasia is more common than simple fusion of pulmonic valve cusps and involves variably thickened, asymmetrical, partially fused leaflets, and a hypoplastic valve annulus (**255**)[1, 36]. RV hypertrophy results from the systolic pressure overload. Myocardial ischemia and its sequelae are likely with severe hypertrophy. Poststenotic dilation of the main pulmonary trunk occurs to a variable degree[36]. Secondary RA and RV dilation are common. Development of tricuspid insufficiency and increased

RV filling pressure predisposes to atrial arrhythmias and congestive failure. Variants of PS, including supravalvular stenosis and a subvalvular RV muscular partition (double chamber RV), are rare[1]. The combination of PS and a patent foramen ovale or ASD can cause right-to-left shunting at the atrial level, but this is uncommon.

A single anomalous coronary artery, thought to contribute to the outflow obstruction, has been described in association with PS in some English Bulldogs and a Boxer[37–39]. Palliative surgical procedures and balloon valvuloplasty have caused death secondary to transection or avulsion of the major left coronary branch in such cases.

CLINICAL FEATURES

PS is more common in small breeds of dogs (*Table 52*, p. 231). Many cases are asymptomatic at the time of diagnosis. Signs of right-sided congestive failure or a history of exercise intolerance or syncope may occur[36, 40], but even in animals with considerable stenosis, these signs may not develop for several years. Sudden death also occurs with severe PS. Physical findings characteristic of moderate to severe stenosis include a prominent right precordial impulse, a thrill high at the left base, normal to slightly diminished femoral pulses, pink mucous membranes, and, sometimes, jugular pulses. The systolic ejection murmur is best heard high at the left base (**256**). The murmur may radiate cranioventrally and to the right in some cases, but usually it is not heard over the carotid arteries. An early systolic click is sometimes

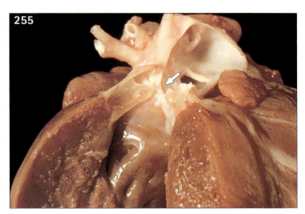

255

the pulmonary artery from a 4-month-old male Miniature Schnauzer with a severely dysplastic pulmonary valve. The thick, malformed valve lacks clearly demarcated leaflets and has only a tiny orifice (arrow). Note the marked RV hypertrophy.

heard, probably resulting from abrupt checking of a fused valve as ejection begins. The murmur of secondary tricuspid insufficiency or arrhythmias may be heard in some cases.

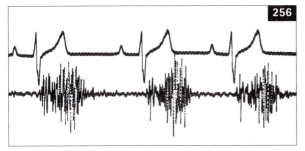

256 Lead II ECG (top) and phonocardiogram (bottom) from a dog with PS demonstrate the systolic ejection murmur and a QRS configuration reflecting right axis deviation from RV hypertrophy.

DIAGNOSIS

Typical radiographic features are outlined in *Table 52* (p. 231). **257–262** illustrate some of the variability in radiographic appearance. Marked RV hypertrophy causes the cardiac apex to be shifted dorsally and to the left. The heart may have a 'reverse D' shape on DV or VD view. A pulmonary trunk bulge (poststenotic dilation) is best seen at the 1 o'clock position on a DV or VD view, but the size of this dilation does not correlate with the severity of the pressure gradient[36]. Dilation of the caudal vena cava is also seen in some animals.

ECG features of moderate to severe PS include a RV hypertrophy pattern, right axis deviation, and, sometimes, a RA enlargement pattern (P pulmonale), tachyarrhythmias, or ST segment elevation (see **111**, p. 62).

Echocardiographic findings with moderate to severe stenosis include RV hypertrophy and enlargement. The interventricular septum often

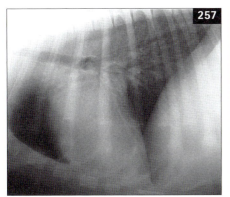 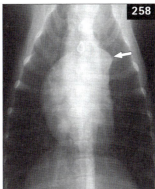 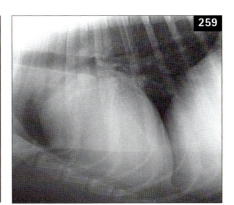
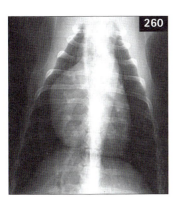 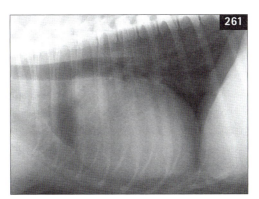 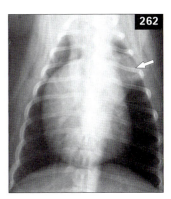

257–262 Examples of variation in the radiographic appearance of PS. (257, 258) RV enlargement appears modest, although there is a clear main pulmonary artery bulge (arrow) on the DV view (258) in a 1-year-old male Vizsla (catheter gradient 80 mm Hg). (259, 260) The lateral view (259) shows nonspecific cardiomegaly, although the DV view (260) indicates right heart enlargement in a 5-year-old male Labrador Retriever with moderately severe PS (Doppler gradient 63 mm Hg); poststenotic dilation of the pulmonary trunk is not clear. (261, 262) Severe PS has caused massive RV enlargement, apex elevation from the sternum (261) and a huge pulmonary trunk bulge (arrow) on the DV view (262) in a 3-year-old female West Highland White Terrier (Doppler gradient 210 mm Hg).

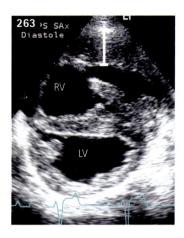

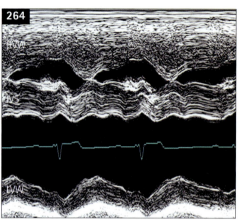

263, 264 (263) Pressure overload from PS causes RV wall hypertrophy (bar), RV dilation, and IVS flattening toward the LV (here in diastole) in a 2-year-old male mixed breed dog (Doppler gradient 126 mm Hg); right parasternal short-axis view. (264) M-mode image from a 3-year-old female Brittany with severe PS shows RV hypertrophy and flattened septal motion. IVS = interventricular septum; LV = left ventricle; LVW = left ventricular wall; RV = right ventricle; RVW = right ventricular wall.

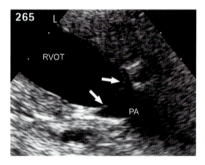

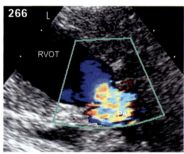

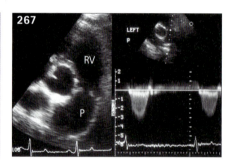

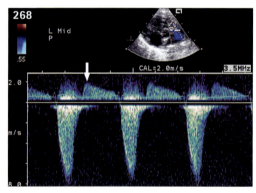

265–268 (265) Systolic doming of the pulmonary valve (arrows) is visualized in the dog in 263; the valve is relatively thin, although the leaflets appear fused. (266) Image plane as in 265; color flow Doppler shows blood flow acceleration proximal to the valve orifice and turbulence distal. (267) 2-D and PW Doppler images from a 5-year-old male Labrador Retriever with moderately severe PS, diagnosed after the recent onset of syncope with exertion. Note the thickened pulmonary valve and modest pulmonary artery dilation. (268) CW Doppler maximal systolic velocity of almost 8 m/sec across the pulmonary valve indicates severe stenosis in an asymptomatic 5-month-old male Pomeranian. Pulmonary regurgitant flow is also seen above the baseline in diastole (arrow). Left cranial short-axis views. P = pulmonary artery; RV = right ventricle.

appears flattened as high RV pressure pushes it toward the left (263, 264). RA enlargement is common. The pulmonic valve usually appears thickened, asymmetrical, or otherwise malformed (265–268), although the outflow area may be narrow and difficult to visualize clearly. Poststenotic dilation of the main pulmonary trunk may also be seen. Pleural effusion and right heart dilation often accompany secondary congestive failure. Paradoxical septal motion (see Chapter 5, p. 78) may be noted in such cases as well. Doppler evaluation, along with anatomic findings, provides an estimate of lesion severity (267, 268). Prominent pulmonary valve insufficiency is common as well.

The systolic pressure gradient across the stenotic valve, the right heart filling pressure, and anatomic features can also be determined by cardiac catheterization and angiocardiography (269–272). Doppler-estimated systolic pressure gradients in unanesthetized animals are usually 40–50% higher than those recorded during cardiac catheterization. PS is generally considered mild if the Doppler-derived gradient is <50 mm Hg and severe if it exceeds (80–)100 mm Hg[1].

MANAGEMENT

The palliation of severe and some cases of moderate stenosis by balloon valvuloplasty is recommended, especially if RV infundibular hypertrophy is not excessive. Balloon valvuloplasty, done in conjunction with cardiac catheterization, is most successful in dogs with simple fusion of the pulmonic valve cusps, although significant reduction in systolic pressure gradient is possible with some dysplastic valves (273–275)[41–47]. Various surgical procedures have been used to palliate moderate to severe PS in dogs as well[48–50]. Usually, balloon valvuloplasty is attempted before surgery because it is generally less risky. In dogs with a single anomalous coronary artery, these procedures are contraindicated[37]. Normal coronary anatomy can be verified using echocardiography or angiography.

Exercise restriction is recommended with moderate to severe stenosis. A beta-blocker may be helpful, especially if infundibular hypertrophy is prominent. Signs of CHF are managed medically (see Chapter 16). Prognosis depends on the severity of the stenosis. Those with mild PS may have a normal life span, but animals with severe stenosis often die within 3 years of diagnosis[36]. Sudden death or the onset of

269–272 (269) ECG (top) and pressure (bottom) trace obtained during cardiac catheterization in a dog with PS. Normal PA pressure is shown on the left. The catheter was pulled back into the RV, which induced a brief paroxysm of ventricular tachycardia and an isolated VPC before the rhythm stabilized and baseline RV systolic pressure was evident (right side of trace). Note the poor systolic pressure generation in response to the ectopic ventricular complexes; subsequent sinus complexes are associated with enhanced RV systolic pressure generation (known as postextrasystolic potentiation; arrows). **(270)** A thickened pulmonary valve is seen as a filling defect (arrow) in this RV angiocardiogram during diastole. **(271)** Doming of the thickened and fused leaflets is seen during systole. Poststenotic dilation of the pulmonary trunk and proximal pulmonary arteries is evident in these images **(270, 271)** from a 1-year-old male Vizsla. **(272)** A thickened, dysplastic pulmonary valve, asymmetrical valve sinuses, a large poststenotic pulmonary trunk dilation, and RV hypertrophy are seen in a 3-year-old female West Highland White Terrier with severe PS.

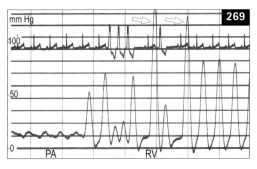
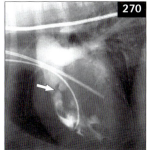
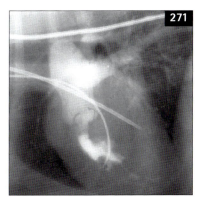
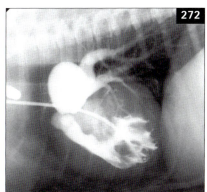

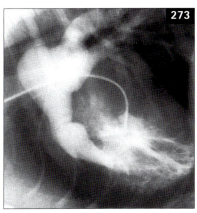
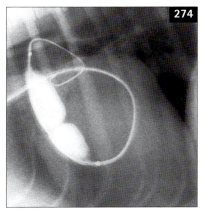
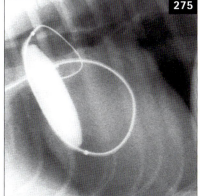

273–275 (273) Baseline RV angiocardiogram from a 1.5-year-old Brittany with severe PS (Doppler gradient ~210 mm Hg). **(274)** A partially filled balloon dilation catheter is in place across the stenotic pulmonary valve, which causes the 'waist' in the balloon. **(275)** The stenotic valve has been dilated by the inflated balloon (Doppler gradient the next day was 75 mm Hg).

CHF is common. Tricuspid regurgitation, AF or other tachyarrhythmias, or CHF worsen the prognosis. Balloon valvuloplasty appears to prolong survival as well as improve clinical signs in dogs with severe PS[51].

PATENT DUCTUS ARTERIOSUS

PATHOPHYSIOLOGY

Functional closure of the ductus arteriosus normally occurs within hours after birth; structural changes over days to weeks cause permanent closure. Animals with inherited PDA have a histologically abnormal ductal wall that is unable to constrict[8, 52]. Closure at only the pulmonary side of the ductus causes a ductus diverticulum from the aorta but no shunt; this 'forme fruste' (incomplete form) of inherited PDA is seen only with angiography or postmortem examination[1, 52]. With a fully patent ductus, blood shunts from the descending aorta to the pulmonary artery during both systole and diastole, because aortic pressure normally is higher throughout the cardiac cycle (276, 277). This left-to-right shunt creates a volume overload on the pulmonary circulation, LA, and LV. Shunt flow depends on the pressure gradient between the two circulations and the ductus diameter. Rarely, an aorticopulmonary window, between the ascending aorta and the pulmonary artery, or other central A-V fistula causes similar hemodynamic and clinical abnormalities[53, 54]. Hyperkinetic arterial pulses are characteristic of PDA because blood run-off from the aorta to the pulmonary system allows diastolic aortic pressure to decrease rapidly and widens pulse pressure (278; see also Chapters 1 and 2).

While compensatory mechanisms (e.g. increased HR, volume retention) maintain systemic blood flow, the hemodynamic burden on the LV can be great because the increased volume must be pumped into the relatively high pressure aorta. LV and mitral annulus dilation in turn cause MR and further volume overload. Excess fluid retention, declining myocardial contractility stemming from the chronic volume overload, and arrhythmias contribute to the development of CHF.

In some cases the excess pulmonary flow induces pulmonary vascular changes, increased resistance, and pulmonary hypertension (see p. 250). If pulmonary artery pressure rises to equal aortic pressure, little shunting occurs; if pulmonary artery pressure exceeds aortic pressure, reversed shunting (right-to-left flow) occurs. Reversed shunt was noted in 15% of dogs with inherited PDA[7]. Female Cocker Spaniels may be at increased risk for reversed PDA.

CLINICAL FEATURES

Left-to-right shunting PDA is by far the most common form[1, 55–57]. Clinical features of reversed PDA are described below (p. 250). The prevalence of PDA is higher in certain breeds of dogs; a polygenic inheritance

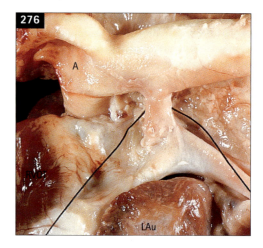

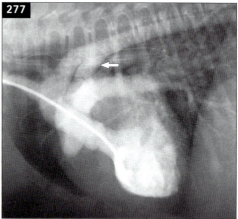

276, 277 (276) A suture passes around the PDA in this necropsy specimen. The ductus connects the proximal descending aorta with the pulmonary artery. A = aorta; LAu = left auricular appendage; RVOT = right ventricular outflow tract. Cranial is to the left of image. (277) LV angiocardiogram highlights a large left-to-right PDA. Dye is seen in the LV, aorta, PDA (arrow), and pulmonary artery; the pulmonary vasculature is engorged. (From Ware WA (2003) Common congenital cardiac anomalies. In Small Animal Internal Medicine (3rd edn). (eds RW Nelson, CG Couto) Mosby, St Louis, p. 155, with permission.)

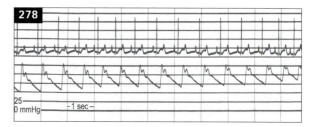

278 ECG trace (top) and femoral arterial pressure (bottom) are shown. At the left side of the trace, a widened pulse pressure caused by PDA is seen. As the ductus is surgically ligated, the pulse pressure narrows (right side of trace). (Courtesy Dr D Riedesel; from Ware WA (2003) Common congenital cardiac anomalies. In Small Animal Internal Medicine (3rd edn). (eds RW Nelson, CG Couto) Mosby, St Louis, p. 154, with permission.)

pattern is thought to be responsible (*Table 51*, p. 228). The incidence is approximately three times greater in female than in male dogs[2, 58]. Many animals with PDA are asymptomatic when first diagnosed, although reduced exercise ability, tachypnea, or cough occurs in some cases. Characteristic physical findings include a continuous murmur (often with a precordial thrill) heard best high at the left base (see **173**, p. 94), hyperkinetic (bounding, 'water hammer') arterial pulses, and pink mucous membranes.

DIAGNOSIS

Radiographic findings include cardiac elongation (left heart dilation), LA and auricular enlargement, and pulmonary overcirculation (*Table 52*, p. 231; see also **54**, p. 42). Often, a bulge is evident in the descending aorta ('ductus bump') or main pulmonary trunk, or both (**279–282**). The triad of all three bulges (i.e. pulmonary trunk, aorta, and left auricle), located in that order from the 1 o'clock to 3 o'clock position on a DV radiograph is infrequently seen[58]. Evidence of pulmonary edema accompanies left-sided heart failure.

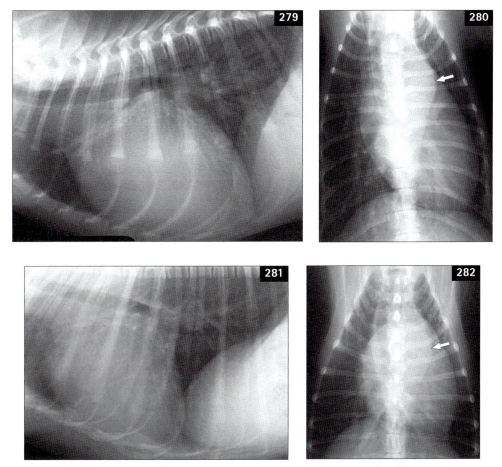

279–282 Examples of variation in the radiographic appearance of PDA. A bulge in the descending aorta (arrow) is seen in both cases on the DV view. (279, 280) Marked elongation of the left heart in a 4-month-old small mixed breed dog. (281, 282) From a 1-year-old female Brussels Griffon.

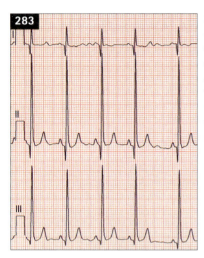

283 Tall QRS complexes with deep Q waves are common with PDA, as seen in this ECG from a small mixed breed dog with 4.8 mV R waves. Leads as marked, 50 mm/sec, 1 cm = 1 mV.

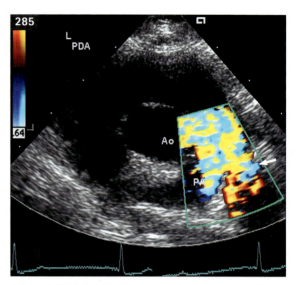

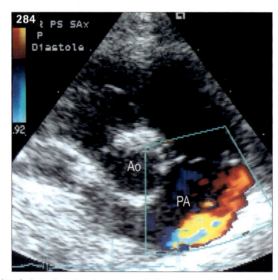

(284) Color flow Doppler shows turbulent flow jet into the dilated pulmonary trunk during diastole in a 4-month-old female Shih Tsu with PDA. Right parasternal short-axis view.

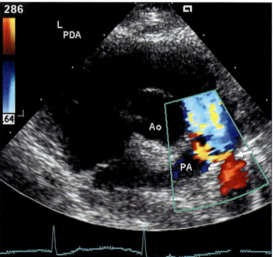

Characteristic ECG findings include wide P waves, tall R waves, and, often, deep Q waves in leads II, aVF, and CV$_6$LL (283). ST-T segment changes secondary to LV enlargement may occur. However, the ECG can be normal.

Left heart and pulmonary trunk dilation are seen with echocardiography. LV fractional shortening may be normal or decreased; the EPSS is often increased. The ductus itself may be visible between the pulmonary artery and descending aorta, especially with the left cranial parasternal or subcostal view. Doppler studies document continuous, turbulent flow into the pulmonary artery (284–287) and allow estimation of aortic to pulmonary artery pressure gradient. Cardiac catheterization, generally done only now in conjunction with an interventional procedure, can demonstrate higher oxygen content in the

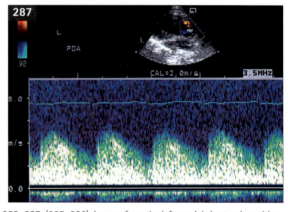

285–287 **(285, 286)** Images from the left cranial short-axis position show flow at the juncture of the PDA and pulmonary artery in systole (285) and diastole (286) in a 5-year-old female Pomeranian. Ao = aortic root; PA = pulmonary artery. **(287)** CW Doppler from the dog in 284 shows continuous flow through the PDA into the pulmonary artery; maximal velocity about 5.5 m/sec (aorta to pulmonary artery gradient ~121 mm Hg) is consistent with normal pulmonary systolic pressure.

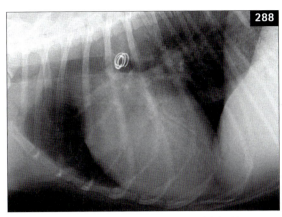

288 A catheter-delivered coil has occluded the PDA in this 10-year-old male Poodle. (Courtesy Dr OL Nelson.)

pulmonary artery than in the right ventricle (oxygen 'step-up') and the wide aortic pressure pulse. Angiocardiography documents left-to-right shunting through the ductus (277).

MANAGEMENT

Closure of the left-to-right PDA is recommended. Several surgical and transcatheter occlusion techniques have been described[7, 58–72]. Surgical ligation is successful in most cases and low complication and mortality rates are reported[58, 73–76]. Transcatheter PDA occlusion methods involve placement of wire coils (with attached thrombogenic tufts; 288) or another vascular occluding device within the ductus. Not all cases are amenable to transcatheter occlusion. Complications associated with this procedure include aberrant coil embolization, ductal reopening, hemolysis, and others, including death. Vascular access is usually via the femoral artery, although some surgeons have used a venous approach to the ductus. Some residual ductal flow is common with transcatheter occlusion, but significant hemodynamic improvement is usual and many such cases develop complete ductal closure over time[77]. After uncomplicated ductal closure, a normal life span can be expected. Concurrent MR usually resolves if the valve is structurally normal.

Some cases require therapy for CHF (see Chapter 16) or arrhythmias (see Chapter 17). Heart failure is the eventual outcome in most cases that do not undergo ductal closure, usually within a year of diagnosis[1]. In animals with pulmonary hypertension and shunt reversal, ductal closure is contraindicated because the ductus acts as a 'pop-off' valve for the high right-sided pressures. Ductal ligation in animals with reversed PDA produces no improvement and promotes the onset of RV failure.

VENTRICULAR SEPTAL DEFECT

PATHOPHYSIOLOGY

VSDs are most often located high in the membranous part of the septum, just below the aortic valve and under the septal tricuspid leaflet (perimembranous VSD); however, other locations in the IVS can be involved[1]. VSDs impose a volume overload on the lungs, LA, LV, and RV outflow tract. Small defects are usually clinically unimportant. Moderate to large defects cause left heart enlargement and, sometimes, left-sided congestive failure. Very large VSDs also cause RV enlargement with both ventricles functioning as a common chamber. Pulmonary hypertension with shunt reversal is more likely to develop with very large defects (see p. 250).

Aortic regurgitation occurs in some animals with VSD, presumably because the deformed septum provides inadequate anatomic support for the aortic root[1, 78]. Aortic regurgitation places an additional volume load on the LV.

CLINICAL FEATURES

Exercise intolerance and signs of left-sided congestive failure are the most common clinical manifestations of VSD, although many animals are asymptomatic. Characteristic physical findings include a holosystolic murmur, usually loudest at the cranial right sternal border (corresponding to the direction of shunt flow). A large shunt volume causes relative or functional PS, with a systolic ejection murmur at the left base. If the VSD is associated with aortic regurgitation, a corresponding diastolic decrescendo murmur may be heard at the left base.

DIAGNOSIS

Radiographic findings depend on VSD size and shunt volume (*Table 52*, p. 231). Large left-to-right shunts cause left heart enlargement and pulmonary overcirculation, but RV enlargement also occurs if pulmonary vascular resistance increases. A large shunt volume can dilate the main pulmonary trunk.

The ECG may be normal or suggest LA or LV enlargement. Sometimes, 'fractionated' or splintered QRS complexes are seen, suggesting intraventricular conduction disturbance. A RV enlargement pattern usually indicates a very large defect, pulmonary hypertension, concurrent RV outflow tract obstruction, or an AV septal defect, although it may also result from right bundle branch block.

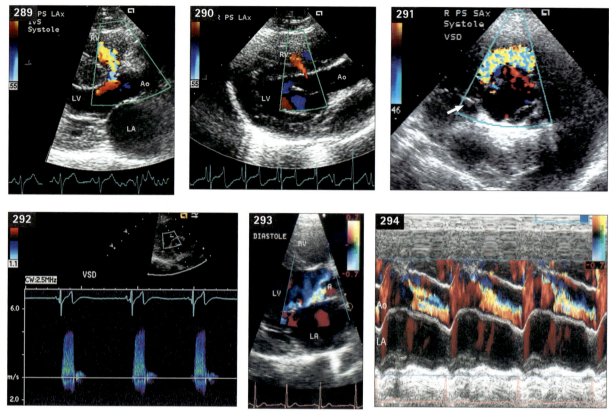

289–294 (289) Color flow Doppler shows abnormal flow from LV to RV through a moderate sized VSD in an 8-year-old female cat; LA enlargement is also present. (290) Small left-to-right VSD flow seen in a 6-month-old female cat. (291) Flow through a perimembranous VSD enters the RV just below the septal tricuspid leaflet (arrow) in this systolic frame from a 4-year-old female English Toy Spaniel. (292) CW Doppler documents high velocity systolic flow across a restrictive VSD in a Border Terrier. Ao = aorta; LA = left atrium; LV = left ventricle; RV = right ventricle. Right parasternal long-axis (289, 290, 292) and short-axis (291) views. 293, 294 A jet of aortic regurgitation is seen with 2-D color flow Doppler (293) and color M-mode (294) in a 1-year-old male English Springer Spaniel with a high VSD. In 294, turbulent flow is only seen in diastole; systolic flow across the aortic valve is normal. Ao = aorta; LA = left atrium; LV = left ventricle; RV = right ventricle.

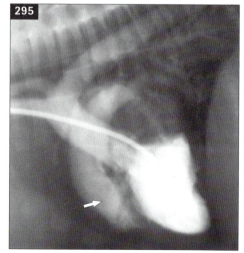

295 LV angiocardiogram shows dye in the RV outflow tract (arrow) and pulmonary arteries as well as in the LV and aorta in a 4-month-old Chow Chow with a VSD.

Echocardiography reveals left heart dilation, with or without RV dilation, in animals with large shunts. Larger defects can usually be visualized just below the aortic valve in the right parasternal long-axis plane. The septal tricuspid leaflet is located to the right of the defect. Because echo 'drop-out' is common at the thin membranous septum, more than one scanning plane should be used to evaluate a suspected VSD. Supporting clinical evidence and a murmur consistent with VSD should also be sought. Doppler studies demonstrate the shunt flow and, in some cases, aortic regurgitation (289–294). Cardiac catheterization, oximetry, and angiocardiography allow measurement of intracardiac pressures, indicate the presence of an oxygen step-up in the RV outflow tract, and show the abnormal blood flow pathway (295).

MANAGEMENT
Dogs and cats with a small to moderate sized defect often have a relatively normal life span. Small defects

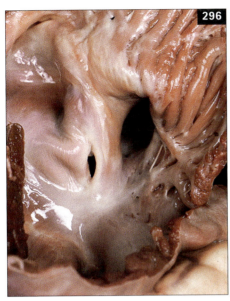

296 Small secundum-type ASD seen from the right in a young dog with multiple cardiac malformations. Right auricle is to upper right; RV is at bottom of the photo.

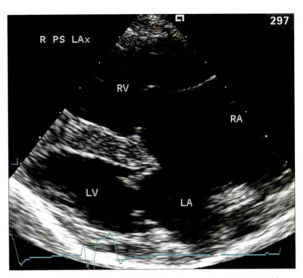

297 Large ASD, with RA and RV dilation, is seen in an 8-year-old female mixed breed dog with concurrent mitral and tricuspid regurgitation.

sometimes close spontaneously within the first 2 years of life, from myocardial hypertrophy around the VSD or by a seal formed by the septal tricuspid leaflet or prolapsed aortic leaflet[1, 79, 80]. Left-sided congestive failure is likely to develop with a large VSD, although pulmonary hypertension with shunt reversal develops in some cases instead, usually at an early age.

Definitive therapy for VSD has required cardiopulmonary bypass or hypothermia and intracardiac surgery; however, transcatheter coil (or other device) occlusion of small perimembranous VSDs is possible in some cases[81, 82]. A large left-to-right shunt is sometimes palliated by placing a constrictive band around the pulmonary trunk to create mild supravalvular PS[83]. This increases RV systolic pressure in response to the increased outflow resistance, reduces the systolic LV to RV pressure gradient, and consequently reduces shunt volume. However, an excessively tight band can cause shunt reversal (functionally analogous to a T of F). Animals that develop left-sided heart failure are managed medically (see Chapter 16). Surgical palliation is contraindicated when pulmonary hypertension and shunt reversal exists.

ATRIAL SEPTAL DEFECT

PATHOPHYSIOLOGY
Ostium secundum ASDs are located in the fossa ovalis region (296). Defects low in the interatrial septum (ostium primum) are likely to be part of an AV septal defect (endocardial cushion defect complex or common A-V canal)[1]. Sinus venosus-type defects, located near the RA–cranial vena cava junction, are rare. ASDs are

more common in cats than in dogs[1]. ASDs are often associated with other cardiac anomalies. In most cases, blood shunts from the left atrium to the right atrium, causing a volume overload to the right heart. If PS or pulmonary hypertension is also present, right-to-left shunting and cyanosis can occur.

CLINICAL FEATURES
The clinical history is usually nonspecific[1, 84–86]. Physical findings may be unremarkable with an isolated ASD, but with a large left-to-right shunt, the murmur of relative PS and fixed splitting of the second heart sound (S_2) (i.e. no respiratory variation) can be heard. Rarely, a soft diastolic murmur of relative tricuspid stenosis might be audible.

DIAGNOSIS
Radiographically, right heart enlargement with or without pulmonary trunk dilation is seen with large shunts (Table 52, p. 231)[86]. The pulmonary circulation may appear increased unless high pulmonary resistance has developed. The left heart is not enlarged unless another defect such as mitral insufficiency is present.

The ECG may be normal or may show RV and RA enlargement patterns. Cats with an AV septal (endocardial cushion) defect may have RV enlargement and a left axis deviation.

RA and RV dilation, with or without paradoxical IVS motion, may be seen with echocardiography. Large ASDs can be visualized (297). But sometimes the thinner fossa ovalis region of the interatrial septum can be confused with a septal defect, because echo dropout also occurs here. Doppler echocardiography may identify smaller shunts that cannot be visualized on 2-D examination (**298**, **299**)[21, 87]. Cardiac catheterization with oximetry shows an oxygen step-up at the level of the RA. The shunt can be demonstrated after injection of contrast material into the pulmonary artery.

MANAGEMENT

Large shunts can be treated surgically, similarly to VSDs. A catheter-delivered occlusive device might be an option, as used in people, but generally, medical management is used if CHF develops. The prognosis is variable and depends on shunt size, presence of other defects, and pulmonary vascular resistance.

MITRAL DYSPLASIA

PATHOPHYSIOLOGY

Congenital malformations of the mitral valve apparatus include shortened or overly elongated chordae tendineae, direct attachment of the valve cusp to a

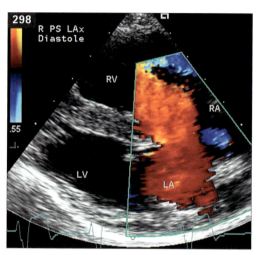
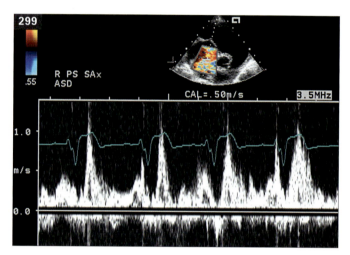

298 Flow from LA to RA is seen in this diastolic frame with color flow Doppler. (**299**) PW Doppler with sample volume placed at the interatrial septum shows variable left-to-right flow throughout the cardiac cycle. Right parasternal long-axis (**297**, **298**) and short-axis (**299**) views. LA = left atrium; LV = left ventricle; RA = right atrium; RV = right ventricle.

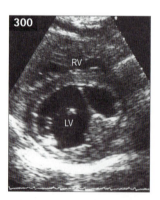
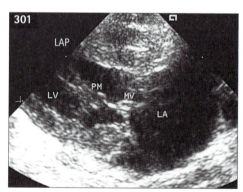
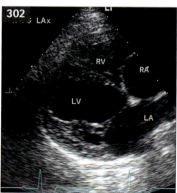
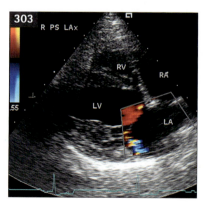

300–303 (**300**) Right parasternal short-axis view of asymmetrical papillary muscles and abnormal chordae in a cat with Mdys. (**301**) Abnormal mitral apparatus and LA enlargement in a 3-week-old Pomeranian with Mdys. (**302**) Shortened mitral chordae with an abnormal papillary muscle in a 2-year-old male Bull Terrier with mild Mdys (**303**) Only minor mitral regurgitation was present in this dog. LA = left atrium; LV = left ventricle; MV = mitral valve; PM = papillary muscle; RV = right ventricle. (**301–303**) Right parasternal long-axis views.

papillary muscle, thickened or cleft or shortened valve leaflets, prolapse of valve leaflets, upwardly displaced or malformed papillary muscles, and excessive dilation of the valve annulus[1, 88, 89]. Valvular regurgitation is the usual functional abnormality and this ranges from mild to severe. The pathophysiology and sequelae are similar to those in animals with acquired MR (see Chapter 19). LV function declines with time[1].

Stenosis of the mitral valve orifice is relatively uncommon[90–92]. It usually coexists with regurgitation. LV inflow obstruction increases the LA pressure and can precipitate pulmonary edema.

CLINICAL FEATURES

Mitral valve dysplasia is most common in large breed dogs and also occurs in cats (*Table 51*, p. 228). Except for the young age of the affected animal, clinical signs seen with mitral dysplasia are similar to those in older dogs with degenerative mitral valve disease. Exercise intolerance, respiratory signs of left-sided CHF, and atrial arrhythmias, especially AF, commonly develop. The systolic murmur of MR is heard at the left apex.

DIAGNOSIS

The radiographic, ECG, echocardiographic, and catheterization findings associated with regurgitant mitral dysplasia are similar to those seen in patients with mitral degenerative disease (see Chapter 19). Echocardiography can identify malformations of the mitral apparatus as well as LV and LA dilation (300–303). Mitral stenosis is characterized by restricted valve opening with a diastolic transmitral pressure gradient, prolonged mitral inflow time (pressure half-time), and increased E and A wave velocities (304–308)[91].

MANAGEMENT

Medical management for CHF as needed is the usual therapy. Animals with only mild to moderate

304–307 (304) Diastolic image shows restricted maximal mitral opening and marked LA enlargement in a 7-year-old female Labrador Retriever with mitral stenosis, AF, and pulmonary edema. (305) Color flow Doppler illustrates diastolic flow acceleration across the stenotic valve in this dog. (306) M-mode at the mitral level from a 6-year-old female Irish Setter shows parallel motion of both mitral leaflets characteristic of mitral stenosis; sinus rhythm with one atrial premature beat is seen. (307) PW Doppler of mitral inflow during one cycle from the dog in 306 demonstrates prolonged transvalvular diastolic pressure gradient (compare with 159 (normal), p. 83). LA = left atrium; LV = left ventricle. 304, 305, and 307 from left apical position.

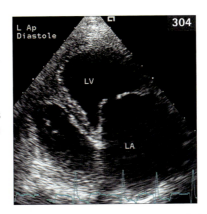

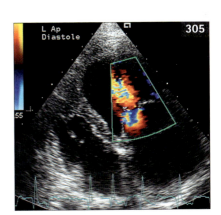

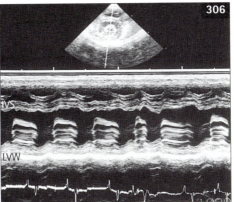

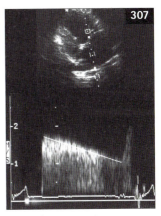

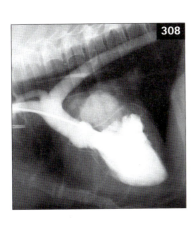

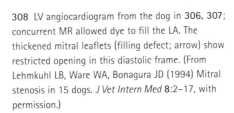

308 LV angiocardiogram from the dog in 306, 307; concurrent MR allowed dye to fill the LA. The thickened mitral leaflets (filling defect; arrow) show restricted opening in this diastolic frame. (From Lehmkuhl LB, Ware WA, Bonagura JD (1994) Mitral stenosis in 15 dogs. *J Vet Intern Med* 8:2–17, with permission.)

malformations do well for years. The prognosis is poor with severe regurgitation or stenosis. Surgical valve reconstruction or replacement is sometimes an option.

TRICUSPID DYSPLASIA

PATHOPHYSIOLOGY

Malformations of the tricuspid valve and its support apparatus are similar to those with mitral valve dysplasia (**309**)[93, 94]. In some cases the tricuspid valve is displaced ventrally into the ventricle (an Ebstein-like anomaly)[95]. The prevalence of ventricular preexcitation (Wolff–Parkinson–White syndrome) may be increased in such animals[96]. The pathophysiologic features relate to right heart volume overload and progressive RA and RV dilation. Increasing end-diastolic pressure eventually results in right-sided congestive failure. Tricuspid stenosis occurs rarely[1, 97].

CLINICAL FEATURES

Tricuspid dysplasia is diagnosed most frequently in large breed dogs; heritability has been demonstrated in Labrador Retrievers[98]. It may occur more often in males[99]. Cats are also affected. The historical signs and clinical findings are similar to those seen with advanced degenerative tricuspid disease[93, 100]. Initially, the animal may be asymptomatic or mildly exercise intolerant, but fatigue, ascites, dyspnea from pleural effusion, anorexia, and cardiac cachexia frequently develop. Physical features include the murmur of tricuspid regurgitation (not always audible) and jugular vein pulsations. Jugular vein distension, muffled heart and lung sounds, and ballotable abdominal fluid develop in animals with congestive failure.

DIAGNOSIS

Right heart enlargement is visible radiographically (see **48, 49**, p. 40). Sometimes, the heart shadow is quite round, similar to that seen with pericardial effusion or DCM. Caudal vena cava distension, pleural or peritoneal effusion, and hepatomegaly are often evident.

The ECG usually shows RV and, occasionally, RA enlargement. The QRS complex may appear splintered (**310**)[94, 99]. Atrial arrhythmias, including AF or atrial tachycardia, commonly develop (**311**). Evidence for ventricular preexcitation is sometimes seen[96].

Echocardiography depicts the often massive right heart dilation. Malformations of the valve apparatus may also be appreciated in multiple views (**312–316**), although the left parasternal apical four-chamber view appears to be especially useful[94]. Intracardiac electrocardiography is necessary to confirm the presence of Ebstein's anomaly, which is suggested by displacement of the tricuspid valve toward the RV. A ventricular electrogram recorded above the tricuspid valve is diagnostic.

MANAGEMENT

CHF and arrhythmias are managed medically (see Chapters 16 and 17). Periodic thoracocentesis may also be required. The prognosis is guarded, especially with marked cardiomegaly; however, some animals survive for years. Tricuspid stenosis has been successfully managed with balloon dilation[97, 101].

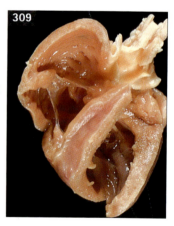

309 Cranioventral view of opened RV (upper left in photo) and LV (lower right) from a Pekingese puppy with bilateral AV valve dysplasia. A large abnormal papillary muscle is fused directly to the parietal tricuspid leaflet.

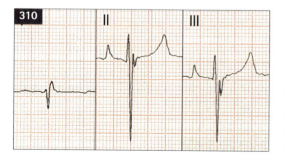

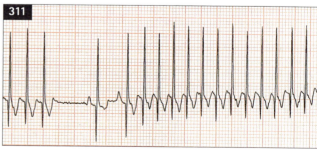

310, 311 (310) QRS complexes appear splintered, especially in leads II and III in a male Labrador Retriever with Tdys. ECG leads as marked; 50 mm/sec, 1 cm = 1 mV. **(311)** Paroxysmal atrial tachycardia in a 3-month-old female Labrador Retriever with Tdys and CHF. Lead II, 25 mm/sec, 1 cm = 1 mV.

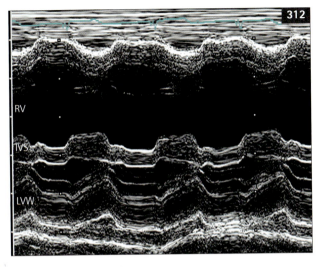

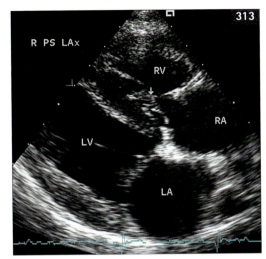

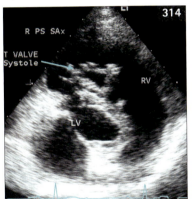

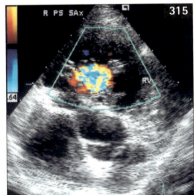

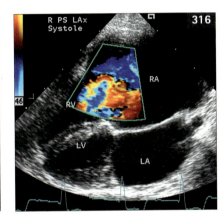

312–316 (312) Marked RV dilation with paradoxical IVS motion is seen in this M-mode echocardiogram from a male cat with Tdys and congestive failure. **(313)** 2-D long-axis image in systole shows an abnormal, tethered-down septal tricuspid leaflet (arrow) that caused moderate tricuspid regurgitation and right heart dilation in a 3-year-old female Labrador Retriever. **(314)** Systolic short-axis view in a 3-year-old male Golden Retriever with Tdys demonstrates a wide gap at the commissure of this closed T valve (arrow). **(315)** Color flow Doppler illustrates regurgitation through the incompetent valve shown in **314**. **(316)** Long-axis image from the cat in **312** shows marked tricuspid regurgitation and a huge RA. Images from right parasternal position. IVS = interventricular septum; LA = left atrium; LV = left ventricle; LVW = left ventricular wall; RA = right atrium; RV = right ventricle.

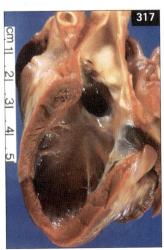

317 The large VSD, with overriding aorta above, is seen from the left in this postmortem specimen from an English Springer Spaniel puppy with T of F.

TETRALOGY OF FALLOT

PATHOPHYSIOLOGY

The anomalies that comprise T of F are VSD, PS, dextropositioning of the aorta, and RV hypertrophy[1]. The VSD is often quite large **(317)**. The PS may involve the valve or infundibular area; sometimes, the pulmonary artery is hypoplastic or atretic (pseudotruncus arteriosus). The rightward shift of the aortic root causes it to override the interventricular septum and facilitates RV-to-aortic shunting. Aortic anomalies also occur in some animals.

RV hypertrophy is secondary to the pressure overload imposed by the PS and systemic arterial circulation. The amount of RV-to-aortic shunting depends on the degree of outflow resistance caused by the fixed PS compared with the degree of systemic arterial resistance, which can vary. Right-to-left shunt volume increases with exercise and other causes of reduced systemic arterial resistance. The pulmonary vascular resistance is normal with T of F.

CLINICAL FEATURES

The inheritance pattern for T of F has been studied in the Keeshond[102, 103]. The defect also occurs in other dog breeds and in cats. A history of syncope, exertional weakness, dyspnea, cyanosis, and stunted growth is common[1, 104]. Physical findings vary with the relative severity of the disease components. Cyanosis is seen at rest in some animals (318); others have pink mucous membranes at rest, but cyanosis usually becomes evident with exercise. The right precordial impulse may be equal to or stronger than that on the left. A precordial thrill may be palpable at the right sternal border or left basilar area, but this is an inconsistent finding. Jugular pulsation may be noted. Auscultation may reveal a holosystolic murmur at the right sternal border compatible with a VSD, or a systolic ejection murmur at the left base compatible with PS, or both. But no murmur is heard in some animals because hyperviscosity associated with polycythemia reduces blood turbulence (see Chapter 1, p. 21).

DIAGNOSIS

Arterial hypoxemia and an elevated PCV are the usual laboratory abnormalities (319).

Cardiomegaly, usually of the right heart, is variably seen on thoracic radiographs (Table 52, p. 231). The main pulmonary artery may appear small, although sometimes a bulge is evident. Pulmonary vascular markings are usually reduced, but a compensatory enhancement of the bronchial circulation will increase overall pulmonary opacity. The malpositioned aorta appears to bulge cranially on lateral views. The thick RV displaces the left heart dorsally, simulating left heart enlargement (320, 321).

The ECG typically indicates RV hypertrophy, although a left axis deviation is occasionally seen in affected cats.

Echocardiography shows the VSD, a large aortic root shifted rightward and overriding the ventricular septum, some degree of PS, and RV hypertrophy (322, 323). Doppler studies reveal the right-to-left shunt and high velocity stenotic pulmonary outflow jet. An echo-contrast study or angiocardiogram also can document the right-to-left shunt (324, 325).

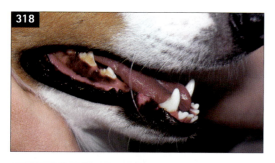

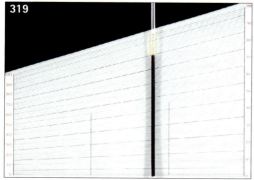

318, 319 (318) Mildly cyanotic tongue in a 2-year-old male Collie with T of F. (Courtesy Dr JO Noxon.) (319) Severe polycythemia (PCV = 0.84 l/l [84%]) was identified in a 3-year-old Lhasa Apso with T of F.

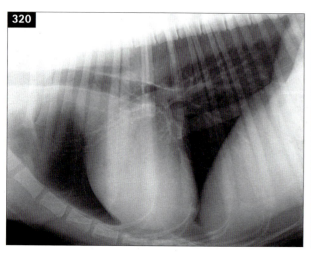

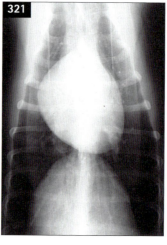

320, 321 Radiographs from the dog in 318 show RV enlargement, a bulge in the area of the aortic arch, and small pulmonary vessels.

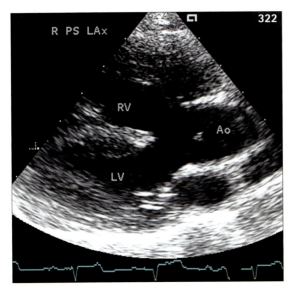

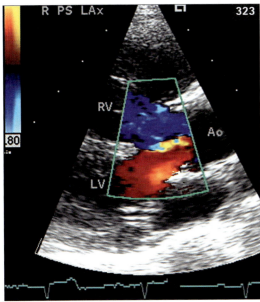

322, 323 (322) Right parasternal long-axis view from the dog in 317 shows the large VSD with wide, overriding aortic root. (323) Color flow Doppler demonstrates flow from both ventricles entering the aorta. Ao = aorta; LV = left ventricle; RV = right ventricle.

MANAGEMENT

Definitive surgical repair requires open-heart surgery[105]. Palliative procedures can increase pulmonary blood flow by surgically creating a left-to-right shunt. Anastomosis of a subclavian artery to the pulmonary artery and the creation of a window between the ascending aorta and pulmonary artery are two techniques that have been used successfully[104, 106].

Periodic phlebotomy has been used to treat severe polycythemia and clinical signs associated with hyperviscosity (e.g. weakness, shortness of breath, seizures). A volume of blood is withdrawn, and sometimes replaced with isotonic fluid, to maintain the PCV at a level where clinical signs are minimal (see p. 253). Further reduction in PCV can exacerbate signs of hypoxia. Alternatively, hydroxyurea might be useful for reducing polycythemia (see p. 254). A beta-adrenergic blocker may help some animals with T of F. Reduction of sympathetic tone, RV contractility, RV (muscular) outflow obstruction, and myocardial oxygen consumption, along with increased peripheral vascular resistance, are thought to be benefits of beta-blocker therapy in children with the disease[1]. Exercise restriction is also important. Systemic vasodilating drugs should not be given.

The prognosis for T of F depends on the degree of PS and polycythemia. Mildly affected animals or those that have undergone successful palliative surgical shunting procedures have lived for years; however, progressive hypoxemia, polycythemia, and sudden death at an earlier age are common[1, 104].

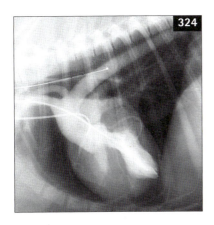

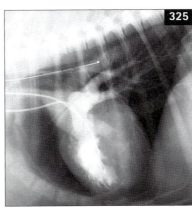

324, 325 Angiocardiograms from the dog in 318. (324) LV injection shows a large aortic root overriding the hypertrophied IVS. Bidirectional shunting is evident from the dye seen in the RV outflow region and pulmonary arteries. The hypertrophied RV has lifted the LV apex dorsally. (325) RV injection via the same catheter as in 324, which was passed from the carotid artery to the ascending aorta then into the RV; dye in the aorta and LV illustrates right-to-left shunting. Poststenotic dilation of the main PA is evident. (Courtesy Drs J O Noxon and S McNeel.)

PULMONARY HYPERTENSION WITH SHUNT REVERSAL

PATHOPHYSIOLOGY

Normally, the low-resistance pulmonary vascular system can accept increased blood flow without marked increase in pulmonary arterial pressure. However, pulmonary hypertension develops in a relatively small percent of dogs and cats with shunts such as PDA, VSD, ASD, AV septal defect, and aorticopulmonary window[107]. The associated defect in these animals is usually large (326–328). Irreversible histologic changes develop in the pulmonary arteries and these increase vascular resistance. These include intimal thickening, medial hypertrophy, and characteristic plexiform lesions[108]. As pulmonary resistance increases, pulmonary artery pressure rises and the left-to-right shunt volume diminishes. If pulmonary pressure exceeds that of the systemic circulation, the shunt reverses direction and unoxygenated blood flows into the aorta. It appears that these changes develop at an early age, although exceptions may occur. The term Eisenmenger's physiology refers to the pulmonary hypertension and shunt reversal that develop.

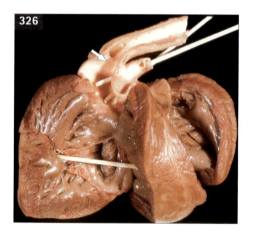 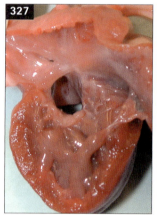 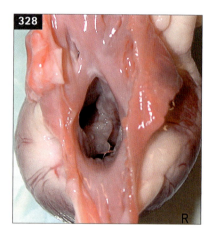

326–328 (326) Speciman from a young female Cocker Spaniel with reversed PDA. The RV is open from inflow to outflow regions; the cut extends into the main pulmonary trunk, through the large PDA (arrow), and into the descending aorta. Two wooden probes are inserted at the pulmonary artery bifurcation. Note the RV hypertrophy and thick ductal wall. (327) View from the right side showing RV hypertrophy and a large AV septal (endocardial cushion) defect with malformed tricuspid valve in a 5-month-old kitten. The enlarged RA and auricle are at the top of the photo. Pulmonary hypertension caused right-to-left shunting. (328) From the kitten in 327: top-down view from the RA through the common AV annulus showing the top of the IVS with malformed septal tricuspid and mitral leaflets. The LV is to the upper left of the septal ridge, the RV opening is below.

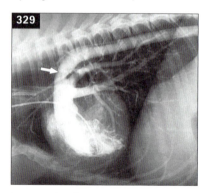 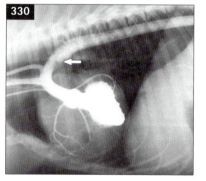 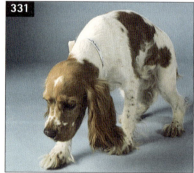

329–331 (329) RV angiocardiogram from an 8-month-old female Cocker Spaniel with reversed PDA. Opacified blood flows from the hypertrophied RV to the dilated pulmonary trunk and into the descending aorta via the large ductus (arrow; see also 326). (330) Relatively small LV appears perched atop the large RV. Note that the brachycephalic and left subclavian arteries exit the aorta upstream from the area of the PDA (arrow). Dye is diluted in the descending aorta because of mixing with unopacified blood entering across the ductus. (331) Hindlimb weakness was the presenting complaint in this dog. (329, 330 from Ware WA (2003) Common congenital cardiac anomalies. In *Small Animal Internal Medicine* (3rd edn). (eds RW Nelson, CG Couto) Mosby, St Louis, p.165, with permission.)

Pathophysiologic and clinical sequelae are similar to those produced by T of F, although the impediment to pulmonary flow occurs at the pulmonary arteriolar level rather than at the pulmonic valve. Hypoxemia, RV hypertrophy and enlargement, polycythemia and its consequences, and increased shunting with exercise occur. Likewise, right-sided congestive failure is uncommon, but may develop in response to secondary myocardial failure or tricuspid insufficiency. The right-to-left shunt may allow venous emboli to cross into the arterial system, causing stroke or other arterial embolization.

CLINICAL FEATURES

The history and clinical presentation are similar to those associated with T of F. Exercise intolerance, shortness of breath, syncope (especially with exercise or excitement), seizures, and sudden death are common. Cough and hemoptysis may also occur. Cyanosis (see 20, p. 29) may be evident only during exercise or excitement. Classically, cyanosis of the caudal mucous membranes alone (differential cyanosis) is caused by reversed PDA[109]. In this case the cranial body receives normally oxygenated blood via the brachycephalic trunk and left subclavian artery, which arise from the aortic arch upstream from the ductus (329–331). Hindlimb weakness is typical in animals with reversed PDA. Intracardiac shunts cause equally intense cyanosis throughout the body.

A murmur typical of the underlying defect, or defects, may be present, but often no murmur or only a very soft systolic murmur is heard because of increased blood viscosity with polycythemia. There is no continuous murmur with reversed PDA. With pulmonary hypertension, the S_2 may be loud and 'snapping' or split (332). A gallop sound is occasionally heard. Other subtle physical examination findings include a pronounced right precordial impulse and jugular pulsations.

DIAGNOSIS

Thoracic radiographs usually show right heart enlargement, a prominent pulmonary trunk, tortuous and proximally widened pulmonary arteries, and, sometimes, a dilated caudal vena cava (333–336, and see 57, p. 43). A bulge in the descending aorta can be seen with reversed PDA. The left heart may also be enlarged with reversed PDA or VSD.

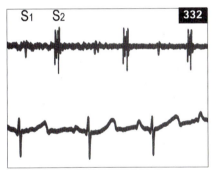

332 Phonocardiogram (top) depicts the snapping, split S_2 sound heard in the dog in 329–331. No murmur was audible. ECG on bottom of trace.

333–334 Chest radiographs from another female Cocker Spaniel with reversed PDA, diagnosed at 3 years of age, show RV enlargement; both a ductus bump (arrowhead) and wide pulmonary trunk bulge (arrow) are seen on the DV view (334).

335, 336 Radiographs from a kitten with a reversed-shunting AV septal defect indicate massive cardiomegaly with right heart predominance. Dilated and tortuous pulmonary vessels are seen on both views, with a bulge in the area of the main pulmonary artery (arrow) seen on the DV view (336).

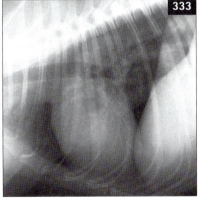

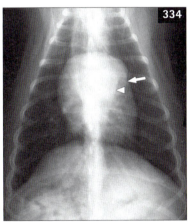

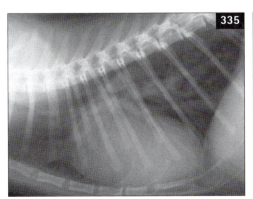

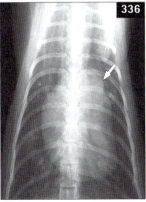

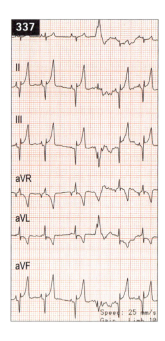

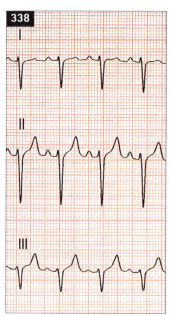

337, 338 (337) ECG from the dog in **333** and **334** shows right axis deviation, sinus rhythm with one VPC (4th complex from left), and mild ST segment elevation in the caudal leads. **(338)** ECG from the kitten in **335** and **336** also shows right axis deviation and sinus rhythm; large QRS complexes and wide P waves are also present. Leads as marked; 25 mm/sec **(337)** and 50 mm/sec **(338)**, 1 cm = 1 mV.

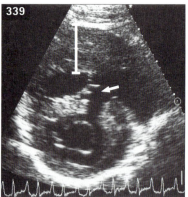

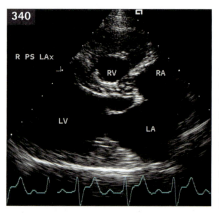

339, 340 (339) Right parasternal short-axis view from a cat with reversed VSD (see also **57**, p. 43 from same case); a large septal defect (arrow) and marked RV wall hypertrophy (bar) are evident. **(340)** Long-axis view from a 2-year-old male Akita with a large ASD, exercise intolerance, and cyanosis (see bubble study in **137**, p. 76). LA = left atrium; LV = left ventricle; RA = right atrium; RV = right ventricle.

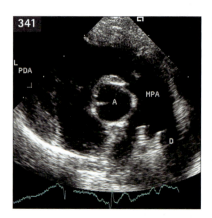

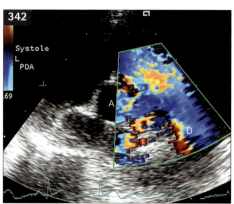

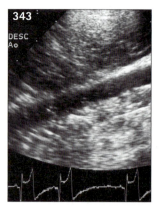

341–343 (341) Left cranial angled 2-D view shows the main pulmonary artery and aortic root in a male Sheltie puppy with reversed PDA. The pulmonary bifurcation is seen, although the echo plane is not optimized for maximal dimension, so that the large ductus can be visualized to the right (D). **(342)** Same view as in **341** with color flow Doppler added showing right-to-left flow through the ductus. **(343)** Echo-contrast study from a female Cocker Spaniel with reversed PDA shows bubbles in the descending aorta after cephalic vein injection of agitated saline. A = aorta; D = ductus; MPA = main pulmonary artery; PDA = patent ductus arteriosis.

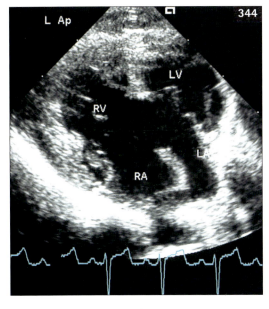

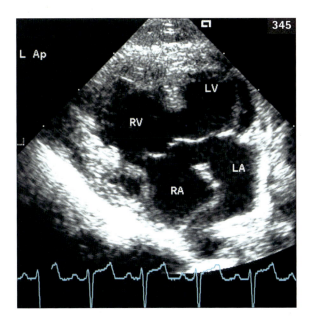

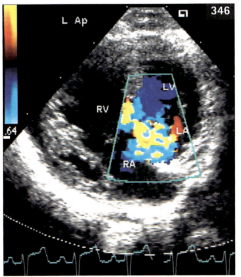

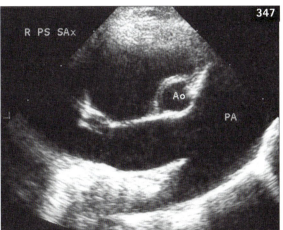

344–347 Left apical 2-D view from the kitten in **335** and **336**. Large primum (low) ASD is seen merged with a high VSD. Malformed AV valves can be seen open in diastole (**344**) and closed in systole (**345**); note also the RV hypertrophy. (**346**) Color flow Doppler demonstrates the right-to-left shunt (systole). (**347**) Massive pulmonary artery dilation (secondary to pulmonary hypertension) is also seen in this case; right short-axis view. Ao = aorta; LA = left atrium; LV = left ventricle; RA = right atrium; RV = right ventricle.

The ECG usually indicates RV and, sometimes, RA enlargement, with a right axis deviation (**337, 338**, p. 252).

Echocardiography demonstrates the RV hypertrophy, a widened pulmonary trunk, and intracardiac anatomic defects. Doppler or echo-contrast study can confirm the presence of an intracardiac right-to-left shunt (**339–347**, pp. 252, 253). Reversed PDA flow can be shown by imaging the abdominal aorta during venous echo-contrast injection (**343**). Measurement of the peak velocity of a tricuspid (or pulmonic) regurgitation jet, allows estimation of RV systolic and, in the absence of PS, pulmonary artery pressure. Cardiac catheterization can confirm the diagnosis and quantify the pulmonary hypertension and systemic hypoxemia (**329–330**, p. 250).

MANAGEMENT

Surgical closure of the reversed shunt is contraindicated. Therapy previously has been limited mainly to exercise restriction and total RBC number reduction to minimize signs of hyperviscosity; however, the phosphodiesterase 5 inhibitor sildenafil citrate reduces pulmonary resistance in at least some cases.

Doses of 0.5–2 mg/kg have been used with anecdotal improvement in clinical signs, although further study is needed (see also Chapter 23, p. 348). Low-dose aspirin (e.g. 5 mg/kg) therapy may also be beneficial.

Periodic phlebotomy to maintain PCV at about 62% has previously been recommended. This can be accomplished by removing 5–10 ml blood/kg body weight and replacing it with an equal volume of isotonic fluid; however, using PCV alone to guide treatment is questionable. Phlebotomy done only when manifestations of hyperviscosity (e.g. hindlimb weakness, shortness of breath, or lethargy) occur has been successful[5]. In the technique described, 10% of circulating blood volume (calculated in ml as 8.5% x body weight (kg) x 1,000 g/kg x 1 ml/g) is removed initially without replacement fluids. After 3–6 hours of cage rest, more blood is removed if the patient's initial PCV was >0.6 l/l (>60%). According to this report, if the PCV initially was between 0.6 l/l and 0.7 l/l (60% and 70%), an additional 5–10% of circulating blood volume is removed; if the initial PCV was >0.7 l/l (>70%), an additional 10–18% is withdrawn[5].

Long-term hydroxyurea therapy (40–50 mg/kg PO q48h or 3 times a week) may be a useful alternative to periodic phlebotomy[110]. A CBC and platelet count should be monitored weekly or biweekly initially, with a suggested target PCV of 0.55–0.6 l/l (55–60%). Potential adverse effects include anorexia, vomiting, bone marrow hypoplasia, alopecia, and pruritus. The dose can be divided twice daily on treatment days, or administered twice a week, or at <40 mg/kg depending on the patient's response. Most vasodilating drugs tend to have systemic effects equal to or greater than their effects on the pulmonary arterial system; therefore, they are of little benefit and possibly detrimental. The prognosis is generally poor, but some cases have done well for several years.

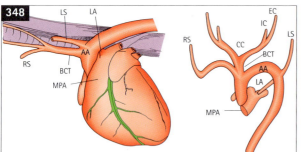

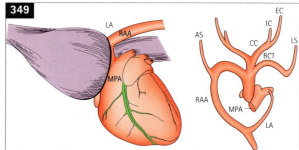

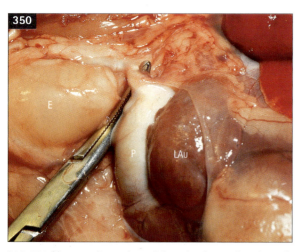

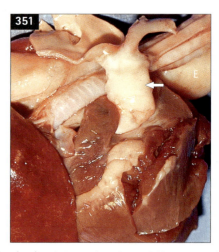

348–351 Diagrams of normal vessel formation from embryonic aortic arches (348) and abnormal, persistent right aortic arch (349). (From Ellison GW (1980) Vascular ring anomalies in the dog and cat. *Compend Cont Educ Pract Vet* 11:693-705, with permission.) (350) Postmortem *in situ* view from the left in a 7-week-old female Chow Chow-cross with PRAA, PDA, and VSD. Hemostat tip is under the PDA; the dilated cranial esophagus is to the left. (351) View from the right shows the right aortic arch (arrow) crossing over the trachea and esophagus; cranial esophageal dilation is to the right in the photo. AA = aortic arch; BCT = brachiocephalic trunk; CC = common carotid; E = esophagus; EC = external carotid; IC = internal carotid; LA = ligamentum arteriosum; Lau = left auricle; LS = left subclavian artery; MPA = main pulmonary artery; P = pulmonary artery; RAA = right aortic arch; RS = right subclavian artery.

VASCULAR RING ANOMALIES

PATHOPHYSIOLOGY

Various malformations of vessels arising from the embryonic aortic arches can occur[111-115]. These may entrap the esophagus and sometimes the trachea within a vascular ring over the heart base. The most common vascular ring anomaly in the dog is the persistent right aortic arch (PRAA), which encloses the esophagus dorsally and to the right with the aortic arch, to the left with the ligamentum arteriosum, and ventrally with the base of the heart (348–351). Additional vascular anomalies, such as a left cranial vena cava or PDA, sometimes coexist with a vascular ring anomaly. Vascular ring anomalies are rare in cats.

CLINICAL FEATURES

Regurgitation and stunted growth commonly develop within 6 months of weaning in affected animals, because the vascular ring prevents solid food from passing normally through the esophagus (352–354). The esophagus dilates cranial to the ring and may retain food. Occasionally, esophageal dilation caudal to the stricture occurs as well, indicating that altered esophageal motility may also be a factor. Respiratory signs such as cough, wheezing, and cyanosis usually signal secondary aspiration pneumonia, although a double aortic arch may cause stridor and other respiratory signs secondary to tracheal stenosis. The animal may appear clinically normal, although thin, but generally becomes progressively debilitated. In some animals a dilated cervical esophagus (containing food or gas) can be palpated at the thoracic inlet. Aspiration pneumonia often causes fever as well as respiratory signs. No murmur is heard unless another cardiac defect is concurrent.

DIAGNOSIS

Leftward deviation of the trachea near the cranial heart border (DV or VD view) is a consistent radiographic sign of PRAA[116]. Focal tracheal narrowing and ventral displacement cranial to the heart (lateral view) as well as cranial mediastinal widening are also common. Air or food may be seen in the cranial esophagus (355) and there may be evidence of aspiration pneumonia. A barium swallow depicts the esophageal stricture over the heart base and cranial esophageal dilation, with or without caudal esophageal dilation (356).

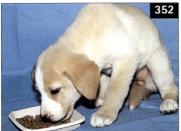

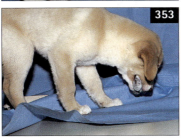

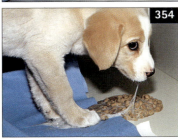

352–354 Eating solid food (352) is soon followed by regurgitation (353, 354) in this puppy with PRAA.

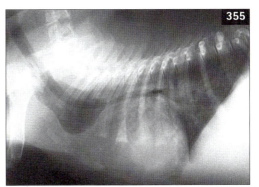

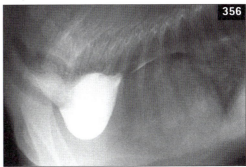

355, 356 (355) An air-filled esophageal dilation cranial to the heart base is seen in this lateral radiograph from a Chow Chow-cross puppy. Cardiomegaly from concurrent PDA and VSD is also evident. (356) Barium swallow illustrates the extent of the esophageal dilation.

MANAGEMENT

Therapy involves surgical division of the ligamentum arteriosum, or other vessel if the anomaly is not a PRAA. Some dogs have a coexisting retroesophageal left subclavian artery or left aortic arch (possibly atretic), which must also be identified and divided for a successful outcome[116]. A thoracoscopic technique also has been reported[117]. Medical management consists of giving frequent, small, semisolid or liquid meals in an upright position for an indefinite time. Most dogs become clinically normal after successful surgery, but some experience persistent regurgitation, indicating a permanent esophageal motility disorder[118].

COR TRIATRIATUM

PATHOPHYSIOLOGY

This uncommon malformation is caused by an abnormal membrane that divides the right (dexter) or left (sinister) atrium into two chambers. There are several reports of cor triatriatum dexter (CTD) in dogs[119-123]. Cor triatriatum sinister has only been described rarely (cat)[1, 124]. The intraatrial membrane of CTD results from failure of the embryonic right sinus venosus valve to regress. The caudal vena cava and coronary sinus empty into the caudal RA chamber; the tricuspid orifice is within the cranial RA chamber. Obstruction to venous flow through the abnormal membrane increases hydrostatic pressure within the caudal vena cava and abdominal structures.

CLINICAL FEATURES

Large to mid-sized breeds of dog are most often affected with CTD. Development of persistent ascites at an early age is the most prominent clinical sign (see 193, p. 121). Exercise intolerance, lethargy, distended cutaneous abdominal veins, and, sometimes, diarrhea are also reported (357). Neither a cardiac murmur nor jugular venous distension are features of this anomaly.

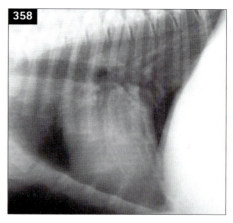

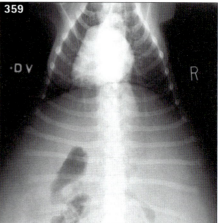

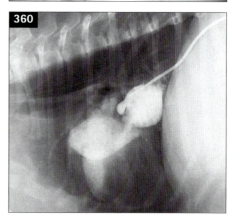

358–360 (358, 359) A normal heart size with caudal vena cava distension and massive ascites are seen in the dog in 357. (360) Caudal vena cava angiogram from a 5-month-old male Pit Bull Terrier with CTD shows a filling defect in the caudal RA caused by the abnormal intra-RA membrane; distension of the caudal RA and proximal caudal vena cava are also evident.

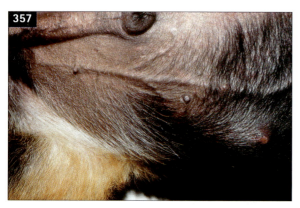

357 Distended abdominal veins and massive ascites are seen in this 5-month-old male Rottweiler with CTD.

DIAGNOSIS

Thoracic radiographs show a distended caudal vena cava without generalized cardiomegaly in CTD. Massive ascites may displace the diaphragm cranially (358–360). The ECG is generally normal. Echocardiography shows the abnormal membrane with prominent caudal RA chamber and vena cava. Doppler studies allow intra-RA pressure gradient estimation and flow disturbance visualization (361–364).

MANAGEMENT

Successful therapy requires enlarging the membrane orifice or excising the abnormal membrane to remove flow obstruction. This can be done surgically[120, 121] or by percutaneous balloon dilation of the membrane orifice[123, 125], as long as a large enough balloon is used. The simultaneous placement of several balloon dilation catheters can be successful in larger dogs.

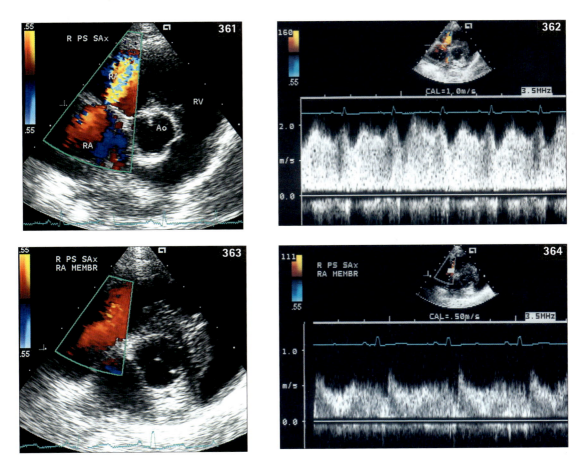

361–364 Right parasternal short-axis images from a 5-month-old Pit Bull Terrier with CTD. (361) The discrete intra-RA membrane obstructs flow from the caudal to the cranial RA, as shown with color flow Doppler. (362) PW Doppler, sampled at the membrane, shows increased flow velocity throughout systole and diastole within the RA (estimated mean gradient ~11 mm Hg). (363) Same view as 361 after triple-balloon dilation of the CTD membrane; low velocity laminar flow is seen. The clinical signs resolved and did not recur. (364) Postdilation PW Doppler shows lower intra-RA velocities (note scale on right; estimated mean gradient ~1 mm Hg).

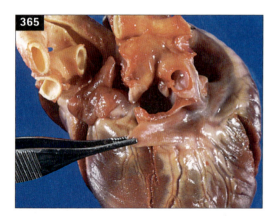

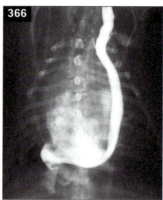

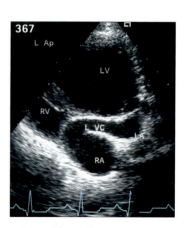

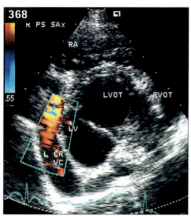

365–368 (365) View from the left dorsal aspect of the heart from an English Springer Spaniel with multiple congenital defects. Forceps grasp the transected edge of a PLCVC. This vessel courses along the AV junction caudal to the LA (cut open above) and enters the caudal RA at the coronary sinus. (366) Left jugular venogram from an old Boston Terrier shows a PLCVC; note the vessel's course to the left and caudal around the LA before entering the RA. A large heart base mass caused tracheal deviation to the right in this dog. (Courtesy Dr E Riedesel) PLCVC = persistent left cranial vena cava. (367) Modified left apical 4-chamber view (angled caudally) in a 9-month-old male Rottweiler shows a PLCVC just caudal to the LA as it enters the RA. (368) Modified right short-axis view with color flow Doppler from the same dog shows flow in the PLCVC at the caudal AV junction toward the RA. LA = left atrium; LV = left ventricle; L VC, L CR VC, and PLCVC = persistent left cranial vena cava; LVOT = left ventricular outflow tract; RA = right atrium; RV = right ventricle; RVOT = right ventricular outflow tract.

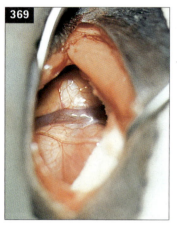

369 Intraoperative view of a PLCVC crossing the heart along the left AV junction in a dog. Cranial is to the left, dorsal at top.

OTHER VASCULAR ANOMALIES

Various venous anomalies have been described, and they are often not clinically relevant. The persistent left cranial vena cava is a fetal venous remnant; it courses lateral to the left AV groove and empties into the coronary sinus of the caudal RA (365–368)[1, 126, 127]. It causes no clinical signs but may complicate surgical exposure of other structures at the left heart base (369). Portosystemic venous shunts, however, are common and can lead to hepatic encephalopathy as well as other signs[128]. These malformations are thought to be more prevalent in the Yorkshire Terrier, Pug, Miniature and Standard Schnauzer, Maltese, Pekingese, Shih Tzu, and Lhasa Apso breeds.

ENDOCARDIAL FIBROELASTOSIS

This congenital abnormality is characterized by diffuse fibrosis and elastic thickening of the endocardium. It more commonly affects cats, especially Burmese and Siamese, but has also been observed rarely in dogs[6, 129, 130]. Left-sided or biventricular heart failure usually develops early in life. The murmur of MR may be present. Criteria for LV and LA enlargement are seen on radiographs, ECG, and echocardiogram. Evidence for reduced LV myocardial function and increased stiffness may be present. Definitive antemortem diagnosis may be difficult.

REFERENCES

1 Bonagura JD, Lehmkuhl LB (1999) Congenital heart disease. In: *Textbook of Canine and Feline Cardiology*, 2nd edn. PR Fox, D Sisson, NS Moise (eds). WB Saunders, Philadelphia, pp. 471–535.

2 Buchanan JW (1999) Prevalence of cardiovascular disorders. In: *Textbook of Canine and Feline Cardiology*, 2nd edn. PR Fox, D Sisson, NS Moise NS (eds). WB Saunders, Philadelphia, pp. 457–470.

3 Lamb CR, Boswood A, Volkman A *et al.* (2001) Assessment of survey radiography as a method for diagnosis of congenital cardiac disease in dogs. *J Small Anim Pract* 42:541–545.

4 Kienle RD, Thomas WP, Pion PD (1994) The natural history of canine congenital subaortic stenosis. *J Vet Intern Med* 8:423–431.

5 Cote E, Ettinger SJ (2001) Long-term clinical management of right-to-left ('reversed') patent ductus arteriosus in 3 dogs. *J Vet Intern Med* 15:39–42.

6 Tidholm A (1997) Retrospective study of congenital heart defects in 151 dogs. *J Small Anim Pract* 38:94–98.

7 Buchanan JW (2003) Patent ductus arteriosus. *Semin Vet Med Surg* 9:168–176.

8 Buchanan JW, Patterson DF (2003) Etiology of patent dutus arteriosus in dogs. *J Vet Intern Med* 17:167–171.

9 Larsson MHMA, Baccaro MR, Pereira L (1997) Endocardial fibroelastosis in a dog. *J Small Anim Pract* 38:168–170.

10 Pyle RL, Patterson DF, Chacko S (1976) The genetics and pathology of discrete subaortic stenosis in the Newfoundland dog. *Am Heart J* 92:324–334.

11 Buoscio DA, Sisson D, Zachary JF *et al.* (1994) Clinical and pathological characterization of an unusual form of subvalvular aortic stenosis in four golden retriever puppies. *J Am Anim Hosp Assoc* 30:100–110.

12 Nakayama T, Wakao Y, Ishikawa R *et al.* (1996) Progression of subaortic stenosis detected by continuous wave Doppler echocardiography in a dog. *J Vet Intern Med* 10:97–98.

13 French A, Luis Fuentes V, Dukes-McEwan J *et al.* (2000) Progression of aortic stenosis in the Boxer. *J Small Anim Pract* 41:451–456.

14 Bonagura JD (2001) Problems in the canine left ventricular outflow tract. Editorial. *J Vet Intern Med* 15:427–429.

15 Pyle RL (2000) Interpreting low-intensity cardiac murmurs in dogs predisposed to subaortic stenosis. Editorial. *J Am Anim Hosp Assoc* 36:379–382.

16 Falk T, Jonsson L, Pedersen HD (2004) Intramyocardial arterial narrowing in dogs with subaortic stenosis. *J Small Anim Pract* 45:448–453.

17 Lehmkuhl LB, Bonagura JD (1994) Comparison of transducer placement sites for Doppler echocardiography in dogs with subaortic stenosis. *Am J Vet Res* 55:192–198.

18 Muna WFT, Ferrans VJ, Pierce JE *et al.* (1978) Discrete subaortic stenosis in Newfoundland dogs: association of infective endocarditis. *Am J Cardiol* 41:746–754.

19 Stepien RL, Bonagura JD (1991) Aortic stenosis: clinical findings in six cats. *J Small Anim Pract* 32:341–350.

20 Lehmkuhl LB, Bonagura JD, Jones DE *et al.* (1995) Comparison of catheterization and Doppler-derived pressure gradients in a canine model of subaortic stenosis. *J Am Soc Echocardiogr* 8:611–620.

21 Bonagura JD, Miller MW, Darke PGG (1998) Doppler echocardiography I. *Vet Clin N Amer* 28:1325–1359.

22 Bussadori C, Amberger C, LeBobinnec G *et al.* (2000) Guidelines for the echocardiographic studies of suspected subaortic and pulmonic stenosis. *J Vet Cardiol* 2:17–24.

23 Abbott JA, Duncan R, Clark EG *et al.* (2001) Aortic valve disease in Boxers with physical and echocardiographic findings of aortic stenosis. Abstract. *J Vet Intern Med* 15:307.

24 Lefbom BK, Rosenthal SL (1998) Left ventricular outflow velocity in 23 miniature Bull Terriers – variation from other breeds. Abstract. *J Vet Intern Med* 12:249.

25 Koplitz SL, Meurs KM, Spier AW *et al.* (2003) Aortic ejection velocity in healthy Boxers with soft cardiac murmurs and Boxers without cardiac murmurs: 201 cases (1997–2001). *J Am Vet Med Assoc* 222:770–774.

26 Belanger MC, DiFruscia R, Dumesnil JG *et al.* (2001) Usefulness of the indexed effective orifice area in the assessment of subaortic stenosis in the dog. *J Vet Intern Med* 15:430–437.

27 Brown DJ, Smith WK (2002) Stenosis hemodynamics: from physical principles to clinical indices. *J Vet Intern Med* 16:650–657.

28 Breznock EM, Whiting P, Pendray D *et al.* (1983) Valved apico-aortic conduit for relief of left ventricular hypertension caused by discrete subaortic stenosis in dogs. *J Am Vet Med Assoc* 182:51–56.

29 Dhokarikar P, Caywood DD, Ogburn PN *et al.* (1995) Closed aortic valvotomy: a retrospective study in 15 dogs. *J Am Anim Hosp Assoc* 31:402–410.

30 Monnet E, Orton EC, Gaynor JS *et al.* (1996) Open resection for subvalvular aortic stenosis in dogs. *J Am Vet Med Assoc* 209:1255–1261.

31 White RN, Boswood A, Garden OA *et al.* (1997) Surgical management of subvalvular aortic stenosis and mitral dysplasia in a Golden Retriever. *J Small Anim Pract* 38:251–255.

32 Orton EC, Herndon GD, Boon JA *et al.* (2000) Influence of open surgical correction on intermediate-term outcome in dogs with subvalvular aortic stenosis: 44 cases (1991–1998). *J Am Vet Med Assoc* 216:364–367.

33 DeLellis LA, Thomas WP, Pion PD (1993) Balloon dilation of congenital subaortic stenosis in the dog. *J Vet Intern Med* 7:153–162.

34 Bonagura JD (2001) Balloon valvuloplasty for congenital aortic stenosis. In: *Proceedings of the 19th ACVIM Forum*, Denver, pp. 154–155.

35 Meurs KM, Lehmkuhl LB, Bonagura JD (2005) Survival times in dogs with severe subvalvular aortic stenosis treated with balloon valvuloplasty or

atenolol. *J Am Vet Med Assoc* 227:420–424.

36 Fingland RB, Bonagura JD, Myer CW (1986) Pulmonic stenosis in the dog: 29 cases. *J Am Vet Med Assoc* 189:218–226.

37 Buchanan JW (1990) Pulmonic stenosis caused by single coronary artery in dogs: four cases (1965–1984). *J Am Vet Med Assoc* 196:115–120.

38 Buchanan JW (2001) Pathogenesis of single right coronary artery and pulmonic stenosis in English Bulldogs. *J Vet Intern Med* 15:101–104.

39 Kittleson M, Thomas WP, Loyer C *et al.* (1992) Letter. *J Vet Intern Med* 6:250–251.

40 Ristic JME, Marin C, Heritage ME (2001) Congenital pulmonic stenosis. A retrospective study of 24 cases seen between 1990–1999. *J Vet Cardiol* 3:13–19.

41 Bussadori C, DeMadron E, Santilli RA *et al.* (2001) Balloon valvuloplasty in 30 dogs with pulmonic stenosis: effect of valve morphology and annular size on initial and 1-year outcome. *J Vet Intern Med* 15:553–558.

42 Johnson MS, Martin M (2003) Balloon valvuloplasty in a cat with pulmonic stenosis. *J Vet Intern Med* 17:928-930.

43 Sisson D, MacCoy DM (1988) Treatment of congenital pulmonic stenosis in two dogs by balloon valvuloplasty. *J Vet Intern Med* 2:92–99.

44 Martin MWS, Godma M, Luis Fuentes V *et al.* (1992) Assessment of balloon pulmonary valvuloplasty in six dogs. *J Small Anim Pract* 33:443–449.

45 Brownlie SE, Cobb MA, Chambers J *et al.* (1991) Percutaneous balloon valvulopasty in four dogs with pulmonic stenosis. *J Small Anim Pract* 32:165–169.

46 Gordon SG, Miller MW, Baig S (2002) A retrospective review of balloon valvuloplasty for the treatment of pulmonic stenosis in 50 dogs. In *Proceedings of the 1st International Symposium for Veterinary Cardiology*, Prague.

47 Estrada A, Moise NS, Renaud-Farrell S (2005) When, how and why to perform a double ballooning

technique for dogs with valvular pulmonic stenosis. *J Vet Cardiol* 7:41–51.

48 Hunt GB, Pearson MRB, Bellenger CR *et al.* (1993) Use of a modified patch-graft technique and valvulectomy for correction of severe pulmonic stenosis in dogs: eight consecutive cases. *Aust Vet J* 70:244–248.

49 Shores A, Weirich WE (1985) A modified pericardial patch graft technique for correction of pulmonic stenosis in the dog. *J Am Anim Hosp Assoc* 21:809–812.

50 Orton EC, Bruecker KA, McCracken TO (1990) An open patch-graft technique for correction of pulmonic stenosis in the dog. *Vet Surg* 19:148–154.

51 Stafford Johnson M, Martin M, Edwards D *et al.* (2004) Pulmonic stenosis in dogs: balloon dilation improves clinical outcome. *J Vet Intern Med* 18:656–662.

52 Gittenberger-De Groot AC, Strengers JLM, Mentink M *et al.* (1985) Histologic studies on normal and persistent ductus arteriosus in the dog. *J Am Coll Cardiol* 6:394–404.

53 Malik R, Bellenger CR, Hunt GB *et al.* (1994) Aberrant branch of the bronchoesophageal artery mimicking patent ductus arteriosus in a dog. *J Am Anim Hosp Assoc* 30:162–164.

54 Nelson AW (1986) Aortiocopulmonary window in a dog. *J Am Vet Med Assoc* 188:1055–1058.

55 Ackerman N, Burk R, Hahn AW (1978) Patent ductus arteriosus in the dog: a retrospective study of radiographic, epidemiologic, and clinical findings. *Am J Vet Res* 39:1805–1810.

56 Cohen JS, Tilley LP, Liu, SK *et al.* (1975) Patent ductus arteriosus in five cats. *J Am Anim Hosp Assoc* 11:95–101.

57 Hitchcock LS, Lehmkuhl LB, Bonagura JD *et al.* (2000) Patent ductus arteriosus in cats: 21 cases. Abstract. *J Vet Intern Med* 14:338.

58 Van Israel N, French AT, Dukes-McEwan J *et al.* (2002) Review of left-to-right shunting patent ductus arteriosus and short term outcome in 98 dogs. *J Small Anim Pract* 43:395–400.

59 Miller MW, Bonagura JD, Meurs KM *et al.* (1995) Percutaneous catheter occlusion of patent ductus arteriosus. In *Proceedings of the 13th ACVIM Forum*, Lake Buena Vista, pp. 308–310.

60 Grifka RG, Miller MW, Frischmeyer KJ *et al.* (1996) Transcatheter occlusion of a patent ductus arteriosus in a Newfoundland pup using the Gianturco–Grifka vascular occlusion device. *J Vet Intern Med* 10:42–44.

61 Fox PR, Bond BR, Sommer RJ (1998) Nonsurgical transcatheter coil occlusion of patent ductus arteriosus in two dogs using a preformed Nitinol snare delivery technique. *J Vet Intern Med* 12:182–185.

62 Stokhof AA, Sreeram N, Wolvekamp WTC (2000) Transcatheter closure of patent ductus arteriosus using occluding spring coils. *J Vet Intern Med* 14:452–455.

63 Schneider M, Hildebrandt N, Schweigl I *et al.* (2001) Transvenous embolization of small patent ductus arteriosus with single detachable coils in dogs. *J Vet Intern Med* 15:222–228.

64 Hogan DF, Green III HW, Gordon S *et al.* (2004) Transarterial coil embolization of patent ductus arteriosus in small dogs with 0.025 inch vascular occlusion coils: 10 cases. *J Vet Intern Med* 18:325–329.

65 Van Israel N, French AT, Wotton PR *et al.* (2001) Hemolysis associated with patent ductus arteriosus coil embolization in a dog. *J Vet Intern Med* 15:153–156.

66 Saunders AB, Miller MW, Gordon SG *et al.* (2004) Pulmonary embolization of vascular occlusion coils in dogs with patent ductus arteriosus. *J Vet Intern Med* 18:663–666.

67 Glaus TM, Berger F, Ammann FW *et al.* (2002) Closure of large patent ductus arteriosus with a self-expanding duct occluder in two dogs. *J Small Anim Pract* 43:547–550.

68 Schneider M, Schneider I, Hildebrandt N *et al.* (2003) Percutaneous angiography of patent ductus arteriosus in dogs: techniques, results and implications for intravascular occlusion. *J Vet Cardiol* 5:21–27.

69 Schneider M, Hildebrandt N (2003) Transvenous embolization of the patent ductus arteriosus with detachable coils in 2 cats. *J Vet Intern Med* **17**:349–353.

70 Sisson D (2003) Use of a self-expanding occluding stent for nonsurgical closure of patent ductus arteriosus in dogs. *J Am Vet Med Assoc* **223**:999–1005.

71 Breznock EM, Wisloh A, Hilwig RW et al. (1971) A surgical method for correction of patent ductus arteriosus in the dog. *J Am Vet Med Assoc* **158**:753–762.

72 Corti LB, Merkley DF, Nelson OL et al. (2000) Retrospective evaluation of occlusion of patent ductus arteriosus with hemoclips in 20 dogs. *J Am Anim Hosp Assoc* **36**:548–55.

73 Eyster GE, Eyster JT, Cords GB et al. (1976) Patent ductus arteriosus in the dog: characteristics of occurrence and results of surgery in one hundred consecutive cases. *J Am Vet Med Assoc* **168**:435–438.

74 Birchard SJ, Bonagura JD, Fingland RB (1990) Results of ligation of patent ductus arteriosus in dogs: 201 cases (1969–1988). *J Am Vet Med Assoc* **196**:2011–2017.

75 Hunt GB, Simpson DJ, Beck JA et al. (2001) Intraoperative hemorrhage during patent ductus arteriosus ligation in dogs. *Vet Surg* **30**:58–63.

76 Bureau S, Monnet E, Orton EC (2005) Evaluation of survival rate and prognostic indicators for surgical treatment of left-to-right patent ductus arteriosus in dogs: 52 cases (1995–2003). *J Am Vet Med Assoc* **227**:1794–1799.

77 Campbell FE, Thomas WP, Miller SJ et al. (2006) Immediate and late outcomes of transarterial coil occlusion of patent ductus arteriosus in dogs. *J Vet Intern Med* **20**:83–96.

78 Sisson D, Luethy M, Thomas WP (1991) Ventricular septal defect accompanied by aortic regurgitation in five dogs. *J Am Anim Hosp Assoc* **27**:441–448.

79 Breznock EM (1973) Spontaneous closure of ventricular septal defects in the dog. *J Am Vet Med Assoc* **162**:399–403.

80 Rausch WP, Keene BW (2003) Spontaneous resolution of an isolated ventricular septal defect in a dog. *J Am Vet Med Assoc* **223**:219–220.

81 Fujii Y, Fukuda T, Machida N et al. (2004) Transcatheter closure of congenital ventricular septal defects in 3 dogs with a detachable coil. *J Vet Intern Med* **18**:911–914.

82 Shimizu M, Tanaka R, Hirao H et al. (2005) Percutaneous transcatheter coil embolization of a ventricular septal defect in a dog. *J Am Vet Med Assoc* **226**:69–72.

83 Eyster GE, Whipple RD, Anderson LK et al. (1977) Pulmonary artery banding for ventricular septal defect in dogs and cats. *J Am Vet Med Assoc* **170**:434–438.

84 Kirberger RM, Berry WL (1992) Atrial septal defect in a dog: the value of Doppler echocardiography. *J So Afr Vet Assoc* **63**:43–48.

85 Eyster GE (1994) Atrial septal defect and ventricular septal defect. *Sem Vet Med Surg* **9**:227–233.

86 Guglielmini C, Diana A, Pietra M et al. (2002) Atrial septal defect in five dogs. *J Small Anim Pract* **43**:317–322.

87 Moise NS (1989) Doppler echocardiographic evaluation of congenital heart disease. *J Vet Intern Med* **3**:195–207.

88 Malik R. Church DB (1988) Congenital mitral insufficiency in Bull Terriers. *J Small Anim Pract* **29**:549–557.

89 Atwell RB, Sutton RH (1998) Atrioventricular valve dysplasia in Dalmations. *Aust Vet J* **76**:249.

90 Fox PR, Miller MW, Liu SK (1992) Clinical, echocardiographic, and Doppler imaging characteristics of mitral valve stenosis in two dogs. *J Am Vet Med Assoc* **201**:1575–1579.

91 Lehmkuhl LB, Ware WA, Bonagura JD (1994) Mitral stenosis in 15 dogs. *J Vet Intern Med* **8**:2–17.

92 Stamoulis ME, Fox PR (1993) Mitral valve stenosis in three cats. *J Small Anim Pract* **34**:452–456.

93 Liu SK, Tilley LP (1976) Dysplasia of the tricuspid valve in the dog and cat. *J Am Vet Med Assoc* **169**:623–630.

94 Wright KN, Bleas ME, Benson DW (2001) Clinical spectrum of congenital tricuspid valve malformations in an extended family of Labrador Retrievers. Abstract. *J Vet Intern Med* **15**:280.

95 Eyster GE, Anderson L, Evans AT et al. (1977) Ebstein's anomaly: a report of 3 cases in the dog. *J Am Vet Med Assoc* **170**:709–713.

96 Atkins CE, Wright KN (1995) Supraventricular tachycardia associated with accessory atrioventricular pathways in dogs. In: *Current Veterinary Therapy XII*. JD Bonagura (ed). WB Saunders, Philadelphia, pp. 807–813.

97 Kunze CP, Abbott JA, Hamilton SM et al. (2002) Balloon valvuloplasty for palliative treatment of tricuspid stenosis with right-to-left arial-level shunting in a dog. *J Am Vet Med Assoc* **220**:491–496

98 Famula TR, Siemens LM, Davidson AP et al. (2002) Evaluation of the genetic basis of tricuspid valve dysplasia in Labrador Retrievers. *Am J Vet Res* **63**:816–820.

99 Kornreich BG, Moise NS (1997) Right atrioventricular valve malformation in dogs and cats: an electrocardiographic survey with emphasis on splintered QRS complexes. *J Vet Intern Med* **11**:226–230.

100 Hoffman G, Amberger CN, Seiler G et al. (2000) Tricuspid valve dysplasia in fifteen dogs. *Schweiz Arch Tierheilkd* **142**:268–277.

101 Brown WA, Thomas WP (1995) Balloon valvuloplasty of tricuspid stenosis in a Labrador Retriever. *J Vet Intern Med* **9**:419–424.

102 Van Mierop LHS, Patterson DF, Schnarr WR (1977) Hereditary conotruncal septal defects in Keeshond dogs: embryologic studies. *Am J Cardiol* **40**:936–937.

103 Patterson DF, Pexieder T, Schanarr WR et al. (1993) A single major gene defect underlying cardiac conotruncal malformations interferes with myocardial growth during embryonic development: studies in the CTD line of Keeshond dogs. *Am J Human Genet* **52**: 388–397.

104 Ringwald RJ, Bonagura JD (1988) Tetralogy of Fallot in the dog: clinical findings in 13 cases. *J Am Anim Hosp Assoc* **24**:33–43.

105 Orton EC, Mama K, Hellyer P *et al.* (2001) Open surgical repair of tetralogy of Fallot in dogs. *J Am Vet Med Assoc* **219**:1089–1093.

106 Eyster GE, Braden TD, Appleford M *et al.* (1977) Surgical management of tetralogy of Fallot. *J Small Anim Pract* **18**:387–394.

107 Oswald GP, Orton CE (1993) Patent ductus arteriosus and pulmonary hypertension in related Pembroke Welsh Corgis. *J Am Vet Med Assoc* **202**:761–764.

108 Nimmo-Wilkie JS, Feldman EC (1981) Pulmonary vascular lesions associated with congenital heart defects in three dogs. *J Am Anim Hosp Assoc* **17**:485–490.

109 Pyle RL, Park RD, Alexander AF *et al.* (1981) Patent ductus arteriosus with pulmonary hypertension in the dog. *J Am Vet Med Assoc* **178**:565–572.

110 Moore KW, Stepien RL (2001) Hydroxyurea for treatment of polycythemia secondary to right-to-left shunting patent ductus arteriosus in 4 dogs. *J Vet Intern Med* **15**:418–421.

111 VanGundy T (1989) Vascular ring anomalies. *Compend Cont Educ Pract Vet* **11**:36–48.

112 Martin DG, Ferguson EW (1983) Double aortic arch in a dog. *J Am Vet Med Assoc* **183**:697–699.

113 Ellison GW (1980) Vacular ring anomalies in the dog and cat. *Comp Cont Educ Pract Vet* **11**:693–706.

114 Fingeroth JM, Fossum TW (1987) Late-onset regurgitation associated with persistent right aortic arch in two dogs. *J Am Vet Med Assoc* **191**:981–982.

115 Hurley K, Miller MW, Willard MD *et al.* (1993) Left aortic arch and right ligamentum arteriosum causing esophageal obstruction in a dog. *J Am Vet Med Assoc* **203**:410–412.

116 Buchanan JW (2004) Tracheal signs and associated vascular anomalies in dogs with persistent right arotic arch. *J Vet Intern Med* **18**:510–514.

117 Isakow K, Fowler D, Walsh P (2000) Video-assisted thoracoscopic division of the ligamentum arteriosum in two dogs with persistent right aortic arch. *J Am Vet Med Assoc* **217**:1333–1336.

118 Muldoon MM, Birchard SJ, Ellison GW (1997) Long-term results of surgical correction of persistent right aortic arch in dogs: 25 cases (1980–1995). *J Am Vet Med Assoc* **210**:1761–1763.

119 Tobias AH, Thomas WP, Kittleson MD *et al.* (1993) Cor triatriatum dexter in two dogs. *J Am Vet Med Assoc* **202**:285–290.

120 Kaufman AC, Swalec KM, Mahafey MB (1994) Surgical correction of cor triatriatum dexter in a puppy. *J Am Anim Hosp Assoc* **30**:157–161.

121 Jevens DJ, Johnston SA, Jones CA *et al.* (1993) Cor triatriatum dexter in two dogs. *J Am Anim Hosp Assoc* **29**:289–293.

122 Fossum TW, Miller MW (1994) Cor triatriatum and caval anomalies. *Semin Vet Med Surg* **9**:177–184.

123 Stafford Johnson M, Martin M, DeGiovanni JV *et al.* (2004) Management of cor triatriatum dexter by balloon dilatation in three dogs. *J Small Anim Pract* **45**:16–20.

124 Wander KW, Monnet E, Orton EC (1998) Surgical correction of cor triatriatum sinister in a kitten. *J Am Anim Hosp Assoc* **34**:383–386.

125 Adin DB, Thomas WP (1999) Balloon dilation of cor triatriatum dexter in a dog. *J Vet Intern Med* **13**:617–619.

126 Jacobs G, Bolton GR, Watrous BJ (1983) Echocardiographic features of dilated coronary sinus in a dog with persistent left cranial vena cava. *J Am Vet Med Assoc* **182**:407–408.

127 DelPalacio MJF, Bayon A, Agut A (1997) Dilated coronary sinus in a dog with persistent left cranial vena cava. *Vet Radiol Ultrasound* **38**:376–379.

128 Johnson SE (2000) Chronic hepatic disorders. In: *Textbook of Veterinary Internal Medicine*, 5th edn. SJ Ettinger, EC Feldman (eds). WB Saunders, Philadelphia, pp. 1311–1319.

129 Lombard CW, Buergelt CD (1984) Endocardial fibroelastosis in four dogs. *J Am Anim Hosp Assoc* **20**:271–278.

130 Paasch LH, Zook BC (1980) The pathogenesis of endocardial fibroelastosis in Burmese cats. *Lab Invest* **42**:197–204.

19
Acquired Valve Diseases

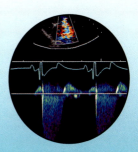

Most acquired valve abnormalities are caused by degenerative disease[1]. Infective disease occurs less often. Reports of traumatic injury and other valve abnormalities are rare.

DEGENERATIVE VALVE DISEASE

OVERVIEW

The most common cause of heart failure in the dog is chronic degenerative AV valve disease, also known as endocardiosis, mucoid or myxomatous valvular degeneration, and chronic valvular fibrosis[1]. The mitral valve is usually affected most, but both AV valves are often involved[2]. Isolated tricuspid valve degenerative disease is uncommon. Aortic or pulmonic valve thickening is seen in some older animals, but insufficiency is usually only mild. Clinically important degenerative valve lesions are rare in cats.

PATHOPHYSIOLOGY

Early lesions appear as small nodules on the free margins of the valve. Progressive collagen degeneration

and accumulation of acid mucopolysaccharides and other substances within the leaflets cause continued nodular thickening, deformity, and weakening of the valve and chordae tendineae (370, 371)[2–5]. Multiple factors involving collagen degeneration, valve leaflet stress, and endothelial function are thought to be involved. Redundant valve tissue between chordal attachments often bulges (prolapses) toward the atrium in systole[2, 6]. Mitral valve prolapse may be important in the pathogenesis of the disease, at least in some breeds. A high prevalence of mitral prolapse is seen in clinically normal dogs of some predisposed breeds and, further, the degree of prolapse has been associated with severity of the disease[6]. Endothelial damage also occurs and may play a role in the pathogenesis of this disease, possibly via ET[5, 7]. Platelet abnormalities have also been identified and are of unclear significance[8]. The valve lesions in dogs with this degenerative disease are similar to those in people with mitral valve prolapse[2, 5]. Valve insufficiency (regurgitation) develops as the lesions progress. This usually worsens slowly, over months to years, which allows mean atrial pressure to remain fairly low unless a sudden, large increase in

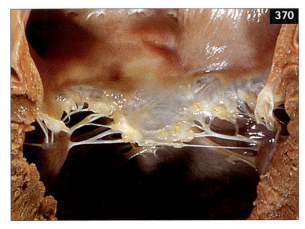
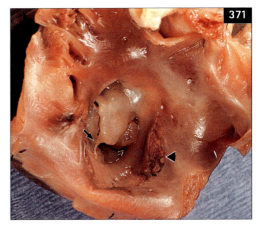

370, 371 (370) Nodular thickening along the free margins of the mitral valve in a Cocker Spaniel with early signs of degenerative AV valve disease. (371) View from the enlarged LA shows marked mitral valve thickening (cranioventral leaflet) with a ruptured chorda tendinea (arrow). A partial thickness LA tear is also seen (arrowhead). The specimen is from a male Chihuahua with advanced endocardiosis that died from fulminant pulmonary edema. (Courtesy Dr M Miller.)

regurgitant volume occurs (e.g. ruptured chordae). Valve regurgitation leads to ipsilateral atrial, ventricular, and valve annulus dilation over time, as compensatory mechanisms augment blood volume to meet the circulatory needs of the body (see Chapter 16) and eccentric hypertrophy develops (see Chapter 1, p. 18). Compensatory changes in blood volume and heart size, along with fairly well-preserved ventricular function, allow most dogs to remain asymptomatic for a prolonged period. Release of ANP may help to counter the effects of RAAS activation in earlier stages of the disease[9, 10]; higher ANP concentrations are associated with marked LA enlargement and severity of congestive failure.

With MR, LA size may become massive before signs of heart failure appear; some dogs never show clinical signs of heart failure. Nevertheless, LA then pulmonary venous and capillary hydrostatic pressures eventually rise in many dogs. Overt pulmonary edema appears when pulmonary lymphatic capacity is exceeded. In some dogs, TR is severe enough to cause right-sided CHF. Increased pulmonary vascular pressure secondary to chronic MR can also contribute to the development of right-sided heart failure.

Atrial jet lesions, endocardial fibrosis, and partial or even full-thickness atrial tears can eventually occur (371). Chronic AV valve disease is also associated with intramural coronary arteriosclerosis, microscopic intramural myocardial infarction, and focal myocardial fibrosis[2]. The extent to which these changes contribute to clinical myocardial dysfunction later in the disease is not clear.

Even with severe signs of CHF, ventricular function appears well-maintained in many dogs[11]. Nevertheless, chronic volume overloading eventually reduces myocyte contractility, although height-ened sympathetic activity can mask this[12–14]. The mechanisms underlying depressed contractility may involve oxygen free radicals as well as NH activation[15]. Long-term beta-blockade has improved myocyte contractility experimentally[16]. Reduced contractility exacerbates ventricular dilation and valve regurgitation and, therefore, may worsen congestive failure. Assessment of myocardial contractility in dogs with MR is difficult. Ejection phase indices, such as fractional shortening and others (see Chapter 5, p. 78), overestimate contractility as MR reduces LV afterload and isovolumetric indices (e.g. dP/dt_{max}) are not truly valid because there is no isovolumetric contraction (regurgitation begins early in systole). Nevertheless, the Doppler-derived MR velocity profile has been used to estimate systolic as well as diastolic function indices[17–19]. The echocardiographic estimation of the end-systolic volume index is also used (see Chapter 5, p. 79). Based on this index, myocardial function appears normal to mildly depressed in most dogs with chronic mitral degeneration, but compensatory mechanisms may mask mild dysfunction[11].

CLINICAL FEATURES

Although the exact cause of endocardiosis is unclear, an hereditary basis is likely[20, 21]. It occurs most commonly in middle-age and older, small to mid-sized breeds[1]. Some large breed dogs are affected with primary mitral valve disease, although the degree of valve thickening and prolapse is less pronounced than in small breed dogs[22, 23]. The German Shepherd Dog may be overrepresented. The prevalence and severity of chronic, degenerative AV valve disease increases with age. More than 30% of small breed dogs older than 10 years are affected[1]. A higher prevalence has been noted in Toy and Miniature Poodles, Miniature Schnauzers, Chihuahuas, Pomeranians, Fox Terriers, Cocker Spaniels, Pekingese, and Boston Terriers in the US, and male Miniature Pinschers, Whippets, and Cavalier King Charles Spaniels in the UK[1]. An especially high prevalence and an early onset of degenerative mitral valve disease is reported in Cavalier King Charles Spaniels in the US, UK, and Sweden[6, 21, 24–28]. In this breed the inheritance may be polygenic, with gender and age influencing expression[21]. The overall prevalence of MR murmurs and degenerative valve disease is similar in males and females. Males showed faster progression, greater severity, and a higher prevalence of congestive failure than females in some studies[21, 25], but not in others[29].

Initial signs of heart failure from MR usually include reduced exercise tolerance and cough or tachypnea with exertion. The resting respiratory rate also increases as pulmonary interstitial edema develops. Coughing typically occurs at night and in the early morning, as well as with activity. Severe edema causes obvious respiratory distress, often with a moist cough. Signs of severe pulmonary edema can develop gradually or acutely. Intermittent episodes of symptomatic pulmonary edema interspersed with periods of compensated heart failure occurring over months to years are also common. Transient weakness or acute collapse (syncope) may occur secondary to arrhythmias, coughing, or an atrial tear. Signs of TR with right-sided heart failure include abdominal distension (ascites, hepatomegaly), respiratory distress from pleural effusion, and, rarely, peripheral tissue edema. GI signs may accompany splanchnic congestion. Arterial pulse strength is usually good, although pulse deficits (see Chapter 2, p. 30) accompany some tachyarrhythmias. Jugular venous distension and pulsations are not expected with MR alone. With TR, jugular pulsations may be seen during ventricular systole and are accentuated after exercise, with excitement, or with hepatojugular reflux testing (see Chapter 2, p. 28).

MR typically causes a holosystolic murmur, best heard at the left apex; the murmur may radiate in any direction (see Chapter 6, p. 94). A murmur heard only in early systole (protosystolic) or no murmur can occur with mild MR[30]. Exercise and excitement increase the intensity of soft MR murmurs. Louder murmurs have been associated with more advanced disease[26]; however, with massive MR and severe heart failure the murmur can be soft or even inaudible. Occasional MR murmurs sound like a musical tone or whoop. Some dogs with degenerative AV valve disease have a mid- to late-systolic click, with or without a murmur (372). In advanced disease, an S_3 gallop may be audible at the left apex. The TR murmur is similar to that of MR, but is loudest at the right apex. The presence of jugular vein pulsations, a precordial thrill over the right apex, and a different quality to the murmur heard over the tricuspid region help the clinician differentiate TR from a MR murmur radiating to the right chest wall.

Harsh breath sounds and end-inspiratory crackles, especially in the ventral lung fields, develop with pulmonary edema. Widespread inspiratory as well as expiratory crackles and wheezes are heard with fulminant pulmonary edema, but primary pulmonary or airway disease also causes abnormal lung sounds in some dogs with MR, and must be differentiated from heart failure. Sinus tachycardia is common with congestive failure because of heightened sympathetic tone; chronic pulmonary disease is frequently associated with marked sinus arrhythmia and a normal heart rate. Pleural effusion causes diminished pulmonary sounds ventrally.

Other diseases that may be confused with symptomatic degenerative AV valve disease include tracheal collapse, chronic bronchitis, bronchiectasis, pulmonary fibrosis, pulmonary neoplasia, pneumonia, pharyngitis, heartworm disease, DCM, and bacterial endocarditis. The cough caused by major airway collapse is often described as a 'honking' cough.

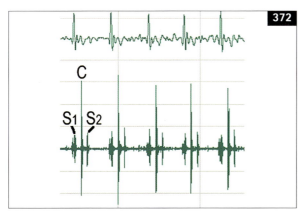

372 Phonocardiogram (bottom) depicts a loud mid-systolic click (C), but no murmur in a 6-year-old female Cavalier King Charles Spaniel with early degenerative mitral disease (ECG trace is on top).

Complicating factors

Certain complicating events can provoke acute clinical signs in dogs with previously compensated disease (*Table 53*). For example, atrial or, less commonly, ventricular tachyarrhythmias can reduce cardiac output, increase myocardial oxygen demand, and precipitate pulmonary edema or syncope. Sudden bradycardia, especially with excitement, may precipitate an exaggerated vasovagal response and

Table 53 Complicating factors with degenerative AV valve disease.

1) Causes of acutely worsened pulmonary edema:
   a) Arrhythmias:
   - Frequent atrial premature complexes.
   - Paroxysmal atrial/supraventricular tachycardia.
   - Atrial fibrillation.
   - Ventricular tachyarrhythmias.
   - Consider drug toxicity (e.g. digoxin).
   b) Ruptured chordae tendineae.
   c) Iatrogenic volume overload:
   - Excessive volumes of IV fluids or blood.
   - High-sodium fluids.
   d) Excessive salt intake (diet, water source).
   e) Erratic or improper medication administration.
   f) Insufficient medication for stage of disease.
   g) Increased cardiac workload:
   - Physical exertion.
   - Anemia.
   - Infections/sepsis.
   - Hypertension.
   - Disease of other organ systems (e.g. pulmonary, renal, liver, endocrine).
   - Hot, humid environment.
   - Excessively cold environment.
   - Other environmental stresses.
   h) Myocardial degeneration and poor contractility.

2) Causes of reduced cardiac output or weakness:
   a) Arrhythmias (see above).
   b) Ruptured chordae tendineae.
   c) Cough-syncope.
   d) Left atrial tear:
   - Intrapericardial bleeding.
   - Cardiac tamponade.
   e) Increased cardiac workload (see above).
   f) Secondary right-sided heart failure.
   g) Myocardial degeneration and poor contractility.

cause weakness or syncope in some dogs. Rupture of diseased chordae tendineae acutely increases regurgitant volume and can also precipitate fulminant pulmonary edema with or without low cardiac output signs. Sometimes, ruptured chordae are an incidental finding on an echocardiogram or at necropsy, especially if 2nd- or 3rd-order chordae are involved[24, 31]. Massive LA enlargement itself can compress mainstem bronchi and stimulate persistent coughing, even in the absence of CHF. A full-thickness LA tear usually causes acute cardiac tamponade. There appears to be a higher prevalence of this complication in male Miniature Poodles, Cocker Spaniels, and Dachshunds[1]. Most of these cases have severe valve disease, marked atrial enlargement, atrial jet lesions, and, often, ruptured first-order chordae tendineae[2, 4]. Pericardiocentesis and surgical repair have been used, but the prognosis is poor[32].

DIAGNOSIS

Clinical laboratory data are often normal, but they may reflect changes consistent with CHF or concurrent extracardiac disease.

Thoracic radiographs are normal early in the disease process. As MR increases, LA and then LV enlargement ensues and gradually pushes the trachea and main bronchi dorsally (373–379 and 44, 45, p. 39). Compression of the left mainstem bronchus occurs,

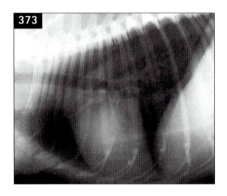
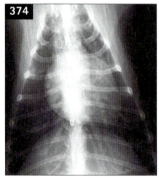

373, 374 Radiographs showing modest LA enlargement but normal overall heart size in a 12-year-old female Schnauzer with MR.

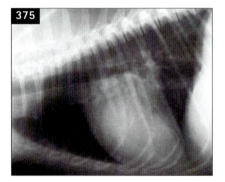
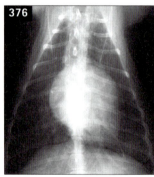

375, 376 More pronounced LA and mild LV enlargement in an 11-year-old female Terrier mix. The carina and RA-caudal vena caval junction are lifted dorsally.

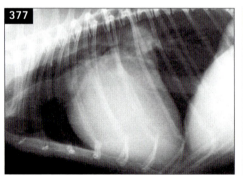
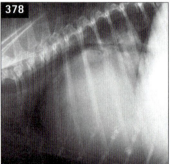
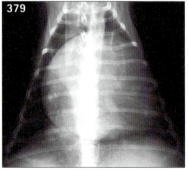

377–379 (377) Lateral radiograph from a 10-year-old Chihuahua with advanced degenerative mitral disease. The dog had persistent coughing, but no evidence for pulmonary edema. Note the marked LA and LV enlargement, narrowed main bronchi, close proximity of the carina to the spine, and incline of the caudal vena cava toward the heart. (378, 379) Besides marked LA enlargement, there is massive generalized cardiomegaly in this 14-year-old female Cockapoo with chronic, severe MR and TR. The trachea is pushed against the spine; pulmonary edema is not evident, although there is some ascites.

especially with severe LA dilation. Fluoroscopy may show dynamic main bronchus collapse associated with coughing or even quiet breathing in such animals (380–382). Variable right heart enlargement occurs with chronic TR. Pulmonary venous congestion (see 56, p. 42) and interstitial edema occur with the onset of left-sided congestive failure; progressive interstitial and alveolar pulmonary edema may follow. Although the radiographic distribution of cardiogenic pulmonary edema in dogs is classically perihilar, dorsocaudal, and bilaterally symmetric, an asymmetrical pattern is seen in some dogs (383, 384 and 58–61, p. 44). The presence and severity of pulmonary edema do not necessarily correlate with the degree of cardiomegaly. Acute, severe MR (e.g. with rupture of chordae tendineae) can produce cardiogenic edema with minimal LA enlargement[31]. Conversely, slowly developing MR can produce massive LA enlargement with no evidence of congestive failure. Early signs of right-sided heart failure include caudal vena caval distension, pleural fissure lines, and hepatomegaly (see 66, p. 45). Overt pleural effusion and ascites occur with advanced failure.

Criteria for LA or biatrial enlargement and LV dilation (see Chapter 4, p. 61) are classic ECG changes, but often the tracing is normal. Occasionally, characteristics of RV enlargement are seen in dogs with severe TR. Arrhythmias are common with advanced disease, especially sinus tachycardia, supraventricular premature complexes, paroxysmal or sustained supraventricular tachycardias, AF, and, sometimes,

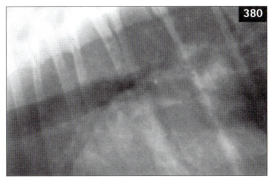

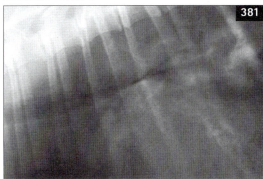

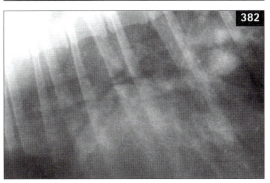

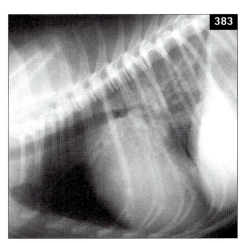

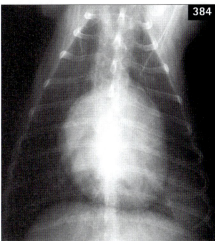

380–382 (380) Fluoroscopic image taken during inspiration in a 9-year-old female Bolognese with chronic MR and cough with excitement. Note the LA enlargement and some main bronchus compression. (381) In early expiration the airways narrow further. (382) Complete expiratory airway collapse follows shortly.

383, 384 Pulmonary interstitial infiltrates of edema are seen in the dorsohilar (383) and left caudal (384) lung regions at initial presentation for heart failure in the dog in 375 and 376. The heart failure was managed medically for 4 more years until the dog died due to chronic renal disease.

VPCs (385–387). These arrhythmias may precipitate clinical signs (*Table 53*, p. 265).

Echocardiography documents the degree of chamber dilation secondary to chronic volume overload. LV wall and septal motion are vigorous, with moderate to marked MR when contractility is normal; little to no EPSS and a high FS are seen (**388–391** and **147**, p. 79). Although the diastolic LV dimension increases, systolic dimension remains normal with good myocardial function. The end-systolic volume index can be used to estimate myocardial function (see Chapter 5, p. 79). Ventricular wall thickness is typically normal. RV and RA dilation develop with TR and increases in pulmonary pressures. Marked RV volume overload sometimes causes paradoxical septal motion (see Chapter 5, p. 78). Pericardial fluid (blood), with or without signs of cardiac tamponade (see Chapter 22), may be evident if a full thickness LA tear

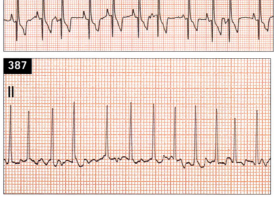

385–387 (385) ECG from a 14-year-old mixed breed dog with chronic MR showing tall R waves and wide QRS complexes, consistent with LV enlargement, and wide P waves, consistent with LA enlargement. One VPC is seen (arrow). **(386)** Sinus rhythm, atrial premature complexes (arrows), and wide P waves are seen in a 9-year-old female Miniature Schnauzer with chronic MR, mild pulmonary edema, and a history of cough and syncope. **(387)** AF in an old dog with chronic MR. All figures leads as marked; 25 mm/sec, 1 cm = 1 mV.

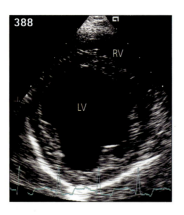

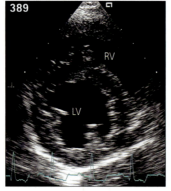

388, 389 (388) End-diastolic 2-D echo frame from an old dog with advanced degenerative MR showing LV dilation with normal wall thickness. **(389)** Systolic frame from the same dog. The vigorous LV motion with normal systolic chamber dimension results from well-preserved LV function and reduced afterload (from the MR).

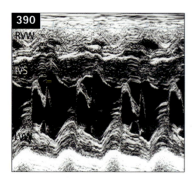

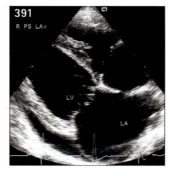

390, 391 (390) M-mode image at the mitral valve level from an 11-year-old Miniature Poodle illustrates thick septal (anterior) mitral leaflet echos with essentially no EPSS (arrow), and good LV motion, as are typical in many cases. **(391)** Early systolic 2-D image showing dilation of all chambers, thick and mildly prolapsed mitral valve, and pericardial effusion (transudate) behind the LV in an old Cockapoo. All images from right parasternal position. IVS = interventricular septum; LA = left atrium; LV = left ventricle; LVW = left ventricular wall; RV = right ventricle; RVW = right ventricular wall.

has occurred. Mild pericardial effusion (transudate) can also develop with right-sided congestive failure. Affected valve cusps are thickened and may appear knobby (392–395). Smooth thickening is characteristic of degenerative disease (endocardiosis), whereas infective endocarditis causes rough and irregular vegetative valve lesions; however, it can be impossible to differentiate between degenerative and infective thickening with echocardiography. Systolic prolapse of one or both valve leaflets into the atrium is common in dogs with degenerative AV valve disease[6]. Sometimes, a ruptured chorda tendinea or flail leaflet tip is seen during systole (395)[31]. LA size correlates well with chronic MR severity.

Color flow Doppler shows the direction and extent of disturbed flow in the atrium (396–399).

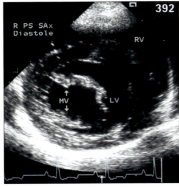 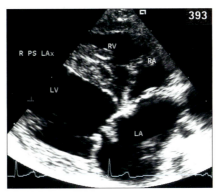 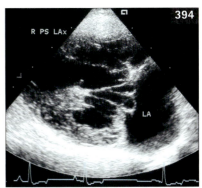

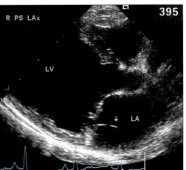

392–395 (392) Thickening along both mitral leaflets is evident in this short-axis 2-D view from a 16-year-old female terrier-cross. (393) Knobby appearance and systolic prolapse of the mitral valve into a markedly enlarged LA in an older Poodle. The tricuspid valve shows similar myxomatous changes. (394) 'Parachute-like' appearance of a prolapsing mitral valve in a terrier-cross. (395) Flail chorda tendinea (arrow) is seen in the LA of a 10-year-old male Maltese with pulmonary congestion. Marked LV dilation is evident in this early systolic frame. All images from right parasternal position. LA = left atrium; LV = left ventricle; MV = mitral valve; RA = right atrium; RV = right ventricle.

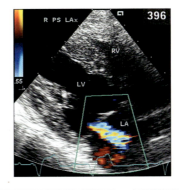 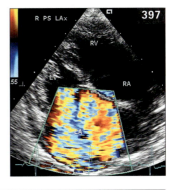

396, 397 (396) Color flow Doppler image from the dog in 373 and 374 shows moderate mitral regurgitation and LA dilation. (397) Systolic frame from the dog in 378 and 379 illustrates severe MR. The turbulent jet angles toward the caudal LA wall before swirling dorsocranially around the huge LA.

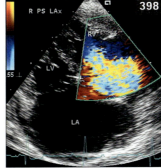 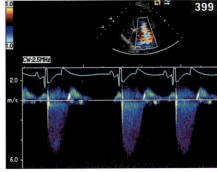

398, 399 (398) Marked TR was also present in this dog. (399) High velocity MR jet from an old dog with chronic AV valve disease. All images from right parasternal position. LA = left atrium; LV = left ventricle; RA = right atrium; RV = right ventricle.

Although there are significant limitations, color flow Doppler allows semiquantitative assessment of MR severity[6, 33]. The PISA method has been described as a more accurate estimate of MR severity than the LA area of disturbed flow[34]. Spectral Doppler interrogation of the high-velocity regurgitant jet allows estimation of the systolic pressure gradient between the affected atrium and ventricle. Indices of LV function can be derived from the MR velocity profile, while the presence/severity of pulmonary hypertension can be estimated from TR jet maximal velocity.

Management

Symptomatic cases are treated medically, although surgical valve repair or replacement is sometimes an option[35–39]. The goals of medical therapy are to control signs of congestion, enhance forward blood flow while reducing regurgitant volume, and modulate excessive NH activation. Drugs that reduce LV size (e.g. diuretics, vasodilators, positive inotropic agents) may reduce regurgitant volume by decreasing mitral annulus size. Arteriolar vasodilators enhance forward cardiac output and reduce regurgitant volume by reducing systemic arteriolar resistance. Clinical compensation for months to years is possible with appropriate therapy, although frequent reevaluation and medication adjustment become necessary as the disease progresses. Many dogs on long-term heart failure therapy have intermittent episodes of decompensation that can be successfully managed. Although congestive signs appear gradually in some dogs, fulminant pulmonary edema or episodes of syncope can develop rapidly. Therapy must be guided by clinical status and the nature of any complicating factors. Categorizing patients into a stage of heart failure (see Chapter 16, p. 170) may be helpful, but the clinical manifestations of heart failure in any individual do not necessarily follow an orderly sequence.

Asymptomatic AV valve regurgitation

Dogs that are asymptomatic do not require drug therapy. There is no convincing evidence for a significant benefit from ACE inhibitor therapy in most asymptomatic dogs[40, 41]. Owner education about the disease process and early signs of heart failure is important. Other recommendations during this preclinical stage include weight reduction for obese dogs, and avoidance of high-salt foods. A diet moderately restricted in sodium chloride may be helpful. Reevaluation at least yearly in the context of a routine preventive health program is advised.

Mild to moderate congestive heart failure

Dogs that develop clinical signs with exercise or activity are treated by several means (Table 54). The aggressiveness of therapy is guided by the individual patient's signs and response. Moderate dietary salt restriction (e.g. diets formulated for geriatric dogs or dogs with kidney disease) is recommended initially. Further salt restriction can be achieved using diets formulated for animals with heart failure.

An ACE inhibitor is recommended for dogs with early signs of failure, although pimobendan is gaining favor in this situation (see Chapter 16, p. 178). Long-term ACE inhibitor therapy improves exercise tolerance, cough, and respiratory effort[42], although the issue of enhanced survival is unclear[43]. Pimobendan appears to have greater benefit than an ACE inhibitor in long-term heart failure management[44]. It is unclear whether a combination of an ACE inhibitor with pimobendan would provide additive benefit. Furosemide is also used for dogs with clinical signs or radiographic evidence of pulmonary edema. Higher and more frequent doses are indicated for more severe edema. When the signs of failure are controlled, the dose and frequency of furosemide are reduced to the lowest effective levels for long-term therapy. Furosemide monotherapy is not recommended for long-term heart failure treatment. When it is unclear whether respiratory signs are caused by heart failure or a noncardiac cause, an initial therapeutic trial of furosemide (e.g. 1–2 mg/kg PO q8–12h) is indicated. Cardiogenic pulmonary edema usually responds rapidly. Pimobendan is also used in areas where it is available[29], and it appears to be well-tolerated in cases of moderately severe heart failure from mitral valve disease.

Digoxin and/or pimobendan, if not already being administered, is advocated in heart failure from advanced AV valve regurgitation (see Chapter 16, p. 180). Digoxin is usually added after ACE inhibitor and furosemide therapy has begun, especially if LV enlargement is marked or myocardial dysfunction is evident. Other indications for digoxin include atrial tachyarrhythmias and recurrent episodes of pulmonary edema despite furosemide and ACE inhibitor treatment. Conservative doses (see Table 44, p. 174) are given and serum concentrations measured to avoid toxicity (see Chapter 16, p. 180). Pimobendan can be used concurrently with digoxin in cases with refractory failure[45].

Exercise should be restricted until signs of failure abate, but mild to moderate regular activity can be beneficial during chronic, compensated disease. Strenuous exercise is best avoided. At-home monitoring is important because decompensation often occurs unexpectedly. A persistent increase in the resting respiratory or heart rate can signal early decompensation. Dogs with a persistent dry cough from mainstem bronchus compression and without pulmonary edema may require antitussive therapy (e.g. hydrocodone bitartrate [0.25 mg/kg PO q8–12h] or butorphanol [0.5 mg/kg PO q6–12h]).

Continued monitoring, especially of renal function and serum electrolyte concentrations, is important.

Table 54 General treatment guidelines for chronic AV valve disease.

1) No clinical signs of disease:

  a) Client education about the disease and early heart failure signs.

  b) Routine health maintenance:
- Maintain (or work toward) normal body weight/condition.
- Regular mild to moderate exercise.
- Avoid excessively strenuous activity.
- Heartworm testing and prophylaxis in endemic areas.

  c) Manage other medical problems.

  d) Avoid high salt foods; consider moderately salt-restricted diet.

2) Mild to moderate signs of CHF:*

  a) Considerations as above, plus:

  b) ACE inhibitor (or pimobendan).

  c) Furosemide, as needed.

  d) +/– digoxin.

  e) +/– additional diuretic (e.g. spironolactone, hydrocholorthiazide).

  f) Antiarrhythmic therapy if necessary.

  g) Complete exercise restriction until signs abate.

  h) Moderate dietary salt restriction.

  i) Resting respiratory (+/– heart) rate monitoring at home.

3) Severe, acute signs of CHF:*

  a) Supplemental oxygen.

  b) Cage rest.

  c) Minimize patient handling.

  d) Furosemide; more aggressive doses, parenterally

  e) Vasodilator:
- Consider IV nitroprusside, or PO hydralazine or amlodipine, +/– topical nitroglycerine.

  f) +/– butorphanol or morphine.

  g) Antiarrhythmic therapy, if necessary.

  h) +/– positive inotropic drug:
- If myocardial failure documented, IV drug can be used (see *Table 43*, p. 171).
- After patient stabilized, can use long-term PO pimobendan +/– digoxin therapy

  i) +/– bronchodilator (e.g. theophylline).

  j) Thoracocentesis, if large volume pleural effusion.

4) Strategies for chronic recurrent or refractory heart failure:*

  a) Increase furosemide dose/frequency; may be able to decrease again in several days after signs abate.

  b) Enforced rest until signs abate.

  c) Add pimobendan, if not currently prescribed.

  d) Increase ACE inhibitor dose/frequency (to q12h from q24h).

  e) Add digoxin, if not currently prescribed. Monitor serum concentration. Only increase dose if subtherapeutic concentration documented.

  f) Further restrict dietary salt intake. Verify that drinking water is low sodium.

  g) Add (or increase dose of) second diuretic (e.g. spironolactone [1–2 mg/kg PO q12–24h], spironolactone/hydrochlorothiazide combination [1–2 mg/kg of the combination 25 mg/25 mg product]).

  h) Add second vasodilator (e.g. amlodipine [0.05–0.2 mg/kg PO q24h] or hydralazine [0.25–0.5 mg/kg PO q12h]). Monitor blood pressure.

  i) Manage arrhythmias, if present.

  j) Periodic thoracocentesis (or abdomincentesis) as needed.

* See *Tables 43, 44,* and *45,* pp. 171, 174, and 187 for further details and doses.

Intermittent arrhythmias can cause decompensated congestive failure as well as episodes of transient weakness or syncope. Cough-induced syncope, atrial rupture, or other causes of reduced cardiac output may also occur. Despite the periodic recurrence of signs of CHF, with proper management, many dogs with chronic AV valve regurgitation enjoy a good quality of life for several years after signs of failure first appear. Dogs with recently diagnosed or decompensated heart failure should be reevaluated more frequently (every few days to every week or so) until their condition is stable (see *Table 45*, p.187); those with chronic heart failure that is well-controlled can be checked less often, usually several times per year.

Severe congestive heart failure

Fulminant pulmonary edema with shortness of breath at rest is a true emergency. Aggressive therapy but gentle handling is crucial in these fragile patients. Cage rest, supplemental oxygen, high-dose (e.g. 2–4 mg/kg q1–4h initially) parenteral furosemide, and vasodilator therapy are indicated (*Table 54* and see Chapter 16, p. 170). Intravenous nitroprusside produces both arteriolar and venous dilation, but blood pressure must be closely monitored to avoid hypotension. Alternatively, hydralazine can be used for acute therapy because of its direct and rapid arteriolar vasodilating effect. A reduced dose is used in animals already receiving an ACE inhibitor (see *Table 44*, p. 174).

Amlodipine is another alternative, although onset of action is slower. Topical nitroglycerin can be used in combination with an arteriolar dilator in an attempt to reduce pulmonary venous pressure by direct venodilation.

Treatment with pimobendan or digoxin can be initiated, if not previously prescribed, once acute dyspnea subsides. Although it takes several days to reach therapeutic digoxin blood concentration with oral maintenance doses, IV digitalization is generally avoided. Diltiazem or a beta-blocker (see *Table 48*, p. 200) can be used instead of or in addition to digoxin for the control of supraventricular tachyarrhythmias. Myocardial function is usually adequate in dogs with chronic AV valve disease but, if poor contractility is documented, other more potent inotropic agents (e.g. dobutamine, dopamine, amrinone) can be given IV (see *Table 43*, p. 171).

Mild sedation is sometimes used to reduce anxiety (e.g. morphine or butorphanol; see *Table 43*, p. 171). Patient handling should be minimized and radiographs and other diagnostic procedures postponed until the dog's respiratory condition is more stable. Bronchodilators (e.g. theophylline, aminophylline) have been used because of possible bronchospasm induced by severe pulmonary edema; although the efficacy of this is unclear, these agents may help support respiratory muscle function. In dogs with moderate to large volume pleural effusion, thoracocentesis is indicated to improve pulmonary function. Ascites severe enough to impede respiration should also be drained. Occasionally, therapy for ventricular tachyarrhythmias is warranted. As always, monitoring for drug toxicities and adverse effects (e.g. azotemia, electrolyte abnormalities, arrhythmias) is important.

After the patient is stabilized, medications are adjusted over several days to weeks to determine the best regimen for long-term treatment. Furosemide is titrated to the lowest dose, and longest interval, that controls signs of congestion. An ACE inhibitor is recommended for chronic therapy if another vasodilator was used initially.

Chronic refractory congestive heart failure
When the patient decompensates, therapy is intensified or adjusted as needed. *Table 54* (p. 271) lists suggestions for modifying therapy.

INFECTIVE ENDOCARDITIS

OVERVIEW
Infection of the cardiac valves or other endocardial tissue is relatively uncommon, but it occurs more often in dogs than in cats[1, 46-50]. Endocarditis usually involves the aortic and/or mitral valves in dogs and cats[1, 46-52]. Bacteremia is a prerequisite for endocarditis; the endocardial surface is infected directly from blood flowing past it. Infections of the skin, mouth, urinary tract, prostate gland, lungs, or other organs can cause recurrent bacteremia[46]. Dentistry procedures are known to cause transient bacteremia in a high percentage of cases, although few individuals develop endocarditis as a consequence[48, 49]. Other procedures (e.g. endoscopy, urethral catheterization, anal surgery, and other 'dirty' procedures) are presumed to cause transient bacteremia in some cases.

Organisms causing endocarditis in dogs and cats have most often been *Streptococcus* species, *Staphylococcus* species, or *Escherichia coli*[46, 48]. Other organisms isolated from infected valves have included *Corynebacterium* (*Arcanobacterium*) species, *Pasteurella* species, *Pseudomonas aeruginosa*, *Erysipelothrix rhusiopathiae* (also identified as *E. tonsillaris*[53]) and others[50, 51, 54]. *Bartonella vinsonii* subsp. *berkhoffii* and other *Bartonella* species have also been identified in dogs with endocarditis[52, 55, 56].

PATHOPHYSIOLOGY
Multiple factors are involved in the development of infective endocarditis, including endothelial damage, disturbed blood flow, immune responses, and bacterial virulence. Highly virulent organisms or a heavy bacterial load increase the risk of cardiac infection, and normal valves can be invaded by virulent bacteria. Previously damaged or diseased valves can become infected after persistent bacteremia. Mechanical trauma can cause such damage (e.g. jet lesions from turbulent blood flow or endocardial injury from a catheter extending into the heart). Diseases that impair immune responses or cause hypercoagulability or endothelial disruption are thought to increase the endocarditis risk[50]. Endocarditis lesions are typically located downstream from disturbed blood flow; common sites include the ventricular side of aortic valve leaflets with subaortic stenosis, the RV side of a ventricular septal defect, and the atrial surface of the mitral valve[48]. Bacterial clumping promoted by agglutinating antibodies may facilitate attachment to the valves. Degenerative mitral valve disease has not been associated with a higher risk for infective endocarditis[47, 48].

Endothelial damage and mechanical valve trauma can also predispose to nonbacterial thrombotic endocarditis, which is a sterile accumulation of platelets and fibrin on the valve surface. Nonseptic (so-called 'bland') emboli may break off from such vegetations and cause infarctions elsewhere. Bacteremia can also cause a secondary infective endocarditis at these sites.

Microbial colonization further damages the endothelium, which stimulates platelet aggregation and coagulation cascade activation and leads to the formation of vegetations. Vegetations consist mainly of aggregated platelets, fibrin, blood cells, and bacteria (**400**). Newer vegetations are more friable; with time, the lesions become fibrous and may calcify[48]. Additional fibrin deposited over bacterial colonies protects them from normal host defenses, as well as many antibiotics. Although vegetations usually involve the valve leaflets, lesions may extend to the chordae tendineae, sinuses of Valsalva, mural endocardium, or adjacent myocardium. Valve leaflet deformity, perforation, or tearing causes valve insufficiency; large vegetations may cause valve stenosis.

CHF commonly results from valve insufficiency and volume overload. Because the mitral and aortic valves are typically affected, pulmonary edema is the usual manifestation. Clinical heart failure can develop rapidly when severe valve destruction, chordae tendineae rupture, multiple valve involvement, or other predisposing factors are present. Extension of infection into the myocardium, or myocardial infarction and abscess formation from coronary embolization, can provoke arrhythmias and compromise cardiac function. Aortic valve endocarditis may extend into the AV node to cause partial or complete AV block. Arrhythmias can cause weakness, syncope, and sudden death, as well as contribute to CHF development.

Fragments of vegetative lesions often break loose and cause infarction or metastatic infection in other body sites. Larger and more mobile vegetations, as assessed echocardiographically, are associated with a higher incidence of embolic events in people and, presumably, in animals[57]. Emboli may be septic or bland. Septic emboli and local abscess formation contribute to recurrent bacteremia and fever. Septic arthritis, diskospondylitis, urinary tract infections, and renal and splenic infarctions are common and contribute to the diverse clinical signs. Both cell-mediated and humoral immune responses are activated[48, 50, 58]. Sterile polyarthritis, glomerulonephritis, vasculitis, and other immune-mediated organ damage are common. Hypertrophic osteopathy has also been associated with bacterial endocarditis[59].

CLINICAL FEATURES

Male dogs are affected more commonly than females, and the prevalence of endocarditis increases with age[46-48, 54]. Most reports suggest German Shepherd Dogs and other large breed dogs are at greater risk[51, 52, 54, 60]. Subaortic stenosis is a known risk factor for aortic valve endocarditis[51, 61]. Immunocompromised animals may possibly also be at greater risk for endocarditis.

The clinical signs are quite variable. Cardiac signs (e.g. those resulting from left-sided congestion or arrhythmias) may predominate or may be overshadowed by systemic signs resulting from infarction, infection, or immune-mediated damage. Nonspecific lethargy, weight loss, inappetence, recurrent fever, and weakness are common. Affected animals may have evidence of past or concurrent infections, although often a clear history of predisposing factors is absent. Infective endocarditis can mimic immune-mediated disease. *Table 55* (p. 274) lists some consequences of infectious endocarditis.

CHF in an unexpected clinical setting or in an animal with a murmur of recent onset could indicate infective endocarditis, especially if other suggestive signs are present. However, a 'new' murmur might indicate noninfective acquired disease (e.g. degenerative valve disease, cardiomyopathy), previously undiagnosed congenital disease, or physiologic alterations (e.g. fever, anemia). Endocarditis can also develop in animals with a known murmur from other cardiac disease. While a change in murmur quality or intensity over a short time frame may indicate active valve damage, physiologic causes of murmur variation are common. However, the onset of a diastolic murmur at the left heart base is suspicious for aortic valve endocarditis, especially if fever or other signs are present.

DIAGNOSIS

Definitive antemortem diagnosis can be difficult. A presumptive diagnosis of infective endocarditis is made based on two or more positive blood cultures in addition to either echocardiographic evidence of vegetations or valve destruction, or the documented recent onset of a regurgitant murmur. Endocarditis is

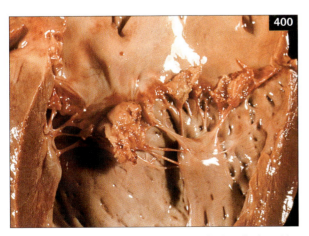

400 Multiple vegetations are seen on the mitral valve of a dog with infective endocarditis. Much of the normal valve structure has been destroyed. (Courtesy Dr R Myers.)

Table 55 Potential sequelae of infective endocarditis.

1) Cardiac:
   a) Valve insufficiency or stenosis:
      ■ Murmur.
      ■ Congestive heart failure.
   b) Coronary embolization (aortic valve*):
      ■ Myocardial infarction.
      ■ Myocardial abscess.
      ■ Myocarditis.
      ■ Decreased contractility (segmental or global).
      ■ Arrhythmias.
   c) Myocarditis (direct invasion by microorganisms):
      ■ Arrhythmias.
      ■ Atrioventricular conduction abnormalities (aortic valve*).
      ■ Decreased contractility.
   d) Pericarditis (direct invasion by microorganisms):
      ■ Pericardial effusion.
      ■ Cardiac tamponade(?).
2) Renal:
   a) Infarction:
      ■ Reduced renal function.
   b) Abscess formation and pyelonephritis:
      ■ Reduced renal function.
      ■ Urinary tract infection.
      ■ Renal pain.
   c) Glomerulonephritis (immune mediated):
      ■ Proteinuria.
      ■ Reduced renal function.
3) Musculoskeletal:
   a) Septic arthritis:
      ■ Joint swelling and pain.
      ■ Lameness.
   b) Immune-mediated polyarthritis:
      ■ Shifting-limb lameness.
      ■ Joint swelling and pain.
   c) Septic osteomyelitis:
      ■ Bone pain.
      ■ Lameness.
   d) Myositis:
      ■ Muscle pain.
4) Nervous system:
   a) Abscesses:
      ■ Associated neurologic signs.
   b) Encephalitis and meningitis:
      ■ Associated neurologic signs.
5) Vascular system:
   a) Vasculitis:
      ■ Thrombosis.
      ■ Petechiae and small hemorrhages (e.g. eye, skin).
   b) Obstruction:
      ■ Ischemia of tissues served, with associated signs.
6) Pulmonary:
   a) Pulmonary emboli (tricuspid or pulmonic valves, rare*).
   b) Pneumonia (tricuspid or pulmonic valves, rare*).
7) General systemic:
   a) Sepsis.
   b) Fever.
   c) Anorexia.
   d) Malaise and depression.
   e) Shaking.
   f) Vague pain.
   g) Inflammatory leukogram.
   h) Mild anemia.
   i) ± positive antinuclear antibody test.
   j) ± positive blood cultures.

* Diseased valve most commonly associated with abnormality.

likely even with negative or intermittently positive blood cultures if there is echocardiographic evidence of vegetations or valve destruction, especially of the aortic valve, combined with other criteria (*Table 56*)[48, 62].

Ideally, several blood samples of at least 10 ml are collected aseptically over 24 hours for bacterial culture, with more than 1 hour elapsing between collections. Different venipuncture sites should be used for each sample. Both aerobic and anaerobic cultures have been recommended, although the value of routine anaerobic culture is questionable. Prolonged incubation (3 weeks) is recommended, because some bacteria are slow growing[48, 60]. Negative culture results do not rule out infective endocarditis, especially with chronic endocarditis, recent antibiotic therapy, intermittent bacteremia, or infection by fastidious or slow growing organisms. Serologic testing and PCR amplification are available for *B. vinsonii*, which is rarely cultured successfully in dogs[56].

Table 56 Criteria for diagnosis of infectious endocarditis*.

1) Definite endocarditis by pathologic criteria:

   a) Pathologic (postmortem) lesions of active endocarditis with evidence of microorganisms in vegetation (or embolus) or intracardiac abscess.

2) Definite endocarditis by clinical criteria:

   a) 2 major criteria (below), or

   b) 1 major and 3 minor criteria, or

   c) 5 minor criteria.

3) Possible endocarditis:

   a) Findings consistent with infectious endocarditis that fall short of 'definite' but not 'rejected'.

4) Rejected diagnosis of endocarditis:

   a) Firm alternative diagnosis for clinical manifestations.

   b) Resolution of manifestations of infective endocarditis with 4 or fewer days of antibiotic therapy.

   c) No pathologic evidence of infective endocarditis at surgery or necropsy after 4 or fewer days of antibiotic therapy.

5) Major criteria:

   a) Positive blood cultures:

     ■ Typical microorganism for infective endocarditis from 2 separate blood cultures.

     ■ Persistently positive blood cultures for organism consistent with endocarditis (samples drawn >12 hours apart or 3 or more cultures drawn at least 1 hour apart).

   b) Evidence of endocardial involvement:

     ■ Positive echocardiogram for infective endocarditis (oscillating mass on heart valve or supportive structure or in path of regurgitant jet; or evidence of cardiac abscess).

     ■ New valvular regurgitation (increase or change in preexisting murmur not sufficient evidence).

6) Minor criteria:

   a) Predisposing heart condition (see text, p. 277).

   b) Fever.

   c) Vascular phenomena: major arterial emboli, septic infarcts.

   d) Immunologic phenomena: glomerulonephritis, positive antinuclear antibody or rheumatoid factor tests.

   e) Microbiologic evidence: positive blood culture not meeting major criterion, above.

   f) Echocardiogram consistent with infective endocarditis but not meeting major criterion, above.

   g) (Rare in dogs and cats: repeated nonsterile IV drug administration).

* Adapted from Durack DT, Lukes AS, Bright DK, and the Duke Endocarditis Service (1994) New criteria for diagnosis of infective endocarditis: utilization of specific echocardiographic findings. *Am J Med* **96(3)**:200–209.

Clinical laboratory findings usually reflect the presence of inflammation[60]. Neutrophilia with a left shift is typical of acute endocarditis; mature neutrophilia with or without monocytosis develops with time. Nonregenerative anemia, thrombocytopenia, azotemia, hyperglobulinemia, hematuria, pyuria, and proteinuria are common as well[48, 60]. Rheumatoid factor and antinuclear antibody tests may be positive in dogs with subacute or chronic bacterial endocarditis[46, 48, 50, 63]. Urine culture may also reveal the causative organism.

The ECG may be normal or document tachyarrhythmias, conduction disturbances, or evidence of myocardial ischemia[48–51, 60].

Radiographic findings may be unremarkable when valve damage is minimal, or show evidence of cardiomegaly, left-sided heart failure, or other organ involvement (e.g. diskospondylitis)[48, 60].

Echocardiography is especially supportive if oscillating vegetative lesions and abnormal valve motion can be identified. Lesion visualization depends on size and location as well as image resolution quality[60]. False negatives and false-positive 'lesions' can appear, so cautious interpretation of images is important. Early lesions consist of valve thickening and/or enhanced echogenicity. Vegetations appear as irregular, dense masses (**401–403**), although degenerative AV valve disease can look similar[60]. As valve destruction progresses, ruptured chordae, flail leaflet tips, or other abnormal valve motion can be seen (**404–406**)[64]. Multiple valves can be involved. Aortic insufficiency can cause visible diastolic flutter of the anterior mitral valve leaflet as the regurgitant jet disturbs this leaflet (see **154–156**, p. 81). Other cardiac sequelae include chamber enlargement from volume overload, myocardial dysfunction, and arrhythmias.

MANAGEMENT

Aggressive therapy with bactericidal antibiotics capable of penetrating fibrin and supportive care is indicated.

Drug choice is ideally guided by culture and sensitivity test results; however, broad-spectrum combination therapy is usually begun immediately after obtaining blood culture samples to avoid treatment delay. Therapy can be altered, if necessary, when culture results are available. Animals with negative culture results should be continued on the broad-spectrum regimen. An initial combination of a cephalosporin, a penicillin, or a synthetic penicillin derivative with an aminoglycoside or a fluoroquinolone is commonly used (*Table 57*). Clindamycin or metronidazole provides added anaerobic efficacy. Azithromycin or, possibly, enrofloxacin or high-dose doxycycline, has been suggested for *Bartonella* species[56]. Antibiotics are best administered IV for the first week or longer to obtain higher and more predictable blood concentrations. Oral therapy can be used thereafter for the sake of practicality, but parenteral administration (SC) is probably better. Antimicrobial therapy is continued for

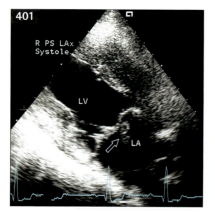 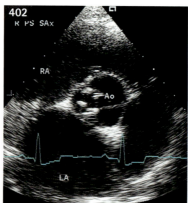 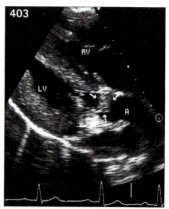

401–403 (401) A large, mobile mitral vegetation (arrow) is seen in the LA during systole in a Great Dane with leptospirosis and endocarditis. (402) Several small nodules were evident on the aortic valve of a 2-year-old female Rottweiler with severe SAS. Reduced exercise tolerance was the only sign of illness in this case. (403) Prominent aortic valve vegetation (arrows) in a 2-year-old male Vizsla with multiple congenital cardiac defects including SAS. All images from right parasternal position. A = aorta; LA = left atrium; LV = left ventricle; RV = right ventricle.

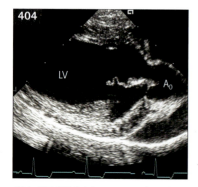 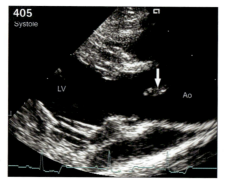 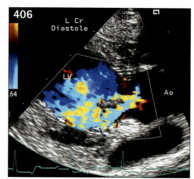

404–406 (404) A long, extremely mobile vegetative lesion was attached to the aortic valve in a 6-year-old Pomeranian with fever, syncope, and hypertension. Right parasternal long-axis view. (405) During systole the vegetation (arrow) extended into the aorta and caused partial obstruction. (406) Color flow Doppler indicated severe aortic regurgitation (seen flowing around the vegetation) during diastole. 405, 406: left cranial long-axis view. Ao = aorta; LV = left ventricle.

1) Initial therapy:

   a) Ampicillin (22 mg/kg IV q6–8h) or cefazolin (22–33 mg/kg IV q8h) with either amikacin (7–10 mg/kg IV q12h [discontinue after 5–7 days]) or enrofloxacin (2.5–5 mg/kg IV q12h).

2) Oral continuation therapy:

   b) Amoxicillin/clavulanate (20–25 mg/kg PO q8h) or cephalexin (25–30 mg/kg PO q8h) with enrofloxacin (2.5–5 mg/kg PO q12h).

* Modify therapy as necessary based on positive blood culture and susceptibility test results. See text for further information.

at least 6 weeks, although therapy for 8 weeks is often recommended; however, aminoglycosides are discontinued after 1 week or sooner if renal toxicity develops. Close monitoring of the urine sediment is indicated to detect early aminoglycoside nephrotoxicity. Repeat serologic testing for *B. vinsonii* (*berkhoffii*) is recommended, probably between 3–6 months after antibiotic therapy[56].

Supportive care includes management of CHF (see Chapter 16) and any arrhythmias (see Chapter 17), as well as complications related to the primary infection source, embolic events, or immune responses. Corticosteroids are contraindicated. The usefulness of aspirin in reducing vegetative lesion growth and incidence of embolic events is questionable. In people, there appears to be no benefit from aspirin or oral anticoagulant use[65]. The potential adverse effects of aspirin must be considered.

The long-term prognosis is generally guarded to poor, especially with echocardiographic evidence of vegetations and volume overload[46, 50, 60]. Aggressive therapy may be successful in the absence of large vegetations and severe valve dysfunction. CHF is the most common cause of death, although sepsis, systemic embolization, arrhythmias, or renal failure may be responsible.

Prophylactic antibiotic use is controversial. Experience in people suggests most infective endocarditis cases are not preventable; the risk of endocarditis involved with a specific (e.g. dental) procedure is very low compared with the cumulative risk associated with normal daily activities[66]. However, in view of the increased incidence of endocarditis with certain cardiovascular malformations, antimicrobial prophylaxis is recommended for animals with such defects prior to dental or other 'dirty' procedures (e.g. ones involving the oral cavity or intestinal or urogenital systems). Besides SAS, endocarditis has occasionally been associated with ventricular septal defect, PDA, and cyanotic congenital heart disease[48]. Antimicrobial prophylaxis should be given to animals with an implanted pacemaker or other device, or with a history of endocarditis, and should be considered in immunocompromised animals as well. Recommendations, extrapolated from human medicine, include administration of high-dose ampicillin or amoxicillin 1 hour prior to, +/– 6 hours after, oral and upper respiratory procedures, and ampicillin with an aminoglycoside, IV, 1/2 hour prior to and 8 hours after GI or urogenital procedures. Ticarcillin or a first generation cephalosporin, IV, 1 hour prior to and 6 hours after the procedure have also been recommended[50].

REFERENCES

1 Buchanan JW (1999) Prevalence of cardiovascular disorders. In *Textbook of Canine and Feline Cardiology*, 2nd edn. PR Fox, D Sisson, NS Moise (eds). WB Saunders, Philadelphia, pp. 457–470.

2 Buchanan JW (1977) Chronic valvular disease (endocardiosis) in dogs. *Adv Vet Sci Comp Med* 21:75–106.

3 Kogure K (1980) Pathology of chronic mitral valvular disease in the dog. *Jpn J Vet Sci* 42:323–335.

4 Sisson D (1987) Acquired valvular heart disease in dogs and cats. In *Contemporary Issues in Small Animal Practice: Cardiology*. JD Bonagura (ed). Churchill Livingstone, New York, pp. 59–116.

5 Corcoran BM, Black A, Anderson H *et al.* (2004) Identification of surface morphologic changes in the mitral valve leaflets and chordae tendineae of dogs with myxomatous degeneration. *Am J Vet Res* 65:198–206.

6 Pedersen HD, Lorentzen KA, Kristensen BO (1999) Echocardiographic mitral prolapse in

Cavalier King Charles Spaniels: epidemiology and prognostic significance for regurgitation. *Vet Rec* **144**:315–320.

7 Mow T, Pedersen HD (1999) Increased endothelin-receptor density in myxomatous canine mitral leaflets. *J Cardiovac Pharmacol* **34**:254–260.

8 Olsen LH, Kristensen AT, Haggstrom J et al. (2001) Increased platelet aggregation response in Cavalier King Charles Spaniels with mitral valve prolapse. *J Vet Intern Med* **15**:209–216.

9 Haggstrom J, Hansson K, Kvart C et al. (1997) Effects of naturally acquired decompensated mitral valve regurgitation on the renin-angiotensin-aldosterone system and atrial natriuretic peptide concentration in dogs. *Am J Vet Res* **58**:77–82.

10 Pedersen HD, Koch J, Poulsen K et al. (1995) Activation of the renin-angiotensin system in dogs with asymptomatic and mildly symptomatic mitral valvular insufficiency. *J Vet Intern Med* **9**:328–331.

11 Kittleson MD, Eyster GE, Knowlen GG et al. (1984) Myocardial function in small dogs with chronic mitral regurgitation and severe congestive heart failure. *J Am Vet Med Assoc* **184**:455–459.

12 Nagatsu M, Zile MR, Tsutsui H et al. (1994) Native β-adrenergic support for left ventricular dysfunction in experimental mitral regurgitation normalizes indexes of pump and contractile function. *Circulation* **89**:818–826.

13 Lord P, Ericksson A, Haggstrom J et al. (2003) Increased pulmonary transit times in asymptomatic dogs with mitral regurgitation. *J Vet Intern Med* **17**:824–829.

14 Pederson HD, Schuett T, Sondergaard R et al. (2003) Decreased plasma concentration of nitric oxide metabolites in dogs with untreated mitral regurgitation. *J Vet Intern Med* **17**:178–184.

15 Prasad K, Gupta JB, Kalra J et al. (1996) Oxidative stress as a mechanism of cardiac failure in chronic volume overload in canine

model. *J Mol Cell Cardiol* **28**:375–385.

16 Tsutsui H, Spinale FG, Nagatsu M et al. (1994) Effects of chronic beta-adrenergic blockade on the left ventricular and cardiocyte abnormalities of chronic canine mitral regurgitation. *J Clin Invest* **93**:2639–2648.

17 Davila-Roman VG, Creswell LL, Rosenbloom M et al. (1993) Myocardial contractile state in dogs with chronic mitral regurgitation: echocardiographic approach to the peak systolic pressure/end systolic area relationship. *Am Heart J* **126**:155–160.

18 Chen C, Rodriguez L, Levine RA et al. (1992) Noninvasive measurement of the time constant of left ventricular relaxation using the continuous-wave Doppler velocity profile of mitral regurgitation. *Circulation* **86**:272–278.

19 Chen C, Rodriguez L, Guerrero JL et al. (1991) Noninvasive estimation of the instantaneous first derivative of left ventricular pressure using continuous-wave Doppler echocardiography. *Circulation* **83**:2101–2110.

20 Olsen LH, Fredholm M, Pedersen HD (1999) Epidemiology and inheritance of mitral valve prolapse in Dachshunds. *J Vet Intern Med* **13**:448–456.

21 Swenson L, Haggstrom J, Kvart C et al. (1996) Relationship between parental cardiac status in Cavalier King Charles Spaniels and prevalence and severity of chronic valvular disease in offspring. *J Am Vet Med Assoc* **208**:2009–2012.

22 de Madron E (1992) Primary acquired mitral insufficiency in adult large breed dogs. *Proceedings of the 10th ACVIM Forum*, pp. 608–609.

23 Borgarelli M, Zini E, D'Agnolo et al. (2004) Comparison of primary mitral valve disease in German Shepherd Dogs and in small breeds. *J Vet Cardiol* **6**:27–34.

24 Beardow AW, Buchanan JW (1993) Chronic mitral valve disease in Cavalier King Charles Spaniels: 95 cases (1987–1991). *J Am Vet Med Assoc* **203**:1023–1029.

25 Haggstrom J, Hansson K, Kvart C et al. (1992) Chronic valvular disease in the Cavalier King Charles Spaniel in Sweden. *Vet Rec* **131**:549–553.

26 Haggstrom J, Kvart C, Hansson K (1995) Heart sounds and murmurs: changes related to severity of chronic valvular disease in the Cavalier King Charles Spaniel. *J Vet Intern Med* **9**:75–85.

27 Malik R, Hunt G, Allan G (1992) Prevalence of mitral valve insufficiency in Cavalier King Charles Spaniels. *Vet Rec* **130**:302–303.

28 Darke PGG (1987) Valvular incompetence in Cavalier King Charles Spaniels. *Vet Rec* **120**:365–366.

29 Smith PJ, French AT, Van Israël N et al. (2005) Efficacy and safety of pimobendan in canine heart failure caused by myxomatous mitral valve disease. *J Small Anim Pract* **46**:121–130.

30 Pedersen HD, Haggstrom J, Falk T et al. (1999) Auscultation in mild mitral regurgitation in dogs: observer variation, effects of physical maneuvers, and agreement with color Doppler echocardiography and phonocardiography. *J Vet Intern Med* **13**:56–64.

31 Jacobs GJ, Calvert CA, Mahaffey MB et al. (1995) Echocardiographic detection of flail left atrioventricular valve cusp from ruptured chordae tendineae in 4 dogs. *J Vet Intern Med* **9**:341–346.

32 Sadanaga KK, MacDonald MJ, Buchanan JW (1990) Echocardiography and surgery in a dog with left atrial rupture and hemopericardium *J Vet Intern Med* **4**:216–221.

33 Muzzi RAL, deAraujo RB, Muzzi LAL et al. (2003) Regurgitant jet area by Doppler color flow mapping: quantitative assessment of mitral regurgitation severity in dogs. *J Vet Cardiol* **5**:33–38.

34 Kittleson MD, Brown WA (2003) Regurgitant fraction measured by using the proximal isovelocity surface area method in dogs with chronic myxomatous mitral valve disease. *J Vet Intern Med* **17**:84–88.

35 Buchanan JW, Sammarco CD (1998) Circumferential suture of the mitral annulus for correction of mitral regurgitation in dogs. *Vet Surg* **27**:182–193.

36 Orton EC (2001) Surgical treament of valvular disease. In *Proceedings of the 19th ACVIM Forum*, Denver, pp. 156–157.

37 Kerstetter KK, Sackman JE, Buchanan JW *et al.* (1998) Short-term hemodynamic evaluation of circumferential mitral annuloplasty for correction of mitral valve regurgitation in dogs. *Vet Surg* **27**:216–223.

38 Griffiths LG, Orton EC, Boon JA (2004) Evaluation of techniques and outcomes of mitral valve repair in dogs. *J Am Vet Med Assoc* **224**:1941–1945.

39 Orton EC, Hackett TB, Mama K *et al.* (2005) Technique and outcome of mitral valve replacement in dogs. *J Am Vet Med Assoc* **226**:1508–1511.

40 Kvart C, Haggstrom J, Pederson HD *et al.* (2002) Efficacy of enalapril for prevention of congestive heart failure in dogs with myxomatous valve disease and asymptomatic mitral regurgitation. *J Vet Intern Med* **16**:80–88.

41 Atkins C (2002) Enalapril monotherapy in asymptomatic mitral regurgitation: results of the VetProof trial. In *Proceedings of the 20th ACVIM Forum*, pp. 75–76.

42 Kitagawa H, Wakamiya H, Kitoh K *et al.* (1997) Efficacy of monotherapy with benazepril, an angiotensin converting enzyme inhibitor, in dogs with naturally acquired chronic mitral insufficiency. *J Vet Med Sci* **59**:513–520.

43 Hamlin RL, Benitz AM, Ericsson GF *et al.* (1996) Effects of enalapril on exercise tolerance and longevity in dogs with heart failure produced by iatrogenic mitral regurgitation. *J Vet Intern Med* **10**:85–87.

44 Lombard CW, Jöns O, Bussadori CM (2006) Clinical effeciency of pimobendan versus benazepril for the treatment of acquired atrioventricular valvular disease in dogs. *J Am Anim Hosp Assoc* **42**:249–261.

45 Haggstrom J, Kvart C (2003) New and old treatment modalities of myxomatous mitral valve disease in dogs. *Proceedings of the 21st ACVIM Forum*, pp. 113–115.

46 Calvert CA, Greene CE, Hardie EM (1985) Cardiovascular infections in dogs: epizootiology, clinical manifestations, and prognosis. *J Am Vet Med Assoc* **187**:612–616.

47 Sisson D (1994) Bacterial endocarditis. *Proceedings of the Waltham/OSU Symposium*, Vernon, pp. 79–87.

48 Miller MW, Fox PR, Saunders AB (2004) Pathologic and clinical features of infectious endocarditis. *J Vet Cardiol* **6**:35–43.

49 Tou SP, Adin DB, Castleman WL (2005) Mitral valve endocarditis after dental prophylaxis in a dog. *J Vet Intern Med* **19**:268–270.

50 Wall M, Calvert CA, Greene CE (2002) Infective endocarditis in dogs. *Compend Contin Educ Pract Vet* **24**:614–625.

51 Sisson D, Thomas WP (1984) Endocarditis of the aortic valve. *J Am Vet Med Assoc* **184**:570-577.

52 MacDonald KA, Chomel BB, Kittleson MD *et al.* (2004) A prospective study of canine infective endocarditis in Northern California (1999–2001): emergence of *Bartonella* as a prevalent etiologic agent. *J Vet Intern Med* **18**:56–64.

53 Takahashi T, Tamura Y, Yoshimura H *et al.* (1993) *Erysipelothrix tonsillarum* isolated from dogs with endocarditis in Belgium. *Res Vet Sci* **54**:264–265.

54 Anderson CA, Dubielzig RR (1984) Vegetative endocarditis in dogs. *J Am Anim Hosp Assoc* **20**:149–152.

55 Breitschwerdt EB, Kordick DL, Malarkey DE *et al.* (1995) Endocarditis in a dog due to infection with a novel *Bartonella* subspecies. *J Clin Microbiol* **33**:154–160.

56 Breitschwerdt EB (2003) *Bartonella* species as emerging vector-transmitted pathogens. *Comp Cont Educ Pract Vet* **25**(Suppl):12–15.

57 DiSalvo G, Habib G, Pergola V *et al.* (2001) Echocardiography predicts embolic events in infective endocarditis. *J Am Coll Cardiol* **37**:1069–1076.

58 Bennett D, Bilbertson EM, Grennan D (1993) Bacterial endocarditis with polyarthritis in two dogs associated with circulating autoantibodies. *J Small Anim Pract* **19**:185–196.

59 Vulgamott JC, Clark RG (1980) Arterial hypertension and hypertrophic pulmonary osteopathy associated with aortic valvular endocarditis in a dog. *J Am Vet Med Assoc* **177**,243–246.

60 Elwood CM, Cobb MA, Stepien RL (1993) Clinical and echocardiographic findings in 10 dogs with vegetative bacterial endocarditis. *J Small Anim Pract* **34**:420–427.

61 Muna WFT, Ferrans VJ, Pierce JE *et al.* (1978) Discrete subaortic stenosis in Newfoundland dogs: association of infective endocarditis. *Am J Cardiol* **41**:746–754.

62 Durack DT, Lukes AS, Bright DK *et al.* (1994) New criteria for diagnosis of infective endocarditis: utilization of specific echocardiographic findings. *Am J Med* **96**:200–209.

63 Smith BE, Tompkins MB, Breitschwerdt EB (2004) Antinuclear antibodies can be detected in dog sera reactive to *Bartonella vinsonii* subsp. *berkhoffii*, *Ehrlichia canis* or *Leishmania infantum* antigens. *J Vet Intern Med* **18**:47–51.

64 Sottiaux J, Franck M (1998) Echocardiographic appearance of flail aortic valve in a dog with infective endocarditis. *Vet Rad Ultrasound* **39**:436–439.

65 Chan KL, Dumesil JG, Cujec B *et al.* (2003) A randomized trial of aspirin on the risk of embolic events in patients with infective endocarditis. *J Am Coll Cardiol* **42**:775–780.

66 Zuckerman JM, Kaye D (2001) Prevention of endocarditis in the dental patient. *Infect Med* **18**:107–113.

20
Myocardial Diseases of the Dog

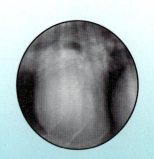

Primary myocardial disease (idiopathic dilated cardiomyopathy) is an important cause of heart failure in large breed dogs. Secondary and infective causes of myocardial disease are documented less often. Hypertrophic cardiomyopathy (HCM) is rare in dogs.

DILATED CARDIOMYOPATHY

OVERVIEW

Dilated cardiomyopathy (DCM) is characterized by impaired myocardial contractility with dilation of the LV or both ventricles[1,2]. Tachyarrhythmias are common. DCM as an entity probably represents the end-stage of different pathologic processes or metabolic defects involving myocardial cells or the intercellular matrix[1,2]. Secondary causes of myocardial failure and cardiac dilation (see below) should be excluded before making a diagnosis of idiopathic DCM.

PATHOPHYSIOLOGY OF DCM

Cardiac chamber dilation follows progressive deterioration of systolic pump function, as cardiac output declines and compensatory volume expansion

mechanisms are activated (**407, 408**). Typically, all chambers dilate, although LA and LV enlargement may predominate. Eccentric hypertrophy causes an increased heart weight:body weight ratio, although LV wall thickness may appear decreased compared with the lumen size[1,3]. Flattened, atrophic papillary muscles and endocardial thickening may be noted. AV valve thickening tends to be only mild, if present at all, although marked degenerative changes can be seen in Cocker Spaniels and some large breed dogs. However, chamber dilation and papillary muscle dysfunction often cause mild to moderate AV valve insufficiency by interfering with mitral and tricuspid leaflet apposition. In advanced disease, increased ventricular diastolic stiffness can contribute to high end-diastolic pressure, venous congestion, and ultimately congestive failure.

Histopathologic findings may be nonspecific and include scattered areas of myocardial necrosis, degeneration, and fibrosis, especially in the LV. Inflammatory cell infiltrates and myocardial hypertrophy are inconsistent features, but active myocarditis is rare[1]. Two distinct types of histopathology are also reported and are thought to relate to underlying mechanisms of disease[2]. The first is characterized by narrowed (attenuated) myocardial cells with a wavy

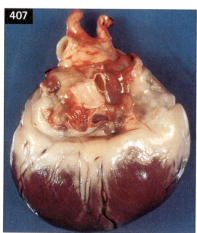

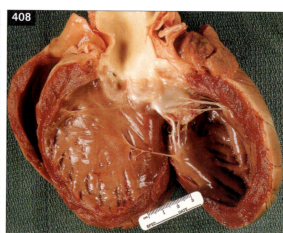

407, 408 Dilated hearts from two large breed dogs with DCM. (**407**) View from caudal right aspect. Courtesy Dr. R. Myers. (**408**) Open LV outflow tract and aorta. Open RV outflow tract is to the left. Courtesy Dr. J. Bonagura.

appearance[4–9]. Such abnormal cells have also been noted in some Newfoundlands predisposed to DCM but without clinical or echocardiographic signs of the disease[4]. The other distinct type is characterized by myofiber degeneration, myocyte atrophy and lysis, fatty infiltration, and fibrosis. This fatty infiltration–degenerative type is described in Boxers[2, 10] and some Doberman Pinschers[11, 12], and is similar to findings in arrhythmogenic RV cardiomyopathy in people (see p. 289)[2].

While underlying mechanisms of the disease are unclear, biochemical defects, nutritional deficiencies, toxins, immunologic mechanisms, and infectious agents may be involved in individual cases[1, 13]. Impaired intracellular energy homeostasis, with reduced myocardial ATP concentrations, has been found in Doberman Pinschers with DCM[14]. Genetic factors are likely involved in many cases. Mutations within several genes that code for cytoskeletal proteins have been identified in people with familial DCM, but similar mutations have yet to be found in dogs[15, 16].

DCM appears to develop insidiously over a prolonged time period. There are no clinical signs during this occult (preclinical) stage. When cardiac output decreases, sympathetic, hormonal, and renal compensatory mechanisms become activated and help maintain cardiac function by increasing HR, peripheral vascular resistance, and volume retention[17]. However, chronic NH activation also contributes to progressive myocardial damage as well as the syndrome of CHF. Right- or left-sided CHF, as well as low-output heart failure, is common in dogs with DCM. Eventually, poor forward blood flow and increased ventricular diastolic pressure can also compromise coronary perfusion, further impair myocardial function, and provoke arrhythmias. Profound myocardial dysfunction may lead to cardiogenic shock.

AF, as well as other atrial and ventricular tachyarrhythmias, are common. Because atrial contraction contributes importantly to ventricular filling at faster HRs, the loss of the 'atrial kick' in AF can markedly reduce cardiac output and precipitate acute clinical decompensation. Persistent tachycardia associated with AF or other arrhythmias may accelerate disease progression[1]. Episodic weakness, syncope, and sudden death are generally associated with tachyarrhythmias, usually of ventricular origin, but paradoxical bradyarrhythmias have also been implicated in Doberman Pinschers[18].

CLINICAL FEATURES

Idiopathic DCM is most common in large and giant breeds of dogs. There is regional variation in prevalence. Doberman Pinschers appear to have a very high prevalence. Other commonly affected breeds include Great Danes, Saint Bernards, Scottish Deerhounds, Irish Wolfhounds, Boxers, Newfoundlands, Afghan Hounds, and Dalmatians[1, 6, 13, 19]. Among smaller breeds, English and American Cocker Spaniels, English Bulldogs, and others are affected, but the disease is rare in dogs weighing less than 12 kilograms. A genetic basis is suspected, especially in breeds with a high prevalence or a familial occurrence of DCM, such as Doberman Pinschers, Boxers, and Cocker Spaniels. Pedigree analysis of a group of Great Danes with DCM suggested inheritance as an X-linked recessive trait[20]. An autosomal dominant inheritance pattern has been found in Boxers with ventricular arrhythmias[21] and Irish Wolfhounds and Doberman Pinschers with DCM[19, 22, 23]; however, a rapidly fatal familial DCM affecting very young Portuguese Water Dogs is thought to have an autosomal recessive inheritance pattern[7, 8].

DCM is most often diagnosed in middle-aged dogs; the prevalence of overt (clinically evident) DCM increases with age. Most reports indicate a male preponderance, especially in dogs with clinical heart failure[1, 11, 13, 19, 24–26]; however, some studies that prospectively screened for DCM found no clear gender predilection appeared once dogs with occult disease were included[1, 2, 19, 21, 27]. Sudden death before the onset of CHF is not uncommon[11, 25].

Preclinical (occult) DCM

The preclinical phase can be prolonged. Ventricular arrhythmias in Doberman Pinschers occur months to several years before echocardiographic or clinical signs of DCM[24–26, 28]. Once LV function begins to deteriorate, the frequency of tachyarrhythmias increases. Progression from silent arrhythmias to overt DCM is thought to occur in Boxers as well[2, 10, 21]. Lone AF precedes overt DCM in some giant breed dogs[2].

The identification of affected dogs before clinical heart failure or sudden death occur is an important issue. 24-hour ambulatory ECG (Holter) recording has been useful for detecting DCM-associated ventricular arrhythmias in Boxers and Doberman Pinschers[10, 21, 24, 25, 29]. An absolute number of VPCs/24 hours that might separate normal from abnormal dogs is not, and may never be, clear. Nevertheless, >50 VPCs/24-hour period is thought to be abnormal in Boxers[21]. Over 50 VPCs/24 hours, or any couplets or triplets, is thought to be predictive of future DCM in Doberman Pinschers[24, 25]; however, dogs with <50 VPCs/24 hours on initial evaluation have also developed cardiomyopathy several years later. The frequency and complexity of ventricular tachyarrhythmias appear to be negatively correlated with FS and sustained ventricular tachycardia has been associated with increased risk of sudden death[11, 25]. There can be large variability in the number of VPCs between repeated Holter recordings in the same dog[30]. There may be other breeds (e.g. Weimeraners, Great Danes) where Holter monitoring might prove useful as a screening tool, but in most breeds the ECG is neither sensitive nor specific enough to be used as a screening tool for preclinical DCM[2]. In-clinic resting ECG recordings are not useful because of their brief duration[31]. Analysis of heart rate variability has not been helpful in differentiating mildly or moderately affected dogs from normal, or in predicting sudden death[32–35]. The technique of signal averaged electrocardiography (SAECG) may be useful if available. The SAECG is abnormal in some but not all Doberman Pinschers with occult DCM that die suddenly[34]. Nevertheless, the presence of ventricular late potentials appears to indicate increased risk for sudden death[36, 37].

Echocardiography is also used to screen dogs thought to be at increased risk for DCM, although abnormalities may be absent in early disease. Ventricular enlargement or depressed FS has been identified in preclinical Newfoundlands and Doberman Pinschers years before overt DCM developed[2, 11, 25, 28]. It is important to note that apparently healthy Doberman Pinschers often have reduced myocardial function compared with what is considered normal for other breeds. The following echocardiographic criteria are thought to be predictors of high risk for overt DCM within 2–3 years in asymptomatic Doberman Pinschers[25, 28]: LVIDd >46 mm (in dogs ≤42 kg) or >50 mm (in dogs >42 kg); LVIDs >38 mm; or VPCs during initial examination, FS <25%, and/or mitral

valve EPSS >8 mm. (LVID = left ventricular internal diameter; d = diastole; s = systole.) Dobutamine stress testing to detect early myocardial dysfunction has been described, but further work is needed to clarify its clinical applicability[38, 39].

The European Society of Veterinary Cardiology (ESVC) has proposed a scoring system for the diagnosis of DCM (*Table 58*)[2]. These guidelines may be useful in identifying dogs warranting serial evaluation (i.e. those that score any points) for progression to DCM, although further investigation of this system is needed.

Overt DCM

The onset of clinical signs may appear sudden despite a protracted preclinical phase, especially in nonworking dogs where early signs may not be noticed. Presenting complaints include any or all of the following: weakness, lethargy, tachypnea or dyspnea, exercise intolerance, cough (sometimes described as 'gagging'), anorexia, abdominal distension (ascites), syncope, and even sudden death. Episodic weakness, syncope, or sudden death may be the only signs in Boxers or other dogs with tachyarrhythmia but relatively well-preserved ventricular function. Loss of muscle mass (cardiac cachexia) may be marked later in the disease, especially in dogs with signs of right-sided heart failure (**409**). Some giant breed dogs with only mild

---

Table 58 European Society for Veterinary Cardiology proposed scoring system for dilated cardiomyopathy diagnosis*.

1) Major criteria (3 points each):**

   a) LV dilation: systolic or diastolic dimension exceeding 95% confidence intervals for the individual or other breed-specific reference ranges.

   b) Increased LV sphericity: ratio of LV diastolic chamber length (from apex to mitral annulus; obtained using right parasternal long axis 4-chamber view) to LV diastolic short-axis dimension (from M-mode) of <1.65.

   c) ■ Reduced LV fractional shortening: <20–25% (depending on breed-specific reference values; M-mode); and/or

      ■ Reduced LV ejection fraction: <40% (from 2-D long-axis view optimized for LV size).

2) Minor criteria (1 point each):

   a) Arrhythmia: where it is strongly associated with DCM in the specific breed (e.g. ventricular ectopy in Boxers or Doberman Pinschers); other causes should be actively excluded.

   b) Atrial fibrillation.

   c) Increased mitral valve EPSS (from M-mode).

   d) Increased preejection PEP:ET ratio: exceeding 95% confidence intervals (e.g. >0.4).

   e) LV fractional shortening in equivocal range: depends on breed-specific reference values (from M-mode).

   f) Left or biatrial enlargement.

Total score of 6 or more points is consistent with DCM once other cardiac and systemic disease is excluded.

Total score of 1 to 5 points should prompt serial reevaluation for evidence of progression.

* Adapted from Dukes-McEwan J, Borgarelli M, Tidholm A *et al.* (2003) Proposed guidelines for the diagnosis of canine idiopathic dilated cardiomyopathy. *J Vet Cardiol* 5:7–19. (Note: These are proposed diagnostic guidelines awaiting further evaluation and refinement. They are not intended as breeding guidelines at this time.)

** Importance of breed specific reference values is stressed. Caution is warranted in assessing very athletic or extreme breeds.

to moderate LV dysfunction are relatively asymptomatic, even in the presence of AF.

Physical findings vary with the degree of cardiac decompensation. Poor cardiac output with high sympathetic tone and peripheral vasoconstriction causes mucous membrane pallor and prolonged CRT. The femoral arterial pulse and precordial impulse are often weak and rapid. Uncontrolled AF and frequent VPCs cause a rapid and irregular heartbeat, with pulse deficits and variable pulse strength (**410**). Pulsus alternans, related to every-other-beat alteration in stroke volume from profound myocardial dysfunction, can also occur[40]. Signs of left- and/or right-sided CHF, such as tachypnea, increased breath sounds, pulmonary crackles, jugular venous distension or pulsations, pleural effusion or ascites, and/or hepatosplenomegaly, are usually present. Heart sounds can be muffled secondary to pleural effusion or poor cardiac contractile strength. An audible third heart sound (S_3 gallop) is a classic finding, although it may be obscured by an irregular heart rhythm. Soft to moderate intensity systolic murmurs of mitral and/or tricuspid regurgitation are common.

Prerenal azotemia (from poor renal perfusion) or mildly increased liver enzyme activities (from passive hepatic congestion) may be present, although clinical laboratory tests are often noncontributory[1, 3]. Severe heart failure can be associated with hypoproteinemia, hyperkalemia, and hyponatremia. Hypothyroidism with hypercholesterolemia occurs in some dogs with DCM, but most have normal TSH and free T_4 concentrations[17]. The prevalence of hypothyroidism in Doberman Pinschers with DCM is not different from those without DCM[41]. Increases in circulating neurohormones can be seen with clinical heart failure[17, 42–45]. Serum cardiac troponin (cTnT or cTnI) concentration elevations occur in some dogs with DCM as well as with other causes of myocyte injury, but markedly increased cTn is not expected with idiopathic DCM[2, 46–48].

Generalized cardiomegaly is usually evident radiographically, although left heart enlargement may predominate (**411–415**). In some Doberman Pinschers and Boxers, LA enlargement without marked

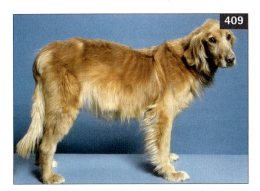

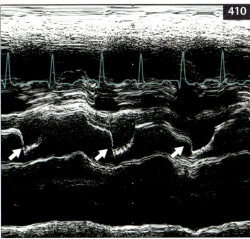

409, 410 (409) Cardiac cachexia in a Golden Retriever with DCM and congestive failure. Loss of muscle mass along the ribs and back is evident; ascites has caused abdominal distension. (410) Presence of pulse deficits is illustrated in this M-mode echo depicting the motion of an aortic valve leaflet. LV systolic pressure generation sufficient to cause ejection (and aortic valve opening [arrows]) only occurs with every other QRS complex. From a Doberman Pinscher with AF and DCM.

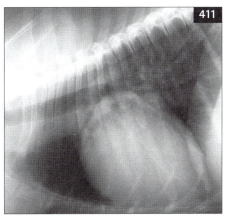

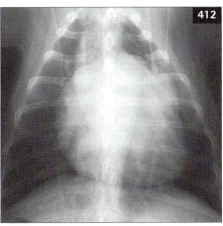

411, 412 Generalized cardiomegaly is seen on lateral (411) and DV (412) views in a 9-year-old female Dalmation with DCM.

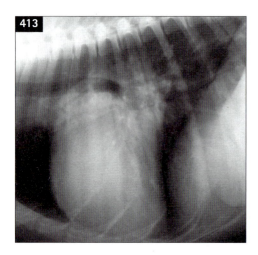

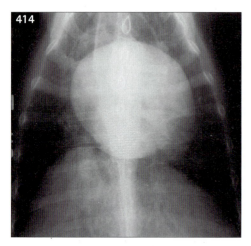

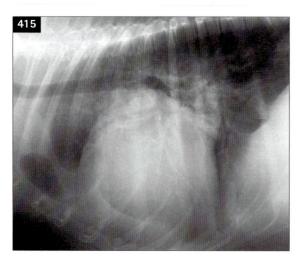

cardiomegaly is seen. Distended pulmonary veins (see 56, p. 42) and pulmonary interstitial or alveolar opacities, especially in the hilar and dorsocaudal regions, accompany left-sided heart failure (416, 417). An asymmetrical or widespread distribution of pulmonary edema infiltrates is evident in some dogs (see 62, 63, p. 44). Pleural effusion, caudal vena cava distension, hepatomegaly, and ascites usually accompany right-sided heart failure.

ECG findings with DCM are variable. The QRS complex voltage can be increased (consistent with LV dilation), normal, or smaller than usual (see 108, p. 59). QRS complex widening, with a sloppy R-wave descent and a slurred ST segment, is

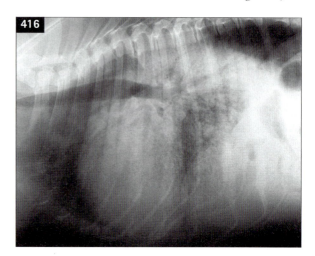

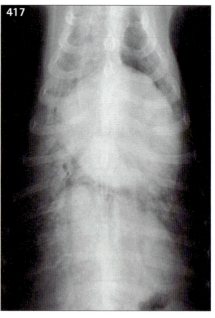

413–415 (413, 414) Prominent LA as well as some LV enlargement is seen in a 6-year-old male Doberman Pinscher with DCM and AF. Minimal peribronchial infiltrate is in the hilar area. (415) Lateral view from the same dog at 8 years of age shows increased cardiomegaly with mild pleural effusion and pulmonary edema; CHF signs resolved with intensified therapy and this dog was still alive a year later.

416, 417 Lateral (416) and DV (417) radiographs from a 6-year-old male Doberman Pinscher with DCM show cardiomegaly and severe interstitial and alveolar infiltrates of edema, especially in the dorsohilar regions.

common (418). A bundle branch block pattern or other intraventricular conduction disturbance is sometimes seen. In dogs with sinus rhythm, P waves are often widened and notched (suggesting LA enlargement). AF is quite common (419, 420; also 87, p. 54), especially in Great Danes and other giant breeds[2, 19]. Uniform or multiform VPCs and paroxysmal ventricular tachycardia, with sinus rhythm or AF, are typical in Doberman Pinschers and Boxers and are also seen frequently in other breeds (421, 422; also 91, 94, and 99, p. 55–57).

Echocardiography is the best clinical means for assessing cardiac function and chamber size, and for excluding other acquired or congenital cardiac disease.

418–420 (418) Sinus tachycardia in a 9-year-old female Doberman Pinscher with DCM and pulmonary edema. The wide P waves are consistent with LA enlargement; wide QRS complexes with slowed and 'sloppy' R wave descent suggest myocardial disease with slowed intraventricular conduction. Leads as marked; 50 mm/sec, 1 cm = 1 mV.
(419) AF with uncontrolled ventricular response rate (~230 beats/minute) in a 3-year-old male Doberman Pinscher with severe signs of heart failure from DCM.
(420) ECG from the same dog as in 419 one month later when signs of congestion were absent. The ventricular rate is well controlled (110 beats/minute); baseline fibrillation waves are clearly evident now. 419, 420: leads as marked; 25 mm/sec, 1 cm = 1 mV.

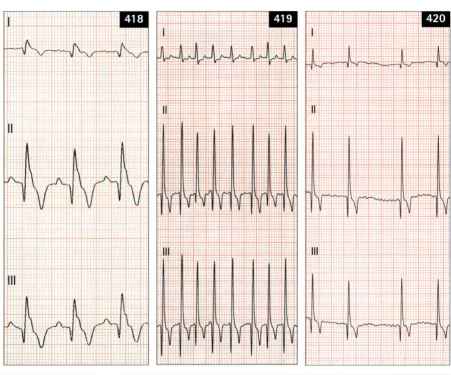

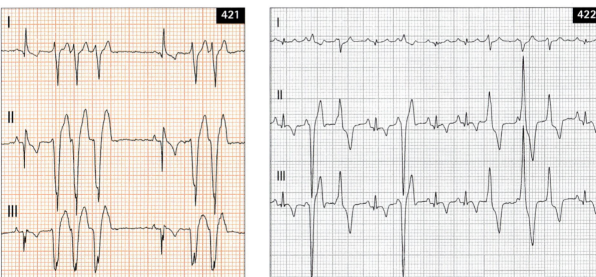

(422) Frequent VPCs, as pairs and triplets, in a 9-year-old female Doberman Pinscher with DCM and clinical heart failure. (422) Multiform VPCs in a 5-year-old male Labrador Retriever with DCM. The QRS compexes are quite small, but no effusion or other cause was evident. The P waves are wide. 421, 422 Leads as marked; 25 mm/sec, 1 cm = 1 mV.

Dilated and rounded cardiac chambers, poor systolic ventricular wall and septal motion, reduced FS (<20–25%) and ejection fraction (EF; <40%), and increased mitral EPSS (>6 mm) are characteristic findings (**423–425**; also **148, 149**, pp. 79, 80). All chambers are usually affected, but the right heart may appear relatively normal, especially in Doberman Pinschers and Boxers. LV free wall and septal thicknesses are normal to decreased. Mild to moderate AV valve regurgitation may be evident with Doppler (**426, 427**). Maximum LV dimensions (from M-mode or 2D) should be compared with breed-specific normals when possible (see *Table 16*, p. 72); a cut-off value for LV enlargement of two standard deviations above mean reference value has been proposed until more specific information is available[2]. The right parasternal long-axis 4-chamber view usually provides a view with maximal LV dimensions, although the left apical view is better in some dogs. LV volumes in diastole and systole (from 2-D images) and EF can then be calculated[2]. Averages from 5 cardiac cycles (10 cycles, if AF is present) obtained from the view

showing maximal LV dimensions have been recommended[2]. LV end-diastolic and end-systolic volumes are normalized to body surface area to yield end-diastolic and end-systolic volume indices (EDVI and ESVI, respectively; see Chapter 5, p. 79). Dogs with overt DCM generally have an ESVI well over 80 ml/m[2]. Increased LV sphericity is a characteristic of DCM; an index of sphericity is proposed to quantify this (*Table 58*, p. 282). Values <1.65 are thought to represent increased sphericity. Other cardiac or systemic disease, including hypertension, must be excluded to make a diagnosis of primary (idiopathic) DCM. Diastolic function is thought to deteriorate only after overt DCM develops. A restrictive transmitral filling pattern and shortened E wave deceleration time have been correlated with increased LV diastolic pressure and poor prognosis in people. Preliminary evidence (restrictive mitral inflow pattern and E wave deceleration <80 m/sec) suggests the same in dogs[49].

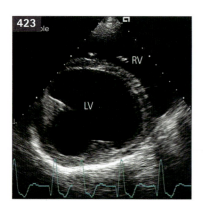
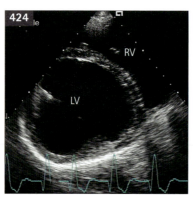
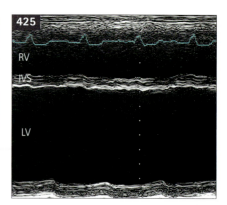

423–425 2-D echo images of the LV at end-diastole (**423**) and maximal systole (**424**) show little change in ventricular size in a 4-year-old male Labrador Retriever with heart failure from DCM. Right parasternal short-axis view. (**425**) M-mode image of the LV from a 7-year-old female Dalmation shows abysmally poor septal and LV free wall motion as well as biventricular dilation. LV = left ventricle; RV = right ventricle; IVS = interventricular septum.

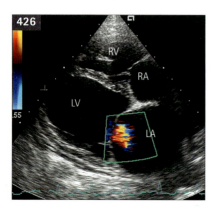
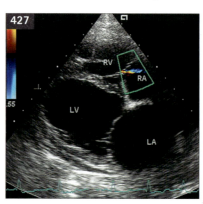

426, 427 (**426**) Color flow Doppler image illustrates mild MR in an 8-year-old female Doberman Pinscher with DCM and AF. All the chambers are dilated. (**427**) Mild TR is also evident in the same dog. Right parasternal long-axis view. LA = left atrium; LV = left ventricle; RA = right atrium; RV = right ventricle.

MANAGEMENT

Preclinical DCM

Dogs with LV dilation or reduced FS are often treated with an ACE inhibitor, although it is unclear whether this delays CHF onset. Experimentally, enalapril has shown a beneficial effect on ventricular remodeling and prevented progression of LV dilation and MR severity[50]. The decision to use antiarrhythmic drug therapy in dogs with ventricular tachyarrhythmias is influenced by whether clinical signs have occurred (e.g. episodic weakness, syncope) as well as the arrhythmia frequency and complexity seen on Holter recording. Various antiarrhythmic drugs have been used but the best regimen(s) and when to institute therapy are still not clear. Drug therapy that successfully reduces the number of VPCs based on Holter recordings may still not prevent sudden death. Drugs or combinations of drugs that increase ventricular fibrillation threshold, as well as reduce arrhythmia frequency and severity, are desired. Sotalol and amiodarone (class III agents) as well as the combination of mexiletine and atenolol hold promise[51]. The combination of procainamide with atenolol has been anecdotally helpful in some dogs. (See Chapter 17 for more information.)

Overt DCM

Therapy is aimed at controlling congestive signs, optimizing cardiac output, managing arrhythmias, improving quality of life, and prolonging survival if possible. Pimobendan (where available) or digoxin, an ACE inhibitor, and furosemide form the core treatment for most dogs. The severity of heart failure signs determines the aggressiveness of therapy. Additional inotropic, diuretic, vasodilator, antiarrhythmic, or other agents are often used for dogs in fulminant heart failure and for chronic management. *Table 59* outlines management strategies for acute CHF as well as chronic treatment of DCM. Additional information can be found in Chapter 16.

Frequent evaluation is important with acute heart failure because clinical status can rapidly deteriorate.

Table 59 General treatment guidelines for overt dilated cardiomyopathy.

1) Mild to moderate signs of CHF:*

   a) ACE inhibitor.

   b) Furosemide.

   c) Pimobendan/digoxin.

   d) Antiarrhythmic therapy, if necessary.

   e) +/– initiate spironolactone.

   f) Complete exercise restriction until signs abate.

   g) Moderate dietary salt restriction.

2) Severe, acute signs of CHF:*

   a) Supplemental O_2.

   b) Furosemide (parenteral).

   c) Inotropic support (e.g. IV dobutamine and/or amrinone with minimal fluid volume; initiate PO pimobendan/digoxin when possible).

   d) ACE inhibitor when possible.

   e) Other vasodilator with caution (e.g. IV nitroprusside, or PO hydralazine, or amlodipine with topical nitroglycerine).

   f) Antiarrhythmic therapy, if necessary.** (With uncontrolled AF, catecholamine infusion can further increase AV conduction and ventricular response rate; if dopamine or dobutamine is necessary, first give digoxin either PO or by **cautious** IV loading, or use IV diltiazem).

   g) +/– bronchodilator (e.g. theophylline).

   h) +/– butorphanol or morphine.

   i) Cage rest.

   j) Minimize patient handling.

   k) Monitor respiratory rate, HR and rhythm, arterial blood pressure, peripheral perfusion, urine output, renal function, serum electrolytes, etc.

3) AF and inadequate heart rate control with digoxin:**

   a) Acute: add IV diltiazem.

   b) Chronic: add PO beta-blocker at low dose or diltiazem; titrate to effect.

4) Chronic DCM management:*

   a) ACE inhibitor.

   b) Furosemide (lowest effective dosage and frequency).

   c) Pimobendan/digoxin.

   d) Spironolactone.

   e) Antiarrhythmic therapy as indicated.

   f) +/– other medications (see p. 288).

   g) +/– carvedilol/metoprolol.

   h) Client education.

   i) Resting respiratory rate (+HR if possible) monitoring at home.

   j) Regular but mild exercise.

   k) Dietary salt restriction.

   l) Routine health maintenance (including heartworm testing and prophylaxis in endemic areas).

   m) Manage other medical problems.

* See text and Chapter 16 for further details.

** See Chapter 17.

Respiratory rate and character, lung sounds, pulse quality, heart rate and rhythm, peripheral perfusion, blood pressure, serum electrolyte and hydration status, renal function, body weight, rectal temperature, and mentation are important parameters. Cardiogenic shock can develop with severe DCM, especially after excessive diuresis and vasodilation. Fluid administration (either SC or IV) may be needed in some dogs, especially after aggressive diuretic therapy. High cardiac filling pressure is often necessary to maintain cardiac output in these dogs. Although venous congestion and edema may be alleviated by diuresis, the resulting preload reduction may cause inadequate cardiac output and hypotension. D5W with potassium chloride added (12 mEq/500 ml), or 0.45% sodium chloride and 2.5% dextrose with potassium chloride added, can be administered at conservative rates (e.g. 15–30 ml/kg/day). Careful monitoring is essential to avoid overhydration and pulmonary edema. Thoracocentesis is indicated for large volume pleural effusion.

When the acute heart failure signs are controlled, long-term oral therapy with pimobendan or digoxin, furosemide, an ACE inhibitor, reduced-sodium diet, and exercise restriction is instituted. Additional therapy (see below) may also be helpful. Client education about the disease process and medications used is important. Home monitoring of resting respiratory and heart rates is advised. The time frame for periodic reevaluation depends on the animal's status; visits once or twice a week may be needed initially.

Digoxin toxicity occurs at relatively low dosages in some dogs, especially Doberman Pinschers. A total maximum daily dose of 0.5 mg for most large and giant breed dogs (0.25–0.375 mg/day for Doberman Pinschers) is recommended. Serum digoxin concentration should be measured 7–10 days after digoxin therapy is initiated or the dose is changed (see Chapter 16, p. 180). The serum electrolyte and creatinine or blood urea nitrogen (BUN) concentrations should be monitored, because hypokalemia and azotemia predispose to the development of digoxin toxicity.

Digoxin is indicated for dogs with AF. If digoxin does not sufficiently reduce the heart rate within 36–48 hours in dogs with AF, a beta-blocker or diltiazem is added (see Chapter 17, p. 205). Because of their potential negative inotropic effect, a low initial dose and gradual dosage titration to effect are advised. Heart rate control in dogs with AF is important. A maximum ventricular rate of 140–150 beats/minute in the hospital (i.e. stressful setting) is the recommended target; lower heart rates (e.g. ~100 beats/minute or less) are expected at home. Because accurate counting of heart rate by auscultation or chest palpation in dogs with AF is difficult, an ECG recording is recommended. Femoral pulses should not be used to assess heart rate in the presence of AF.

Spironolactone is recommended as an additional diuretic and because of its action as an aldosterone antagonist. Not only can insufficient suppression of aldosterone develop despite ACE inhibition (so-called aldosterone escape), aldosterone can also promote collagen synthesis and contribute to abnormal cardiac remodeling. In people with myocardial dysfunction, the addition of spironolactone to standard therapy reduces mortality[52]; therefore, the addition of spironolactone earlier in the course of therapy may be advantageous.

A small percentage of dogs have shown marked clinical improvement in response to oral L-carnitine supplementation[1, 53, 54], but high doses of L-carnitine in the absence of myocardial deficiency are unlikely to be beneficial. Nevertheless, because carnitine supplementation does not appear to cause serious adverse effects, a 3-month to 6-month therapeutic trial is reasonable (see p. 290).

Taurine deficiency is part of the DCM syndrome in some dogs, especially American Cocker Spaniels[55, 56], although breeds commonly affected with DCM generally have normal taurine levels and do not respond to supplementation[57]. Measurement of plasma or whole blood taurine concentration is recommended in this breed as well as other breeds not usually affected by DCM[56, 57]. Supplemental taurine is advised when the plasma concentration is <25 µmol/l (<25 nmol/ml) (see p. 292). In the absence of plasma measurement, empirical taurine and carnitine supplementation may be beneficial in American Cocker Spaniels with DCM.

The use of other nutritional supplements is controversial. Preliminary evidence suggests that omega-3 fatty acid supplementation in the form of fish oil capsules may help reduce cytokine (e.g. tumor necrosis factor) production associated with cardiac cachexia. Oxygen free-radical damage can also contribute to myocardial dysfunction[58]. There is experimental evidence in other species that antioxidant vitamins reduce oxidative stress and possibly attenuate associated myocardial and endothelial dysfunction. Whether supplementation with vitamin C or other antioxidant vitamins would have a measurable benefit in canine DCM remains to be seen.

Long-term, low-dose beta-blocker therapy with carvedilol or metoprolol is probably beneficial over time if the individual can tolerate the drug. This therapy is used only in dogs with chronic, stable DCM; it must be initiated with very low doses and titrated upward slowly (see Chapter 16, p. 184). Caution is necessary to avoid clinical decompensation. Further study and clinical experience in dogs is needed.

Surgical treatment modalities have been explored, including dynamic cardiomyoplasty, where a surgically transposed latissimus dorsi muscle is wrapped around the heart[1, 59], and others[60]. Such procedures have had mixed results and are not in common use. Biventricular pacing has had positive results in people, but its effectiveness in dogs has not been studied.

The prognosis with DCM has historically been guarded to poor. Most Doberman Pinschers have not survived longer than 3 months following the clinical manifestations of heart failure[26]. But about 25–40% of affected dogs of all breeds live longer than 6 months if the initial response to therapy is good[1]. The probability of survival for 2 years is estimated at 7.5–28%[3, 26, 61]. Most symptomatic dogs are between 5 and 10 years old at the time of death. However, with recent treatment advances, survival times are increasing; some dogs live well for several years after initial decompensation. Sudden death is common. An estimated 20–40% of affected Doberman Pinschers experience sudden death, often before clinical heart failure develops[11, 25, 26, 28].

Initial echo estimates of myocardial function do not consistently correlate with survival, but an ESVI >140 ml/m^2 is associated with reduced survival[62]. Young age at CHF onset, ascites, and dyspnea were independent risk factors for shorter survival in one study, but ACE inhibitors were not then in common use[3]. Other studies suggest a worse prognosis with right-sided CHF signs or if AF is present with CHF[26, 61]. A restrictive transmitral flow pattern on Doppler examination has been identified as the most important negative prognostic indicator, and is evidence that diastolic dysfunction is an important factor in DCM[62].

ARRHYTHMOGENIC RIGHT VENTRICULAR CARDIOMYOPATHY

BOXER MYOCARDIAL DISEASE
Disease features and histopathology in Boxers with myocardial disease resemble those of arrhythmogenic right ventricular cardiomyopathy (ARVC) in people[1, 30, 63]. Renaming Boxer cardiomyopathy as Boxer ARVC has been proposed. Myocardial histologic changes are more extensive in Boxers than in most other dogs with DCM and include myofiber atrophy, fibrosis, and fatty infiltration. Focal areas of myocytolysis, necrosis, hemorrhage, and mononuclear cell infiltration are also common[10]. Clinical findings vary and three disease categories have been described[10]: 1) asymptomatic dogs with ventricular tachyarrhythmia; 2) dogs with normal heart size and LV function, but with syncope or weakness from paroxysmal or sustained ventricular tachycardia; 3) Boxers with poor myocardial function and CHF, as well as ventricular arrhythmias. The prognosis is especially poor in the last category. There is geographical variation in the prevalence of these clinical presentations. Ventricular tachyarrhythmias with normal LV FS and chamber size is the more common presentation in the US[21], while a more

classical DCM presentation with CHF predominates in Europe[64]. Progression through the disease categories may occur if sudden death does not intercede[1, 10, 21].

Clinical signs can appear at any age, but a mean age of 8.5 years is reported[1]. The most consistent clinical finding is cardiac arrhythmia[30]. Spontaneous variability in the number of VPCs/day in dogs with >500 VPCs/24 hours was ≤80% in one study, but the severity grade of the arrhythmia was fairly consistent[30]. When CHF occurs, left-sided signs are more common; many Boxers also develop a mitral insufficiency murmur. Radiographic findings vary from normal (categories 1 and 2) to evidence of cardiomegaly and pulmonary edema (category 3). Sinus rhythm is usually evident on ECG, but the characteristic finding is ventricular ectopy. Supraventricular tachyarrhythmias, including AF, and other ECG abnormalities also occur but are less common[10, 65]. VPCs occur singly, in pairs, in short runs, or as sustained ventricular tachycardia (**428**; also **91**, p. 55). Most ectopic ventricular complexes appear upright in leads II and aVF, suggesting an RV origin[30, 66]. Some Boxers have multiform VPCs. 24-hour Holter monitoring is recommended to screen dogs for this disease (see p. 281), as well as to evaluate antiarrhythmic drug efficacy. Frequent VPCs and ventricular tachycardia are thought to signal increased

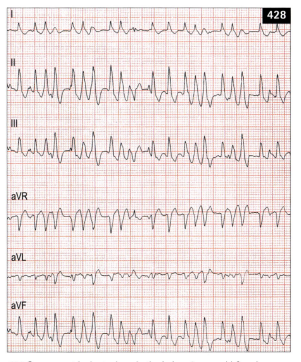

428 Severe ventricular tachyarrhythmia in a 3-year-old female Boxer with reduced LV function and signs of congestive failure. Sudden death occurred a short time later. Leads as marked; 25 mm/sec, 0.5 cm = 1 mV.

risk for syncope and sudden death. Echocardiographic findings vary from normal cardiac size and function to chamber dilation with poor FS (**429**). Therapy for symptomatic Boxers with normal LV size and function is usually limited to antiarrhythmic drugs[51]. Dogs with CHF are treated as described for other dogs with DCM. Digoxin is used sparingly if at all when ventricular tachyarrhythmias are prominant. Myocardial carnitine deficiency has been documented in some Boxers with DCM and heart failure[53, 67].

ARRHYTHMOGENIC RIGHT VENTRICULAR CARDIOMYOPATHY IN OTHER DOGS

A rare cardiomyopathy limited mainly to the RV and similar to ARVC in people and cats (see Chapter 21, p. 316) has been reported[1, 68]. Pathologic changes are characterized by widespread and extensive replacement of the RV myocardium by fibrous and fatty tissue, to a greater degree than in most Boxers. Clinical manifestations are largely related to right-sided CHF, with marked right heart dilation, and severe ventricular tachyarrhythmias. Sudden death is a common outcome in people with the disease. A possible differential diagnosis in certain geographical areas could be trypanosomiasis.

SECONDARY MYOCARDIAL DISEASES

A variety of agents and conditions are known to harm myocardial function (*Table 60*). DCM has been associated with prior viral infection in people; however, based on PCR analysis of myocardial samples from a

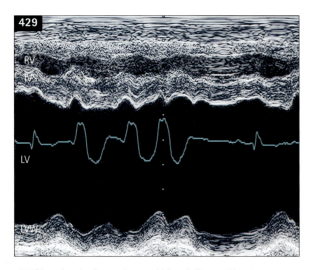

429 M-mode echo from a 4-year-old female Boxer with cardiomyopathy shows LV dilation and reduced FS. The VPCs have the typical 'upright' configuration common in Boxers. Note the arrhythmia's effect on LV motion. RV = right ventricle; IVS = interventricular septum; LV = left ventricle; LVW = left ventricular wall.

small number of DCM affected dogs, viral agents appear to be rarely associated with DCM in this species[69].

DOXORUBICIN

The antineoplastic drug doxorubicin induces both acute (arrhythmias and anaphylaxis) and chronic cardiotoxicity[1, 70]. Histamine, secondary catecholamine release, and free-radical production appear to be involved in the pathogenesis of myocardial injury[70]. Myocyte degeneration, reduced cardiac output, and arrhythmias result. Infranodal AV and bundle branch blocks, and ventricular and supraventricular tachyarrhythmias can occur. ECG changes do not necessarily precede clinical heart failure[70]. Progressive myocardial damage and fibrosis develop with cumulative doses >160 mg/m^2 and sometimes as low as 100 mg/m^2, but in dogs with normal pretreatment cardiac function, clinical cardiotoxicity may not appear until the cumulative dose exceeds 240 mg/m$^{2, 70}$. Breeds with a higher prevalence of idiopathic DCM and dogs with underlying cardiac disease are thought to be at greater risk for doxorubicin-induced cardiotoxicity. Clinical features are similar to those of idiopathic DCM. Circulating cardiac troponin concentrations may become useful in monitoring for doxorubicin-induced myocardial injury.

METABOLIC/NUTRITIONAL DEFICIENCIES
L-carnitine
DCM has been associated with L-carnitine–linked defects in myocardial metabolism in some dogs[1, 53, 54]. Inherited or acquired metabolic defects, rather than simple L-carnitine deficiency, are suspected. L-carnitine is an essential component of the mitochondrial membrane transport system for fatty acids, which are the heart's primary energy source. It also binds with and transports potentially toxic metabolites out of the mitochondria; excess production of such metabolites can result in L-carnitine depletion. L-carnitine is present mainly in foods of animal origin. DCM has developed in some dogs fed strict vegetarian diets. An association between DCM and carnitine deficiency may exist in some families of Boxers, Doberman Pinschers, Great Danes, Irish Wolfhounds, Newfoundlands, and Cocker Spaniels[53]. Plasma carnitine concentration is not a sensitive indicator of myocardial carnitine deficiency, although it is specific (at <8 mmol/l free carnitine)[53]. Most dogs with myocardial carnitine deficiency or abnormal esterified:free carnitine ratio confirmed on endomyocardial biopsy, have had normal or high plasma carnitine concentrations[53, 67]. Furthermore, the response to oral carnitine supplementation is inconsistent and few dogs have echocardiographic evidence of improved function. L-carnitine supplementation does not suppress preexisting arrhythmias or prevent sudden death. The recommendations for L-carnitine

Table 60 Causes of secondary myocardial disease and myocarditis.

1) Cardiac toxins:

   a) Anesthetic drugs.

   b) Antineoplastic drugs (e.g. doxorubicin [see p.290]; potentially also cyclophosphamide, 5-fluorouracil, interleukin-2, alpha-interferon).

   c) Catecholamines (endogenous [e.g. brain–heart syndrome] or exogenous amphetamines).

   d) Cobalt.

   e) Cocaine.

   f) Ethyl alcohol (e.g. when administered rapidly or undiluted for ethylene glycol toxicity).

   g) Heavy metals (e.g. arsenic, lead, mercury).

   h) Insect toxins (e.g. wasp or scorpion stings, spider bites).

   i) Ionophores (e.g. monensin).

   j) Other drugs (e.g. lithium, thyroid hormone).

   k) Plant toxins (e.g. *Taxus* species, foxglove, black locust, buttercups, lily-of-the-valley, gossypol).

   l) Snake venom.

2) Myocardial infection:

   a) Bacterial (e.g. *B. burgdorferi*, *Bartonella* species, other, see p. 294).

   b) Protozoal (e.g. *T. cruzi*, *T. gondii*, *B. canis*, other, see p. 294).

   c) Rickettsial and other organisms (see p. 295).

   d) Viral (e.g. parvovirus, other, see p. 293).

3) Myocardial inflammation:

   a) Antimicrobial and diuretic drugs (hypersensitivity myocarditis documented in people).

   b) Immunologic responses to infectious agents.

   c) Various systemic immune-mediated diseases (documented in people).

4) Myocardial ischemia/infarction (see p. 292):

   a) Coronary atherosclerosis.

   b) Coronary thromboembolic disease.

   c) Intramural coronary arteriosclerosis.

5) Neoplastic or other infiltrative disease:

   a) Nutritional/metabolic deficiency (see p. 290) (L-carnitine, taurine)

6) Other metabolic or endocrine disease:

   a) Diabetes mellitus.

   b) Glycogen storage disease.

   c) Hyperthyroidism.

   d) Hypothyroidism.

   e) Muscular dystrophies.

   f) Pheochromocytoma.

7) Persistent tachycardia (tachycardia induced cardiomyopathy).

8) Physical injury:

   a) Blunt or sharp trauma.

   b) Electric shock.

   c) Hyperthermia.

   d) Hypothermia.

   e) Ionizing radiation.

supplementation are:
- Use only L-carnitine.
- Dose at 1 g (for dogs <25 kg) to 2 g (for dogs 25–40 kg) mixed with food, q8h. Up to 200 mg/kg PO q8h has also been recommended. 1 g is about 1/2 teaspoonful of pure substance.
- Dogs that respond show improved activity within 1–4 weeks; echocardiographic improvement appears in some dogs after 2–3 months of supplementation, although a response plateau is reached in 6–8 months. Medication for CHF is usually still needed[51].

Taurine

Low plasma taurine, and sometimes carnitine, concentrations have been found in American Cocker Spaniels with DCM[55, 56, 71]. Oral supplementation of these two amino acids has improved LV function and reduced the need for heart failure medication in this breed[55]. Taurine supplementation alone is useful in some but not all of these dogs[72]. Other dogs with DCM, including some Golden Retrievers, Labrador Retrievers, Dalmations, St. Bernards, and others, also have had low plasma taurine concentrations, even with normally adequate dietary levels of taurine[56, 71]. However, the role of taurine supplementation and its possible effect on survival time in such dogs is not clear[56]. Several dogs eating commercial lamb meal and rice-based diets as well as home-made low protein vegetarian diets have developed DCM with low blood taurine concentrations[73]. Low blood taurine has been found in some Newfoundlands without clinical DCM that were eating lamb and rice diets[74]. High-fat/low-protein diets can also cause decreased blood and plasma taurine[75]. Therefore, in any atypical breed or mixed breed dog with DCM, measurement of taurine in blood and plasma and/or supplemental taurine for at least 4 months is recommended. The laboratory used should be consulted for specific collection and submission requirements; heparin is the recommended anticoagulant. Plasma taurine concentrations <25 (to 40) µmol/l (<25[to 40] nmol/ml) and blood taurine

concentrations <200 (or 150) µmol/l (<200 [or 150] nmol/ml) are considered deficient[13, 57, 73]. The recommendations for taurine supplementation are:
- 0.5–1 g (for dogs <25 kg) to 1–2 g (for dogs 25–40 kg) PO q12h or q8h (can mix with food).
- Three to four months of supplementation are needed to determine if echocardiographic improvement will occur.

Other conditions
The extent to which free radicals cause clinical myocardial injury is not clear. Evidence for increased oxidative stress occurs in dogs as well as people with CHF and myocardial failure. A negative correlation between disease severity and plasma vitamin E concentration has been noted in dogs with DCM[58].

Reduced myocardial function has been associated with diseases such as hypothyroidism, pheochromocytoma, and diabetes mellitus, but clinical heart failure in dogs secondary to these conditions alone is unusual[76]. Excessive sympathetic stimulation from brain or spinal cord injury causes myocardial hemorrhage, necrosis, and arrhythmias (brain–heart syndrome). Muscular dystrophy of the fasciohumoral type (reported in Springer Spaniels) can result in atrial standstill and heart failure. Canine X-linked (Duchenne's) muscular dystrophy in Golden Retrievers and other breeds has also been associated with myocardial fibrosis and mineralization. Rarely, non-neoplastic (e.g. glycogen storage disease) and neoplastic (metastatic and primary) infiltrative myocardial diseases interfere with normal myocardial function. Immunologic mechanisms may also play an important role in the pathogenesis of myocardial dysfunction in some dogs. Autoantibodies directed against the heart are found in some DCM dogs[1].

ISCHEMIC HEART DISEASE
Acute myocardial infarction from coronary embolization occurs uncommonly in dogs[77–79]. Most cases have an underlying disease associated with a tendency for embolus and/or thrombus formation, such as bacterial endocarditis, neoplasia, severe renal disease, immune-mediated hemolytic anemia, acute pancreatitis, DIC, and/or corticosteroid use[78]. Myocardial infarction has also occurred with congenital ventricular outflow obstructions, PDA, MR, and HCM[78, 80, 81]. Although atherosclerosis of major coronary arteries is rare in dogs, it can accompany hypercholesterolemia of severe hypothyroidism and diabetes mellitus and occasionally lead to acute myocardial infarction as well as thrombosis and infarction of other tissues[77, 82–84]. The abrupt onset of arrhythmias, pulmonary edema, marked ST segment changes on ECG, along with regional or widespread myocardial dysfunction evident on an echocardiogram, would be likely with acute obstruction of a major coronary artery. Increased circulating cardiac troponin and CK concentrations are expected with myocardial injury and necrosis.

Nonatherosclerotic narrowing of small coronary arteries is more clinically important than previously appreciated. Hyalinization of small intramural coronary vessels and intramural myocardial infarctions occur with chronic degenerative AV valve disease, but are also seen in older dogs without endocardiosis[77]. Fibromuscular arteriosclerosis of small coronary vessels is also described. These mural changes cause luminal narrowing and can impair resting coronary blood flow as well as vasodilatory responses. Small myocardial infarctions, focal myocardial necrosis, and secondary fibrosis can lead to deterioration of myocardial function and a variety of tachyarrhythmias and conduction disturbances[77, 78]. One study of dogs with histopathologically confirmed intramural coronary arteriosclerosis, with or without multiple chronic or acute infarctions, found almost half of the cases died from CHF[77]. An additional 20% of cases died suddenly; most of these had hyaline arteriosclerosis without degenerative valve disease. Another 15% of cases died during or after general anesthesia. A moderate decrease in contractility was seen in most of the cases that had an echocardiogram. The majority of dogs in this study were of larger breeds; Cocker Spaniels and Cavalier King Charles Spaniels were the most common small breeds[77]. Myocardial necrosis has also been associated with some drugs, CNS lesions, trauma, stress, pancreatitis, gastric dilatation/volvulus, viral infections, splenic masses, IMHA, renal disease, and neoplasia[78, 80].

TACHYCARDIA–INDUCED CARDIOMYOPATHY
Rapid, incessant tachycardia leads to progressive myocardial dysfunction, activation of NH compensatory mechanisms, and CHF. This is known as tachycardia-induced cardiomyopathy (TICM). The myocardial failure is sometimes reversible if the heart rate can be normalized. TICM has been described in dogs with AV nodal reciprocating tachycardias associated with accessory conduction pathways bypassing the AV node (e.g. Wolff–Parkinson–White, see Chapter 4, p. 59)[85]. Rapid artificial ventricular pacing (e.g. >200 beats/minute) is a common model for inducing experimental myocardial failure that simulates DCM[1].

HYPERTROPHIC CARDIOMYOPATHY

HCM is rare in dogs. Although its cause is unknown, a genetic basis is suspected. It may be that several disease processes produce similar ventricular changes.

PATHOPHYSIOLOGY

Abnormal and excessive myocardial hypertrophy characterizes HCM and causes diastolic dysfunction by increasing ventricular stiffness. The hypertrophy is usually symmetrical, but regional variation in wall or septal thickness can occur. Severe ventricular hypertrophy is likely to compromise coronary perfusion, which can cause myocardial ischemia, exacerbate arrhythmias, slow ventricular active relaxation, and further impair filling. Increased LV filling pressure leads to pulmonary congestion and edema. These abnormalities are magnified as heart rate increases. Besides impaired diastolic function, systolic dynamic LV outflow obstruction occurs in some dogs. Malposition of the mitral apparatus may contribute to abnormal systolic mitral valve motion and outflow obstruction as well as to mitral regurgitation[1]. Asymmetrical septal hypertrophy also contributes to outflow obstruction in some dogs. LV outflow obstruction increases ventricular wall stress and myocardial oxygen requirement, but it also impairs coronary flow and worsens ischemia. Whether dynamic LV outflow obstruction results from a congenital abnormality (of LV outflow tract or mitral valve apparatus) or is a form of primary myocardial disease may be unclear in a particular individual.

CLINICAL FEATURES

Young to middle-age, large breed dogs are more commonly diagnosed with HCM, although various breeds and a wide age distribution are affected. Males may be affected more often. Clinical signs of heart failure, episodic weakness, and syncope (presumably from ventricular ectopy) develop in some dogs, but sudden death can occur before other signs. A systolic murmur of LV outflow obstruction or mitral insufficiency may be heard. The ejection-type outflow obstruction murmur is accentuated when ventricular contractility is increased (e.g. by exercise or in the heartbeats after VPCs) or when systemic arterial pressure is decreased (by a vasodilator). An atrial gallop sound (S_4) is heard in some affected dogs.

Thoracic radiographs may be normal or indicate LA and LV enlargement, with or without pulmonary edema. Ventricular tachyarrhythmias and conduction abnormalities, including complete heart block, 1st degree AV block, and fascicular blocks, appear to be common ECG findings. Criteria for LV enlargement are variably present[1]. An abnormally thick LV, sometimes with LV outflow area narrowing and asymmetrical septal hypertrophy, and LA enlargement are characteristic echo findings[1]. MR may be evident on Doppler studies. Dynamic outflow obstruction is associated with SAM of the mitral valve and partial systolic aortic valve closure. Other causes of LV hypertrophy that should be excluded include congenital SAS, hypertensive renal disease, thyrotoxicosis, and pheochromocytoma.

MANAGEMENT

Treatment goals are to enhance myocardial relaxation and ventricular filling, control pulmonary edema, and suppress arrhythmias. A beta-blocker (see Chapter 17, p. 214) or calcium channel-blocker (see Chapter 17, p. 217) is used to lower HR, prolong ventricular filling time, and reduce myocardial oxygen requirement. Beta-blockers also reduce outflow obstruction and may prevent sympathetically-mediated arrhythmias, whereas calcium channel-blockers may facilitate myocardial relaxation. Resolution of dynamic LV outflow obstruction with atenolol therapy was reported in several young dogs, although the exact cause of obstruction was unclear[86]. Diltiazem, with a lesser negative inotropic effect, would be less useful for dynamic outflow obstruction, especially in view of its vasodilating effect. The beta-blocker and calcium channel-blocker drugs can worsen any AV conduction abnormalities that may exist. A diuretic and ACE inhibitor are indicated for congestive signs. Digoxin is avoided because it may worsen any outflow obstruction, increase myocardial oxygen need, and predispose to arrhythmias. Exercise restriction is advised.

INFECTIVE MYOCARDITIS

Many agents affect the myocardium, but disease manifestations in other organ systems often predominate. Direct invasion by an infective agent, elaborated toxins, or host immune responses can cause myocardial injury. Cardiac arrhythmias and impaired myocardial function are potential consequences of myocarditis. An association between acute (viral) myocarditis and subsequent DCM has long been recognized in people, but similar evidence from dogs is weak[69]. Active myocarditis appears to be uncommon in dogs with DCM[87].

PATHOPHYSIOLOGY

Viral myocarditis

Lymphocytic myocarditis occurs in experimental animals and in people with acute viral infections. The individual's immune response to viral and nonviral antigens can cause persistent inflammation and myocardial damage[88]. A syndrome of parvoviral myocarditis was widely recognized 25–30 years ago, although it is uncommon today, probably as a result of maternal antibody production. It was characterized by peracute necrotizing myocarditis and sudden death, with or without signs of acute respiratory distress, usually in 4–8-week-old puppies. Necropsy findings included cardiac dilation with pale myocardial streaks, gross evidence of congestive failure, large basophilic or amorphophilic intranuclear inclusion bodies, myocyte degeneration, and focal mononuclear cell infiltrates. Parvovirus was suspected to cause a form of DCM in young dogs that survive neonatal infection. Canine distemper virus can cause myocarditis in young puppies, but multisystemic signs usually predominate. Myocardial histologic changes are mild compared with those in acute parvovirus myocarditis. Herpesvirus infection of pups *in utero* also can cause fatal necrotizing myocarditis with intranuclear inclusion bodies.

Bacterial myocarditis

Bacteremia and bacterial endocarditis or pericarditis sometimes causes suppurative myocardial inflammation or abscessation. Malaise, weight loss, arrhythmias and cardiac conduction abnormalities are common, but murmurs are rare unless concurrent valvular endocarditis or another underlying cardiac defect is present. Fever is an inconsistent finding. Serial bacterial, or fungal, blood cultures may allow identification of the organism. *Bartonella vinsonii* subsp. *berkhoffii* and related species have been associated with cardiac arrhythmias, myocarditis, endocarditis, and sudden death in dogs[89].

Lyme disease

Lyme borrelosis is recognized in certain geographic areas, especially the northeastern and north central US, as well as in Europe, Japan, and other areas. The spirochete *Borrelia burgdorferi*, or a closely related species, is transmitted to dogs by ticks, especially of the genus *Ixodes*[90]. Small mammals and birds serve as reservoir hosts[90]. High-grade AV block is a manifestation of Lyme carditis in people; 3rd degree (complete) and high-grade 2nd degree heart block have been identified in dogs with Lyme disease[91]. Syncope, CHF, impaired myocardial contractility, and ventricular arrhythmias have also been identified in affected dogs. Histopathologic findings of myocarditis with infiltrates of plasma cells, macrophages, neutrophils, and lymphocytes, in conjunction with areas of myocardial necrosis, are similar to those seen in human Lyme carditis. A presumptive diagnosis is made on the basis of positive (or increasing) serum titers and concurrent signs of myocarditis, with or without other systemic signs. Endomyocardial biopsy, if available, may be helpful in confirming the diagnosis. Antibiotics (e.g. doxyclycline, azithromycin) are used in treatment. Cardiac drugs are used as necessary.

Protozoal myocarditis

The protozoal organisms *Trypanosoma cruzi*, *Toxoplasma gondii*, *Neosporum caninum*, *Babesia canis*, and *Hepatozoon canis* can affect the myocardium. Trypanosomiasis (Chagas disease) is an important cause of myocarditis in people in Central and South America. In the US it has occurred mainly in young dogs in Texas, Louisiana, Oklahoma, Virginia, and other southern states[92–94]. The organism is carried by bloodsucking insects of the family Reduviidae and is enzootic in wild animals of the region. Zoonotic transmission via infected blood or tissue is possible. Amastigotes of *T. cruzi* cause myocarditis with a mononuclear cell infiltrate and disruption and necrosis of myocardial fibers. Acute, latent, and chronic phases of Chagas myocarditis have been described. Lethargy, depression, and other systemic signs, as well as various tachyarrhythmias, AV conduction defects, and sudden death, have been observed in dogs with acute trypanosomiasis, although clinical signs are sometimes subtle[95]. In the acute stage, trypomastigotes may be found in thick peripheral blood smears; the organism can be isolated in cell culture or by inoculation into mice. Survivors of the acute phase enter a latent phase of variable duration, in which parasitemia resolves and antibodies develop against the organism as well as components of the heart. Chronic Chagas disease is characterized by progressive, right-sided or generalized cardiomegaly and arrhythmias[93, 95]. Ventricular tachyarrhythmias are most notable, but supraventricular tachyarrhythmias, right bundle branch block, and AV conduction disturbances are also reported[93]. Ventricular dilation and myocardial dysfunction are usually evident on echocardiograms, and clinical signs of biventricular failure are common. Serologic testing may allow antemortem diagnosis in chronic cases. Therapy in the acute stage is aimed at eliminating the organism and minimizing myocardial inflammation; several treatments have been tried with variable success[93, 94]. The therapy for chronic Chagas disease is directed at supporting myocardial function, controlling congestive signs, and suppressing arrhythmias.

Toxoplasmosis and neosporiosis occasionally cause clinical myocarditis as part of a generalized systemic process, especially in the immuno-compromised animal[96]. After the initial infection, the organism becomes encysted in the heart and various other body tissues. When these cysts rupture, expelled bradyzoites induce hypersensitivity reactions and tissue necrosis. Other systemic signs often predominate over signs of myocarditis. Immunosuppressed dogs with chronic toxoplasmosis (or neosporiosis) may be at risk for active disease, including clinically relevant myocarditis, pneumonia, chorioretinitis, and encephalitis. Therapy with appropriate antiprotozoal agents may be successful.

Babesiosis has sometimes been associated with cardiac lesions in dogs, including myocardial hemorrhage, inflammation, and necrosis. Pericardial effusion and variable ECG changes are also noted in some cases[97]. A correlation between plasma cTnI concentration and clinical severity, survival, and cardiac histologic changes has been reported in dogs with babesiosis[98]. Myocardial involvement with *H. canis* infection has been found in dogs along the Texas coast in the US. Infection results from ingestion of the organism's definitive host, the brown dog tick (*Rhipicephalus sanguineus*). Reported clinical signs include stiffness, anorexia, fever, neutrophilia, and periosteal new bone reaction.

Miscellaneous causes
In rare instances, fungi (*Aspergillus*, *Cryptococcus*, *Coccidioides*, *Histoplasma*, and *Paecilomyces* species), rickettsiae (*Rickettsia rickettsii*, *Ehrlichia canis*, *Bartonella elizabethae*), algae-like organisms (*Prototheca* species), and nematode larval migration (*Toxocara* species) cause myocarditis[99]. Affected animals are usually immunosuppressed and have systemic signs of disease. Rocky Mountain spotted fever (*R. rickettsii*) occasionally causes fatal ventricular arrhythmias, along with necrotizing vasculitis, myocardial thrombosis, and ischemia. *Angiostrongylus vasorum* infection in association with immune-mediated thrombocytopenia has, rarely, caused myocarditis, thrombosing arteritis, and sudden death[100].

CLINICAL FEATURES
The classic clinical presentation of acute myocarditis involves the unexplained onset of arrhythmias or heart failure after a recent episode of infective disease or drug exposure, however, findings are often nonspecific. (See above for other signs associated with specific organisms.)

DIAGNOSIS
A CBC, serum biochemical profile including CK activity, circulating cardiac troponin concentrations, urinalysis, and thoracic and abdominal radiographs are recommended as part of a broad database. There may be nonspecific ECG changes (e.g. ST segment shifts, T wave or QRS voltage changes, AV conduction abnormalities) as well as tachyarrhythmias. Poor regional or global wall motion, altered myocardial echogenicity, or pericardial effusion are sometimes found on ultrasound examination. In dogs with persistent fever, serial blood cultures may be rewarding. Serologic screening for known infective causes is occasionally helpful; however, inconsistent clinical presentation and lack of specific noninvasive tests makes establishing a definitive diagnosis difficult. The diagnostic criteria for myocarditis are histologic and include the finding of inflammatory infiltrates with myocyte degeneration and necrosis[88, 101]. Endomyocardial biopsy specimens are currently the only means of obtaining a definitive antemortem

diagnosis, but the findings may not be diagnostic if the lesions are focal.

MANAGEMENT
Therapy for suspected myocarditis is largely supportive unless a specific etiology can be identified and treated. Strict rest, antiarrhythmic therapy as needed (see Chapter 17), an ACE inhibitor with or without digoxin for reduced myocardial function, a diuretic for signs of congestion or edema (see Chapter 1), and other support are used as indicated. Corticosteroids have not been proven clinically beneficial in dogs with myocarditis and, considering the possible infective causes, they are not recommended as nonspecific therapy. Immunosuppressive therapy appears of little benefit in most human myocarditis cases, but exceptions include confirmed immune-mediated disease, drug related or eosinophilic myocarditis, and patients with confirmed myocarditis that fails to resolve[88].

NONINFECTIVE MYOCARDITIS

Drugs, toxins, immunologic responses, and trauma can cause myocardial inflammation. Although there is little clinical documentation for many of these in animals, many potential causes have been identified in people (*Table 60*, p. 291). Immune-mediated diseases and pheochromocytoma can cause myocarditis. Hypersensitivity reactions to antiinfective agents and other drugs are known to cause myocarditis in people. Eosinophilic and lymphocytic infiltrates characterize drug-related myocarditis[88].

TRAUMATIC MYOCARDITIS
Blunt trauma to the chest and heart is more common than penetrating wounds in dogs and cats. Post-traumatic cardiac arrhythmias are common, especially in dogs. Mechanisms of myocardial injury and subsequent arrhythmias could include compression or acceleration-deceleration forces, autonomic imbalance, ischemia, reperfusion injury, or electrolyte and acid-base disturbances. Arrhythmias usually appear within 24–48 hours after trauma. VPCs, ventricular tachycardia, and accelerated idioventricular rhythms (at 60–100 beats/minute or slightly faster) are more common than supraventricular tachyarrhythmias or bradyarrhythmias[102]. The percentage of dogs with frequent VPCs and ventricular tachycardia appears small[102]. Accelerated idioventricular rhythms are often evident only when the sinus rate slows (see **97**, p. 57). They are usually benign and tend to disappear in a week or so in animals with a functionally normal heart.

ECG, radiographs, serum biochemical tests, including cardiac troponin concentrations, and echocardiography are useful for assessing these patients and defining preexisting cardiac disease and myocardial function[46, 102]. Antiarrhythmic therapy for post-traumatic accelerated idioventricular rhythm is usually unnecessary, but the animal should be monitored closely. If more serious arrhythmias (e.g. faster rate or multiform configuration) or hemodynamic deterioration develops, antiarrhythmic therapy may be indicated (see Chapter 17).

Traumatic avulsion of papillary muscles, septal perforation, and rupture of the heart or pericardium have also been reported. Acute low-output failure and shock, or rapid onset congestive failure, as well as arrhythmias, can result.

REFERENCES

1 Sisson DD, Thomas WP, Keene BW (2000) Primary myocardial diseases in the dog. In: *Textbook of Veterinary Internal Medicine*, 5th edn. SJ Ettinger, EC Feldman (eds.) WB Saunders, Philadelphia, pp. 874–895.

2 Dukes-McEwan J, Borgarelli M, Tidholm A *et al.* (2003) Proposed guidelines for the diagnosis of canine idiopathic dilated cardiomyopathy. *J Vet Cardiol* 5:7–19.

3 Tidholm A, Svensson H, Sylven C (1997) Survival and prognostic factors in 189 dogs with dilated cardiomyopathy. *J Am Anim Hosp Assoc* 33:364–368.

4 Tidholm A, Haggstrom J, Jonsson L (2000) Detection of attenuated wavy fibers in the myocardium of Newfoundlands without clinical or echocardiographic evidence of heart disease. *Am J Vet Res* 61:238–241.

5 Tidholm A, Haggstrom J, Jonsson L (1998) Prevalence of attenuated wavy fibers in myocardium of dogs with dilated cardiomyopathy. *J Am Vet Med Assoc* 212:1732–1734.

6 Tidholm A, Jonsson L (1996) Dilated cardiomyopathy in the Newfoundland: a study of 37 cases (1983–1994). *J Am Anim Hosp Assoc* 32:465–470.

7 Dambach DM, Lannon A, Sleeper MM *et al.* (1999) Familial dilated cardiomyopathy of young Portuguese Water Dogs. *J Vet Intern Med* 13:65–71.

8 Sleeper MM, Henthorn PS, Vijayasarathy C *et al.* (2002) Dilated cardiomyopathy in juvenile Portuguese Water Dogs. *J Vet Intern Med* 16:52–62.

9 Vollmar AC, Fox PR, Meurs KM *et al.* (2003) Dilated cardiomyopathy in juvenile Doberman Pinscher dogs. *J Vet Cardiol* 5:23–27.

10 Harpster NK (1991) Boxer cardiomyopathy. *Vet Clin North Am: Small Anim Pract* 21:989–1009.

11 Calvert CA, Hall G, Jacobs G *et al.* (1997) Clinical and pathological findings in Doberman Pinschers with occult cardiomyopathy that died suddenly or developed congestive heart failure: 54 cases (1984–1991). *J Am Vet Med Assoc* 210:505–511.

12 Everett RM, McGann J, Wimberly HC *et al.* (1999) Dilated cardiomyopathy of Doberman Pinschers: retrospective histomor-phologic evaluation on hearts from 32 cases. *Vet Pathol* 36:221–227.

13 Freeman LM, Michel KE, Brown DJ *et al.* (1996) Idiopathic dilated cardiomyopathy in Dalmatians: nine cases (1990–1995). *J Am Vet Med Assoc* 209:1592–1596.

14 O'Brien PJ (1997) Deficiencies of myocardial troponin-T and creatine kinase MB isoenzyme in dogs with idiopathic dilated cardiomyopathy. *Am J Vet Res* 58:11–16.

15 Spiers AW, Meurs, KM, Coovert DD *et al.* (2001) Use of western immunoblot for evaluation of myocardial dystrophin, α-sarcoglycan, and β-dystroglycan in dogs with idiopathic dilated cardiomyopathy. *Am J Vet Res* 62:67–71.

16 Meurs KM, Magnon AL, Spier AW *et al.* (2001) Evaluation of cardiac actin gene in Doberman Pinschers with dilated cardiomyopathy. *Am J Vet Res* 62:33–36.

17 Tidholm A, Haggstrom J, Hansson K (2001) Effects of dilated cardiomyopathy on the renin-angiotensin-aldosterone system, atrial natriuretic peptide activity, and thyroid hormone concentrations in dogs. *Am J Vet Res* 62:961–967.

18 Calvert CA, Jacobs GJ, Pickus CW (1996) Bradycardia-associated episodic weakness, syncope, and aborted sudden death in cardiomyopathic Doberman Pinschers. *J Vet Intern Med* 10:88–93.

19 Vollmar AC (2000) The prevalence of cardiomyopathy in the Irish Wolfhound: a clinical study of 500 dogs. *J Am Anim Hosp Assoc* 36:126–132.

20 Meurs KM, Miller MW, Wright NA (2001) Clinical features of dilated cardiomyopathy in Great Danes and results of a pedigree analysis: 17 cases (1990–2000). *J Am Vet Med Assoc* 218:729–732.

21 Meurs KM, Spier AW, Miller MW *et al.* (1999) Familial ventricular arrhythmias in Boxers. *J Vet Intern Med* 13:437–439.

22 Cobb MA, Brownlie SE, Pidduck HG *et al.* (1996) Evidence for genetic involvement in dilated cardiomyopathy in the Irish Wolfhound. In: *Proceedings of the BSAVA Annual Congress*, Birmingham, p. 215.

23 Hammer TA, Venta PJ, Eyster GE (1996) The genetic basis of dilated cardiomyopathy in Doberman Pinschers. Abstract. *Anim Genet* 27(suppl 2), 109.

24 Calvert CA, Jacobs GJ, Smith DD (2000) Association between results of ambulatory electrocardiography and development of cardiomyopathy during long-term follow-up of Doberman Pinschers. *J Am Vet Med Assoc* 216:34–39.

25 Calvert CA, Jacobs G, Pickus C *et al.* (2000) Results of ambulatory electrocardiography in overtly healthy Doberman Pinschers with echocardiographic abnormalities. *J Am Vet Med Assoc* 217:1328–1332.

26 Calvert CA, Pickus CW, Jacobs CJ *et al.* (1997) Signalment, survival, and prognostic factors in Doberman Pinschers with end-stage cardiomyopathy. *J Vet Intern Med* **11**:323–326.

27 O'Grady MR, Horne R (1998) The prevalence of dilated cardiomyopathy in Doberman Pinschers: a 4.5 year follow-up. In: *Proceedings of the 16th ACVIM Forum*, p. 689.

28 O'Grady MR, Horne R (1995) Outcome of 103 asymptomatic Doberman Pinschers: incidence of dilated cardiomyopathy in a longitudinal study. Abstract. In: *Proceedings of the 13th ACVIM Forum*, p. 1014.

29 Calvert CA, Meurs KM (2000) Doberman Pinscher occult cardiomyopathy. In: *Kirk's Current Veterinary Therapy XIII*. JD Bonagura (ed). WB Saunders, Philadelphia, pp. 756–760.

30 Spier AW, Meurs KM (2004) Evaluation of spontaneous variability in the frequency of ventricular arrhythmias in Boxers with arrhythmiogenic right ventricular cardiomyopathy. *J Am Vet Med Assoc* **24**:538–541.

31 Meurs KM, Spier AW, Wright NA *et al.* (2001) Comparison of in-hospital versus 24-hour ambulatory electrocardiography for detection of ventricular premature complexes in mature Boxers. *J Am Vet Med Assoc* **218**:222–224.

32 Calvert CA Wall M (2001) Effect of severity of myocardial failure on heart rate variability in Doberman Pinschers with and without echocardiographic evidence of dilated cardiomyopathy. *J Am Vet Med Assoc* **219**:1084–1088.

33 Calvert CA, Jacobs GJ (2000) Heart rate variability in Doberman Pinschers with and without echocardiographic evidence of dilated cardiomyopathy. *Am J Vet Res* **61**:506–511.

34 Spier AW, Meurs, KM (2004) Assessment of heart rate variability in Boxers with arrhythmogenic right ventricular cardiomyopathy. *J Am Vet Med Assoc* **224**:534–537.

35 Minors SL, O'Grady MR (1997) Heart rate variability in the dog: is it too variable? *Can J Vet Res* **61**:134–144.

36 Calvert CA, Jacobs GJ, Kraus M (1998) Possible ventricular late potentials in Doberman Pinschers with occult cardiomyopathy. *J Am Vet Med Assoc* **213**:235–239.

37 Spier AW, Meurs KM, Muir WW *et al.* (2001) Correlation of QT dispersion with indices used to evaluate the severity of familial ventricular arrhythmias in Boxers. *Am J Vet Res* **62**:1481–1485.

38 McEntee K, Clercx C, Soyeur D *et al.* (2001) Usefulness of dobutamine stress tests for detection of cardiac abnormalities in dogs with experimentally induced early left ventricular dysfunction. *Am J Vet Res* **62**:448–455.

39 Minors SL, O'Grady MR (1998) Resting and dobutamine stress echocardiographic factors associated with the development of occult dilated cardiomyopathy in healthy Doberman Pinscher dogs. *J Vet Intern Med* **12**:369–380.

40 Moneva-Jordan A, Lius Fuentes V, Corcoran B *et al.* (2002) Pulsus alternans in English Cocker Spaniels with dilated cardiomyopathy. *J Small Anim Pract* **43**:410.

41 Calvert CA, Jacobs GJ, Medleau L, Pickus CW *et al.* (1998) Thyroid-stimulating hormone stimulation tests in cardiomyopathic Doberman Pinschers: a retrospective study. *J Vet Intern Med* **12**:343–348.

42 Borgarelli M, Tarducci A, Tidholm A *et al.* (2001) Canine idiopathic dilated cardiomyopathy. Part II: pathophysiology and therapy. *Vet J* **162**:182–195.

43 Ware WA, Lund DD, Subieta AR *et al.* (1990) Sympathetic activation in dogs with congestive heart failure caused by chronic mitral valve disease and dilated cardiomyopathy. *J Am Vet Med Assoc* **197**:1475–1481.

44 Koch J, Pedersen HD, Jensen AL *et al.* (1995) Activation of the renin-angioensin system in dogs with asymptomatic and symptomatic dilated cardiomyopathy. *Research in Vet Sci* **59**:172–175.

45 Roche BM, Schwartz D, Lehnhard RA *et al.* (2002) Changes in concentrations of neuroendocrine hormones and catecholamines in dogs with myocardial failure induced by rapid ventricular pacing. *Am J Vet Res* **63**:1413–1417.

46 Schober KE, Kirbach B, Cornand C *et al.* (2001) Circulating cardiac troponins in small animals. In: *Proceedings of the 19th ACVIM Forum*, Denver, pp. 91–92.

47 DeFrancesco TC, Atkins CE, Keene BW *et al.* (2002) Prospective clinical evaluation of serum cardiac troponin T in dogs admitted to a veterinary teaching hospital. *J Vet Intern Med* **16**:553–557.

48 Sleeper MM, Clifford CA, Laster LL (2001) Cardiac troponin I in the normal dog and cat. *J Vet Intern Med* **15**:501–503.

49 Borgarelli M, Tarducci A, Santilli RA *et al.* (2000) Echo prognostic indicators for DCM. In: *Proceedings of the 18th ACVIM Forum*, pp. 78–80.

50 Shimoyama H, Sabbah, HN, Rosman H *et al.* (1995) Effects of long-term therapy with enalapril on severity of functional mitral regurgitation in dogs with moderate heart failure. *J Am Coll Cardiol* **25**:768–772.

51 Meurs, KM, Spier AW, Wright NA *et al.* (2002) Comparison of the effects of four antiarrhythmic treatments for familial ventricular arrhythmias in Boxers. *J Am Vet Med Assoc* **221**:22–527.

52 Weber KT (2001) Aldosterone in congestive heart failure. *New Engl J Med* **345**:1689–1697.

53 Keene BW (2000) Carnitine supplementation: what have we learned? In: *Proceedings of the 18th ACVIM Forum*, pp. 105–106.

54 Carroll MC, Cote E (2001) Carnitine: a review. *Compend Cont Educ Pract Vet* **23**:45–52.

55 Kittleson MD, Keene B, Pion PD *et al.* (1997) Results of the multicenter spaniel trial (MUST): taurine- and carnitine-responsive dilated cardiomyopathy in American Cocker Spaniels with decreased plasma taurine concentration. *J Vet Intern Med* **11**:204–211.

56 Freeman LM, Rush JE, Brown DJ et al. (2001) Relationship between circulating and dietary taurine concentration in dogs with dilated cardiomyopathy. *Vet Ther* 2:370–378.

57 Pion PD, Sanderson SL, Kittleson MD (1998) The effectiveness of taurine and levocarnitine in dogs with heart disease. *Vet Clin North Am: Small Anim Pract* 28:1495–1514.

58 Freeman LM, Brown DJ, Rush JE (1999) Assessment of degree of oxidative stress and antioxidant concentration in dogs with idiopathic dilated cardiomyopathy. *J Am Vet Med Assoc* 215:644–646.

59 Orton EC, Monnet E, Brevard SM et al. (1994) Dynamic cardiomyoplasty for treatment of idiopathic dilatative cardiomyopathy in a dog. *J Am Vet Med Assoc* 205:1415–1419.

60 de Andrade JNBM, Camacho AA, Santos PSP et al. (2005) Plication of the free wall of the left ventricle in dogs with doxorubicin-induced cardiomyopathy. *Am J Vet Res* 66:238–243.

61 Monnet E, Orton EC, Salman M et al. (1995) Idiopathic dilated cardiomyopathy in dogs: survival and prognostic indicators. *J Vet Intern Med* 9:12–17.

62 Borgarelli M, Santilli RA, Chiavegato D et al. (2006) Prognostic indicators for dogs with dilated cardiomyopathy. *J Vet Intern Med* 20:104–110.

63 Gemayel C, Pelliccia A, Thompson PD (2001) Arrhythmogenic right ventricular cardiomyopathy. *J Am Coll Cardiol* 38:1773–1781.

64 Wotton PR (1999) Dilated cardiomyopathy in closely related Boxer dogs and its possible resemblance to arrhythmogenic right ventricular cardiomyopathy in humans. In: *Proceedings of the 17th ACVIM Forum*, pp. 88–89.

65 Baumwart RD, Meurs KM, Atkins CE et al. (2005) Clinical, echocardiographic, and electrocardiographic abnormalities in Boxers with cardiomyopathy and left ventricular systolic dysfunction: 48 cases (1985–2003). *J Am Vet Med Assoc* 226:1102–1104.

66 Kraus MS, Moise NS, Rishniw M et al. (2002) Morphology of ventricular arrhythmias in the Boxer as measured by 12-lead electrocardiography with pace-mapping comparison. *J Vet Intern Med* 16:153–158.

67 Keene BW, Panciera DP, Atkins CE et al. (1991) Myocardial L-carnitine deficiency in a family of dogs with dilated cardiomyopathy. *J Am Vet Med Assoc* 201:647–650.

68 Bright JM, McEntee M (1995) Isolated right ventricular cardiomyopathy in a dog. *J Am Vet Med Assoc* 207:64–66.

69 Maxson TR, Meurs KM, Lehmkuhl LB et al. (2001) Polymerase chain reaction analysis for viruses in parraffin-embedded myocardium from dogs with dilated cardiomyopathy or myocarditis. *Am J Vet Res* 62:130–135.

70 Mauldin GE, Fox PR, Patnaik AK (1992) Doxorubicin-induced cardiotoxicosis: clinical features in 23 dogs. *J Vet Intern Med* 6:82–88.

71 Kramer GA, Kittleson MD, Fox PR et al. (1995) Plasma taurine concentrations in normal dogs and in dogs with heart disease. *J Vet Intern Med* 9:253–258.

72 Gavaghan BJ, Kittleson MD (1997) Dilated cardiomyopathy in an American Cocker Spaniel with taurine deficiency. *Aust Vet J* 75:862–868.

73 Fascetti AJ, Reed JR, Rogers QR et al. (2003) Taurine deficiency in dogs with dilated cardiomyopathy:12 cases (1997–2001). *J Am Vet Med Assoc* 223:1137–1141.

74 Backus RC, Cohen G, Pion PD et al. (2003) Taurine deficiency in Newfoundlands fed commercially available complete and balanced diets. *J Am Vet Med Assoc* 223:1130–1136.

75 Sanderson SL, Gross KL, Ogburn PH et al. (2001) Effects of dietary fat and L-carnitine on plasma and whole blood taurine concentrations and cardiac function in healthy dogs fed protein-restricted diets. *Am J Vet Res* 62:1616–1623.

76 Panciera DL (1994) An echocardiographic and electrocardiographic study of cardiovascular function in hypothyroid dogs. *J Am Vet Med Assoc* 205:996–1000.

77 Falk T, Jonsson L (2000) Ischaemic heart disease in the dog: a review of 65 cases. *J Small Anim Pract* 41:97–103.

78 Driehuys S, Van Winkle TJ, Sammarco CD et al. (1998) Myocardial infarction in dogs and cats: 37 cases (1985–1994). *J Am Vet Med Assoc* 213:1444–1448.

79 Kelley DF (1995) Myocardial infarction (MI) in dogs. Abstract. *Vet Pathol* 32:550

80 Kidd L, Stepien RL, Amrheiw DP (2000) Clinical findings and coronary artery disease in dogs and cats with acute and subacute myocardial necrosis: 28 cases. *J Am Anim Hosp Assoc* 36:199–208.

81 DeFrancesco TC, Atkins CE, Keene BW (1996) Myocardial infarction complicating management of congestive heart failure in a dog. *J Am Anim Hosp Assoc* 32:68–72.

82 Hess RS, Kass PH, Van Winkle TJ (2003) Association between diabetes mellitus, hypothyroidism or hyperadrenocorticism and atheroslerosis in dogs. *J Vet Intern Med* 17:489–494.

83 Liu SK, Tilley LP, Tappe JP et al. (1986) Clinical and pathological findings in dogs with atherosclerosis: 21 cases (1970–1983). *J Am Vet Med Assoc* 189:227–232.

84 Zeiss CJ, Waddle G (1995) Hypothyroidism and atherosclerosis in dogs. *Compend Cont Educ Pract Vet* 17:1117–1128.

85 Wright KN, Mehdirad AA, Giacobbe P et al. (1999) Radiofrequency catheter ablation of atrioventricular accessory pathways in 3 dogs with subsequent resolution of tachycardia-induced cardiomyopathy. *J Vet Intern Med* 13:361–371.

86 Connolly DJ, Boswood A (2003) Dynamic obstruction of the left ventricular outflow tract in four young dogs. *J Small Anim Pract* 44:319–325.

87 Keene BW (1993) Evidence for the

role of myocarditis in the pathophysiology of dilated cardiomyopathy. In: *Proceedings of the 11th ACVIM Forum*, Washington DC, pp. 565–567.

88 Pisani B, Taylor DO, Mason JW (1997) Inflammatory myocardial diseases and cardiomyopathies. *Am J Med* **102**:459–469.

89 Breitschwerdt EB, Atkins CE, Brown TT *et al.* (1999) *Bartonella vinsonii* subsp. *berkhoffii* and related members of the alpha subdivision of the Proteobacteria in dogs with cardiac arrhythmias, endocarditis, or myocarditis. *J Clin Microbiol* **37**:3618–3626.

90 Fritz CL, Kjemtrup AM (2003) Lyme borreliosis. *J Am Vet Med Assoc* **223**:1261–1270.

91 Levy, SA, Harrison P (1998) Complete heart block in a dog seropositive with *Borrelia burgdorferi*. *J Vet Intern Med* **2**:138–144.

92 Bradley KK, Bergman DK, Woods JP *et al.* (2000) Prevalence of American trypanosomiasis (Chagas disease) among dogs in Oklahoma. *J Am Vet Med Assoc* **217**:1853–1857.

93 Meurs KM, Anthony MA, Slater, M *et al.* (1998) Chronic *Trypanosoma cruzi* infection in dogs: 11 cases (1987–1996). *J Am Vet Med Assoc* **213**:497–500.

94 Barr SC, Van Beek O, Carlisle-Novak MS *et al.* (1995) *Trypanosoma cruzi* infection in Walker Hounds from Virginia. *Am J Vet Res* **56**:1037–1044.

95 Barr SC, Holmes RA, Klei TR (1992) Electrocardiographic and echocardiographic features of trypanosomiasis in dogs inoculated with North American *Trypanosoma cruzi* isolates. *Am J Vet Res* **53**:521–527.

96 Barber JS, Trees AJ (1996) Clinical aspects of 27 cases of neosporosis in dogs. *Vet Rec* **139**:439–443.

97 Dvir E, Lobetti RG, Jacobson LS *et al.* (2004) Electrocardiographic changes and cardiac pathology in canine babesiosis. *J Vet Cardiol* **6**:15–23.

98 Lobetti R, Dvir, E, Pearson J (2002) Cardiac troponins in canine babesiosis. *J Vet Intern Med* **16**:63–68.

99 Meurs KM, Atkins CE, Khoo L *et al.* (1994) Aberrant migration of *Toxocara* larvae as a cause of myocarditis in the dog. *J Am Anim Hosp Assoc* **30**:580–582.

100 Gould SM, McInnes EL (1999) Immune-mediated thrombocytopenia associated with *Angiostrongylus vasorum* infection in a dog. *J Small Anim Pract* **40**:227–232.

101 Aretz HT, Billingham ME, Edwards WD *et al.* (1987) Myocarditis. A histopathologic definition and classification. *Am J Cardiovasc Pathol* **1**:3–14.

102 Snyder PS, Cooke KL, Murphy ST *et al.* (2001) Electrocardiographic findings in dogs with motor vehicle-related trauma. *J Am Anim Hosp Assoc* **37**:55–63.

21
Myocardial Diseases of the Cat

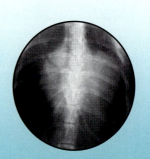

Myocardial diseases (cardiomyopathies) cause a spectrum of pathophysiologic and structural abnormalities in cats[1–3]. As a group, they are the most common cause of heart disease in cats[2, 4]. Myocardial disease occurs secondary to an identifiable cause in some cats, but the disease is idiopathic in many. General categories of myocardial disease are hypertrophic, restrictive, dilated, and arrhythmogenic right ventricular cardiomyopathy (ARVC)[1, 3]. Features of more than one category can coexist in an individual, and some cats are considered to have 'indeterminate' or unclassified myocardial disease. Systemic thromboembolism (TE) remains a troubling complication in cats with myocardial disease.

HYPERTROPHIC CARDIOMYOPATHY

OVERVIEW

Idiopathic (primary) HCM is the most common type of myocardial disease in cats[1, 2, 5–8]. It is characterized by excessive LV hypertrophy without dilation. Secondary myocardial hypertrophy also occurs frequently (see p. 309), but this is not considered to be HCM. Although the cause of HCM in cats is unknown, a genetic basis is thought to underlie many cases[5, 9, 10]. An autosomal dominant inheritance pattern is found in some breeds. Most HCM in people is familial; many different mutations in genes coding for myocardial proteins have been identified in various kindreds (extended families). Reduced myomesin (a sarcomeric protein) content and a missense mutation in the cardiac myosin binding protein C gene have been identified in affected Maine Coon cats[11, 12]. Other mutations will likely be identified in the future. Besides mutations of genes that code for myocardial contractile or regulatory proteins, postulated causes of HCM include increased myocardial sensitivity to, or excessive production of, catecholamines; abnormal hypertrophic response to myocardial ischemia, fibrosis, or trophic factors; primary collagen abnormality; or abnormal myocardial calcium-handling processes[1]. Myocardial hypertrophy, but infrequent congestive failure, is known to occur

with hypertrophic feline muscular dystrophy, an X-linked recessive dystrophin deficiency similar to Duchenne muscular dystrophy in people[13]. Whether viral myocarditis has a role in the pathogenesis of feline cardiomyopathy is not clear. In one study of formalin-fixed cardiomyopathic feline hearts, 55% of HCM samples showed evidence of myocarditis; panleukopenia virus DNA was documented in some[14].

PATHOPHYSIOLOGY

LV free wall and/or IVS hypertrophy is seen grossly with HCM; the heart weight:body weight ratio is increased (430, 431)[15]. The extent and distribution of hypertrophy is variable[1, 6, 16, 17]; it may encompass the entire ventricle symmetrically or involve only certain regions. Asymmetrical septal thickening is common. Hypertrophy in some cats is limited to portions of the LV wall or papillary muscles. LA enlargement varies from mild to massive, depending largely on the severity of diastolic dysfunction. The LV lumen

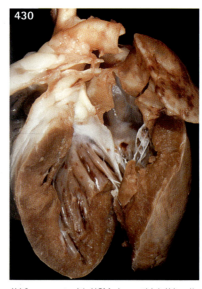

430 Open LV from a cat with HCM shows thick LV wall and enlarged LA (upper right).

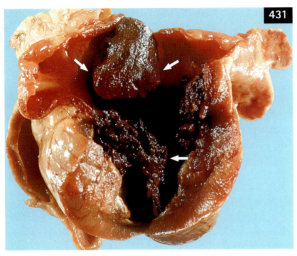

431 Large thrombi (arrows) were present in both the LA (top) and LV in this cat with HCM.

usually appears small. Myocyte hypertrophy is evident histologically. Focal or diffuse areas of fibrosis within the endocardium, conduction system, or myocardium and narrowing of small intramural coronary arteries can be seen[1, 5, 6, 15]. Areas of myocardial infarction may be present. Myocardial fiber disarray, common in people with HCM, is also found in many cats [1, 5, 6, 15]. On necropsy, over half of affected cats have pulmonary edema; fewer show pleural effusion[1]. A thrombus is sometimes found within the LA or attached to the ventricular wall (**431**). Evidence for arterial TE is common.

Myocardial hypertrophy promotes diastolic dysfunction as ventricular stiffness increases and relaxation abnormalities develop; however, these are not always correlated to the degree or distribution of hypertrophy[1, 18]. When ventricular distensibility is reduced, LV filling is impaired and higher diastolic pressures are required. Fibrosis and disorganized myocardial cell structure contribute to abnormal ventricular stiffness. LV relaxation abnormalities with or without increased LV filling pressure have been documented in feline HCM[18–20]. Slowed or incomplete early (active) relaxation prolongs IVRT (see Chapter 1, p. 17), reduces early LV filling, and increases the importance of atrial contraction. Myocardial ischemia promotes these relaxation abnormalities. Factors that contribute to myocardial ischemia in cats with HCM include intramural coronary artery narrowing, decreased coronary artery perfusion pressure because of increased LV filling pressure, and myocardial capillary density inadequate for the degree of hypertrophy. Ischemia not only impairs active ventricular relaxation, long term it leads to myocardial fibrosis. It is also thought to predispose to lethal arrhythmias and possibly thoracic pain. Ischemia and diastolic dysfunction are exacerbated by tachycardia.

Increasing LV stiffness causes progressively higher LA and LV diastolic pressures. LA enlargement buffers this, but eventually pulmonary congestion and edema result from increasing LA pressure. Geometric changes in the LV and papillary muscles as well as abnormal systolic mitral valve motion can interfere with normal valve closure. Secondary MR exacerbates the increased LA volume and pressure. LV volume is normal or decreased; reduced ventricular volume results in lower stroke volume and may contribute to NH activation. Higher HRs further interfere with LV filling, exacerbate myocardial ischemia, and promote pulmonary venous congestion and edema by shortening the diastolic filling period. Contractility (systolic function) is usually normal in affected cats, but some cats show regional LV systolic dysfunction, likely from myocardial infarction or fibrosis. Progression to ventricular systolic failure and LV dilation occasionally develops as end-stage changes[2, 21].

Systolic dynamic LV outflow obstruction (i.e. functional SAS or hypertrophic obstructive cardiomyopathy [HOCM]) occurs in many cats with HCM and causes a systolic pressure gradient across the LV outflow tract[1, 5, 6]. Excessive diffuse or focal hypertrophy of the basilar IVS may be evident echocardiographically or at necropsy. Another important component of the obstruction is SAM of the septal (anterior) mitral valve leaflet. Several mechanisms may underlie SAM, including myocardial hypertrophy, structural abnormalities of the mitral apparatus, and a suction (Venturi) effect pulling the mitral leaflet toward the IVS during ejection[1]. SAM may cause endocardial scar tissue on the IVS opposite the mitral leaflet. LV outflow gradients tend to increase with stress and excitement; a gradient may or may not be present at rest. Systolic outflow obstruction increases LV pressure, wall stress, and myocardial oxygen demand and promotes myocardial ischemia. Mild to moderate functional MR is associated with SAM. MR severity tends to parallel the degree of SAM and LV outflow obstruction[1, 6]. Dynamic RV outflow obstruction has also been reported in cats, but this is not always associated with HOCM and tends to be mild [1, 22]. Some degree of tricuspid regurgitation is also common in HCM.

In addition to pulmonary edema, pleural effusion also develops in some cats as a manifestation of heart failure. A modified transudate is typical, although the effusion often becomes chylous. RAAS activation and variably elevated plasma TNF concentrations have been shown in cats with CHF [23, 24]. Increased cTnI also occurs in cats with moderate to severe HCM, with higher levels associated with CHF signs[25].

Thrombi may form within the heart, especially a dilated LA, and cause systemic TE if dislodged. Marked LA enlargement and secondary blood stasis are considered risk factors for TE (see Chapter 15).

CLINICAL FEATURES

There may be a higher prevalence in breeds such as the Maine Coon, Ragdoll, American Shorthair, and, possibly, Persian[5, 9, 11, 26]. HCM is also reported in littermates and other closely related DSH cats[1, 10, 21]. An autosomal dominant inheritance pattern has been found in the families studied, similar to the most common inheritance pattern in people[5, 9].

HCM is reported most often in middle-aged male cats, but it can occur in young as well as geriatric cats[1, 8]. Cats with mild disease may be asymptomatic for years. Clinically ill cats most commonly show respiratory signs from pulmonary edema, including tachypnea, panting with activity, and overt dyspnea. Coughing, sometimes misinterpreted as vomiting, occurs only rarely. The onset of CHF may seem acute in sedentary cats, even though pathologic changes have developed gradually. Acute signs of thromboembolism (see Chapter 15, p. 152) occur in some cats. Others experience syncope or, occasionally, sudden death without other signs[5, 6, 7, 21]. Lethargy or anorexia is the only evidence of disease in some cats. Stress from anesthesia and surgery, fluid administration, systemic illness (e.g. fever or anemia), and even boarding can precipitate CHF in an otherwise compensated cat[7]. The disease is sometimes discovered by detecting a murmur or gallop sound on auscultation.

A systolic murmur of either MR or LV outflow tract obstruction is common, but some cats have no murmur, even with marked ventricular hypertrophy. With dynamic LV outflow obstruction, murmur intensity varies with the degree of obstruction. The murmur may be very soft or inaudible in the relaxed cat, especially with beta-blocker therapy. The murmur becomes louder as dynamic obstruction worsens with increased sympathetic tone (increased HR,

contractility, vasodilation). A diastolic gallop sound (usually S_4) may be heard, especially if heart failure is evident or imminent. Cardiac arrhythmias are relatively common. Femoral pulses are usually strong, unless distal aortic thromboembolism has occurred. A vigorous precordial impulse is often palpable. Prominent lung sounds, pulmonary crackles, and, sometimes, cyanosis accompany severe pulmonary edema; pleural effusion usually attenuates ventral lung sounds. Physical examination findings can be normal in the absence of CHF.

DIAGNOSIS

Radiographic features of advanced HCM include a prominent LA with variable LV enlargement (432–437; also 46, 47, p. 39). The classic valentine-shaped appearance of the heart on DV or VD view (435) is not always present, but usually the point of the LV apex is maintained. Mild to moderate pericardial effusion can increase the cardiomegaly in some cats with CHF. The cardiac silhouette appears normal in most cats

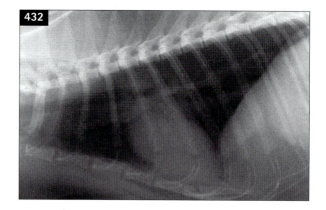

432

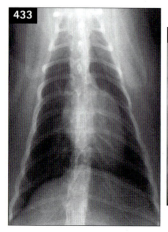

433

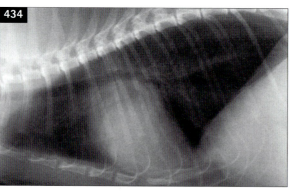

434

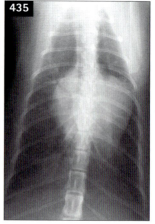

435

432–435 (432, 433) Mild cardiomegaly in a 5-year-old DSH cat with early hypertrophic obstructive cardiomyopathy. (434, 435) More prominent cardiomegaly is evident in an 11-year-old cat with HCM and marked LA enlargement. The heart appears 'valentine-shaped' on the DV view (435).

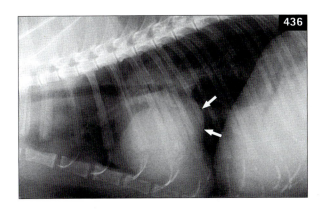

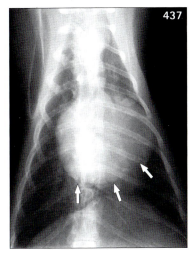

436, 437 Massive LA enlargement causes a caudal bulge on the lateral view (436, arrows) and a double-shadow effect on the DV view (437 arrows). Large caudal pulmonary veins (436) indicate chronically high LA pressure. The LV apex point is maintained in this 15-year-old cat with HCM.

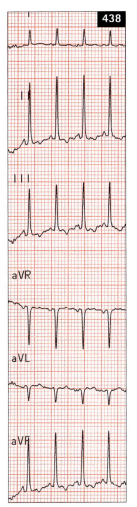

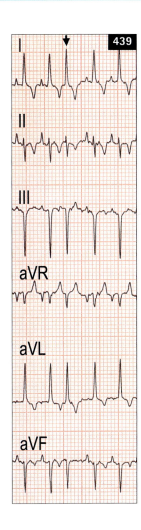

438, 439 (438) Tall and wide R waves on this ECG suggest LV enlargement in a cat with cardiomyopathy. Sinus rhythm and a normal electrical axis are seen. Leads as marked; 25 mm/sec; 1 cm = 1 mV. (439) Left axis deviation as well as an atrial premature complex (arrow) are present in a 16-year-old DSH cat with HCM. Leads as marked; 25 mm/sec, 2 cm = 1 mV.

with mild HCM. Enlarged, tortuous pulmonary veins indicate chronically high LA and pulmonary venous pressures. A variable degree of patchy interstitial or alveolar infiltrate develops with pulmonary edema (see 64, 65, p. 45). The distribution of these infiltrates can be focal or diffuse throughout the lung fields, in contrast to the characteristic perihilar distribution of cardiogenic pulmonary edema in dogs. Pleural effusion is common in advanced left or biventricular failure (see 67–68, p. 45).

ECG abnormalities are common with HCM, although the ECG is unremarkable in many cats. Criteria for LA and LV enlargement, ventricular and/or, less often, supraventricular tachyarrhythmias, and left axis deviation are seen most often (see 438, 439; also 89, p. 55). AF occurs in some cats (see 88, p. 55)[27]. Occasionally, an AV conduction delay, complete AV block, or sinus bradycardia is found (see 105, p. 58).

Echocardiography is the best means of diagnosis and noninvasive differentiation of HCM from other myocardial disorders. 2-D echocardiography shows the extent and distribution of hypertrophy within the ventricular wall, septum, and papillary muscles, and helps characterize systolic and diastolic functional abnormalities (see Chapter 5). Nonselective angiocardiography is an alternative means of diagnosis, but it poses a greater risk to the cat and is rarely used now. Hypertrophy is commonly widespread, but often asymmetrically distributed among LV wall, IVS, and papillary muscle locations

(440–444)[1, 6, 17, 25]. Focal hypertrophy also occurs. Use of 2-D–guided M-mode is important to ensure proper beam position. Standard M-mode views and measurements are obtained, but thickened areas outside these standard positions should also be measured (445, 446). The upper limit of normal for diastolic LV wall and IVS thickness is usually considered to be 5.0–5.5 mm. The diagnosis may be questionable in cats with mild or only focal thickening; furthermore, falsely increased LV wall and IVS thickness measurements (pseudo-hypertrophy) can occur with dehydration and, sometimes, with tachycardia[28]. Cats with severe HCM may have diastolic LV wall or IVS thicknesses of 8 mm or more, but the degree of hypertrophy is not necessarily correlated with the severity of clinical signs[1, 17]. Marked papillary muscle hypertrophy and systolic LV cavity obliteration are observed in some cats. Increased echogenicity (brightness) of papillary muscles and subendocardial areas is thought to be a marker for chronic myocardial ischemia and subsequent fibrosis. LV fractional shortening is generally normal to increased; however, some cats have mild to moderate LV dilation and contractility reduction (e.g. FS ~23–29%). RV enlargement and pericardial (see 488, p. 324) or pleural effusion are sometimes detected[1, 2, 6].

Doppler-derived measures of diastolic function, such as mitral and pulmonary venous inflow patterns and IVRT, are being used more commonly[1, 18, 29]. Mitral inflow pattern alterations seen with HCM include reduced maximal velocity of early filling (E) wave, slowed E wave deceleration rate, increased A wave maximal velocity, reduced E/A ratio, and prolonged IRVT (447–449)[18, 29]. The A wave peak velocity is greater than that of the E wave in some cases.

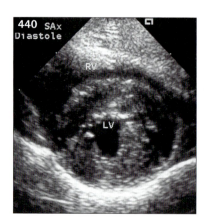
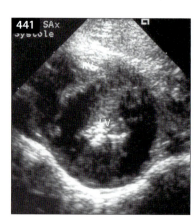

440–442 2-D echocardiographic examples of variation in distribution of hypertrophy with HCM. Symmetrical LV wall and septal hypertrophy with thick papillary muscles in diastole (440) and systole (441). The LV lumen is virtually obliterated in systole; increased subendocardial brightness is evident.

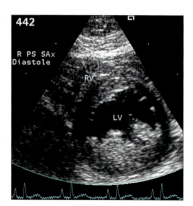
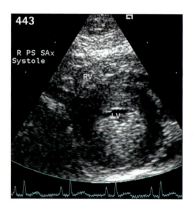
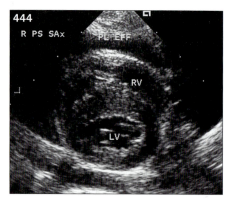

442–444 (442, 443) Hypertrophy is localized to the LV wall and papillary muscles in diastole (442) and systole (443) in an old DSH cat. The hypertrophied area shows increased brightness consistent with chronic ischemia and fibrosis in the subendocardial and mid-ventricular regions. (444) Diastolic frame from a 4-year-old cat with asymmetrical hypertrophy of the dorsal septum. Right parasternal short-axis views. RV = right ventricle; LV = left ventricle.

These mitral inflow changes are consistent with delayed myocardial relaxation (**448**). A 'pseudonormal' mitral inflow pattern occurs in the face of abnormal diastolic function when LV stiffness causes increased LA pressure, which then increases early filling velocity. The pseudonormal pattern is transitional between the impaired relaxation pattern and restrictive pattern. An abnormal pulmonary venous inflow pattern can help differentiate pseudonormal from true normal mitral filling[29]. The restrictive filling pattern is characterized by a shortened IVRT, a tall narrow mitral E wave, and a small blunted A wave (**449**)[2, 18]. PW Doppler tissue

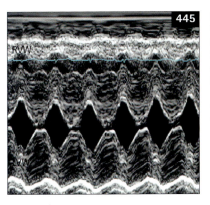

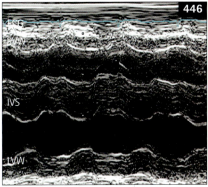

445, 446 (**445**) This M-mode echocardiogram from a 16-year-old male DLH cat with symmetrical LV hypertrophy shows typical vigorous systolic motion and normal RV size. (**446**) Marked septal hypertrophy is seen in a 4-year-old female DSH with hypertrophic obstructive cardiomyopathy. ECG = electrocardiogram; IVS = interventricular septum; RVW = right ventricular wall; LVW = left ventricular wall.

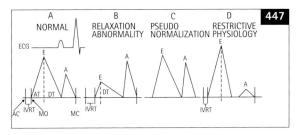

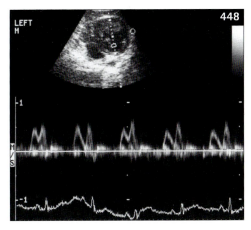

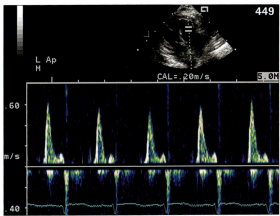

447–449 (**447**) Diagram of normal and abnormal PW Doppler transmitral inflow patterns. Normal pattern shows higher velocity early diastolic filling wave (E wave) compared with the late diastolic, atrial contraction wave (A wave); the E/A ratio is generally 1.0–2.0. The IVRT is an index of active myocardial relaxation; it occurs between the time of aortic valve closure (AC) and mitral valve opening (MO). Impaired relaxation may cause lower E wave velocity and accentuated A wave velocity (E/A < 1.0), as well as prolonged IVRT, reduced flow acceleration time (AT), and prolonged deceleration time (DT). Diastolic LV pressure may be increased. 'Pseudonormalization' of the mitral inflow pattern represents a transition between relaxation abnormality and restrictive patterns, as either increasing LA pressure or declining LV compliance complicate delayed myocardial relaxation. Restrictive physiology is associated with a very tall E wave, related to high LA pressure, and a small A wave because poor LV compliance allows little filling in late diastole. Both IVRT and DT are shortened. (From Fox PR (1999) Feline cardiomyopathies. In *Textbook of Canine and Feline Cardiology* (2nd edn). (eds PR Fox, DD Sisson, NS Moise) WB Saunders, Philadelphia, p. 624, with permission.) (**448**) Doppler echo of mitral inflow from a 2-year-old Manx with HCM shows reduced E and accentuated A wave velocities, typical of LV relaxation abnormality. (**449**) Restrictive mitral inflow pattern from a 5-year-old DSH cat with chronic HCM.

imaging, ratios involving mitral E wave compared with early diastolic peak annulus velocity or flow propagation velocity, M-mode derived global LA shortening fraction, and other measures have also been described in the evaluation of LV diastolic function[30–34]. Indices derived from such techniques may provide important diagnostic and prognostic information, although their clinical usefulness remains to be clarified.

With dynamic LV outflow tract obstruction, mitral SAM (450–453; also 152, 153, p. 81) or mid-systolic partial aortic valve closure is often evident on M-mode scans. Doppler modalities can demonstrate MR and increased LV outflow velocity in mid-systole (452, 453). Optimal beam alignment with the maximal velocity outflow jet may be difficult and, along with the dynamic nature of HOCM, makes accurate systolic gradient estimation challenging.

LA enlargement ranges from mild to marked; the LA wall may look hypertrophied[1, 2, 6]. Spontaneous contrast (swirling, 'smokey' echos) is visible within the enlarged LA of some cats (454). This is thought to result from blood stasis with cellular aggregates and to be a harbinger of TE[35]. A thrombus is occasionally visualized within the LA, usually in the auricle (455).

Other causes of myocardial hypertrophy (see p. 309) should be excluded before a diagnosis of idiopathic HCM is made. Myocardial thickening can also result from infiltrative disease. Variation in myocardial echogenicity or wall irregularities may be evident in such cases. Excess moderator bands, which may represent a congenital anomaly[36], appear as bright, linear echos within the LV cavity.

MANAGEMENT

The main goals of therapy are to facilitate LV filling, relieve congestion, control arrhythmias, minimize ischemia, and prevent thromboembolism (*Table 61*). Treatment is guided by the underlying pathophysiology as revealed by echo findings. Ventricular filling is improved by slowing the HR and enhancing relaxation. Stress and activity level should be minimized toward

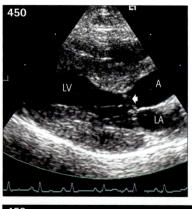

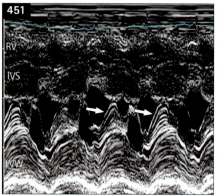

450, 451 (450) Long-axis 2-D echo image in systole from a DSH cat with dynamic LV outflow obstruction shows the anterior mitral leaflet pulled toward the IVS (arrow). A = aorta; LA = left atrium; LV = left ventricle. (451) M-mode echo from a different cat with dynamic LV outflow obstruction also shows this abnormal SAM (arrows) of the mitral valve. IVS = interventricular septum; LVW = left ventricular wall; RV = right ventricle.

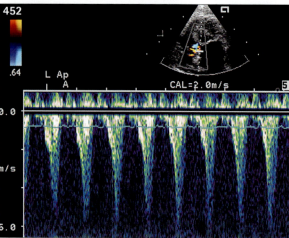

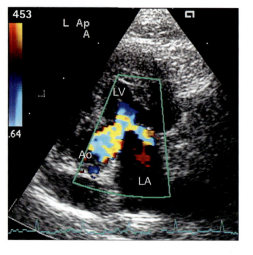

452, 453, (452) CW Doppler of aortic flow from a 4-year-old Persian cat with dynamic LV outflow obstruction shows the pattern of mid-systolic flow acceleration, as the obstruction worsens, and high peak velocity. (453) Systolic color flow image from the same cat as in 452 illustrates turbulent flow into the aorta and mild MR related to SAM. Left apical view. Ao = aorta; LA = left atrium; LV = left ventricle.

this end. Diltiazem or a beta-blocker (see Chapter 16, p. 186 and *Table 44*, p. 174) has historically been the foundation of long-term oral therapy[2, 37]. The decision to use one drug over another is influenced by the specific abnormalities in the individual or the response to medication. Situations where a beta-blocker has been preferred include suspected myocardial infarction (used with an ACE inhibitor also), LV outflow obstruction, tachyarrhythmias, and syncope. A beta-blocker can also be used in some cases of severe hypertrophy, although diltiazem is also recommended for this. Beta-blockers are relatively contraindicated with

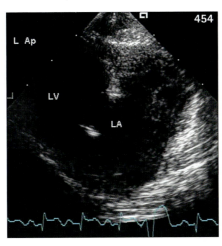

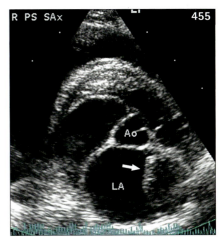

454, 455 (454) Ill-defined 'smoke-like' echos are seen in the large LA of a 5-year-old male DSH cat with chronic cardiomyopathy and biventricular heart failure. Left apical view. **(455)** A large thrombus (arrow) is seen in the left auricle of a female DSH cat with hypertrophic obstructive cardiomyopathy. Right parasternal short-axis view. Ao = aorta; LA = left atrium; LV = left ventricle.

Table 61 General treatment guidelines for hypertrophic cardiomyopathy in the cat.

1) Mild to moderate signs of CHF:*
   a) Beta-blocker (e.g. atenolol) or diltiazem.
   b) Furosemide.
   c) +/– ACE inhibitor.
   d) Antithrombotic prophylaxis (e.g. aspirin, warfarin, LMWH).**
   e) Exercise restriction.
   f) Moderate dietary salt restriction, if accepted.

2) Severe, acute signs of CHF:*
   a) Supplemental O_2.
   b) Cage rest.
   c) Minimize patient handling.
   d) Furosemide (parenteral).
   e) Thoracocentesis, if pleural effusion.
   f) Heart rate control and antiarrhythmic therapy, if indicated; can use IV diltiazem or esmolol; avoid IV propranolol (nonselective beta-blocker) when possible if pulmonary edema present.***
   g) +/– nitroglycerin (cutaneous).
   h) +/– bronchodilator (e.g. aminophylline or theophylline).
   i) +/– acepromazine or other sedation.

j) Monitor: respiratory rate, HR and rhythm, arterial blood pressure, renal function, serum electrolytes, etc.

3) Chronic HCM management:*
   a) Beta-blocker (e.g. atenolol) or diltiazem.
   b) Furosemide (lowest effective dosage and frequency).
   c) +/– ACE inhibitor.
   d) +/– spironolactone and/or hydrochlorothiazide.
   e) Antithrombotic prophylaxis (e.g. aspirin, warfarin, LMWH).**
   f) Thoracocentesis as needed.
   g) +/– concurrent beta-blocker and diltiazem therapy.
   h) +/– additional antiarrhythmic drug therapy, if indicated.
   i) Client education.
   j) Resting respiratory rate (+HR if possible) monitoring at home.
   k) Dietary salt restriction, if accepted.
   l) Monitor renal function, electrolytes, etc.
   m) Manage other medical problems (rule out hyperthyroidism and hypertension if not done previously).
   n) +/– digoxin (only for deteriorating systolic function without LV outflow obstruction).

* See text and Chapters 16 and 17 for further details.

** See Chapter 15 for further details.

*** See Chapter 17 for additional ventricular antiarrhythmic drug therapy.

bradycardia or severe contractility failure. ACE inhibitors may help reduce LV remodeling and NH activation, but this awaits clarification.

There is debate about whether, and how, asymptomatic cats with HCM should be treated. It is unclear whether disease progression can be slowed or survival prolonged by initiating drug therapy before the onset of clinical signs. Nevertheless, some cats anecdotally have shown increased activity or subjective improvement after a beta-blocker or diltiazem was given based on abnormal echo findings in the absence of overt CHF signs. Antithrombotic prophylaxis is prudent for cats with marked LA enlargement, especially with spontaneous echocontrast ('smoke'), whether CHF signs are present or not (see Chapter 15, p. 160).

Mild signs of congestive heart failure

Furosemide (e.g. 1 mg/kg q8–12h) is used to treat pulmonary edema and mild pleural effusion; dosing is guided by severity. Once congestive signs have resolved and other therapy is initiated, furosemide dosage is tapered to the lowest effective level. Some cats can be weaned off furosemide once a beta-blocker or diltiazem therapy is in place. Close monitoring for recurrence of congestive signs is necessary.

Beta-blockers can provide greater HR control than diltiazem, as well as help control tachyarrhythmias, reduce systolic outflow obstruction, and lessen myocardial oxygen demand[38]. Diminished HR and myocardial ischemia from beta-blocker therapy may also indirectly enhance LV compliance and filling, although beta-blockers do not directly enhance relaxation. Atenolol is often used because it is beta$_1$ selective and can be dosed q8h or q24h. Nonselective agents such as propranolol may stimulate bronchoconstriction, by blocking airway beta$_2$-receptors, especially when CHF is present. However, the advantages of slowing sinus tachycardia and minimizing ventricular arrhythmias may outweigh the risk of bronchospasm, even with propranolol. Some cats do not tolerate propranolol well (e.g. lethargy, depressed appetite), and it requires more frequent dosing. Other beta-blockers can also be used. It should be noted that there is controversy over beta-blocker use in cats with prior congestive failure.

Diltiazem is effective in many cases. The author chooses diltiazem over a beta-blocker in HCM cats without LV outflow obstruction, tachyarrhythmias, or suspected myocardial infarction. Diltiazem promotes coronary vasodilation and may enhance ventricular relaxation. The drug mildly decreases heart rate and contractility, and may also reduce systolic outflow gradients if peripheral vasodilation does not enhance ventricular shortening. Hypotension is generally not a problem. Longer-acting diltiazem products are more convenient for long-term use, but serum concentrations are not consistent from cat to cat. (see Chapter 17, p. 217)

Fulminant/severe congestive heart failure signs

Parenteral furosemide (e.g. 1–2 mg/kg q1–4h or PRN) is given for severe respiratory distress. Initial IM dosing is used unless or until IV access can be established with minimal patient stress (*Table 61*, p. 307; also *Table 43*, p. 171). If large volume pleural effusion is present, or suspected, thoracocentesis is performed expediently, with the cat restrained gently in a sternal position. Nitroglycerin ointment (see *Tables 43* and *44*, pp. 171 and 174) can be applied for the first 24–36 hours (usually a 12 hour on/12 hour off schedule), although no studies of its efficacy in this situation have been done. Some cats require therapy for serious arrhythmias such as ventricular tachycardia (see Chapter 17). Once initial medications have been given, the cat should be allowed to rest, preferably with supplemental oxygen. The respiratory rate is noted initially, then every 30 minutes or so without disturbing the cat. Catheter placement, blood sampling, radiographs, and other tests and therapies are delayed until the cat appears more stable. Airway suctioning and mechanical ventilation with positive end-expiratory pressure can be considered in extreme cases. The bronchodilating and mild diuretic effects of aminophylline (see *Table 43*, p. 171) may be helpful in cats with severe pulmonary edema, as long as the drug does not increase the heart rate. Acepromazine has been used to reduce anxiety and promote the peripheral redistribution of blood by its alpha-adrenergic-blocking effects, but preexisting hypothermia can be exacerbated by peripheral vasodilation. Combination with butorphanol can be helpful. Morphine should not be used in cats.

When the respiratory distress is alleviated, furosemide can be continued at reduced doses q8–12h; diuretic therapy is guided by the animal's respiratory rate and effort. Once pulmonary edema is controlled, furosemide is given PO and tapered to the lowest dose and longest dosing interval that is effective.

Complications of excessive diuresis include azotemia, anorexia, electrolyte disturbances, especially hypokalemia, and suboptimal LV filling pressure. Cautious fluid administration may be needed in some cats after excessive diuresis (e.g. 15–20 ml/kg/day of 1/2 strength saline, D5W, or other low-sodium fluid).

Chronic congestive heart failure management

Beta-blocker or diltiazem therapy is generally continued, although evidence for a long-term survival benefit appears lacking and these recommendations may change. Furosemide is adjusted to find the current optimal dosage. Some cats only need furosemide a couple times per week or less, while others require it several times per day. An ACE inhibitor appears to be helpful, presumably by modulating NH activation, especially in cats with refractory CHF. ACE inhibitor therapy may also mitigate AT II-mediated ventricular hypertrophy (remodeling). Preliminary evidence suggests ACE inhibitors might reduce LA size and ventricular/septal wall thickness in some cats[39]. Enalapril and benazepril are used most commonly, and others are available (see Chapter 16, p. 178 and *Table 44*, p. 174); however, further study in cats with HCM is needed to determine if there is enhanced survival with ACE inhibitors.

Sometimes, a beta-blocker is added to diltiazem therapy (or vice versa) if CHF is hard to control or if the HR in cats with AF remains uncontrolled, but caution must be used to avoid bradycardia or hypotension. Some cats may require additional therapy to control tachyarrhythmias.

Certain drugs are relatively contraindicated with HCM. These include digoxin and other positive inotropic agents, which increase myocardial oxygen demand and can worsen dynamic LV outflow obstruction. Any drug that accelerates the HR is potentially detrimental, because tachycardia decreases filling time and predisposes to myocardial ischemia. Arterial vasodilators can cause hypotension and reflex tachycardia, because cats with HCM have little preload reserve. Hypotension also exacerbates dynamic outflow obstruction. Although ACE inhibitors also have this potential, their vasodilating effects are usually mild. One study showed no increase in LV outflow gradient with ACE inhibitor (benazepril) use[40].

Refractory pulmonary edema or pleural effusion can be difficult to manage, especially with disease progression to restrictive pathophysiology. Moderate to large pleural effusions should be drained. Other strategies in chronic cases include increasing furosemide dosage (up to 4 mg/kg q8h); adding an ACE inhibitor; maximizing the dose of ACE inhibitor, diltiazem or beta-blocker; and adding another diuretic such as spironolactone, with or without hydrochlorothiazide (see *Table 44*, p. 174). Frequent monitoring of renal function and serum electrolytes is warranted. Digoxin can also be considered for the treatment of refractory pleural effusion in the absence of LV outflow obstruction.

The development of progressive LV dilation and myocardial systolic failure is difficult to manage successfully. Besides an ACE inhibitor, digoxin can also be added. Blood taurine concentration should be measured and oral supplementation initiated if needed (see p. 315).

Long-term therapy also includes prophylaxis against TE (e.g. aspirin, warfarin, or a low molecular weight heparin) (see Chapter 15, p. 160). If possible, exercise and dietary sodium restrictions are also recommended.

The prognosis for cats with HCM is quite variable and influenced by factors such as response to therapy, occurrence of thromboembolic events, disease progression, and development of arrhythmias[7]. Clinically normal cats with only mild to moderate LV hypertrophy and LA enlargement often live well for years. Greater hypertrophy, marked LA enlargement, older patient age, AF, pleural effusion, and TE have been variably associated with worse prognosis[6–8, 16]. Cats presented with TE generally survive less than 6 months[8]. Some do well for a time if congestive signs can be controlled and infarction of vital organs has not occurred, but recurrent TE is common.

SECONDARY HYPERTROPHIC MYOCARDIAL DISEASE

Myocardial hypertrophy is a compensatory response to certain stresses or disease. Such cases are not considered to be idiopathic HCM. Secondary causes should be ruled out when LV hypertrophy is identified.

Testing for hyperthyroidism is indicated in cats 6 years of age or older with myocardial hypertrophy. Thyroid hormone affects the heart directly as well as indirectly through sympathetic nervous system effects on the heart and circulation. Cardiac effects include myocardial hypertrophy and enhanced heart rate and contractility[41–43]. Hyperthyroidism creates a hyperdynamic circulatory state characterized by increased cardiac output, oxygen demand, blood volume, and heart rate. Associated systemic hypertension can further stimulate myocardial hypertrophy. Multisystemic signs of weight loss, polyphagia, vomiting, polydipsia, polyuria, and hyperactivity occur in most cats, although a small minority shows depression and anorexia[43]. Clinical cardiovascular signs often include a systolic murmur, hyperdynamic precordial and arterial impulses, tachycardia and arrhythmias, and evidence of LV enlargement or hypertrophy seen on ECG, thoracic radiographs, or echocardiogram[16, 43–45]. A gallop sound is heard in about 15% of hyperthyroid cats[45]. Some develop CHF, usually with normal to high FS, but a few have poor contractile function. In addition to antithyroid treatment, other therapy may be needed to manage cardiac complications of hyperthyroidism. A beta-blocker can temporarily control adverse cardiac effects of excess thyroid hormone, especially tachyarrhythmias. Diltiazem is an alternative therapy, although a beta-blocker is preferred. CHF signs are treated as described for HCM. The rare hypodynamic (dilated) cardiac failure is treated as for DCM (see p. 314). However, beta-blocker or other cardiac therapy is not a substitute for antithyroid treatment. Cardiac changes usually regress or normalize after the cat becomes euthyroid[43].

LV concentric hypertrophy is the expected response to increased ventricular systolic pressure (afterload) created by systemic arterial hypertension (see Chapter 25). Increased LV systolic pressure also occurs because of fixed (e.g. congenital SAS, see Chapter 18) or dynamic LV outflow tract obstruction (see p. 301). Cardiac hypertrophy develops in cats with hypersomatotropism (acromegaly) as a result of growth hormone's trophic effects on the heart[46, 47]. CHF occurs in some of these cats. Increased myocardial thickness occasionally results from infiltrative myocardial disease (e.g. lymphoma).

RESTRICTIVE CARDIOMYOPATHY

OVERVIEW

Cardiomyopathy characterized by restrictive pathophysiology is seen less often than HCM[48]. The etiology is unknown but probably multifactorial, as there is a spectrum of pathophysiologic findings. Restrictive cardiomyopathy (RCM) may be a sequela of endomyocarditis, either infectious or immune mediated, or represent the end-stage of myocardial failure and infarction from HCM[2, 21, 48].

PATHOPHYSIOLOGY

RCM may be associated with extensive endocardial, subendocardial, or myocardial fibrosis. A prominent pathologic feature is marked atrial enlargement and hypertrophy. LV chamber size is usually normal or slightly decreased, but there can be mild LV dilation. LV wall hypertrophy is variably present, and can be regional[2]. An endomyocardial form of RCM, also known as endomyocardial fibrosis, is characterized by extensive LV endocardial scarring and chamber deformity. The mitral valve apparatus and papillary muscles may be distorted and fused to surrounding structures. Fibrous tissue bridging between the LV wall and septum can cause intraventricular obstruction[48]. Thrombi are commonly found within the LA, LV, or systemic vasculature. Histopathologic changes include endocardial and myocardial fibrosis, intramural coronary arteriosclerosis, hypertrophied myocytes, areas of myocardial degeneration and necrosis, and, sometimes, endomyocardial cellular infiltrates[2, 48]. Excess moderator bands (branching, fibrous bands extending along or between the LV wall and septum) are found in some cats, but their role in the development of myocardial disease and CHF is unclear. They may represent a congenital anomaly, because they have been identified in young kittens as

well as old cats[36]. Secondary RCM occasionally results from neoplastic (e.g. lymphoma) or other infiltrative or infectious diseases.

Ventricular filling is impeded (restricted) because of abnormal ventricular stiffness. Contractility is normal or mildly reduced in most affected cats; contractility may decline with time as more functional myocardium is lost. Regional LV dysfunction occurs in some cats, which reduces overall systolic function, but these cases are perhaps better called unclassified rather than restrictive. MR may exist but it is usually mild and does not explain the degree of LA enlargement, which is often massive. LA enlargement is secondary to the progressively increasing pressure needed to fill the stiff LV. Arrhythmias, ventricular dilation, and myocardial ischemia or infarction also contribute to diastolic dysfunction. Chronic elevation of left heart filling pressure in combination with compensatory NH activation leads to left-sided or biventricular congestive failure. Blood stasis, especially in the enlarged LA, predisposes to thrombus formation and TE.

CLINICAL FEATURES

RCM appears most often in middle-aged or older cats, although cats under 1 year old have been affected. No gender or breed predilection is apparent. Clinical signs are variable but usually reflect the presence of pulmonary edema, pleural effusion, or both. Signs are often precipitated by stress or concurrent disease, which increases demand on the CV system. Signs are likely to develop or worsen suddenly. Thromboembolic events are common. Inactivity, poor appetite, vomiting, and weight loss may be part of the cat's recent history. Sometimes, preclinical disease is discovered by finding abnormal heart sounds or radiographic evidence of cardiomegaly.

Cats with RCM often have a soft systolic murmur of MR or TR, a gallop sound, or arrhythmias, but some have no abnormal sounds. Abnormal or muffled lung sounds may be heard with pulmonary edema or pleural effusion, respectively. Femoral arterial pulses are normal or slightly weak. Jugular vein distension and pulsation are associated with high right heart filling pressure. Signs of distal aortic, or other, TE may be present (see Chapter 15). Cats with CHF are often hypothermic.

DIAGNOSIS

As for cats with HCM, clinicopathologic findings are nonspecific. Pleural effusions usually are a modified transudate or chyle. Plasma taurine concentration is low in some affected cats and should be measured if decreased contractility is identified.

Radiographs show LA or biatrial enlargement, and LV or generalized cardiomegaly (456-459)[48].

Mild to moderate pericardial effusion may magnify the cardiomegaly. Proximal pulmonary veins may be dilated and tortuous. Infiltrates of pulmonary edema, pleural effusion, and, sometimes, hepatomegaly are seen in cats with CHF.

The ECG is often abnormal. Wide QRS complexes, tall R waves, evidence of disturbed intraventricular conduction, wide P waves, and atrial tachyarrhythmias or fibrillation are common (460, 461)[27].

Echocardiographic features include marked left and, sometimes, right atrial enlargement, variable LV free wall and IVS thickening, and normal to mildly depressed wall motion (FS usually exceeds 25%)[2].

456–459 (456, 457) Massive LA enlargement, common with chronic RCM, is apparent radiographically in an 8-year-old male cat. The LV apex is shifted into the right hemithorax (457). (458, 459) Pulmonary edema has developed 9 months later in this cat.

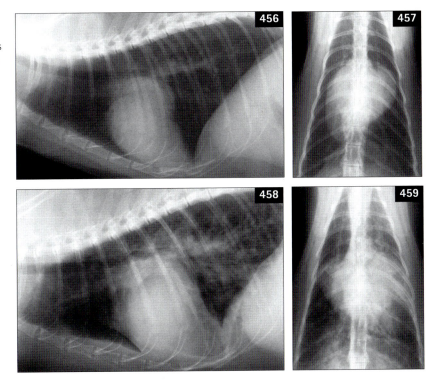

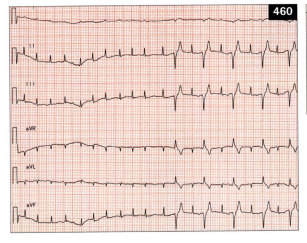

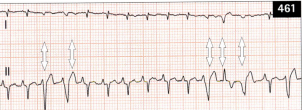

460, 461 (460) The underlying rhythm in this cat with RCM is AF, which suggests marked LA enlargement. VPCs occur in a bigeminal pattern on the right side of this ECG strip. (461) Sinus rhythm with multiform VPCs (arrows) in a cat with RCM. The negative sinus QRS configuration in lead II is due to a right axis deviation. 460, 461: leads as marked; 25 mm/sec, 1 cm = 1 mV.

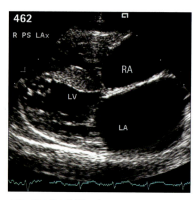
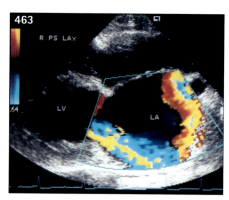
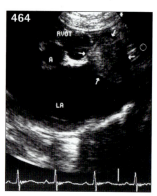

462–464 (462) Fibrotic areas are seen as multiple irregular and bright echos near the LV apex in a cat with RCM. Note the absence of significant hypertrophy and the marked LA enlargement. The RA is also moderately enlarged. (463) A jet of MR swirls around the large LA of a 10-year-old DSH cat with RCM (see also ECG in 460). (464) Massive LA enlargement with an auricular thrombus (arrows) in an older cat with RCM. A = aorta; LA = left atrium; LV = left ventricle; RA = right atrium; RVOT = right ventricular outflow tract.

Hyperechoic areas of fibrosis may appear within the LV wall and/or endocardial areas (462–464). Endocardial scarring can be extensive and bridge to the septum, contricting portions of the LV lumen[48]. Extraneous intraluminal echos representing excess moderator bands are occasionally seen. Right ventricular dilation is common with CHF. Sometimes, an intracardiac thrombus is found, usually in the left auricle or atrium, but occasionally in the LV. Doppler evaluation may show mild MR or TR as well as a restrictive mitral inflow pattern (see p. 305). Cats with endomyocardial fibrosis may have a mitral inflow pattern of restrictive filling, relaxation abnormality, or pseudonormal flow[48]. Nonselective angiocardiography reveals the anatomic findings and highlights distended pulmonary veins.

Some cats have marked regional wall dysfunction, especially of the LV free wall, which depresses FS, along with mild LV dilation. These may represent cases of myocardial infarction or unclassified cardiomyopathy rather than RCM.

MANAGEMENT

Therapy for acute CHF is as for cats with HCM (see p. 308 and *Table 61*). Treatment for TE is outlined in Chapter 15 (p. 157). Cats that require inotropic support can be given dobutamine by CRI acutely or digoxin long term (see Chapter 16, p. 173). Dietary taurine supplementation is also advised.

Long-term therapy for heart failure includes furosemide at the lowest effective dose; resting respiratory rate, activity level, and radiographic findings are used to monitor dosage efficacy. An ACE inhibitor is also used (see Chapter 16, p. 178). Refractory heart failure with pleural effusion is difficult to manage. Besides repeated thoracocentesis, ACE inhibitor and furosemide dosages can be increased cautiously, and spironolactone, alone or with hydrochlorothiazide, and

nitroglycerin ointment can be added to the regimen. Renal function and serum electrolyte concentrations as well as blood pressure should be monitored. Diuretic and/or ACE inhibitor dosages are reduced if hypotension or azotemia develops. Some cats with refractory azotemia require SC fluid support (e.g. 20–50 ml/kg/day of 0.45% NaCl/2.5% dextrose with 8–12 mEq KCl/500 ml added).

A beta-blocker is usually used for tachyarrhythmias or if myocardial infarction is suspected. Alternatively, diltiazem can be used, although its value in the face of marked fibrosis is uncertain. Cats with refractory failure or reduced systolic function are also given digoxin (see *Table 44*, p. 174). Prophylaxis against thrombo-embolism is recommended (see Chapter 15 p. 160), and a low-sodium diet is fed, if accepted.

The overall prognosis for cats with heart failure from RCM is guarded to poor, although occasional cats live well for more than a year after diagnosis. The time course of subclinical RCM is unknown. Thromboembolism and refractory pleural effusion commonly occur.

DILATED CARDIOMYOPATHY

OVERVIEW

Taurine deficiency was discovered to be a major cause of feline DCM in the late 1980s[49–54]. The taurine content of commercial feline diets was subsequently increased, and clinical DCM is now uncommon in cats. Because not all cats fed taurine-insufficient diets develop DCM, more than simple deficiency of this essential amino acid is likely involved, such as genetic factors and a possible link with potassium depletion[55, 56]. The few DCM cases identified now are usually not taurine deficient and may be the end-stage of another myocardial metabolic abnormality, toxicity, or infection.

Doxorubicin causes characteristic myocardial histologic lesions in cats as well as dogs; however, cats appear fairly resistant to clinical dilated myocardial failure. Some cats show echocardiographic changes consistent with DCM after receiving cumulative doses of doxorubicin of 170–240 mg/m^2 [57].

PATHOPHYSIOLOGY

The features of DCM in cats are similar to those in dogs (see Chapter 20). Poor myocardial contractility is the hallmark, with dilation of all cardiac chambers (**465**). Mild to moderate AV valve regurgitation develops secondary to chamber enlargement and papillary muscle atrophy. Compensatory NH mechanisms are activated as cardiac output decreases, leading to clinical manifestations of CHF. Arrhythmias and pleural effusion are common in cats with DCM. Signs of low output failure and cardiogenic shock sometimes occur.

CLINICAL FEATURES

Affected cats tend to be older, although DCM occurs in cats of all ages with no breed or gender predilection. Increased respiratory effort, lethargy, anorexia, dehydration, and hypothermia are frequent findings. Subtle evidence of poor ventricular function may be found. Jugular venous distension, a weak precordial impulse, weak femoral pulses, a gallop sound (usually S$_3$), and a left or right apical systolic murmur (of MR or TR) are common. Although many cats have normal sinus rhythm, bradycardia and arrhythmias are frequently auscultated. Increased lung sounds and pulmonary crackles are heard in some cats. Pleural effusion may muffle ventral lung

sounds. Signs of arterial thromboembolism may be evident (see Chapter 15, p. 152).

DIAGNOSIS

Pleural fluid in cats with DCM is usually a modified transudate, although chylous effusions occur. Prerenal azotemia, mildly increased liver enzyme activity, and a stress leukogram are common clinicopathologic findings. High serum muscle enzyme activities, an abnormal blood clotting profile, and DIC often occur with thromboembolism. Plasma or blood taurine concentration should be measured. Plasma taurine concentrations are influenced by the amount of taurine in the diet, the type of diet, and the time of sampling in relation to eating; however, a plasma taurine concentration of 20–30 µmol/l (20–30 nmol/ml) or less in a cat with DCM is considered diagnostic for taurine deficiency. Nonanorexic cats with a plasma taurine concentration of less than 60 µmol/l (60 nmol/ml) probably should receive taurine supplementation or have their diet changed. Results are more consistent if whole blood samples rather than plasma samples are used for taurine determinations. Normal whole blood taurine

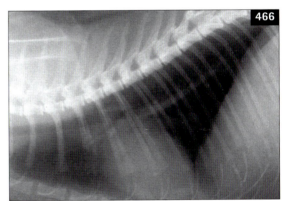

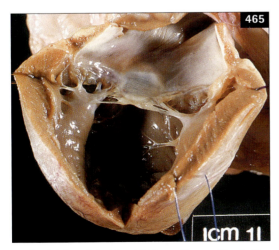

465 Caudal view of the LA and LV from a 9-year-old male Siamese cat with DCM and low blood taurine. Note the chamber dilation without hypertrophy.

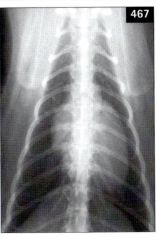

466, 467 Cardiomegaly with apex rounding is seen radiographically in a 12-year-old female DSH cat with DCM.

concentrations are >200 µmol/l (>200 nmol/ml); <140 µmol/l (<140 nmol/ml) is considered deficient.

Generalized cardiomegaly with rounding of the cardiac apex is a typical radiographic finding (**466, 467**). Pleural effusion is common and may obscure the heart shadow and any evidence of pulmonary edema or venous congestion. Hepatomegaly and, occasionally, ascites may be seen. An LV enlargement pattern, AV conduction disturbances, and arrhythmias are frequent ECG findings.

Definitive diagnosis is best made using echocardiography (**468–471**). Findings may be analogous to those in dogs with DCM (see Chapter 20, pp. 285, 286), but some cats have focal areas of hypertrophy, or either IVS or LV wall hypokinesis with relatively hyperdynamic motion of the opposite wall. FS, EF, and LV ejection time are reduced and the preejection period is prolonged[2]. A thrombus may be identified within the LA. Nonselective angiocardiography, although not usually done now, characteristically illustrates generalized chamber enlargement, atrophied papillary muscles, a decreased aortic diameter, and a slow circulation time (**472, 473**). Complications of angiography, especially in cats with poor myocardial function or decompensated CHF, include vomiting with aspiration, arrhythmias, and cardiac arrest.

MANAGEMENT

Treatment goals are the same as for dogs with DCM. Pleural fluid is drained by thoracocentesis. For acute CHF, furosemide is given as described earlier for

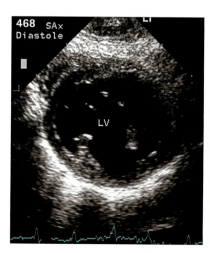
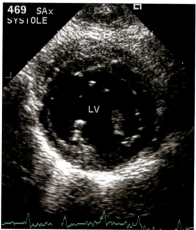

468,469 2-D echo frames in diastole (**468**) and systole (**469**) from a female DSH cat show LV dilation with normal wall thickness and little change in volume through the cardiac cycle. Right parasternal short-axis views.

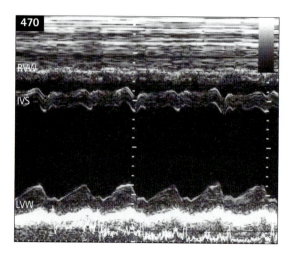
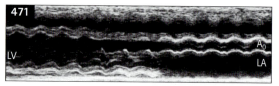

470,471 (**470**) M-mode echo at the ventricular level documents poor systolic motion (FS ~18%) in the cat in figure **465**. IVS = interventricular septum; LVW = left ventricular wall; RVW = right ventricular wall. (**471**) M-mode sweep from another cat with DCM illustrates LV dilation and reduced FS at the ventricular level (to the left), increased EPSS at the mitral level (center), and LA enlargement below the aortic root echos (to the right). Ao = aorta; LA = left atrium; LV = left ventricle; RV = right ventricle.

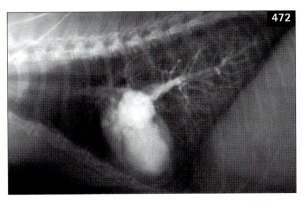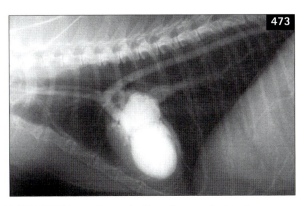

472, 473 Nonselective angiocardiogram from a 13-year-old Siamese cat with DCM. (472) Image 3 seconds after radiopaque dye injection highlights the pulmonary venous bed and dilated LA and LV. (473) Remarkably slow circulation time is documented by this image 13 seconds post injection; much of the dye is still in the left heart. (From Ware WA (2003) Myocardial diseases of the cat. In *Small Animal Internal Medicine* (3rd edn). (eds RW Nelson, GC Couto), Mosby, St Louis, p. 131, with permission.)

HCM; however, overly aggressive diuresis can adversely affect cardiac output because of the poor systolic function (see below). Supplemental O_2 may be needed. The venodilator nitroglycerin may be helpful in cats with severe pulmonary edema. Vasodilators (e.g. hydralazine, an ACE inhibitor, or amlodipine) may increase cardiac output, although with the risk of hypotension (see *Table 44*, p. 174). Blood pressure, hydration, renal function, electrolyte balance, and peripheral perfusion should be monitored closely. Hypothermia is common in cats with decompensated DCM; external warming should be provided as needed. Supportive therapy for cats with TE is described in Chapter 15 (p. 157). Once pulmonary edema is controlled, furosemide is tapered to the lowest effective dosage.

Positive inotropic support is indicated. A dobutamine or dopamine infusion (see Chapter 16, p. 173 and *Table 43*, p. 171) can be used for critical cases. Adverse effects of dobutamine can include seizures or tachycardia; if these occur, the infusion rate is decreased by 50% or the drug discontinued. Adverse effects of dopamine usually occur at higher doses and include tachycardia and increased peripheral vascular resistance (alpha-adrenergic effect). Dopaminergic effects may increase renal blood flow at low infusion rates. Amrinone (see Chapter 16, p. 175) or pimobendan might be tried, although the dosage for cats is not well established. Digoxin PO (see Chapter 16, p. 179 and *Table 44*, p. 174) is used for maintenance therapy. The tablet form is usually used because digoxin elixir is generally distasteful to cats. Toxicity occurs easily, especially when other drugs are used concurrently. Periodic serum digoxin concentration measurement is recommended (see Chapter 16, p. 180).

Furosemide and vasodilating agents reduce cardiac filling and can predispose to cardiogenic shock in cats with DCM. Fluids may be needed to support blood pressure (e.g. 0.45% NaCl with 2.5% dextrose, or other low-sodium fluids, IV at 15–35 ml/kg/day in several divided doses or by CRI); potassium supplementation may be needed. SC fluid administration can be used if necessary, although absorption from the extravascular space may be impaired.

Long-term therapy for DCM in cats includes PO furosemide, an ACE inhibitor, digoxin, antithrombotic prophylaxis, and (if taurine deficient) taurine supplementation or a high-taurine diet. Taurine supplementation (250–500 mg PO q12h) should be instituted as soon as possible in cats with low or unmeasured plasma taurine concentrations[2, 50, 51]. Clinical improvement, if seen, follows 1–2 weeks of supplementation, so supportive cardiac care is important. Echocardiographic evidence of improved systolic function is seen in most taurine-deficient cats within 6 weeks of starting supplementation. Some cats can be weaned from drug therapy after 6–12 weeks, although resolution of pleural effusion and pulmonary edema should be confirmed radiographically before reducing medication dosages. When LV systolic function is at or near normal, taurine supplementation can be decreased and perhaps eventually discontinued, as long as a diet known to support adequate plasma taurine concentration (e.g. most branded commercial foods) is fed. Dry diets with 1,000–1,200 mg of taurine per kilogram of dry weight and canned diets with 2,000–2,500 mg of taurine per kilogram of dry weight are thought to maintain normal plasma taurine concentrations in adult cats. Plasma taurine concentration measurement 2–4 weeks after supplement discontinuation is advised.

Taurine deficient cats that survive a month after initial diagnosis appear to have about a 50% chance for 1-year survival[50]. The prognosis for cats not taurine supplemented or not responsive to taurine is guarded to poor. TE is a grave sign.

ARRHYTHMOGENIC RIGHT VENTRICULAR CARDIOMYOPATHY

An idiopathic cardiomyopathy mainly involving the RV, similar to ARVC in people, also occurs in cats[58, 59]. Moderate to severe dilation of the RV chamber, with either focal or diffuse RV wall thinning, is characteristic. RV wall aneurysm is also common. RA and, less often, LA dilation may occur. Histologic findings include myocardial atrophy with fatty and/or fibrous replacement tissue, focal myocarditis, and evidence of apoptosis. These are most prominent in the RV wall. Fibrous tissue or fatty infiltration is sometimes found in the LV and LA walls[58].

The clinical presentation is usually that of right-sided congestive failure, with labored respirations, jugular venous distension, ascites or hepato-splenomegaly, and, occasionally, syncope. Presenting signs can also be lethargy and inappetence without overt heart failure[58].

Thoracic radiography demonstrates right heart and sometimes LA enlargement. Pleural effusion is common; ascites, caudal vena caval distension, and evidence for pericardial effusion may also be noted. Various arrhythmias have been documented on ECG in affected cats, including VPCs, ventricular tachycardia, AF, and supraventricular tachyarrhythmias. A right bundle branch block pattern appears to be common; AV block occurs in some cats[58, 59]. Echocardiography shows severe RA and RV enlargement. Other echo findings can include abnormal muscular trabeculation, aneurysmal dilation, areas of dyskinesis, and paradoxical IVS motion[58]. TR appears to be a consistent finding on Doppler examination.

The prognosis is guarded once signs of heart failure appear. Recommended therapy includes diuretics as necessary, digoxin, and an ACE inhibitor. Additional therapy for specific arrhythmias may be needed (see Chapter 17). In people with similar disease, both supraventricular and ventricular tachyarrhythmias are prominent and sudden death is common.

CORTICOSTEROID-ASSOCIATED CONGESTIVE HEART FAILURE

CHF signs occasionally develop subsequent to corticosteroid administration in cats[7, 60]. This may represent a previously unrecognized form of feline heart failure, unrelated to preexisting HCM,

hypertension, or hyperthyroidism. Subclinical HCM may exist in some cases. Affected cats experience acute onset of lethargy, anorexia, tachypnea, and respiratory distress. Auscultatory abnormalities are described in a minority of cases. The heart rate is not elevated in most cats, and blood pressure may be low[60]. Moderate cardiomegaly, moderate to severe diffuse pulmonary infiltrates, and mild/moderate pleural effusion are noted radiographically. Reported ECG findings include sinus bradycardia, intraventricular conduction abnormalities, atrial standstill, AF, and VPCs[60]. Echocardiographically, most cats show some increase in IVS and LVW diastolic thickness and LA diameter; AV valve insufficiency or SAM are described in some. Cats that survive the initial episode of CHF seem to experience at least partial resolution of abnormal cardiac findings. Gradual withdrawal of all cardiac medications without recurrence of CHF is described in these long-term survivors[60].

MYOCARDITIS

Inflammation of the myocardium and adjacent structures occurs in cats (see also Chapter 20, p. 293). Histologic evidence of myocarditis has been identified in myocardial samples from 58% of cardiomyopathic cats, but none from control cats; in almost one third of the cases, panleukopenia viral DNA was amplified by PCR techniques[14]; however, the possible role of viral myocarditis in the pathogenesis of cardiomyopathy is not clear. CHF or fatal arrhythmias can result from severe, widespread myocarditis. Cats with focal myocardial inflammation may be asymptomatic. Acute and chronic cases of suspected viral myocarditis and pericarditis–epicarditis (e.g. coronavirus) have been described, although a viral cause is rarely documented[61, 62].

Endomyocarditis has been found histologically, mostly in young cats. Acute death, with or without signs of pulmonary edema lasting for 1–2 days, is the most common presentation. Histopathologic characteristics of acute endomyocarditis include focal or diffuse lymphocytic, plasmacytic, and histiocytic infiltrates with a few neutrophils. Degenerative and lytic changes are seen in adjacent myocytes. Chronic endomyocarditis has been associated with a minimal inflammatory response but much myocardial degeneration and fibrosis. It is speculated that RCM represents the end-stage of nonfatal endomyocarditis[61, 63]. Therapy involves the management of congestive signs and arrhythmias as well as other supportive care.

Bacterial myocarditis may result from sepsis or from bacterial endocarditis or pericarditis, as it does in dogs. Subclinical lymphoplasmacytic myocarditis has been found in cats with experimental *Bartonella* species infections, but it is unclear whether natural infections have any role in the development of cardiomyopathy[64]. Myocarditis caused by *Toxoplasma gondii* also occurs occasionally, usually in immunosuppressed cats as part of a generalized disease process. Traumatic myocarditis is infrequently recognized in cats.

REFERENCES

1 Fox PR (2003) Hypertrophic cardiopathy. Clinical and pathologic correlates. *J Vet Cardiol* 5:39–45.

2 Fox, PR (1999) Feline cardiopathies. In *Textbook of Canine and Feline Cardiology*, 2nd edn. PR Fox, DD Sisson, NS Moise (eds). WB Saunders, Philadelphia, pp. 621–678.

3 Richardson P, McKenna W, Bristow M *et al.* (1996) Report of the 1995 World Health Organization/International Society and Federation of Cardiology Task Force on the definition and classification of cardiomyopathies. *Circulation* 93:841–842.

4 Ferasin L. Sturgess CP, Cannon MJ *et al.* (2003) Feline idiopathic cardiomyopathy: a retrospective study of 106 cats (1994–2001). *J Feline Med Surg* 5:151–159.

5 Kittleson MD, Meurs KM, Munro, MJ *et al.* (1999) Familial hypertrophic cardiomyopathy in Maine Coon cats: an animal model of human disease. *Circulation* 99:3172–3180.

6 Fox PR, Liu SK, Maron BJ (1995) Echocardiographic assessment of spontaneously occurring feline hypertrophic cardiomyopathy: an animal model of human disease. *Circulation* 92:2645–2651.

7 Rush JE, Freeman LM, Fenollosa NK *et al.* (2002) Population and survival characteristics of cats with hypertrophic cardiomyopathy: 260 cases (1990–1999). *J Am Vet Med Assoc* 220:202–207.

8 Atkins CE, Gallo AM, Kurzman ID *et al.* (1992) Risk factors, clinical signs, and survival in cats with a clinical diagnosis of idiopathic hypertrophic cardiomyopathy: 74 cases (1985–1989). *J Am Vet Med Assoc* 201:613–618.

9 Meurs KM, Kittleson MD, Towbin J *et al.* (1997) Familial systolic anterior motion of the mitral valve and/or hypertrophic cardiomyopathy is apparently inherited as an autosomal dominant trait in a family of American shorthair cats. Abstract. *J Vet Intern Med* 11:138.

10 Kraus MS, Calvert CA, Jacobs, GJ (1999) Hypertrophic cardiomyopathy in a litter of five mixed-breed cats. *J Am Anim Hosp Assoc* 35:293–296.

11 Meurs KM, Kittleson MD, Reiser PF *et al.* (2001) Myomesin, a sarcomeric protein is reduced in Maine Coon cats with familial hypertrophic cardiomyopathy. *J Vet Intern Med* 15:281.

12 Meurs KM, Sanchez X, David RM *et al.* (2005) A cardiac myosin binding protein C mutation in the Maine Coon cat with familial hypertrophic cardiomyopathy. *Hum Mol Genet* 14:3587–93

13 Gaschen L, Lang J, Lin S *et al.* (1999) Cardiomyopathy in dystrophin-deficient hypertrophic feline muscular dystrophy. *J Vet Intern Med* 13:346–356.

14 Meurs KM, Fox PR, Magnon AL *et al.* (2000) Molecular screening by polymerase chain reaction detects panleukopenia virus DNA in formalin-fixed hearts from cats with idiopathic cardiomyopathy and myocarditis. *Cardiovasc Pathol* 9:119–126.

15 Liu SK, Roberts WC, Maron BJ (1993) Comparison of morphologic findings in spontaneously occurring hypertrophic cardiomyopathy in humans, cats, and dogs. *Am J Cardiol* 72:944–951.

16 Peterson EN, Moise NS, Brown CA *et al.* (1993) Heterogeneity of hypertrophy in feline hypertrophic heart disease. *J Vet Intern Med* 7:183–189.

17 Moise NS, Dietze AE, Mezza LE *et al.* (1986) Echocardiography, electrocardiography, and radiography of cats with dilatation cardiomyopathy, hypertrophic cardiomyopathy, and hyperthyroidism. *Am J Vet Res* 47:1476–1486.

18 Bright JM, Herrtage ME, Schneider JF (1999) Pulsed Doppler assessment of left ventricular diastolic function in normal and cardiomyopathic cats. *J Am Anim Hosp Assoc* 35:285–291.

19 Bright JM, Mears E (1997) Chronic heart disease and its management. *Vet Clin North Am: Small Anim Pract* 27:1305–1329.

20 Golden AL, Bright JM (1990) Use of relaxation half-time as an index of ventricular relaxation in clinically normal cats and cats with hypertrophic cardiomyopathy. *Am J Vet Res* 51:1352–1356.

21 Baty CJ, Malarkey DE, Atkins CE *et al.* (2001) Natural history of hypertrophic cardiomyopathy and aortic thromboembolism in a family of domestic shorthair cats. *J Vet Intern Med* 15:595–599.

22 Rishniw M, Thomas WP, Kienle RD (2002) Dynamic right ventricular outflow obstruction: a new cause of systolic murmurs in cats. *J Vet Intern Med* 16:547–552.

23 Taugner FM (2001) Stimulation of the renin-angiotensin system in cats with hypertrophic cardiomyopathy. *J Comp Path* 125:122–129.

24 Meurs KM, Fox PR, Miller MW *et al.* (2002) Plasma concentration of tumor necrosis factor-α in cats with congestive heart failure. *Am J Vet Res* 63:640–642.

25 Herndon WE, Kittleson MD, Sanderson K *et al.* (2002) Cardiac troponin I in feline hypertrophic cardiomyopathy. *J Vet Intern Med* 16:558–564.

26 Lefbom BK, Rosenthal SL, Tyrrell WD *et al.* (2001) Severe hypertrophic cardiomyopathy in 10 young Ragdoll

cats. Abstract. *J Vet Intern Med* **15**:308.

27 Cote E, Harpster NK, Laste NJ *et al.* (2004 Atrial fibrillation in cats: 50 cases (1979–2002). *J Am Vet Med Assoc* **225**:256–260.

28 Campbell FE, Kittleson MD (2005) Effect of hydration status on echocardiographic measures of the left heart in normal cats. Abstract. *J Vet Intern Med* **19**:931.

29 Luis Fuentes V, Schober KE (2001) Diastology: theory and practice II. In: *Proceedings of the 19th ACVIM Forum*, Denver, pp. 142–144.

30 Gavaghan BJ, Kittleson MD, Fisher KJ *et al.* (1999) Quantification of left ventricular diastolic wall motion by Doppler tissue imaging in healthy cats and cats with cardiomyopathy. *Am J Vet Res* **60**:1478–1486.

31 Strickland KN (2001) Left atrial global shortening fraction in cats with cardiomyopathy. In: *Proceedings of the 19th ACVIM Forum*, Denver, pp. 86–87.

32 Ohad DG (2005) Spontaneous feline cardiomyopathy as a model for diastolic heart failure (DHF): is color M-mode transmitral flow propagation velocity sensitive enough? Abstract. *J Vet Intern Med* **19**:931.

33 Schober KE, Bonagura JD (2005) Doppler echocardiographic assessment of E:Ea and E:Vp as indicators of left ventricular filling pressure in normal cats and cats with hypertrophic cardiomyopathy. Abstract. *J Vet Intern Med* **19**:931.

34 Koffas H, Dukes-McEwan J, Corcoran BM *et al.* (2006) Pulsed tissue Doppler imaging in normal cats and cats with hypertrophic cardiomyopathy. *J Vet Intern Med* **20**:65–77.

35 Schober KE, Maerz I (2006) Assessment of left atrial appendage flow velocity and its relation to spontaneous echocardiographic contrast in 89 cats with myocardial disease. *J Vet Intern Med* **20**:120–130.

36 Liu SK, Fox PR, Tilley LP (1982) Excessive moderator bands in the left ventricle of 21 cats. *J Am Vet Med Assoc* **180**:1215–1219.

37 Bright JM, Golden AL, Gompf RE *et al.* (1991) Evaluation of the calcium channel–blocking agents diltiazem and verapamil for treatment of feline hypertrophic cardiomyopathy. *J Vet Intern Med* **5**:272–282.

38 Bonagura JD, Stepien RL, Lehmkuhl LB (1991) Acute effects of esmolol on left ventricular outflow tract obstruction in cats with hypertrophic cardiomyopathy: a Doppler-echocardiographic study. Abstract. *J Vet Intern Med* **5**:123.

39 Rush JE, Freeman LM, Brown DJ *et al.* (1998) The use of enalapril in the treatment of feline hypertrophic cardiomyopathy. *J Am Anim Hosp Assoc* **34**:38–41.

40 Oyama MA, Gidlewski J, Sisson DD (2003) Effect of ACE inhibition on dynamic left ventricular obstruction in cats with hypertrophic obstructive cardiomyopathy. Abstract. *J Vet Intern Med* **17**:372.

41 Jacobs G, Panciera D (1992) Cardiovascular complications of feline hyperthyroidism. In *Kirk's Current Veterinary Therapy XI*. JD Bonagura, RW Kirk RW (eds). WB Saunders, Philadelphia, pp. 756–759.

42 Bond BR, Fox PR, Peterson ME *et al.* (1988) Echocardiographic findings in 103 cats with hyperthyroidism. *J Am Vet Med Assoc* **192**:1546–1549.

43 Fox PR, Broussard JD, Peterson ME (1999) Hyperthyroidism and other high output states. In: *Textbook of Canine and Feline Cardiology*, 2nd edn. PR Fox, DD Sisson, NS Moise (eds). WB Saunders, Philadelphia, pp. 781–793.

44 Moise NS, Dietze AE (1986) Echocardiographic, electrocardiographic, and radiographic detection of cardiomegaly in hyperthyroid cats. *Am J Vet Res* **47**:1487–1494.

45 Broussard JD, Peterson ME, Fox PR (1995) Changes in clinical and laboratory findings in cats with hyperthyroidism from 1983 to 1993. *J Am Vet Med Assoc* **206**:302–305.

46 Peterson ME, Taylor RS, Greco DS *et al.* (1990) Acromegaly in 14 cats. *J Vet Intern Med* **4**:192–201.

47 Kittleson MD, Pion PD, DeLellis LA *et al.* (1992) Increased serum growth hormone concentration in feline hypertrophic cardiomyopathy. *J Vet Intern Med* **6**:320–324.

48 Fox PR (2004) Endomyocardial fibrosis and restrictive cardiomyopathy: pathologic and clinical features. *J Vet Cardiol* **6**:25–31.

49 Pion PD, Kittleson MD, Rogers QR *et al.* (1987) Myocardial failure in cats associated with low plasma taurine: a reversible cardiomopathy. *Science* **237**:764–768.

50 Pion PD, Kittleson MD, Thomas WP (1992) Response of cats with dilated cardiomyopathy to taurine supplementation. *J Am Vet Med Assoc* **201**:275–284.

51 Pion PD, Kittleson MD, Thomas WP *et al.* (1992) Clinical findings in cats with dilated cardiomyopathy and relationship of findings to taurine deficiency. *J Am Vet Med Assoc* **201**:267–274.

52 Sisson, DD, Knight DH, Helinski, C *et al.* (1991) Plasma taurine concentrations and M-mode echocardiographic measures in healthy cats and in cats with dilated cardiomyopathy. *J Vet Intern Med* **5**:232–238.

53 Fox PR, Trautwein EA, Hayes KC *et al.* (1993) Comparison of taurine, α-tocopherol, retinol, selenium, and total triglycerides and cholesterol concentrations in cats with cardiac disease and in healthy cats. *Am J Vet Res* **54**: 563–569.

54 Novotny MJ, Hogan PM, Flannigan G (1994) Echocardiographic evidence for myocardial failure induced by taurine deficiency in domestic cats. *Can J Vet Res* **58**:6–12.

55 Lawler DF, Templeton AJ, Monti KL (1993) Evidence for genetic involvement in feline dilated cardiomyopathy. *J Vet Intern Med* **7**:383–387.

56 Dow SW, Fettman MJ, Smith KR *et al.* (1992) Taurine depletion and cardiovascular disease in adult cats fed a potassium-depleted acidified diet. *Am J Vet Res* **53**:402–405.

57 O'Keefe DA, Sisson DD, Gelberg HB *et al.* (1993) Systemic toxicity associated with doxorubicin administration in cats. *J Vet Intern Med* **7**:309–317.

58 Fox PR, Maron BJ, Basso C *et al.* (2000) Spontaneously occurring

arrhythmogenic right ventricular cardiomyopathy in the domestic cat: a new animal model similar to the human disease. *Circulation* **102**:1863–1870.

59 Harvey AM, Battersby IA, Faena M *et al.* (2005) Arrhythmogenic right ventricular cardiomyopathy in two cats. *J Small Anim Pract* **46**:151–156.

60 Smith SA, Tobias AH, Fine DM *et al.* (2004) Corticosteroid-associated congestive heart failure in 12 cats. *Intern J Appl Res Vet Med* **2**:159–170.

61 Liu SK (1985) Myocarditis and cardiomyopathy in the dog and cat. *Heart Vessels Supp* **1**:122–126.

62 Liu SK, Keene BW, Fox PR (1995) Myocarditis in the dog and cat. In *Kirk's Current Veterinary Therapy XII.* JD Bonagura (ed). WB Saunders, Philadelphia, pp. 842–845.

63 Stalis IH, Bossbaly MJ, Van Winkle TJ (1995) Feline endomyocarditis and left ventricular endocardial fibrosis. *Vet Pathol* **32**:122–126.

64 Kordick DL, Brown TT, Shin K *et al.* (1999) Clinical and pathologic evaluation of chronic *Bartonella henselae* or *Bartonella clarridgeiae* infection in cats. *Clin Microbiol* **37**:1536–1547.

22
Pericardial Diseases and Cardiac Tumors

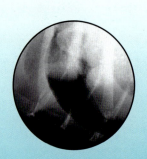

The pericardium forms a double-layered sac around the heart and is attached to the great vessels at the heart base. There is an outer fibrous layer (parietal pericardium) and an inner serous membrane covering the heart (visceral pericardium or epicardium)[1]. A small volume (~0.25 ml/kg) of serous fluid, normally between these layers, serves as a lubricant. The pericardium helps balance the output of the right and left ventricles, limits acute distension of the heart, and maintains normal cardiac position within the chest. The pericardium also provides a barrier to infection or inflammation of surrounding structures[2].

Diseases involving the pericardium and intrapericardial space can disrupt normal cardiac function. Excess or abnormal fluid accumulation is the most common pericardial disorder. This occurs most often in dogs[3]. Constrictive pericardial disease is occasionally recognized in dogs (see p. 329)[4, 5]. Acquired pericardial diseases causing clinical signs are uncommon in cats, but of these, pericardial effusion from feline infectious peritonitis was identified most often in one survey[6]. Pericardial effusions secondary to CHF (especially HCM), lymphoma, systemic infections, and, rarely, renal failure are also found in cats. Cardiac tumors occur relatively infrequently in dogs and rarely in cats[7, 8]. Many heart tumors cause pericardial effusion with tamponade (see below, p. 332), but some do not. Peritoneopericardial diaphragmatic hernia (PPDH) is the most common congenital pericardial malformation in dogs and cats (see p. 330)[4, 5]. Other congenital defects of the pericardium are quite rare; most are discovered on postmortem examination.

ACQUIRED PERICARDIAL EFFUSIONS

OVERVIEW

Most pericardial effusions in dogs are serosanguineous or sanguineous, and are of neoplastic or idiopathic ('benign' idiopathic pericarditis, idiopathic hemorrhagic pericardial effusion, and similar terms) origin[9]. Transudates, modified transudates, and exudates are found occasionally in both dogs and cats.

Hemorrhagic effusions

The fluid usually is dark red (**474**), with a PCV > 0.07 l/l (>7%), a specific gravity >1.015, and a protein concentration >30 g/l (>3 g/dl)[10, 11]. Mostly RBCs are found on cytology, but reactive mesothelial, neoplastic, or other cells may be seen. The fluid does not clot unless hemorrhage was very recent.

Older dogs are more likely to have neoplastic hemorrhagic effusion. Hemangiosarcoma (HSA) is most commonly involved (see p. 332), but hemorrhagic effusion also results from heart base tumors and pericardial mesothelioma. HSAs usually arise within the right heart, especially the right auricular appendage[12, 13]. The most common heart base tumor is chemodectoma, arising from chemoreceptor cells at the base of the aorta[9, 14]. Other heart base tumors include thyroid, parathyroid, lymphoid, or connective tissue neoplasms. Pericardial mesotheliomas are occasionally reported in the dog and cat[15, 16]. Pericardial effusion secondary to tumor metastasis develops rarely[17].

Idiopathic pericardial effusion occurs most often in medium to large breeds of dogs[16, 18–21]. Dogs of any age can be affected; however, the median age appears to be about 6–7 years. Histologic evidence of mild inflammation with areas of hemorrhage and diffuse pericardial fibrosis, especially perivascular, has been described[20]. Less common causes of intrapericardial

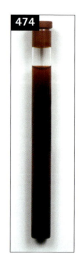

474 Most pericardial effusions in dogs are hemorrhagic, as is this fluid from a dog with 'benign' idiopathic pericardial effusion.

hemorrhage include LA rupture from severe mitral insufficiency, coagulopathy, and penetrating trauma (including iatrogenic laceration of a coronary artery during pericardiocentesis).

Transudative effusions

Pure transudates are clear, with a low cell count (usually <1,000 cells/microliter), specific gravity <1.012, and protein content <25 g/l (<2.5 g/dl). Modified transudates may appear slightly cloudy or pink tinged; cellularity is low (~1,000–8,000 cells/microliter) but specific gravity (1.015–1.030) and total protein concentration (25–50 g/l [2.5-5.0 g/dl]) are higher than those of a pure transudate[11]. Transudative effusions (475) can be caused by CHF, PPDH (see p. 330), hypoalbuminemia, pericardial cysts, or toxemias that increase vascular permeability, including uremia. Usually, these conditions are associated with a small volume of pericardial effusion and cardiac tamponade rarely develops.

Exudates

Exudates appear cloudy to opaque or serofibrinous to serosanguineous. They are characterized by a high nucleated cell count (well over 3,000 cells/microliter), a protein concentration usually much higher than 30 g/l (3 g/dl), and a specific gravity >1.015[11]. Cytologic findings are related to the etiology. Exudative pericardial effusions are rare in small animals. Infectious causes have usually been related to plant awn migration, bite wounds, or extension of infection in nearby structures[4, 5, 22]. Various aerobic and anaerobic bacteria, actinomycosis, coccidioidomcosis, disseminated tuberculosis, and, rarely, systemic protozoal infections have been identified[5]. Sterile exudative effusions have occurred with leptospirosis, canine distemper, and idiopathic pericardial effusion in dogs, and with feline infectious peritonitis and toxoplasmosis in cats[5, 6]. Chronic uremia occasionally causes a sterile, serofibrinous or hemorrhagic effusion[23].

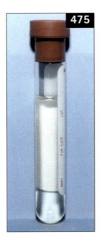

475 Transudative pericardial effusion from a dog with chronic AV valve insufficiency and CHF.

PATHOPHYSIOLOGY

Pericardial effusion impairs cardiac function by restricting filling[2, 4, 5], but if the effusion accumulates slowly, sufficient pericardial enlargement may occur to accommodate the increased volume at low intrapericardial pressure. As long as intrapericardial pressure is low, cardiac filling and output remain relatively normal and clinical signs are absent; however, pericardial tissue is relatively noncompliant. Rapid pericardial fluid accumulation or a large volume effusion causes intrapericardial pressure to rise markedly, which impedes ventricular filling. This condition is known as cardiac tamponade[4, 5]. Fibrosis and thickening further limit the compliance of pericardial tissue. Pericardial fibrosis and inflammatory cell infiltrates are described with idiopathic as well as neoplastic causes of effusion[20, 21, 24].

Large volume pericardial effusions occasionally cause clinical signs by virtue of their size, even in the absence of cardiac tamponade. Lung and/or tracheal compression can cause dyspnea and cough; esophageal compression can cause dysphagia or regurgitation.

Cardiac tamponade

Cardiac tamponade develops when intrapericardial pressure rises toward and exceeds normal cardiac diastolic pressure[25]. This compresses the heart externally and progressively limits RV then LV filling. Systemic venous pressure increases while cardiac output falls. Diastolic pressures in all the cardiac chambers and great veins eventually become equilibrated (476). The NH compensatory mechanisms of heart failure are activated as cardiac output falls[26, 27].

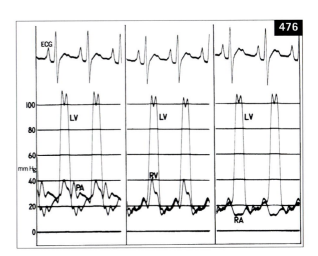

476 Simultaneous pressure recordings from the LV and pulmonary artery (PA), LV and RV, and LV and RA. Note the elevated end-diastolic pressure (20-25 mm Hg), which is equilibrated across the heart; the PA and RV systolic pressures are also mildly increased (40 mm Hg). From Thomas WP (1983) Pericardial disease. In: *Textbook of Veterinary Internal Medicine* (2nd edn). (ed. SJ Ettinger) WB Saunders, Philadelphia, p. 1082, with permission.)

Signs of systemic venous congestion become especially prominent with time. Although myocardial contractility is not directly affected by pericardial effusion, reduced coronary perfusion during tamponade can impair both systolic and diastolic function. Low cardiac output, arterial hypotension, and poor perfusion of other organs as well as the heart can ultimately lead to cardiogenic shock and death. The rate of pericardial fluid accumulation and the distensibility of the pericardial sac determine whether and how quickly cardiac tamponade develops. Rapid accumulation of even a small volume (e.g. 50–100 ml) can markedly raise intrapericardial pressure because the pericardium can stretch only slowly. A large volume of pericardial fluid implies a gradual process. Cardiac tamponade is relatively common in dogs, but rare in cats.

Cardiac tamponade causes an exaggerated respiratory variation in arterial blood pressure, called pulsus paradoxus. Inspiration lowers intrapericardial and RA pressures, which facilitates right heart filling and pulmonary blood flow. Simultaneously, left heart filling is reduced as more blood is held in the lungs and the IVS bulges leftward from the inspiratory increase in RV filling. Consequently, left heart output and systemic arterial pressure decrease during inspiration. Tamponade exaggerates this inspiratory reduction in cardiac output, causing a ≥10 mm Hg fall in arterial pressure during inspiration in patients with pulsus paradoxus (**477**)[28, 29].

CLINICAL FEATURES

Clinical findings associated with cardiac tamponade generally reflect poor cardiac output and congestion behind the right heart. Although right-sided congestive signs predominate, signs of biventricular failure may exist. Nonspecific signs such as lethargy, weakness, poor exercise tolerance, inappetence, or other GI signs may also occur before obvious ascites develops. Loss of lean body mass (cachexia) is seen in some chronic cases (see **16**, p. 27). Rapid pericardial fluid accumulation can cause acute tamponade, shock, and death. In such cases, pulmonary edema, jugular venous distension, and hypotension may be evident without signs of pleural effusion, ascites, or radiographic cardiomegaly.

Historical findings of weakness, exercise intolerance, abdominal enlargement, tachypnea, syncope, and cough are typical. Jugular vein distension and/or positive hepatojugular reflux, hepatomegaly, ascites, labored respiration, and weakened femoral pulses are common physical examination findings[5, 9, 19, 30, 31]. Collapse is more likely in dogs with a cardiac mass than in those without; ascites is more prevalent in dogs without an identifiable mass lesion[31]. Pulsus paradoxus is sometimes discernable by femoral pulse palpation. High sympathetic tone commonly produces sinus tachycardia, pale mucous membranes, and prolonged CRT. The precordial impulse is palpably weak with a large pericardial fluid volume. Heart sounds are muffled by moderate to large pericardial effusions[4, 9, 31]. Lung sounds are muffled ventrally with pleural effusion. Although pericardial effusion does not cause a murmur, concurrent cardiac disease may do so. Fever may accompany infectious pericarditis.

DIAGNOSIS

Radiography depicts enlargement of the cardiac silhouette caused by pericardial fluid accumulation[4, 5, 10, 16]. Massive pericardial effusion causes the

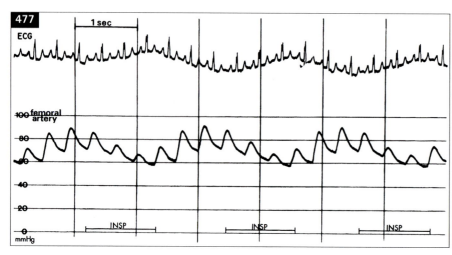

477 Pulsus paradoxus caused by cardiac tamponade. Directly measured femoral arterial pressure shows an exaggerated fall in mean pressure (15–20 mm Hg) and a markedly decreased pulse pressure during normal inspiration (INSP). (From Thomas WP (1983) Pericardial disease. In: *Textbook of Veterinary Internal Medicine* (2nd edn). (ed. SJ Ettinger) WB Saunders, Philadelphia, p. 1089, with permission.)

'classic' globoid-shaped cardiac shadow ('basketball heart') seen on both lateral and DV views (478–481); however, a large, rounded heart shadow can also be caused by DCM or tricuspid dysplasia. Smaller volumes of pericardial fluid allow some cardiac contours to be identified, especially those of the atria. Other findings associated with tamponade include pleural effusion, caudal vena cava distension, hepatomegaly, and ascites (482, 483). Pulmonary opacities of edema and distended pulmonary veins are noted only occasionally. Some heart base tumors cause deviation of the trachea or a soft tissue mass effect. Metastatic lung lesions are common in dogs with HSA.

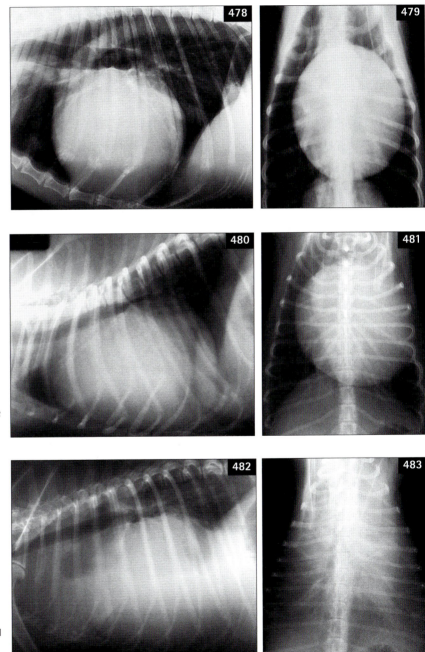

478–481 (478, 479) Pericardial effusion caused the classic 'basketball-shaped' cardiac silhouette in an Afghan Hound. (480, 481) The huge size of the cardiac silhouette in this 6-year-old male Maltese indicates chronic, slow pericardial fluid accumulation.

482, 483 Chronically high systemic venous pressure secondary to cardiac tamponade caused considerable pleural fluid accumulation in a 10-year-old female Miniature Schnauzer with a heart base tumor. Although the enlarged heart shadow is obscured by pleural fluid, dorsal tracheal displacement is evident.

ECG findings (484–487) might include diminished amplitude QRS complexes (less than 1 mV in dogs), electrical alternans, and ST segment elevation, suggesting an epicardial injury current[9, 32]. Electrical alternans is a recurring, beat-to-beat alteration in the size or configuration of the QRS complex and, sometimes, the T wave. It is most often seen with large volume pericardial effusion and results from the heart swinging back and forth within the pericardium[31]. Electrical alternans may be more evident at heart rates between 90–140 beats/minute or in certain body positions (e.g. standing). Sinus tachycardia is common with cardiac tamponade. Atrial and/or ventricular tachyarrhythmias also occur in some cases[31].

Echocardiography is highly sensitive for detecting even small volume pericardial effusion and may document an underlying neoplasm or other cardiac condition[4, 5, 9, 33]. It is, therefore, the diagnostic test of choice. Pericardial effusion appears as an echo-free space between the bright parietal pericardium and the epicardium (488–492). Abnormal cardiac wall motion and chamber shape, and intrapericardial or intracardiac mass lesions can also be imaged (493–496)[33–36]. Diastolic compression or collapse of the RA, and sometimes the RV, is consistent with cardiac tamponade (492)[34]. Idiopathic pericardial effusion is diagnosed only after infectious and neoplastic causes have been excluded. Unfortunately, some mass lesions are not easily visualized.

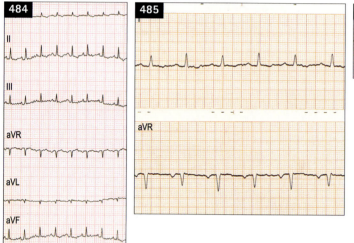

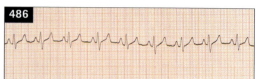

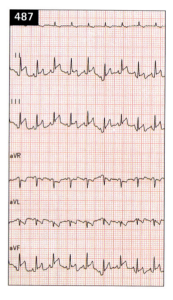

484–487 (484) Sinus tachycardia in a 9-year-old female Miniature Schnauzer with idiopathic pericardial effusion. Note the small QRS voltage. Baseline muscle tremor artifact is present. Leads as marked; 25 mm/sec, 1 cm = 1 mV. (485) Electrical alternans is seen in some ECG leads from an 11-year-old Dalmation with a large volume of pericardial effusion and cardiac tamponade. Sinus rhythm: leads I and aVR (not simultaneous); 50 mm/sec, 1 cm = 1 mV. (486) More subtle electrical alternans is seen in this ECG from a 7-year-old male Labrador Retriever with pericardial effusion. Sinus rhythm: lead II; 50 mm/sec, 1 cm = 1 mV. (487) ST-segment elevation, as well as dampened QRS complex size, is evident in this ECG of a 10-year-old mixed breed dog with pericardial effusion from a large tumor on the lateral RA and RV walls. Sinus rhythm: leads as marked; 25 mm/sec, 1 cm = 1 mV.

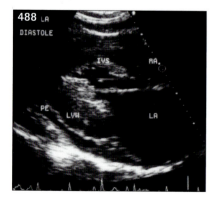

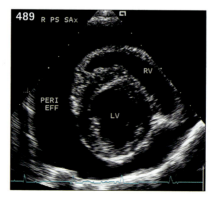

488, 489 (488) Even a small volume of pericardial effusion (PE) can be identified with echocardiography, as seen in this cat with HCM. Right parasternal long-axis view. (489) Fairly large volume pericardial effusion (PERI EFF) in a 2-year-old female Labrador Retriever. In this unusual case the fluid was chylous and caused by systemic blastomycosis. Right parasternal short-axis view.

Mesothelioma without a discrete mass lesion cannot be reliably distinguished by noninvasive tests[15, 16]. Sometimes, pleural effusion, marked LA enlargement, a dilated coronary sinus, or persistent left cranial vena cava (see p. 258) can be confused with pericardial effusion. Identification of the parietal pericardium in relation to the echo-free fluid helps in differentiating pleural from pericardial effusion. The pericardium generally produces the brightest echos, so it is the structure seen most persistently when the echocardiographer progressively damps returning echo signals. Most pericardial fluid accumulates near the cardiac apex; because the pericardium adheres to the heart base, there is usually little fluid behind the LA. Furthermore, evidence of collapsed lung lobes or pleural folds can often be seen within pleural effusion.

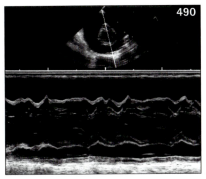 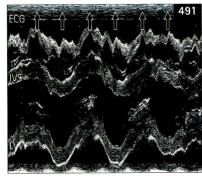 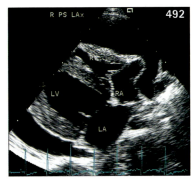

490–492 (490) A large echolucent space surrounds the heart in this duplex 2-D/M-mode view at the ventricular level from the dog in 482 and 483. (491) Large volume pericardial effusion allows the heart to swing back and forth within the pericardial sac on alternating heartbeats, which causes the electrical alternans seen on ECG in some dogs. This M-mode echo from a Labrador Retriever demonstrates this motion. Note how the relative position of the heart shifts with every QRS complex (arrows). (492) Cardiac tamponade causes RV compression as well as RA wall collapse, seen here at the onset of diastole. ECG = electrocardiogram; IVS = interventricular septum; LA = left atrium; LV = left ventricle; LVW = left ventricular wall; RA = right atrium; RV = right ventricle; RVW = right ventricular wall. (492) right parasternal long-axis view; (490, 491) right parasternal short-axis view.

493, 494 (493) A large soft tissue mass is evident near the RV wall and ascending aorta in a 10-year-old male Keeshond with cardiac tamponade. The origin of the mass is not clear from this right parasternal long-axis view. (494) The tumor mass in the dog in 493 is seen to arise from the right auricle, as is common for HSA. This view from the left cranial transducer position is the most reliable for evaluating the right auricular appendage.

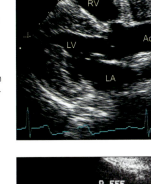 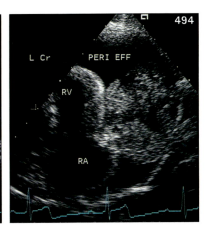

495, 496 (495) A smaller HSA is seen at the tip of the right auricle in another dog with cardiac tamponade. This tumor was not visible on any other view. (496) An aortic body tumour is seen at the heart base, nestled between the aortic root, left auricle, and origin of the main pulmonary artery. Ao = aorta; LA = left atrium; LV = left ventricle; PERI EFF and P EFF = pericardial effusion; RA = right atrium; RV = right ventricle.

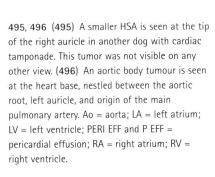 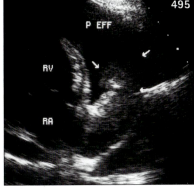 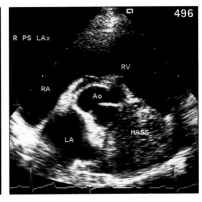

Other diagnostic techniques are used less commonly. Fluoroscopy shows diminished to absent motion of the cardiac shadow, since the heart is surrounded by fluid. Angiocardiography, now rarely used to diagnose pericardial effusion and cardiac neoplasia, typically reveals increased endocardial to pericardial distance[37]. Cardiac tumors can displace normal structures and cause filling defects and angiographic vascular 'blushing'. Echocardiography has also essentially replaced the use of pneumo-pericardiography, which employs CO_2 or air injected into the drained pericardial sac to outline the heart (497). The left lateral and DV radiographic views are most helpful because they allow injected gas to outline the RA and heart base areas, respectively, where tumors are most common[38].

CVP measurement may be a useful diagnostic aid, especially if the jugular veins are difficult to assess or it is unclear whether right heart filling pressure is elevated. A CVP >10–12 cm H_2O is common with cardiac tamponade; normally CVP is <8 cm H_2O. Tamponade alters the CVP (and RA) waveform by markedly diminishing the *y* descent (during ventricular relaxation). This occurs during tamponade because ventricular diastolic expansion immediately raises intrapericardial pressure, which then raises atrial pressure and impairs caval flow into the RA. The curtailed atrial filling prevents the normal early diastolic decrease in CVP (*y* descent), but blood flow into the RA (and *x* descent on the CVP waveform) continues to occur during ventricular contraction.

Nonregenerative or poorly regenerative anemia is common in dogs with benign as well as neoplastic effusions; less often, hypoproteinemia is seen[31].

Management

It is important to differentiate cardiac tamponade from other causes of right-sided heart failure signs because its treatment is different. Diuretics and vasodilators can further decrease cardiac output and exacerbate hypotension by reducing cardiac filling pressure; the compressed ventricles require high venous pressure in order to fill. Positive inotropic drugs do not improve cardiac output or ameliorate the signs of tamponade because the underlying pathophysiology is impaired cardiac filling, not poor contractility.

Immediate pericardiocentesis is the initial therapeutic procedure for tamponade (498, 499). It can also provide some diagnostic information. Signs of CHF usually resolve after intrapericardial pressure is reduced by fluid removal. In some animals a modest dose of diuretic is useful after pericardiocentesis. Determining the underlying cause for pericardial effusion is important to guide further management. Pericardial effusion secondary to other acquired or congenital causes of CHF or to hypoalbuminemia does not usually cause tamponade and often resolves with management of the underlying disease.

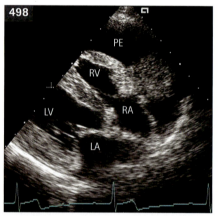

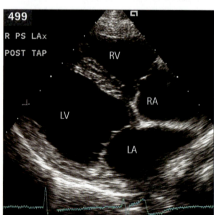

498, 499 (498) Long-axis echo from a dog with cardiac tamponade shows reduced filling of all the cardiac chambers; a mass (HSA) is seen adjacent to the RA. (499) Same view of the dog in 498 after removal of 300 ml pericardial fluid. Note the markedly improved filling of both left and right heart chambers. LA = left atrium; LV = left ventricle; PE = pericardial effusion; RA = right atrium; RV = right ventricle.

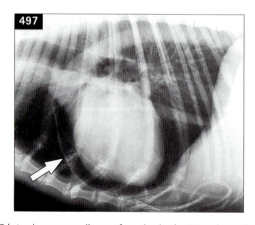

497 Lateral pneumocardiogram from the dog in 478 and 479 shows the pericardium (arrow) distended with air and normal cardiac contours with no evidence of a mass. The intrapericardial catheter is seen ventral and cranial to the heart.

Pericardiocentesis

Pericardiocentesis is a relatively safe procedure when performed carefully. Sedation may be helpful depending on the clinical status and temperament of the animal. ECG monitoring during the procedure is important; needle/catheter contact with the heart commonly causes ventricular arrhythmias. Pericardiocentesis is usually done from the right side of the chest to minimize the risk of trauma to the lung (by using the cardiac notch area) and major coronary vessels, located mostly on the left (500, 501). The patient is usually placed in left lateral or sternal recumbency to allow more stable restraint. Alternatively, good success can be had using an elevated echocardiography table with a large cut-out; the animal is placed in right lateral recumbency and the tap is performed from underneath. The advantage of this method is that gravity pulls fluid down to the right side; however, if adequate space is not available for wide sterile skin preparation or

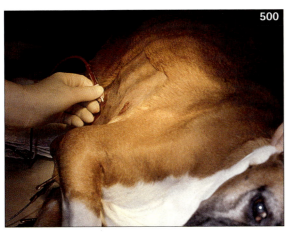

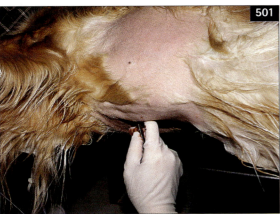

500, 501 (500) Pericardiocentesis was carried out on this Boxer in left lateral recumbency. Note the typically hemorrhagic fluid in the extension tubing; this dog had an aortic body tumor. (501) Gravity can facilitate drainage of pericardial effusion when the animal is placed in right lateral recumbency on a table with a large cut-out. This Golden Retriever had cardiac tamponade from a large right atrial HSA.

needle/catheter manipulation, this approach is not advised. Echo-guidance can be used, but is not necessary unless the effusion is of very small volume or appears compartmentalized. Sometimes, needle pericardiocentesis can be successfully performed on the standing animal, but the risk of injury is increased if the patient moves suddenly.

A variety of equipment can be used to drain the pericardial space. A butterfly needle or appropriately long hypodermic or spinal needle attached to extension tubing is adequate in emergency situations. A safer alternative is an over-the-needle catheter system (e.g. 18–20 gauge, 3.75–5.0 cm [1.5–2.0 in] long or larger). The needle-catheter unit must be advanced far enough into the pericardial space so that the catheter is not deflected by the pericardium as the needle stylet is removed. Larger over-the-needle catheter systems (e.g. 12–16 gauge, 10–15 cm [4–6 in]) allow for faster fluid removal in large dogs; a few extra small side holes can be cut (smoothly) near the tip of the catheter to facilitate flow. During initial catheter placement the extension tubing is attached to the needle stylet; after the catheter is advanced into the pericardial space and the needle removed, the extension tubing is attached directly to the catheter. For all methods a three-way stopcock is placed between the tubing and a collection syringe.

The skin is shaved and surgically prepared over the right precordium, from about the third to seventh intercostal spaces and from sternum to costochondral junction. Using sterile gloves and aseptic technique, the puncture site is located by palpating for where the cardiac impulse is strongest, usually between the 4th and 6th rib just lateral to the sternum. Local anesthesia is necessary when using a larger catheter and is recommended for needle pericardiocentesis. Two percent lidocaine is infiltrated (with sterile technique) at the skin puncture site, underlying intercostal muscle, and into the pleura. A small stab incision is made in the skin to allow catheter entry. Care should be taken to avoid the intercostal vessels just caudal to each rib when entering the chest.

Once the needle has penetrated the skin, an assistant should gently apply negative pressure to the attached syringe as the operator slowly advances the needle toward the heart. This way, any fluid will be detected as soon as it is encountered. Pleural fluid, usually straw-colored, may enter the tubing first. It is helpful to aim the needle tip toward the patient's opposite shoulder. The pericardium creates increased resistance to needle advancement and may produce a subtle scratching sensation when contacted. The needle is advanced with gentle pressure through the pericardium; a loss of resistance may be noted with needle penetration and pericardial fluid, usually dark red, will appear in the tubing. With a catheter system, after the needle/stylet is well within the pericardial space the catheter is advanced, the stylet removed, and the extension tubing attached to the catheter. Initial pericardial fluid samples are saved in sterile EDTA and serum (no anticoagulant) tubes for evaluation; as much fluid as possible is then drained.

A scratching or tapping sensation is usually felt if the needle contacts the heart. Also, the needle may move with the heartbeat and VPCs are often provoked – the needle should be retracted slightly to avoid cardiac trauma. Care should be taken to minimize extraneous needle movement within the chest. If it is unclear whether pericardial fluid or intracardiac blood (from cardiac penetration) is being aspirated, a few drops can be placed on the table or into a serum tube and a sample spun in a hematocrit tube (502). Pericardial fluid does not clot (unless associated with very recent hemorrhage), the PCV is usually much lower than peripheral blood, and the supernatant appears yellow-tinged (xanthochromic). Furthermore, as pericardial fluid is drained, the patient's ECG complexes usually increase in amplitude, tachycardia diminishes, and the animal often takes a deep breath and appears more comfortable.

Complications of pericardiocentesis

Ventricular premature beats occur commonly from direct myocardial injury or puncture; these are usually self-limiting when the needle is withdrawn. Coronary artery laceration with myocardial infarction or further bleeding into the pericardial space can occur, but is uncommon especially when pericardiocentesis is done from the right side. Lung laceration causing pneumothorax and/or hemorrhage is also a potential complication during the procedure. In some cases, dissemination of infection or neoplastic cells into the pleural space may be facilitated.

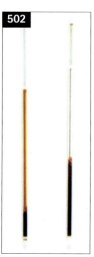

502 When spun in a hematocrit tube, hemorrhagic pericardial effusion (left) usually has a lower PCV than peripheral blood (right). RBC break down in the effusion produces a yellow-tinged (xanthochromic) supernatant.

Pericardial fluid evaluation

Cytologic evaluation helps characterize the fluid, although differentiating sanguinous neoplastic effusions from benign hemorrhagic pericarditis is usually impossible on the basis of cytology alone[39]. Reactive mesothelial cells within the effusion often resemble neoplastic cells; furthermore, common tumors such as chemodectoma and HSA may not shed cells into the effusion. Effusion related to cardiac lymphoma tends to be serous, with neoplastic lymphocytes apparent on cytologic examination[40].

Neoplastic (and other noninflammatory) effusions tend to have a pH of 7.0 or greater, and inflammatory effusions (e.g. benign idiopathic pericarditis) tend to have lower pH values[41]; however, there is too much overlap between these groups for pericardial fluid pH to be a reliable discriminator[42]. If cytology and fluid pH suggest an infectious/inflammatory cause, the pericardial fluid should be cultured. Fungal titers (e.g. coccidioidomyosis) or other serologic tests can be helpful in some patients. It is unclear how useful the measurement of cardiac troponin or other substances within pericardial fluid will be for differentiating underlying etiologies[43].

Therapy after pericardiocentesis

Idiopathic pericarditis is generally treated conservatively at first. Therapy may consist of a glucocorticoid (e.g. prednisone, 1 mg/kg/day PO tapering over 2–4 weeks) after ruling out infectious causes by pericardial fluid analysis; however, the efficacy of glucocorticoid therapy in preventing recurrent idiopathic pericardial effusion is not known. A 1–2 week course of broad-spectrum antibiotic is sometimes used in conjunction. Periodic reevaluation of these dogs by radiography or echocardiography is advised to detect recurrence. Effusion recurs in up to 64% of idiopathic cases[2, 9, 10, 31]; persistent recurrence (e.g. after 2–3 pericardiocenteses) is usually treated with subtotal pericardiectomy[9, 19–21, 44]. Removal of the pericardium ventral to the phrenic nerves allows drainage to the larger absorptive surface of the pleural space. Significantly increased long-term survival after subtotal pericardiectomy is reported in dogs with idiopathic pericardial effusion, although perioperative mortality was 13%[31]. Undetected mesothelioma may underlie some recurrent effusions[16]. Thorascopic partial pericardiectomy has been successfully used for idiopathic as well as some cases of neoplastic pericardial effusion[45, 46]. Percutaneous balloon pericardiotomy is a less invasive means of providing long-term continuous pericardial drainage[47–49], but premature closure of the pericardial opening may lead to recurrent tamponade in some cases. Balloon pericardiotomy, done under general anesthesia with fluoroscopic guidance, involves placing a needle or short catheter into the pericardial space, followed by a guide wire. The needle is then replaced with a percutaneous sheath introducer, through which the balloon dilation catheter is inserted. The balloon is positioned so that when inflated, it stretches the hole in the parietal pericardium.

Neoplastic effusions are also initially drained to relieve cardiac tamponade. Therapy may involve attempted surgical resection or surgical biopsy[14, 50–52], partial pericardiectomy, chemotherapy[53–56], or conservative therapy until episodes of cardiac tamponade become unmanageable. Surgery can be associated with significant morbidity and mortality, and is usually only palliative[44]. Prognosis is generally poor in dogs with HSA or mesothelioma[16, 57]. Heart base tumors (e.g. chemodectoma) tend to be slow growing, so partial pericardiectomy may prolong survival for months to years[58, 59]. Percutaneous balloon pericardiotomy may be an effective palliative procedure in some cases.

CONSTRICTIVE PERICARDIAL DISEASE

Constrictive pericardial disease occurs when visceral and/or parietal pericardial thickening and scarring restrict ventricular diastolic filling. Usually, the entire pericardium is involved symmetrically. Fusion of the parietal and visceral pericardial layers can occur and obliterate the pericardial space. In some cases the visceral layer (epicardium) alone is involved. A small amount of pericardial effusion may be present (constrictive–effusive pericarditis). Constrictive pericardial disease is diagnosed occasionally in dogs and rarely in cats. Histopathologically, increased fibrous connective tissue and variable amounts of inflammatory and reactive infiltrates are seen in the pericardium. Pericardial mineralization occurs rarely[60, 61]. The etiology of constrictive pericardial disease is often unknown. Specific causes identified in some dogs include recurrent idiopathic hemorrhagic effusion, infectious pericarditis (e.g. actinomycosis, mycobacteriosis, coccidioidomycosis), a metallic foreign body in the pericardium, neoplasia, including mesothelioma, and idiopathic osseous metaplasia and/or fibrosis of the pericardium[5, 60–63].

PATHOPHYSIOLOGY
Pericardial fibrosis creates a stiff shell around the heart. With advanced constrictive disease, ventricular filling is essentially limited to early diastole, before ventricular expansion is curtailed (503). Any further filling occurs only at high venous pressures. The compromised filling reduces cardiac output. Compensatory NH mechanisms cause fluid retention, tachycardia, and vasoconstriction.

CLINICAL FEATURES
Large to medium-sized, middle-aged dogs are most often affected; males and German Shepherd Dogs may be at higher risk[60, 61]. Clinical signs of right-sided CHF predominate. Client complaints include abdominal distension (ascites), dyspnea or tachypnea, tiring, syncope, weakness, and weight loss. Signs can develop over weeks to months[60]. Occasionally, there is a history of pericardial effusion. As for cases of cardiac tamponade, ascites and jugular venous distension are the most consistent clinical findings. Weakened femoral pulses and muffled heart sounds are also detected in many cases. An audible pericardial 'knock', caused by the abrupt deceleration of ventricular filling in early diastole, has been described in people, but has not been commonly identified in dogs[60]. A systolic murmur or click, probably caused by valvular disease not associated with the pericardial pathology, may be heard.

DIAGNOSIS
Constrictive pericardial disease can be a diagnostic challenge. Radiographic findings include mild to moderate cardiomegaly, pleural effusion, and caudal vena cava distension. Reduced cardiac motion may be evident on fluoroscopy. ECG abnormalities

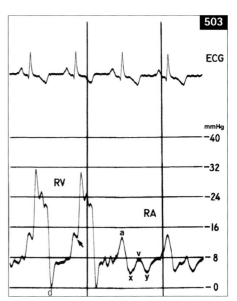

503 RV and RA pressure recordings from a dog with constrictive pericardial disease. A characteristic early diastolic dip (d) when most filling occurs, mid-diastolic plateau, and elevated end-diastolic pressure of 14 mm Hg (arrow) are seen in the RV pressure trace. On the RA tracing, a tall 'a' wave (corresponding to the high end-diastolic RV pressure) and prominent 'x' and 'y' descents are seen. (From Thomas WP, Reed JR, Bauer TG et al. (1984) Constrictive pericardial disease in the dog. *J Am Vet Med Assoc* 184: 546–553, with permission.)

have included sinus tachycardia, P wave prolongation, and small QRS complexes[60]. Constrictive pericardial disease can produce subtle but suggestive echocardiographic changes, such as flattening of the left ventricular free wall in diastole and abnormal septal motion. The pericardium may appear thickened and intensely echogenic, but differentiation of this finding from normal pericardial echogenicity may be difficult. Doppler findings include marked respiratory fluctuation in flow velocities across the mitral and tricuspid valves and into both atria.

Invasive hemodynamic studies are most diagnostic. CVPs over 15 mm Hg and high mean atrial and diastolic ventricular pressures are common. In contrast to the CVP (atrial) waveform seen with cardiac tamponade (see p. 322), constrictive pericarditis is associated with a prominent y descent. Classically, there is an early diastolic dip in ventricular pressure, followed by a mid-diastolic plateau as filling is curtailed, but this is not found consistently in dogs with constrictive pericardial disease. Angiocardiography may show atrial and vena caval enlargement with increased endocardial to pericardial distance, although images can be normal.

MANAGEMENT

Surgical pericardiectomy is necessary to improve ventricular filling. The procedure is most likely to be successful if only the parietal pericardium is affected. Visceral pericardial involvement requires epicardial stripping, which increases the difficulty and associated complications of surgery. Pulmonary thrombosis, sometimes massive, is reported as a relatively common postoperative complication[60]. Tachyarrhythmias are another complication. Moderate doses of diuretic may be helpful postoperatively. The effectiveness of ACE inhibition is unclear, but positive inotropic and arteriolar vasodilating drugs are not indicated. Without surgical intervention, disease progression and death are expected.

CONGENITAL PERICARDIAL MALFORMATIONS

PERITONEOPERICARDIAL DIAPHRAGMATIC HERNIA

PPDH is the most common pericardial malformation in dogs and cats[5]. Abnormal embryonic development, probably of the septum transversum, allows persistent communication between the pericardial and peritoneal cavities at the ventral midline. The pleural space is not involved. Other congenital defects such as umbilical hernia, sternal malformations, and cardiac anomalies may coexist. Although the peritoneal–pericardial communication is not trauma-induced, trauma can facilitate movement of abdominal contents through a preexisting defect.

Clinical features

Males appear to be affected more frequently than females, and Weimaraners may be predisposed. The malformation is common in cats as well; Himalayan and DLH cats may be predisposed[64]. The initial onset of clinical signs from PPDH can occur at any age, but the majority of cases are diagnosed during the first 4 years of life, usually within the first year. Some animals never develop clinical signs and PPDH is an incidental finding[64]. Clinical signs are variable and result from herniation of abdominal contents into the pericardial space. Signs are usually GI or respiratory[5, 64–67]. Vomiting, diarrhea, anorexia, weight loss, abdominal pain, cough, dyspnea, and wheezing are most often reported; shock and collapse can also occur. Physical examination may reveal muffled heart sounds on one or both sides of the chest, displacement or attenuation of the apical precordial impulse, an 'empty' feel on abdominal palpation, with herniation of many organs, and, rarely, signs of cardiac tamponade.

Diagnosis

Thoracic radiography is often diagnostic or highly suggestive of PPDH[5, 65, 67]. Characteristic findings include enlargement of the cardiac silhouette with dorsal tracheal displacement, overlap of the diaphragmatic and caudal heart borders, and abnormal fat and/or gas densities within the cardiac silhouette (504, 505). A pleural fold is usually evident, extending between the caudal heart shadow and the diaphragm ventral to the caudal vena cava on lateral view. Gas-filled loops of bowel crossing the diaphragm into the pericardial sac, a small liver, and few organs within the abdominal cavity may also be evident. Pectus excavatum or other thoracic skeletal deformity is occasionally present as well[64]. Echocardiography can be useful in confirming the diagnosis (506, 507)[67, 68]. A GI barium series is diagnostic if stomach and/or intestines are in the pericardial cavity (508, 509). Fluoroscopy, nonselective angiography, especially if only falciform fat or liver has herniated (510), positive contrast peritoneography, or pneumopericardiography can also be performed for diagnosis. ECG changes are inconsistent; decreased amplitude complexes and axis deviations caused by a shift in the cardiac position sometimes occur.

Management

In symptomatic animals, therapy involves surgical closure of the peritoneal–pericardial defect after viable organs are returned to their normal location[64, 69]. The presence of other congenital or acquired abnormalities and the animal's clinical signs may influence the decision to operate. The prognosis in uncomplicated cases is excellent, although minor complications from surgery are common[64]. Animals without clinical signs,

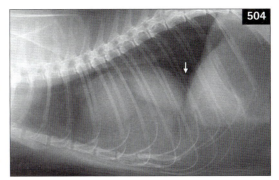
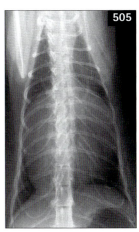

504, 505 Lateral (504) and DV (505) radiographs from a 3-year-old female DSH cat with recent onset vomiting and lethargy. The massive cardiac silhouette is caused by a PPDH. Note the caudal pleural fold (arrow) between the pericardium and diaphragm on the lateral view and lack of pericardial-diaphragmatic separation on the DV view. There is also variable opacity within the cardiac silhouette caused by fat (abdominal) as well as soft tissue densities.

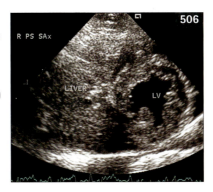
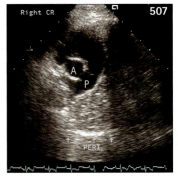

506, 507 (506) Echo image from a 1-year-old male DSH cat with PPDH and dyspnea. A liver lobe is seen next to the normal heart. LV = left ventricle. (507) Echo from an asymptomatic 7-year-old female Miniature Schnauzer referred for evaluation of cardiomegaly. A large amount of soft tissue (liver) and some fat lies next to the heart within the pericardium (PERI, arrows) because of PPDH. A = aorta; P = pulmonary artery. Right parasternal long-axis view at the heart base.

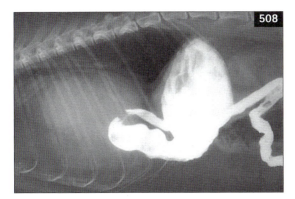
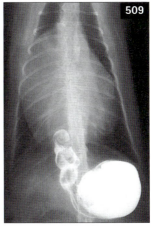
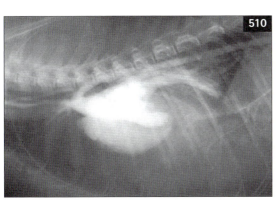

508–510 (508, 509) PPDH can be demonstrated after barium administration when the stomach or intestines have crossed the hernia. This 5-year-old male Persian cat had a history of exercise-induced respiratory difficulty. (510) Nonselective angiocardiography can also be used to diagnose PPDH. The normal heart has been displaced dorsally by liver and omental fat in this cat.

and some with mild signs, often do well without surgery[64]. Trauma to organs chronically adhered to the heart or pericardium during attempted repositioning is of concern.

OTHER PERICARDIAL ANOMALIES

Pericardial cysts are rare anomalies thought to originate from abnormal fetal mesenchymal tissue development or from incarcerated omental or falciform fat secondary to a small PPDH[4]. The pathophysiologic signs and clinical presentation of these cases are similar to those of animals with pericardial effusion. The cardiac shadow may appear enlarged and deformed radiographically. Echocardiography or pneumopericardiography provides the diagnosis. Surgical removal of the cyst in conjunction with partial pericardiectomy has usually resulted in cure[4].

Congenital defects of the pericardium itself are extremely rare in dogs and cats; most are discovered incidentally on postmortem examination. Instances of partial (usually on the left side) and complete absence of the pericardium have been reported. A possible complication of partial absence of the pericardium is herniation of a portion of the heart; this could cause syncope, embolic disease, or sudden death. Echocardiography or angiocardiography should facilitate antemortem diagnosis[5].

CARDIAC TUMORS

OVERVIEW

The overall prevalence of cardiac tumors in dogs is estimated at 0.19%; 90 breeds were affected in a large database survey[7]. Cats are less likely to be affected with cardiac tumors than dogs[8, 70]. The estimated occurrence rate in cats is <0.03%[8]. Although cardiac metastases occur in people much more frequently than primary heart tumors[71], this does not appear to be true in dogs. In a database survey, approximately 84% of heart tumors were identified as primary to the heart, while only 16% were identified as metastatic[7]. Of histologically identified cardiac metastases, >33% were HSAs (angiosarcoma, malignant hemangioendothelioma) and about 20% were adenocarcinomas[7]. Other metastatic tumors found in

the heart have included osteosarcoma, various other sarcomas, lymphoma, and mast cell tumors[7].

Primary cardiac tumors are usually malignant[7]. Most primary cardiac tumors in dogs involve the right side of the heart[7, 13, 36]. HSA is the most common cardiac tumor in dogs (**511**)[7, 9, 12, 13, 53, 72]. Of cardiac tumors identified as to histologic type, 69% were HSAs[7]. HSA is a highly malignant tumor and is in general more common in the dog than other species. The heart, especially the right auricle, is one of the most common primary sites for this tumor; other common locations include the spleen, subcutaneous tissues, and liver. Aortic body tumors (ABT) (chemodectomas, nonchromaffin paragangliomas) have also been reported relatively frequently in dogs; these develop at the aortic root or heart base[7, 73–76]. ABT is the second-most common tumor of the heart or heart base structures. Approximately 8% of heart tumors histologically identified were ABTs[7]. They arise from chemoreceptor cells, which are sensitive to blood oxygen and carbon dioxide tensions, as well as other factors. Clusters of these cells are located near the aortic root (aortic bodies), carotid bifurcations (carotid bodies), and elsewhere, but tumors most often develop in the aortic bodies (rather than other sites) in dogs[73]. ABTs are usually locally invasive, although they sometimes metastasize. Unless symptomatic pericardial effusion or dysfunction of surrounding structures results, they may be only an incidental finding. Occasional cases of ectopic thyroid or parathyroid tumors also occur at the heart base. Mesotheliomas are infrequently reported, but may be more common in certain geographic locations[15, 16, 77]. Only sporadic cases of cardiac myxoma, various (nonhemangio-) sarcomas, and other neoplasms have been reported in dogs.

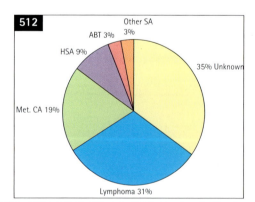

511 Chart illustrates the occurrence rate of various cardiac tumors in dogs from a large database survey. A histologic diagnosis was not reported in 33% of the cases. ABT = aortic body tumor; CA = carcinoma; HSA = hemangiosarcoma. (From Ware WA, Hopper DL (1999) Cardiac tumors in dogs: 1982-1995. *J Vet Intern Med* **13**:95–103, with permission.)

512 Occurrence rate of various cardiac tumors in cats. Based on a survey of the Veterinary Medical Database at Purdue University from 1982 to 1993. A histologic diagnosis was not reported in 35% of the cases. ABT = aortic body tumor; Met. CA = metastatic carcinomas; HSA = hemangiosarcoma; SA = sarcomas. (From Ware WA (2001) Cardiac tumors. In *Manual of Canine and Feline Cardiology* (3rd edn). (eds LP Tilley, JK Goodwin) WB Saunders, Philadelphia, p. 266, with permission.)

The most common cardiac tumor in cats is lymphoma, accounting for 31% of cases in one study (512)[8]. Various carcinomas, mostly metastatic, occur in 19% of cases[8]. Cardiac HSAs (8.6%), ABTs, and fibrosarcomas are uncommon in cats[6, 8, 78].

PATHOPHYSIOLOGY

Cardiac tumors cause a variety of effects, depending on their anatomic location and consequent hemodynamic disturbances. In general, physiologic disturbances relate to either external cardiac compression that impedes filling (e.g. pericardial effusion and resulting cardiac tamponade; see p. 321), obstruction of blood flow either into or out of the heart, and/or disruption of normal heart rhythm or contractility from myocardial infiltration or ischemia. Most reports describe tumors causing pericardial effusion and cardiac tamponade; the majority of these are HSAs or ABTs (513–515).

Intracardiac tumors of various histologic types cause signs of congestive or low output heart failure by obstructing blood flow and/or by inducing arrhythmias, rather than by causing pericardial effusion (516–519, p. 334). The location as well as the size of the tumor influence the degree of functional disruption[7, 8, 36, 50, 79]. RV inflow obstruction is most common, although RV and, occasionally, LV outflow obstruction occurs.

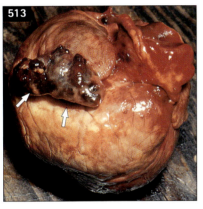
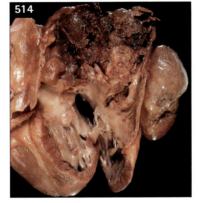
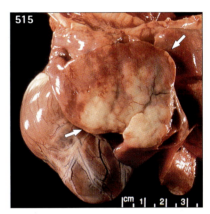
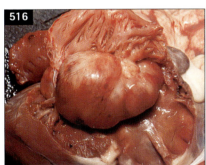
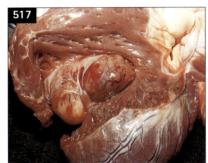
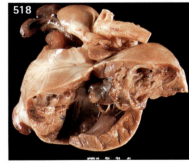
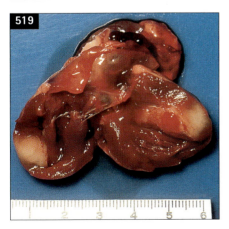

513–519 (513) HSA (arrows) originating at the right auricle in a German Shepherd Dog. View from the cranial aspect of heart; note the small left auricle seen to the right of the photo. (514) A large HSA almost obliterates the RA and protrudes outside the heart (at right of photo) in an older Beagle. View from the caudal aspect of the open RA (top) and RV (bottom). (515) A chemodectoma (ABT, arrows) extends from the heart base caudally and to the left in an older Schnauzer. View from left side; the tumor mass also invaded the lung (pushed caudally) and LA. (516) An intracardiac sarcoma arising from the lateral RA wall occupies most of that chamber; it obstructed venous return to the heart, but did not cause pericardial effusion. View from the open RA. (517) This tumor (as in 516) bulged into the tricuspid orifice during diastole. View from the open RV shows the tumor mass straddling the parietal tricuspid leaflet, chordae, and a papillary muscle. (518) An intracardiac rhabdomyosarcoma extensively infiltrated the RV and LV myocardium and protruded from the LV apex in a young female Golden Retriever with syncope, malignant ventricular tachyarrhythmias, and a systolic murmur. The tumor formed bulbous projections that obstructed both the RV (top left) and LV (central) outflow regions. View from the left cranial aspect; left apex to lower left of photo, open LV in center, open RV at top. (519) Myocardial lymphoma seen as focal pale areas in the open LV and RV (top) of a cat. (Courtesy Dr. JO Noxon.)

CLINICAL FEATURES

Cardiac tumors are more common in middle-aged to older dogs (7–15 years old). The highest occurrence rate is in dogs 10–15 years of age, although a low rate was reported in dogs over 15 years old. About 55% of dogs with cardiac HSAs or ABTs are 10–15 years old and about 35% are 7–10 years old[7]. Pericardial mesothelioma is also most common in middle-aged dogs[16]. In contrast to other heart tumors, lymphoma occurs more often in dogs 7 years and younger[7]. Almost 28% of cats with a heart tumor are 7 years old or younger, which likely reflects the greater percentage of lymphoma cases. At least two thirds of cats with heart tumors are >7 years old[8].

Although equal numbers of male and female dogs are affected, reproductive status has a significant effect on relative risk for cardiac tumor[7]. Spayed females appear to have an overall 4 times greater risk of cardiac tumor than intact females (5 times for HSA); the risk for castrated males is about 1.6 times that of intact males, and for intact males is about 2.4 times greater than for intact females[7]. The overall relative risk of cardiac tumor appears similar between spayed females and neutered males. In a database survey, 53% of affected cats were female and 47% were male, but the effect of reproductive status is not known[8].

Breed predilections have been identified for some cardiac tumors in dogs[7]. Breeds that had higher rates of HSA, as well as of all cardiac tumors, included the Afghan Hound, English Setter, German Shepherd Dog, and Golden Retriever. Other breeds that appear to have increased risk for HSA include the American Cocker Spaniel, Doberman Pinscher, Labrador Retriever, and Miniature Poodle. The majority of canine ABTs reported in the literature have been in brachycephalic breeds, specifically Boxers, Boston Terriers, and Bulldogs[73, 75, 76, 80]; however, not all dogs diagnosed with ABT are of brachycephalic breeds[7]. Conversely, some breeds appear to have a significantly lower prevalence of cardiac tumors[7].

Signs of right-sided CHF are common with tumors that obstruct blood flow within the RA or RV, or that cause pericardial effusion and cardiac tamponade. These signs include ascites, pleural effusion, jugular vein distension, abnormal jugular pulsations, and, occasionally, subcutaneous edema. Weakness and syncope with exertion or excitement are also common signs. These signs of low cardiac output can result from cardiac tamponade, blood flow obstruction, arrhythmias, or impaired myocardial function. Lethargy or collapse can occur with bleeding tumors (e.g. HSA) that may also be present in extracardiac locations. Abnormal heart sounds can include a murmur caused by blood flow obstruction, a murmur of unrelated disease (e.g. degenerative mitral insufficiency), or unusual transient sounds (e.g. clicks, gallops). Muffled heart sounds are common with large volume pericardial effusion. Some cases have no auscultable abnormalities.

DIAGNOSIS

Radiographic evidence of pericardial effusion or cardiac tamponade may be found (see p. 322). Dorsal deviation of the trachea and increased perihilar opacity are seen with some heart base tumors (520, 521). Large heart base masses create unusual bulges at the dorsal aspect of the heart shadow, with or without the presence of pericardial effusion. Intracardiac masses can enlarge or create an unusual contour of the chamber(s) they affect (522, 523). Pulmonary metastases may be seen with some primary or secondary (metastatic) cardiac neoplasms (524, 525). Caudal vena caval distension, pleural effusion, and/or ascites commonly occur with RV inflow or outflow obstruction. Some intracardiac tumors cause no noticeable radiographic changes.

The ECG might suggest pericardial effusion (see p. 324). Atrial or ventricular tachyarrhythmias such as premature complexes and paroxysmal tachycardias can result from tumor infiltration (526). Varying degrees of bundle branch or A–V block and symptomatic bradycardia can result from conduction system infiltration (527, 528). Intracardiac tumors that obstruct RV outflow can cause a right axis shift and RV hypertrophy pattern on the ECG. Other chamber enlargement or abnormal conduction patterns could result, depending on the tumor location and hemodynamic sequelae.

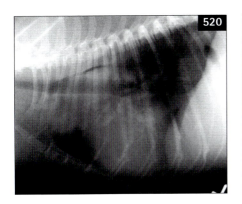
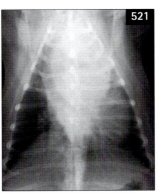
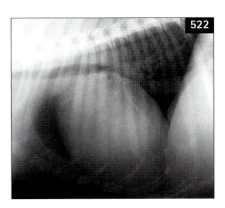

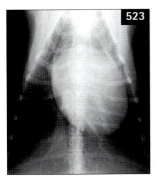
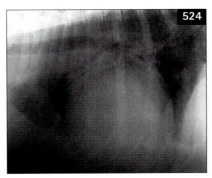
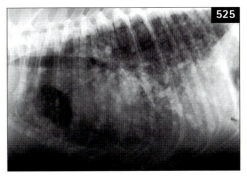

520–525 (520, 521) A large soft tissue mass extends from the heart base into the cranial left mediastinum in a 12-year-old female Cocker Spaniel with a 3-month history of cough. The trachea is pushed to the right (521). Mild cardiomegaly was caused by concurrent degenerative mitral valve disease; there was no pericardial effusion. (522, 523) Generalized cardiomegaly, without pericardial effusion, was observed in the dog in 518. (524) Large volume pericardial effusion and small pulmonary nodules were found in an 8-year-old male Great Dane with signs of cardiac tamponade from a right atrial HSA. (525) Evidence of widespread pulmonary metastases was present in a 9-year-old male Husky with a 1-week history of cough; a right auricular HSA was found.

526 Paroxysmal ventricular tachycardia was recorded in a 17-year-old female Keeshond with recent onset of weakness and acute collapsing episodes. An LV mass was identified with echocardiography (see 534 and 535, p. 336).

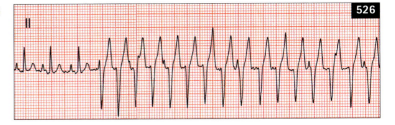

527, 528 (527) Variable AV conduction block was found in a 17-year-old female mixed breed dog with a recent onset of collapsing episodes. This continuous lead II ECG shows sinus tachycardia (tall P waves) with complete AV block. No ventricular activity is seen until ventricular escape complexes (arrows) finally appear in the middle of the bottom strip. (528) A small HSA (arrow) was found within the high ventricular septum, the region of the AV conduction system, of the dog in 527. No other cardiac lesions were seen.

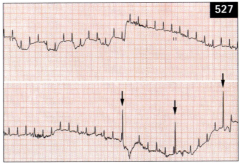
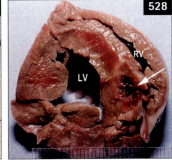

Echocardiography is a sensitive tool for identifying cardiac neoplasia as well as the presence or absence of pericardial effusion (**529–535**)[4, 5, 33, 36, 50, 79]. Non-neoplastic masses occur rarely[81]. The presence of pericardial effusion aids in the visualization of heart base and other tumors that extend into the pericardial space. The location and extent of mass lesions can be assessed and hemodynamic effects surmised with echocardiography. Secondary changes in chamber size, wall thickness, and valve motion may be observed. Doppler echocardiography can define blood flow abnormalities (**532**). Assessment of the location, size, attachment (pedunculated or broad-based), and extent (superficial or deeply invading adjacent myocardium) of the cardiac tumor(s) is valuable in determining whether surgical resection or biopsy may be possible.

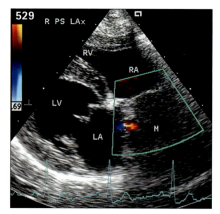

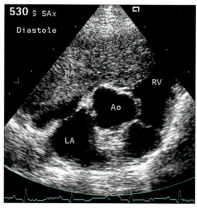

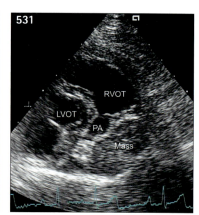

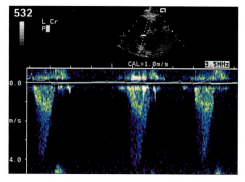

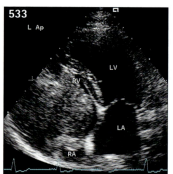

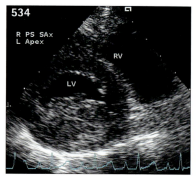

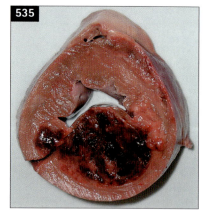

529–535 (529) Color flow, long-axis echo image from the dog in 520 and 521 shows the large mass over the heart base. Flow is seen in an abnormal vessel between the tumor and the dorsal LA. No pericardial effusion is seen. (530) An extensive soft tissue mass is seen within the RA of a 16-year-old male Cockapoo with ascites and hindlimb weakness. The mass bulges through the tricupid orifice into the RV in this diastolic image. In systole the mass moved back into the RA as the tricuspid valve closed. The heart size was radiographically normal and there was no pericardial effusion. Right parasternal short-axis view. (531) A mass within the pericardium compressed the RV outflow tract/main PA area in a 9-year-old male Keeshond, causing a systolic ejection murmur and compensatory RV hypertrophy. There was no pericardial effusion. Right parasternal short-axis view. (532) CW Doppler recording of the dog in 531 shows increased pulmonary velocity to about 4 m/sec (estimated gradient of 64 mm Hg) caused by the RV outflow obstruction. (533) Large mass involving the RA and RV walls obliterates much of the lumen in a 10-year-old female Golden Retriever with a history of weight loss, weakness, and ascites. The mass was an undifferentiated sarcoma. Left apical view. (534) A soft tissue mass in the LV apical area invades the free wall myocardium and extends into the lumen; from the dog whose ECG is in 526. No pericardial effusion was noted. Right parasternal short-axis view. (535) Cut section of lower LV from the dog in 534 shows a dark tumor mass, which was identified histologically as HSA. This tumor is rarely found in the left heart. Ao = aortic root; LA = left atrium; LV = left ventricle; LVOT = left ventricular outflow tract; M = mass; PA = (main) pulmonary artery; RA = right atrium; RV = right ventricle; RVOT = right ventricular outflow tract.

Other diagnostic techniques such as pneumo-pericardiography and angiocardiography may be helpful in identifying cardiac tumors, although echocardiography has largely replaced these tests (536, 537). Although differentiation of neoplastic effusions from benign hemorrhagic pericarditis is usually not possible by cytology alone, because of reactive mesothelial cells in the effusion[39], lymphoma and some other tumors can occasionally be diagnosed by pericardial fluid evaluation.

MANAGEMENT

Pericardiocentesis is indicated immediately for cardiac tamponade (see p. 327). Conservative management, with pericardiocentesis as needed, is used in some patients until episodes of cardiac tamponade become unmanageable. Whether antiinflammatory doses of a glucocorticoid are of benefit is unclear. Surgical subtotal pericardiectomy prevents recurrent tamponade but may facilitate metastatic dissemination throughout the thoracic cavity; however, this does not appear to affect survival time with HSA or mesothelioma[57]. Balloon pericardiotomy (see p. 328) may provide a less invasive alternative to surgery in some patients, but this procedure is not recommended with HSA, as this tumor is quite friable. Because heart base tumors (e.g. chemodectoma) tend to be slow growing, partial pericardiectomy, or pericardiotomy, may prolong survival of affected dogs for months to years. Because of local invasion with this and other tumors, complete surgical resection is rarely possible. Nevertheless, some tumors may be amenable to surgical resection, depending on their location and invasiveness[50–52]. Surgical biopsy of a nonresectable mass may be helpful if chemotherapy is being contemplated. While many cardiac tumors appear to be fairly unresponsive to chemotherapy, some are treated, with short-term success[53–55]. Specific sources for antineoplastic drug protocols should be consulted as needed. The long-term prognosis for animals with cardiac tumors is generally guarded to poor.

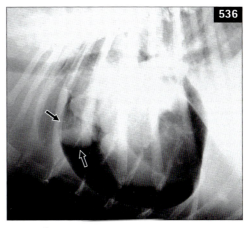

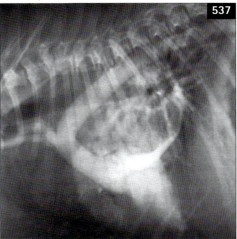

536, 537 (536) Lateral pneumopericardiogram from an older Boxer with cardiac tamponade shows abnormal soft tissue opacity (arrows) at the cranial heart base, consistent with an ABT. Compare with the normal study in **497**. **(537)** Levo-phase of nonselective angiocardiogram shows dye in the left heart and aorta; dye is seen faintly in the pulmonary artery. A large heart base mass has compressed the LA and pushed the carina and descending aorta dorsally. From a 9-year-old Boston Terrier. (Courtesy Dr. E Riedesel.)

REFERENCES

1 Dyce KM, Sack WO, Wensing CJG (1996) *Textbook of Veterinary Anatomy*. WB Saunders, Philadelphia, pp. 219–220.

2 Bouvy BM, Bjorling DE (1991) Pericardial effusion in dogs and cats. Part I. Normal pericardium and causes and pathophysiology of pericardial effusion. *Compend Contin Educ Pract Vet* 13:417–424.

3 Buchanan JW (1992) Causes and prevalence of cardiovascular disease.

In: *Current Veterinary Therapy XI.* W Kirk, JD Bonagura (eds). WB Saunders, Philadelphia, 647–654.

4 Sisson D, Thomas WP (1999) Pericardial disease and cardiac tumors. In: *Textbook of Feline and Canine Cardiology*, 2nd edn. PR Fox, D Sisson, NS Moise (eds). WB Saunders, Philadelphia, pp. 679–701.

5 Miller MW, Sisson D (2000) Pericardial disorders. In: *Textbook of Veterinary Internal Medicine*, 5th

edn. SJ Ettinger, EC Feldman (eds). WB Saunders, Philadelphia, pp. 923–936.

6 Rush JE, Keene BW, Fox PR (1990) Pericardial disease in the cat: a retrospective evaluation of 66 cases. *J Am Anim Hosp Assoc* 26:39–46.

7 Ware WA, Hopper DL (1999) Cardiac tumors in dogs: 1982–1995. *J Vet Intern Med* 13:95–103.

8 Ware WA (1995) Cardiac neoplasia. In *Current Veterinary Therapy XII.*

JD Bonagura (ed). WB Saunders, Philadelphia, pp. 873–876.

9 Berg RJ (1984) Pericardial effusion in the dog: a review of 42 cases. *J Am Anim Hosp Assoc* **20**:721–730.

10 Bouvy BM, Bjorling DE (1991) Pericardial effusion in dogs and cats. Part II. Diagnostic approach and treatment. *Compend Contin Educ Pract Vet* **13**:633–641.

11 Alleman AR (2003) Abdominal, thoracic, and pericardial effusions. *Vet Clin North Am: Small Anim Pract* **33**:89–118.

12 Aronsohn M (1985) Cardiac hemangiosarcoma in the dog: a review of 38 cases. *J Am Vet Med Assoc* **187**:922–926.

13 Kleine LJ, Zook BC, Munson TO (1970) Primary cardiac hemangiosarcoma in dogs. *J Am Vet Med Assoc* **157**:326–337.

14 Berg J (1994) Pericardial disease and cardiac neoplasia. *Semin Vet Med Surg* **9**:185–191.

15 McDonough SP, MacLachlan NJ, Tobias AH (1992) Canine pericardial mesothelioma. *Vet Path* **29**:256–260.

16 Stepien RL, Whitley NT, Dubielzig RR (2000) Idiopathic or mesothelioma-related pericardial effusion: clinical findings and survival in 17 dogs studied retrospectively. *J Small Anim Pract* **41**:342–347.

17 Kirsch JA, Dhupa S, Cornell KK (2000) Pericardial effusion associated with metastatic disease from an unknown primary tumor in a dog. *J Am Anim Hosp Assoc* **36**:121–124.

18 Berg RJ (1984) Idiopathic hemorrhagic pericardial effusion in eight dogs. *J Am Vet Med Assoc* **185**:988–992.

19 Gibbs C, Gaskell CJ, Darke PGG *et al.* (1982) Idiopathic pericardial haemorrhage in dogs: a review of fourteen cases. *J Small Anim Pract* **23**:483–500.

20 Aronsohn MG, Carpenter JL (1999) Surgical treatment of idiopathic pericardial effusion in the dog: 25 cases (1978–1993). *J Am Anim Hosp Assoc* **35**:521–525.

21 Mattiesen DT, Lammerding J (1985) Partial pericardiectomy for idiopathic hemorrhagic pericardial effusion in the dog. *J Am Anim Hosp Assoc* **21**:41–47.

22 Aronson LR, Gregory CR (1995) Infectious pericardial effusions in five dogs. *Vet Surg* **24**:402–407.

23 Madewell BR, Norrdin RW (1975) Renal failure associated with pericardial effusion in a dog. *J Am Vet Med Assoc* **167**:1091–1093.

24 Day MJ, Martin MWS (2002) Immunohistochemical characterization of the lesions of canine idiopathic pericarditis. *J Small Anim Pract* **43**:382–387.

25 Cohen ML (1990) Experimental cardiac tamponade: correlation of pressure, flow velocity, and echocardiographic changes. *J Appl Physiol* **69**:924–931.

26 Kaszaki J, Nagy S, Tarnoky K *et al.* (1989) Humoral changes in shock induced by cardiac tamponade. *Circ Shock* **29**:143–153.

27 Stokhof AA, Overduin LM, Mol JA *et al.* (1994) Effect of pericardiocentesis on circulating concentrations of atrial natriuretic hormone and arginine vasopressin in dogs with spontaneous pericardial effusion. *Eur J Endocrinol* **130**:357–360.

28 Fitchett DH, Sniderman AD (1990) Inspiratory reduction in left heart filling as a mechanism of pulsus paradoxus in cardiac tamponade. *Can J Cardiol* **6**:348–354.

29 Savitt MA, Tyson GS, Elbeery JR *et al.* (1993) Physiology of cardiac tamponade and paradoxical pulse in conscious dogs. *Am J Physiol* **265**: H1996–H2008.

30 Vogtli T, Gaschen F, Vogtli-Burger R *et al.* (1997) Hemorrhagic pericardial effusion in dogs. A retrospective study of 10 cases (1989–1994) with a review of the literature. *Schweiz Arch Tierheilkd* **139**:217–224.

31 Stafford Johnson M, Martin M, Binns S *et al.* (2004) A retrospective study of clinical findings, treatment and outcome in 143 dogs with pericardial effusion. *J Small Anim Pract* **45**:546–552.

32 Bonagura JD (1981) Electrical alternans associated with pericardial effusion in the dog. *J Am Vet Med Assoc* **178**:574–579.

33 Thomas WP, Sisson D, Bauer TG *et al.* (1984) Detection of cardiac masses in dogs by two-dimensional echocardiography. *Vet Radiol* **25**:65–72.

34 Berry CR, Lombarde CW, Hager DA *et al.* (1988) Echocardiographic evaluation of cardiac tamponade in dogs before and after pericardiocentesis: four cases (1984–1986). *J Am Vet Med Assoc* **192**:1597–1603.

35 Cobb MA, Brownlie SE (1992) Intrapericardial neoplasia in 14 dogs. *J Small Anim Pract* **33**:309–316.

36 Atkins CE, Badertscher RR, Greenlee P *et al.* (1984) Diagnosis of an intracardiac fibrosarcoma using two-dimensional echocardiography. *J Am Anim Hosp Assoc* **20**:131–137.

37 Cantwell HD, Blevins WE, Weirich WE (1982) Angiographic diagnosis of heart base tumor in the dog. *J Am Anim Hosp Assoc* **18**:83–87.

38 Thomas WP, Reed JR, Gomez JA (1984) Diagnostic pneumopericardiography in dogs with spontaneous pericardial effusion. *Vet Radiol* **25**:2–16.

39 Sisson D, Thomas WP, Ruehl WW *et al.* (1984) Diagnostic value of pericardial fluid analysis in the dog. *J Am Vet Med Assoc* **184**:51–55.

40 Sims CS, Tobias AH, Hayden DW *et al.* (2003) Pericardial effusion due to a primary cardiac lymphosarcoma in a dog. *J Vet Intern Med* **17**:923–927.

41 Edwards NJ (1996) The diagnostic value of pericardial fluid pH determination. *J Am Anim Hosp Assoc* **32**:63–67.

42 Fine DM, Tobias AH, Jacob KA (2003) Use of pericardial fluid pH to distinguish between idiopathic and neoplastic effusions. *J Vet Intern Med* **17**:525–529.

43 Schober KE, Kirbach B, Cornand C *et al.* (2001) Circulating cardiac troponins in small animals. In: *Proceedings of the 19th Annual ACVIM Forum*, Denver, pp. 91–92.

44 Kerstetter KK, Krahwinkel DJ, Millis DL *et al.* (1997) Pericardiectomy in dogs: 22 cases (1978–1994). *J Am Vet Med Assoc* **211**:736–740.

45 Jackson J, Richter KP, Launer DP (1999) Thoracoscopic partial pericardiectomy in 13 dogs. *J Vet Intern Med* **13**:529–533.

46 Sobel DS (2000) Video-assisted thoracoscopic pericardiectomy in dogs using a paraxyphoid approach. Abstract. *J Vet Intern Med* **14**:374.

47 Cobb MA, Boswood A, Griffin GM *et al.* (1996) Percutaneous balloon pericardiotomy for the management of malignant pericardial effusion in two dogs. *J Small Anim Pract* **37**:549–551.

48 Glaus TM (2000) Balloon pericardiotomy for treating recurring idiopathic pericardial effusion in 2 dogs. Abstract. *J Vet Intern Med* **14**:231.

49 Sidley JA, Atkins CE, Keene BK *et al.* (2002) Percutaneous pericardiotomy as a treatment for recurrent pericardial effusion in 6 dogs. *J Vet Intern Med* **16**:541–546.

50 Ware WA, Merkley DF, Riedesel DH (1994) Intracardiac thyroid tumor in a dog: diagnosis and surgical removal. *J Am Anim Hosp Assoc* **30**:20–23.

51 Wykes PM, Rouse GP, Orton EC (1986) Removal of five canine cardiac tumors using a stapling instrument. *Vet Surg* **15**:103–106.

52 Brisson BA, Holmberg DL (2001) Use of pericardial patch graft reconstruction of the right atrium for treatment of hemangiosarcoma in a dog. *J Am Vet Med Assoc* **218**:723–725.

53 Ogilvie GK, Powers BE, Mallinckrodt CH *et al.* (1996) Surgery and doxorubicin in dogs with hemangiosarcoma. *J Vet Intern Med* **10**:379–384.

54 deMadron E, Helfand SC, Stebbins KE (1987) Use of chemotherapy for treatment of cardiac hemangiosarcoma in a dog. *J Am Vet Med Assoc* **190**:887–891.

55 Hammer AS, Couto CG (1992) Diagnosing and treating canine hemangiosarcoma. *Vet Med* **87**:188–201.

56 Closa JM, Font A, Mascort J (1999) Pericardial mesothelioma in a dog: long-term survival after pericardiectomy in combination with chemotherapy. *J Small Anim Pract* **40**:383–386.

57 Dunning D, Monnet E, Orton EC *et al.* (1998) Analysis of prognostic indicators for dogs with pericardial effusion: 46 cases (1985–1996).

J Am Vet Med Assoc **212**:1276–1280.

58 Ehrhart N, Ehrhart EJ, Willis J *et al.* (2002) Survival of dogs with aortic body tumors. *Vet Surg* **31**:44–48.

59 Vicari ED, Brown DC, Holt DE *et al.* (2001) Survival times of and prognostic indicators for dogs with heart base masses: 25 cases (1986–1999). *J Am Vet Med Assoc* **219**:485–487.

60 Thomas WP, Reed JR, Bauer TG *et al.* (1984) Constrictive pericardial disease in the dog. *J Am Vet Med Assoc* **184**:546–553.

61 Wright KN, DeNovo RC, Patton CS *et al.* (1996) Effusive-constrictive pericardial disease secondary to osseous metaplasia of the pericardium in a dog. *J Am Vet Med Assoc* **209**:2091–2095.

62 Schwartz A, Wilson GP, Hamlin RL *et al.* (1971) Constrictive pericarditis in two dogs. *J Am Vet Med Assoc* **159**:763–776.

63 Fife TD, Finegold SM, Grennan T (1991) Pericardial actinomycosis: case report and review. *Rev Infect Dis* **13**:120–126.

64 Reimer SB, Kyles AE, Filipowicz DE *et al.* (2004) Long-term outcome of cats treated conservatively or surgically for peritoneopericardial diaphragmatic hernia: 66 cases (1987–2002). *J Am Vet Med Assoc* **224**:728–732.

65 Evans SM, Biery DO (1980) Congenital peritoneopericardial diaphragmatic hernia in the dog and cat: a literature review and 17 additional case histories. *Vet Radiol* **21**:108–116.

66 Neiger R (1996) Peritoneopericardial diaphragmatic hernia in cats. *Compend Cont Educ Pract Vet* **18**:461–479.

67 Hay WH, Woodfield JA, Moon MA (1989) Clinical, echocardiographic, and radiographic findings of peritoneopericardial diaphragmatic hernia in two dogs and a cat. *J Am Vet Med Assoc* **195**:1245–1248.

68 Lamb CR, Mason GC, Wallace MK (1989) Ultrasonographic diagnosis of peritoneopericardial diaphragmatic hernia in a Persian cat. *Vet Rec* **125**:186.

69 Wallace J, Mullen HS, Lesser MB (1992) A technique for surgical

correction of peritoneal pericardial diaphragmatic hernia in dogs and cats. *J Am Anim Hosp Assoc* **28**:503–510.

70 Tilley LP, Bond B, Patnaik AK *et al.* (1981) Cardiovascular tumors in the cat. *J Am Anim Hosp Assoc* **17**:1009–1021.

71 Colucci WS, Braunwald E (1992) Primary tumors of the heart. In: *Heart Disease: A Textbook of Cardiovascular Medicine*, 4th edn. E Braunwald (ed). WB Saunders, Philadelphia, pp. 1451–1464.

72 Hirsch VM, Jacobsen J, Mills JHL (1981) A retrospective study of canine hemangiosarcoma and its association with acanthocytosis. *Can Vet J* **22**:152–155.

73 Hayes HM (1975) An hypothesis for the aetiology of canine chemoreceptor system neoplasms, based upon an epidemiological study of 73 cases among hospital patients. *J Small Anim Pract* **16**:337–343.

74 Kurtz HJ, Finco DR (1969) Carotid and aortic body tumors in a dog. *Am J Vet Res* **30**:1247–1251.

75 Johnson KH (1968) Aortic body tumors in the dog. *J Am Vet Med Assoc* **152**:154–160.

76 Patnaik AK, Liu SK, Hurvitz AI *et al.* (1975) Canine chemodectoma (extra-adrenal paragangliomas) – a comparative study. *J Small Anim Pract* **16**:785–801.

77 Harbison ML, Godleski JJ (1983) Malignant mesothelioma in urban dogs. *Vet Pathol* **20**:531–540.

78 Paola JP, Hammer AS, Smeak DD *et al.* (1994) Aortic body tumor causing pleural effusion in a cat. *J Am Anim Hosp Assoc* **30**:281–285.

79 Bright JM, Toal RL, Blackford LM (1990) Right ventricular outflow obstruction caused by primary cardiac neoplasia. *J Vet Intern Med* **4**:12–16.

80 Richards MA, Mawdesley-Thomas LE (1969) Aortic body tumors in a boxer dog with a review of the literature. *J Pathol* **98**:283–288.

81 Simpson DJ, Hunt GB, Church DB *et al.* (1999) Benign masses in the pericardium of two dogs. *Aust Vet J* **77**:225–229.

23
Pulmonary Hypertension

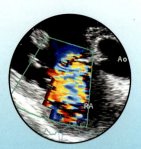

OVERVIEW

The pulmonary circulation is normally a low pressure, low resistance, high capacitance system. Normal pulmonary arterial (PA) pressures in dogs are about 25 mm Hg systolic, 8 mm Hg diastolic, and 12–15 mm Hg mean. These low PA pressures minimize RV workload and maintain optimal RV myocardial blood flow[1, 2]. Increases in pulmonary blood flow are usually accommodated with minimal increase in PA pressure because of the highly distensible thin-walled pulmonary vasculature, recruitment of underperfused vessels, and a large pulmonary capillary surface area[1, 3]. In dogs with normal lungs, up to 60% of the pulmonary vascular bed can be lost before pulmonary hypertension develops[1].

Pulmonary hypertension (PH) is generally defined as a mean PA pressure >25 mm Hg or systolic PA pressure >35 mm Hg[1–5]. Although somewhat higher systolic PA pressures occur in some athletic, geriatric, and obese people without clinical consequence[4], whether the same occurs in dogs is unknown. Pulmonary compliance and airway resistance may also influence PA pressure because of the interdependence of the pulmonary parenchyma and vasculature[2, 6]. A number of underlying disorders are associated with PH in dogs (Table 62). Reports of PH in cats are rare[2, 5]. PH can exacerbate the clinical manifestations and mortality associated with the underlying disease process. In one report, almost half of PH cases in dogs were associated with either hypoxic pulmonary disease or vascular obstructive disease[5]. Pulmonary thromboembolism (PTE) can develop when hypercoagulability, endothelial damage, or blood stasis occurs. Various clinical conditions have been associated with PTE in dogs and cats (see Chapter 15 and Table 62)[2, 7–11]. Chronically elevated pulmonary venous pressure may lead to almost one quarter of cases of PH in dogs[5]. PH secondary to left-sided CHF and chronic pulmonary disease tends to be mild to moderate in most affected animals and people. Eisenmenger's syndrome involves systemic to PA connections that lead to PH development and result in right-to-left or bi-directional shunting[12]. The PA changes observed are similar to those found in idiopathic PH[12, 13]. PH is also associated with certain drugs in people, especially appetite suppressants (including fenfluramine, phenyl-propanolamine) and other amphetamines[3, 12, 14]. It also occurs in some people with liver disease and portal hypertension, HIV, and connective tissue diseases. Although primary (idiopathic or familial) PH is well known in people, documentation for it in animals is rare[2, 15]. People with severe PH in association with other disease, previously known as secondary PH, tend to have marked vascular changes similar to those in idiopathic PH; the pathobiology may be similar in animals[13, 16, 17]. The greatly increased pulmonary vascular resistance (PVR) that underlies severe PH involves structural changes in the vasculature, not merely pulmonary vasoconstriction. Endothelial dysfunction plays a key role, and individual predisposition is thought to be important in the development of severe PH[3, 12, 18]. Thrombosis in situ can also be a factor[18–22].

PATHOPHYSIOLOGY

Increased PVR raises PA pressure according to the relationship: cardiac output = pressure/resistance (see Chapter 1, p. 21). PA vasoconstriction in response to hypoxia and other stimuli increases PVR, but the development of severe PH also involves angioproliferative changes that permanently reduce vascular compliance and lumen size[18, 19]. Because PVR is related inversely to the total cross-sectional area of the resistance vessels, when enough of these vessels are narrowed or destroyed and when their capacity to dilate is impaired by disease, even a normal cardiac output generates increased PA pressure.

Pulmonary arterial vasoconstriction is a normal response to alveolar hypoxia, although response magnitude varies among species[23, 24]. Usually this helps optimize ventilation/perfusion balance by preferentially perfusing well-ventilated lung regions.

Table 62 Diseases associated with pulmonary arterial hypertension.

1) Alveolar hypoxia with pulmonary vasoconstriction/remodeling:

  a) Interstitial pulmonary disease/fibrosis.

  b) Chronic obstructive pulmonary disease.

  c) Pneumonia.

  d) Tracheobronchial disease.

  e) Pulmonary mineralization.

  f) Neoplasia.

  g) (?) High altitude disease.

2) Pulmonary vascular obstructive disease:

  a) Heartworm disease (see Chapter 24).

  b) Pulmonary thromboembolism (see Chapter 15) (e.g. immune-mediated hemolytic anemia, protein-losing nephropathy, neoplasia, sepsis, hyperadrenocorticism or long-term exogenous glucocorticoids, cardiac disease, pancreatitis, DIC, protein-losing enteropathy, possibly trauma or major surgery).

  c) Pulmonary endarteritis.

3) Pulmonary overcirculation:*

  a) Large congenital shunts (e.g. atrial or ventricular septal defects, PDA) (see Chapter 18, p. 250).

4) High pulmonary venous pressure:

  a) Mitral valve regurgitation (see Chapter 19).

  b) Mitral valve stenosis (see Chapter 18, p. 244).

  c) Dilated cardiomyopathy (see Chapter 20).

  d) Other causes of left-sided heart failure.

5) Idiopathic.*

*Included in the 2003 World Health Organization classification of pulmonary hypertension under the broad category of 'pulmonary arterial hypertension', which also includes familial PH and PH associated with collagen vascular disease, portal hypertension, HIV infection, drugs/toxins, and certain other disorders. These conditions have in common the development of a pulmonary arteriopathy induced by various, sometimes unknown, stimuli in susceptible individuals [12, 18].

Hypoxia-induced pulmonary vasoconstriction is thought to occur with chronic obstructive pulmonary disease, lung lobe torsion, airway collapse or obstruction, hypoventilation, and low inspired O_2 concentrations. However, the prevalence of clinically important PH with these conditions is not known. Normal dogs exposed to lower inspired O_2 at high altitudes typically show only mild pulmonary vasoconstriction[24]. Erythrocytosis is absent and the associated mild PH does not appear to be clinically important[15, 24]; however, such hypoxia can cause or contribute to reactive PH in people and may be a factor in some dogs as well[5]. Increases in erythropoietin, endothelin, and vascular endothelial growth factor have been found in dogs living at high altitude, despite the absence of erythrocytosis[25].

Severe pulmonary parenchymal disease or fibrosis can destroy normal pulmonary vascular structure as well as stimulate regional hypoxic vasoconstriction, thereby further increasing PVR. The development of PH associated with chronic lung disease may be related to hypoxia, inflammation, and increased sheer stress in vessels, leading to pulmonary vascular morphologic changes[1, 5, 26, 27]. Restrictive pulmonary diseases, including chronic interstitial pulmonary disease and fibrosis, decrease dynamic lung compliance and can also contribute to PH because of abnormal pulmonary mechanics[2, 28].

Abnormal endothelial function is involved in the pathogenesis of vascular changes associated with PH[16, 20]. These include smooth muscle hypertrophy, intimal proliferation and fibrosis, and increased extracellular matrix deposition[1, 18, 26, 27]. Chronic vasoconstriction can provoke such vascular remodeling, perhaps related to persistent pulmonary inflammation with exuberant expression of growth factors and increased release of vasoactive mediators[5, 29]. Individual genetic predisposition likely plays an important role in cases of severe PH. Endothelial cells normally modulate vascular smooth muscle cell activity through production of both vasodilator/antimitotic (e.g. prostacyclin and nitric oxide) and vasoconstrictor/mitogenic (e.g. thromboxane A2 and endothelin) substances. Nitric oxide is produced from L-arginine by the action of nitric oxide synthases. Nitric oxide directly promotes vascular smooth muscle relaxation via increased intracellular cyclic guanylate monophosphate (cGMP) production[19]. Prostacyclin, produced from arachidonic acid, induces smooth muscle relaxation via cyclic adenylate monophosphate (cAMP) production. Prostacyclin also inhibits growth of smooth muscle cells and inhibits platelet aggregation. Excessive vasoconstrictor production with relative vasodilator deficiency, leads to abnormal endothelial–smooth muscle interactions, which promote pulmonary vasoconstriction and vascular remodeling[5, 29]. Endothelin induces vascular remodeling with various causes of PH, including PTE[16, 30]. Besides vasoconstriction, endothelin stimulates smooth muscle proliferation, collagen production, and platelet aggregation; it also has proinflammatory actions[16, 19, 31]. Other mediators include serotonin, known to be a potent vasoconstrictor, which can stimulate platelet aggregation as well as pulmonary smooth muscle proliferation[12, 18].

Pulmonary vascular obstructive disease (obliterative pulmonary arterial hypertension) can result from PTE (see Chapter 15, p. 151), in situ pulmonary thrombosis, as well as heartworm disease (HWD)[7, 21, 22, 32, 33]. Vascular obstruction reduces total cross-sectional pulmonary vascular area by mechanically obstructing vessels and provoking local hypoxic pulmonary vasoconstriction as well as other reactive changes. Associated pulmonary parenchymal disease can contribute to reduced vascular area. HWD is a common cause of PH in dogs and, sometimes, cats (see Chapter 24). Proliferative intimal lesions of the pulmonary arteries, obstructions from dead worms, and inflammation of surrounding parenchyma damage the vasculature and cause sustained PH[5]. PTE not associated with HWD can be large enough to obstruct a major vessel(s); alternatively, numerous small emboli may block many arteries and capillaries[7]. Flow obstruction occurs directly and also by the effects of vasoactive amines[1, 5]. Abnormal pulmonary blood flow and endothelial dysfunction promote platelet aggregation, activation of the clotting cascade, and elaboration of vasoconstrictor substances such as endothelin, thromboxane A2, and serotonin. Nitric oxide production is decreased and endothelial-mediated vasodilation is impaired[34]. These factors promote further vascular obstruction; in addition, a PA wall baroreflex may contribute to vasoconstriction as pulmonary pressure increases[35]. Acute PTE may resolve spontaneously and is sometimes subclinical, but in some individuals, incomplete resolution, recurrent PTE, or in situ thrombosis lead to chronic disease with vascular remodeling and development of progressive PH, RV failure, and ultimately death[36]. Prognosis has been negatively correlated with PA pressure in people[36].

Pulmonary overcirculation related to a congenital cardiac shunt can lead to pulmonary arterial remodeling[17]. Increased blood flow can raise perfusion pressure and damage pulmonary vessels[2, 13]. Dysfunction of mechanisms involved in pulmonary vasorelaxation occurs with high pulmonary blood flow[37], and increased endothelin levels have been identified in animal models of overcirculation-induced PH[16]. The size of the shunt and individual susceptibility play a role in whether PH develops. The PA changes observed with Eisenmenger's syndrome include medial hypertrophy, intimal proliferation and fibrosis, occlusion of small vessels, and eventually, plexiform lesions similar to those of idiopathic PH[12, 13]. Increased pulmonary vascular resistance is exacerbated by reactive polycythemia[18].

Chronic pulmonary venous hypertension can also induce structural changes in pulmonary capillaries and increase the muscularity of resistance arterioles[5, 38]. Pulmonary edema or congestion associated with high venous pressure could contribute to increasing pulmonary vascular resistance by reducing lung compliance and increasing resistance to air flow[2]. Endothelin is also thought to contribute to PH associated with left-sided heart failure[39].

PH imposes a systolic pressure overload on the right heart, resulting in both RV dilation and hypertrophy (**538, 539**)[27, 40]. The degree of hypertrophy varies; marked RV wall thickening is more common in young animals[5]. RV diastolic pressure also increases as RV function deteriorates. This leads to systemic venous hypertension and, eventually, signs of right-sided CHF. The term cor pulmonale refers to the right heart changes resulting from PH caused by pulmonary vascular and/or parenchymal disease. Cardiac output progressively declines as the RV fails. Inadequate cardiac output generation during exercise leads to exertional dyspnea, fatigue, and syncope[20].

CLINICAL FEATURES

Signs of PH are often subtle and nonspecific, increasing the challenge of diagnosis. PH should be suspected when persistent respiratory difficulty, fatigue, or exercise intolerance occurs without apparent cause. Animals with mild to moderate PH may be asymptomatic. PH can develop in dogs of any age, but middle-aged to geriatric dogs are most often affected[5]. There seems to be no sex predilection. Breeds affected are often those in which airway or pulmonary disease and degenerative AV valve disease are common. Younger dogs with PH are more likely to have congenital heart disease or pneumonia; these are often of larger breeds[5]. A small minority of dogs with PH had a history of HWD in one survey[5].

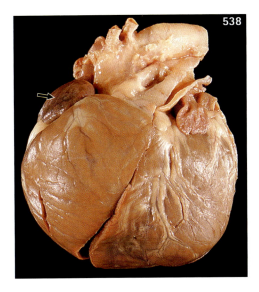

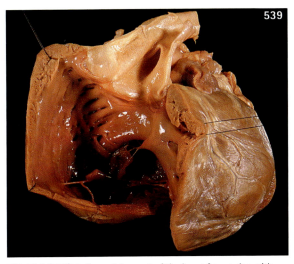

538, 539 (538) Left cranial aspect of the heart from a dog with severe PH as well as tricuspid insufficiency. Enlargement of the RV, as well as the right auricular appendage (arrow) is seen. (539) Open RV outflow tract and main PA from the same dog. There is prominent dilation of the RV and pulmonary trunk, but hypertrophy is minimal in this dog. The LV apex is at the lower right of the image.

The most commonly reported presenting complaints in one study included exercise intolerance (in 45% of cases), cough (30%), respiratory difficulty (28%), and syncope (23%)[5]. The mechanism for syncope may be related to the underlying disease process, as well as an inability to increase cardiac output in response to peripheral vasodilation during exercise. In addition to the above, other signs reported in people include hoarseness (from recurrent laryngeal nerve compression by the enlarged pulmonary artery) and rare but potentially fatal hemoptysis[18].

Clinical signs of PTE can be difficult to differentiate from those of other cardiopulmonary diseases[7]. Acute onset of respiratory difficulty is a classic manifestation of PTE, but is not always present. Exercise-induced dyspnea in people with chronic thromboembolic PH is thought to involve impaired cardiac performance caused by the increased PVR as well as increased ventilatory needs because of greater alveolar dead space[36]. Other signs reported with PTE in dogs include tachycardia, lethargy, altered mentation, and, occasionally, vomiting or coughing[7]. Lethargy, anorexia, weight loss, difficult breathing, and, occasionally, vomiting or coughing, dehydration, hypothermia, and icterus have been reported in cats[11]. A history of an indwelling venous catheter is common[7, 11]. Dry cough, especially with exertion, and occasionally hemoptysis are also reported in people with chronic PTE- induced PH[36].

Physical findings with PH include a systolic heart murmur in many cases[5]. Localization to the mitral or tricuspid valve area is most common, but aortic and pulmonic murmurs are also reported. A pulmonary diastolic murmur is heard rarely[5]. With severe PH especially, a loud, snapping or split S_2 may be heard. An S_4 gallop over the RV is described in people[36]. An S_3 gallop sound, especially during inspiration, is also described in people with RV dysfunction from PH; the prevalence of this in dogs is unknown[2, 36].

Signs of right-sided heart failure can be a manifestation of either underlying cardiac disease or cor pulmonale. Ascites was reported in 26% of PH cases; other right-sided congestive signs (jugular venous distension and subcutaneous edema) were noted less often in one study[5]. Pulmonary crackles or wheezes are common in animals with underlying pulmonary disease. Abnormal lung sounds were present in 23% and cyanosis in 15% of PH cases[5]. Increased inspiratory or expiratory respiratory effort may be observed, depending on the underlying disease.

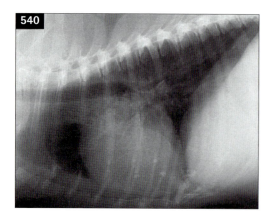

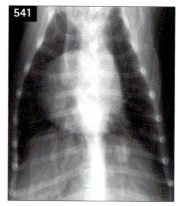

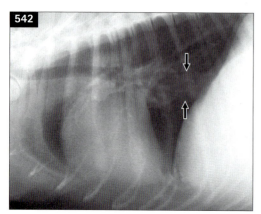

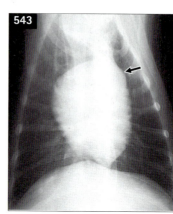

540–543 (540, 541) Lateral and DV radiographs from a 14-year-old male Shih Tzu with Doppler-estimated systolic pulmonary artery pressure [sPAP] of ~98 mm Hg, multiple neoplasia, and hypoproteinemia. Marked RV enlargement is apparent on both views. (542, 543) Lateral and DV radiographs from a young Chow Chow with histoplasmosis and Doppler-estimated sPAP of ~90 mm Hg. The caudal vena cava is distended (arrows, 542). A modest RV enlargement pattern and small bulge in the main PA region are seen (arrow, 543). Mild pleural effusion and ascites were also present.

DIAGNOSIS
Presence of PH

The diagnostic process involves identifying that PH is present, as well as defining any associated condition. Radiographic findings that suggest severe PH include cardiomegaly, especially right-sided cardiomegaly, and enlarged pulmonary arteries (540–543). Pulmonary parenchymal infiltrates are common and generally reflect underlying disease. Evidence of right-sided congestive failure (i.e. pleural effusion, large caudal vena cava, hepatomegaly) occurs in some advanced cases. Large pulmonary veins suggest high pulmonary venous pressure in dogs with underlying left-sided CHF. Radiographs can be unremarkable in mild to moderate PH.

The ECG may show evidence of RA or RV enlargement (see Chapter 4, p. 61), but this is inconsistent[5]. AF, atrial or ventricular tachyarrhythmias, and, occasionally, bradycardia or slowed AV conduction have been observed[5].

2-D and M-mode echocardiographic findings are variable and include RV chamber dilation, hypertrophy (RV wall thickness greater than half that of the LV wall), and pulmonary artery dilation (544–549); however, in about half of the cases in one study, RV size and wall thickness were normal[5]. RV dilation was graded as moderate in 22% of the cases and severe in 31% and did not correlate well with the severity of PH; moderate RV hypertrophy was seen in 39% of the cases and severe hypertrophy in 10%[5]. Severe hypertrophy was seen only in dogs under one year of age[5]. Flattened or paradoxical septal motion occurs in some cases. Reduced LV lumen size with pseudohypertrophy can be seen; this is thought to be a poor prognostic sign, associated with decreased output from a failing RV. A large pulmonary thrombus or heartworms are sometimes visualized in the proximal pulmonary artery. If a patent foramen ovale, or other intracardiac shunt, is present, right-to-left shunting may be evident on echo-bubble study (see 137, p. 76).

Noninvasive estimation of PA pressures is possible with CW Doppler echocardiography when pulmonic stenosis (or other RV outflow obstruction) is absent and when TR or pulmonary valve regurgitation (PR) is present. Color flow Doppler helps identify the presence of a regurgitant jet when an audible murmur is absent and guide CW Doppler cursor placement. Maximum TR jet velocity allows estimation of the systolic pressure gradient between the RV and the RA using the modified Bernoulli relationship (see Chapter 5, p. 86; 550, 551; also 562, p. 357). This gradient, plus about 8–10 mm Hg (or

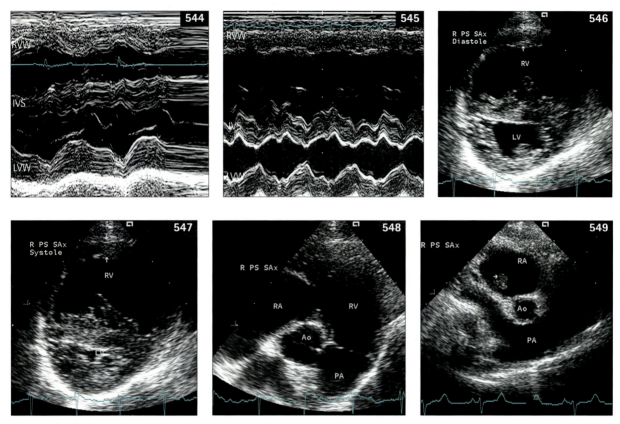

544–549 (544) M-mode echo image at the ventricular level from a 13-year-old male Yorkshire Terrier with Doppler-estimated sPAP of ~130 mm Hg, diabetes mellitus, and protein-losing nephropathy. The RV is moderately dilated and hypertrophied. Mitral valve echoes are seen within the LV. (545) M-mode echo from a 3-year-old female Cocker Spaniel with pulmonary thromboembolism (Doppler-estimated sPAP of ~145 mm Hg). The RV is markedly dilated. (546, 547) Diastolic (546) and systolic (547) 2-D echo frames from the dog in 545 show RV hypertrophy (arrows) and dilation. The ventricular septum is flattened toward the left because of high RV pressure. Poor filling of the left heart is indicated by the small LV lumen size and relatively thickened walls (pseudohypertrophy). (548) 2-D image at the heart base, from the same dog (545–547), demonstrates RV outflow tract and PA dilation common with PH. The diameter of the main PA is not normally larger than that of the aortic root. RA dilation is also seen in this image. (549) 2-D echo image from a 13-year-old female Yorkshire Terrier with severe PH and right-sided heart failure. PA dilation is striking compared with the size of the aorta. Part of an intracardiac thrombus (arrow) is seen within the dilated RA. Right parasternal short-axis position. Ao = aorta; IVS = interventricular septum; LV = left ventricle; LVW = left ventricular wall; PA = pulmonary artery; RA = right atrium; RV = right ventricle; RVW = right ventricular wall.

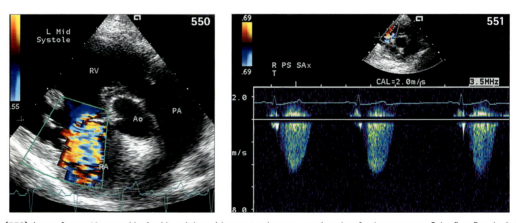

550, 551 (550) Image from a 10-year-old mixed breed dog with severe pulmonary arteriopathy of unknown cause. Color flow Doppler indicates moderate tricuspid insufficiency; RV hypertrophy and dilation and PA dilation are also evident. Doppler-estimated sPAP of ~94 mm Hg. LV filling was poor in this dog, which died a short time later. Left cranial short-axis position. Ao = aorta; PA = pulmonary artery; RA = right atrium; RV = right ventricle. (551) CW Doppler from the dog in 544 indicates a peak tricuspid regurgitation jet velocity of 5.45 m/sec. Right parasternal short-axis view.

the measured CVP) to account for RA pressure, approximates RV systolic pressure and, therefore, PA systolic pressure. Likewise, the diastolic pressure gradient between the PA and the RV is calculated from maximal PR jet velocity; this gradient, plus the estimated RV diastolic pressure, represents PA diastolic pressure. PH is associated with peak TR velocities >2.8 m/second or peak PR velocities >2.2 m/second[5, 41]. PH severity has been categorized, based on Doppler RV to RA systolic pressure gradients, as mild (~35–50 mm Hg; TR maximum velocity of 2.9–3.5 m/sec), moderate (~51–75 mm Hg; TR maximum velocity 3.6–4.3 m/sec), and severe (>75 mm Hg; TR maximum velocity >4.3 m/sec)[4, 5].

The PW Doppler pulmonary velocity profile also shows characteristic changes associated with PH[5, 42, 43]. Elevated PA pressure causes more rapid pulmonary flow acceleration, similar to the normal aortic flow profile (552; also 563, p. 357). Severe PH can also cause a midsystolic notch in the PA flow profile, as well as delayed deceleration. Right heart systolic time intervals (e.g. RV preejection period, RV ejection time, time to peak flow) can be measured with Doppler echocardiography and these have also been used to characterize PH in people[5, 43]; however, the clinical usefulness of this in dogs is unclear. Without measurable TR, Doppler echo measures of pulmonary flow, as well as systolic and diastolic ventricular function, have not allowed reliable differentiation of mild or moderate PH from normal[44].

Cardiac catheterization is necessary for direct measurement of PA pressures. A Swan–Ganz type catheter, with an end hole and inflatable balloon near its tip, is used to measure pressures within the RA, RV,

and main PA. When the balloon is inflated and the catheter gently advanced into the PA until it (temporarily) obstructs a smaller branch, the pressure recorded here reflects pressure in the pulmonary capillaries (pulmonary capillary wedge pressure [PCWP]). PCWP approximates LA pressure, assuming no pulmonary venous obstruction exists. If PH is secondary to high pulmonary venous pressure from left-sided heart failure (postcapillary cause), PCWP is elevated. When PH is caused by pulmonary vascular, bronchopulmonary, or other disease (with precapillary pulmonary vascular remodeling), PCWP is substantially lower than PA diastolic pressure[20]. Right heart catheterization can also be used to evaluate acute pulmonary vasoreactivity in response to vasodilator drugs (see p. 347)[2]. Responsiveness is defined in people as a decrease in mean PA pressure of at least 10 mm Hg, to a level of 40 mm Hg or lower[4].

Underlying disease
Clinical laboratory and pulmonary radiographic findings generally reflect underlying disease processes. Diagnostic tests used to evaluate pulmonary or vascular causes of PH may include thoracic radiography, fluoroscopy (to document dynamic airway collapse), arterial blood gas analysis or pulse oximetry, routine blood and urine analyses, tracheal or bronchoalveolar washings, pulmonary nuclear perfusion scintigraphy, pulmonary angiography, CT, D-dimer assay, and other tests of coagulation or immune system function. Pulmonary function testing, although not widely available, may also help characterize underlying disease. Hypoxemia is common with most causes of PH. Nucleated RBCs, often seen with chronic hypoxia, were found in 28% of dogs with PH[5]. Mild leukocytosis was found in a similar percentage of dogs with PH and in most dogs with PTE[7]. PTE causes varied radiographic abnormalities, although radiographs are sometimes normal[7, 11] (see Chapter 15, p. 155). Peripheral noncircumscribed consolidations are observed in some patients[11]. Uneven pulmonary vascular diameter and blood flow distribution between lung lobes, proximal PA dilation with abrupt tapering, and pleural effusion have also been described[11]. HWD should be excluded by serologic testing, at minimum (see Chapter 24). Evidence for primary heart disease as a cause for PH either from pulmonary overcirculation (with shunt reversal; see Chapter 18, p. 250) or pulmonary venous congestion (see Chapters 18–20) should be sought.

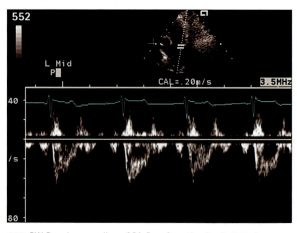

552 PW Doppler recording of PA flow from the dog in **545** shows rapid rate of systolic flow acceleration and slight notching during deceleration. Maximal systolic velocity is attenuated in this dog. See text for further information. Left cranial short-axis position.

MANAGEMENT
There is no cure and few treatment options for severe PH, although sildenafil citrate (see p. 348) is helpful in some cases. The high PVR is largely 'fixed' because

of vascular morphologic changes, and there is usually limited capacity for pulmonary vasodilation. The potential for concurrent systemic vasodilation and significant hypotension must be considered when vasodilator drugs are used. Underlying disease should be managed as possible and exercise restriction imposed.

Supplemental O_2 administration is recommended in acute care settings. Benefits include a degree of pulmonary vasodilation in actively constricted vessels, reduced acidosis and ischemia, and improved right heart function[2]. Whether nocturnal O_2 supplementation at home is of any long-term benefit is unknown. No effect of such therapy on survival or quality of life was found in people with Eisenmenger's syndrome, and controlled studies with other causes of PH are unavailable[45].

Diuretics (see Chapter 16, p. 176) are useful in reducing blood volume in animals with CHF, but extensive diuresis can further reduce cardiac output in patients with poor RV function, where RV output is dependent on preload. If chronic obstructive pulmonary disease underlies PH, diuretics can further impair gas exchange by drying secretions and facilitating mucous plug formation within bronchi[2].

The positive inotropic agent digoxin (see Chapter 16, p. 179) has been used occasionally in an attempt to improve RV function, but it is not generally used in dogs with chronic obstructive pulmonary disease or PH[2]. In addition to the potential risk of toxicity, digoxin can increase PA pressures along with cardiac output. Acute pulmonary vasoconstriction has been reported[27]. Furthermore, digoxin-related cardiac arrhythmias may be more likely in patients with concurrent hypoxia or acidosis[46].

Methyxanthine bronchodilators might help some animals with PH. Theophylline and related drugs have mild positive inotropic effects on the heart. In people with chronic obstructive pulmonary disease, theophylline has produced long-term pulmonary vasodilation and enhanced right heart function[2]. Theophylline improves diaphragmatic contractile strength and reduces respiratory muscle fatigue in dogs[2]. In addition, bronchodilation and improved intrathoracic pressure gradients may reduce the tendency for airway collapse in patients with bronchiectasis or tracheal collapse[2]. Sustained release theophylline can be used (20 mg/kg q12h in dogs), although some dogs show adverse sympathomimetic effects at this dose. Beta$_2$-agonist bronchodilators (e.g. terbutaline) may also improve pulmonary hemodynamics, but this is not well studied. Terbutaline can be used (1.25–5 mg/kg q8–12h in dogs; 1.25 mg/kg q12h in cats).

Oral calcium channel-blockers or other vasodilators may reduce pulmonary vasoconstriction in patients capable of a vasodilatory response. High doses of Ca^{++} channel-blocking agents (see Chapter 17, p. 217), hydralazine (see Chapter 16, p. 182), ACE inhibitors (see Chapter 16, p. 178), and others have been used in people[2, 19, 45], but there is no good way to predict response except with acute therapeutic testing during cardiac catheterization. In the absence of acute vasodilatory response, such agents are unlikely to have long-term benefit and, furthermore, they create the potential for systemic hypotension, and increased right-to-left shunting, when present. Only about half of dogs with experimental heartworm-induced PH showed significant decrease in PA pressure and PVR in response to hydralazine[2, 47].

Acute pulmonary vasoreactivity

Some potentially therapeutic agents can be administered during cardiac catheterization to assess whether improvement in PA pressure, cardiac output, and PVR occurs. Patients that demonstrate acute pulmonary vasodilation may respond to long-term vasodilator therapy; however, vasodilatory response is likely to be minimal or absent with severe PH. Intravenous response testing has been done using aminophylline (10 mg/kg), terbutaline (0.01 mg/kg), hydralazine (1 mg/kg), verapamil (0.05 mg/kg), and nifedipine (<0.1 mg/kg); marked systemic hypotension can occur with some agents[1, 2]. In people, acute trials with IV epoprostenol (a synthetic prostacyclin), inhaled nitric oxide, IV adenosine, or inhaled iloprost (a prostacyclin analog) may predict hemodynamic response to long-term oral calcium channel-blocker therapy[4, 48, 49]. Long-term calcium channel-blocker treatment yields hemodynamic and functional improvement in <10% of people with primary PH[45]; however, with newer oral and inhaled treatments that combine vasodilatory and antiproliferative properties, the usefulness of invasive testing for drug-induced vasoreactivity is not clear[4]. These therapies include endothelin-receptor antagonists, other prostacyclin analogs, and phosphodiesterase (PDE) type 5 inhibitors. The ACE inhibitors may also have beneficial effects by reducing vascular remodeling and improving nitric oxide production[50].

The rationale for therapy with prostacyclin analogs relates to the increased production of vasoconstrictors, including thromboxane A_2, and relative deficiency of prostacyclin in patients with PH. Prostacyclin analogs may also decrease endothelin release. Improvement in exercise capacity, hemodynamics, and survival time have been shown in people, but long-term use is complicated by the need to administer by constant infusion techniques or inhalation, depending on the drug, and a possibly limited duration of effectiveness[45]. Beraprost, a new orally effective prostacyclin analog, appears to improve survival time as well as hemodynamics in people, and is relatively selective for pulmonary vasodilation in experimental vasoconstrictive PH in dogs[45, 51, 52]; however, clinical experience is lacking.

Endothelin-receptor antagonists may prove to be useful agents in treating chronic PH. Bosentan is an orally administered dual endothelin A- and endothelin B-receptor antagonist. It improves exercise capacity and hemodynamic parameters in people, but is potentially hepatotoxic[16, 31, 45]. Combination therapy with bosentan and epoprostenol also appears promising[45].

Various PDE inhibitors, besides the xanthine bronchodilators, present other therapeutic possibilities. Amrinone and milrinone (PDE type 3 inhibitors) have reduced vasoconstriction, although to a lesser degree than bronchoconstriction, experimentally in dogs with serotonin-induced PH and PTE, but systemic vascular resistance was reduced as well[53, 54]. Sildenafil citrate is a selective PDE type 5 inhibitor (cGMP specific) that is thought to enhance nitric oxide-dependent pulmonary vasodilation[19]. It appears to be useful for improving symptoms, exercise capacity, and hemodynamics in primary and secondary PH in people[19, 45, 55]. Although experience in animals is limited, initial reports are encouraging. Definitive dosing recommendations have not been established. Doses of 0.5–2(–3) mg/kg q12h or q8h appear to be well-tolerated and produce some reduction in Doppler-estimated PA pressure, as well as clinical improvement in a majority of dogs evaluated[57]. Pentoxifylline (and similar drugs) is a xanthine-derivative PDE inhibitor with bronchodilatory effects that also increases RBC flexibility and reduces viscosity[56, 58]. It may also have some vasodilatory effect. Although there is anecdotal evidence of clinical improvement with Eisenmenger's syndrome, the potential usefulness for acquired PH as well as PH secondary to large cardiac shunts is unclear.

Evidence-based treatment protocols for idiopathic PH and drug or immunologic disease-induced PH in people have been evaluated and summarized into the following guidelines, which may or may not be useful in dogs: oral anticoagulant for all patients; a diuretic for patients with fluid retention; supplemental O_2 for hypoxemic patients; high-dose calcium channel-blocker only for the minority responding to acute vasoreactivity testing.

For patients without a positive vasodilatory response, treatment with either an endothelin-receptor antagonist or a prostanoid, or a PDE type 5 inhibitor may be useful; combination therapy may be helpful in some patients[45]. In people, indomethacin can exacerbate PH. It is not known whether the use of selective cyclooxygenase-2 inhibitors might lead to increased endothelin production, with consequent vascular remodeling in susceptible individuals[59].

The prognosis is guarded for animals with severe PH. While some appear to respond to medical therapy for a time, many die within a few months of diagnosis. In one study of dogs with PH, median survival time after diagnosis was only 3–4 days; the disease course did not seem related to Doppler-estimated RV–RA gradient[5]. Parameters correlated with survival times in people with idiopathic PH include exercise capacity, acute pulmonary vasoreactivity, hemodynamic characteristics, RV function, and plasma concentrations of BNP, NE, endothelin-1, uric acid, and troponin[4].

REFERENCES

1 Perry LA, Dillon AR, Bowers TL (1991) Pulmonary hypertension. *Compend Cont Educ Pract Vet* **13**: 226–233.

2 Johnson LR, Hamlin RL (1995) Recognition and treatment of pulmonary hypertension. In: *Kirk's Current Veterinary Therapy XII*. JD Bonagura (ed). WB Saunders, Philadelphia, pp. 887–892.

3 Kim NHS (2004) Diagnosis and evaluation of the patient with pulmonary hypertension. *Cardiol Clin* **22**:367–373.

4 Barst RJ, McCoon M, Torbicki A *et al.* (2004) Diagnosis and differential assessment of pulmonary arterial hypertension. *J Am Coll Cardiol* **43**:40S–47S.

5 Johnson L, Boon J, Orton EC (1999) Clinical characteristics of 53 dogs with Doppler-derived evidence of pulmonary hypertension: 1992–1996. *J Vet Intern Med* **13**:440–447.

6 West JB (2003) *Pulmonary Pathophysiology: The Essentials*, 6th edn. Lippincott Williams & Wilkins, Philadelphia, pp. 101–121.

7 Johnson LR, Lappin MR, Baker DC (1999) Pulmonary thromboembolism in 29 dogs: 1985–1995. *J Vet Intern Med* **13**:338–345.

8 Klein MK, Dow SW, Rosychuk RAW (1989) Pulmonary thromboembolism associated with immune-mediated hemolytic anemia in dogs: ten cases (1982–1987). *J Am Vet Med Assoc* **195**:246–250.

9 LaRue MJ, Murtaugh RJ (1990) Pulmonary thromboembolism in dogs: 47 cases (1986–1987). *J Am Vet Med Assoc* **197**:1368–1382.

10 Ritt MG, Rogers KS, Thomas JS (1997) Nephrotic syndrome resulting in thromboembolic disease and disseminated intravascular coagulation in a dog. *J Am Anim Hosp Assoc* **33**:385–391.

11 Norris CR, Griffey SM, Samii VF (1999) Pulmonary thromboembolism in cats: 29 cases (1987–1997). *J Am Vet Med Assoc* **215**:1650–1654.

12 McLaughlin VV (2004) Classification and epidemiology of pulmonary hypertension. *Cardiol Clin* **22**:327–341.

13 Oswald GP, Orton CE (1993) Patent ductus arteriosus and pulmonary hypertension in related Pembroke Welsh Corgis. *J Am Vet Med Assoc* **202**:761–764.

14 Barst RJ, Abenhaim L (2004) Fatal pulmonary hypertension associated with phenylpropanolamine exposure. *Heart* **90**:e42.

15 Glaus TM, Soldati G, Maurer R *et al.* (2004) Clinical and pathological characterization of primary pulmonary hypertension in a dog. *Vet Rec* **154**:786–789.

16 Galie N, Manes A, Branzi A (2004) The endothelin system in pulmonary hypertension. *Cardiovasc Res* **61**:227–237.

17 Turk JR, Miller JB, Sande RD (1982) Plexogenic pulmonary arteriopathy in a dog with ventricular septal defect and pulmonary hypertension. *J Am Anim Hosp Assoc* **18**:608–612.

18 Nauser TD, Stites SW (2003) Pulmonary hypertension: new perspectives. *Congest Heart Fail* **9**:155–162.

19 Humbert M, Sitbon O, Simonneau G (2004) Treatment of pulmonary arterial hypertension. *N Engl J Med* **351**:1425–1436.

20 Voelkel NF, Cool C (2004) Pathology of pulmonary hypertension. *Cardiol Clin* **22**:343–351.

21 Pyle RL, King MD, Saunders GK *et al.* (2004) Pulmonary thrombosis due to idiopathic main pulmonary artery disease. *Vet Med* **99**:836–842.

22 Karlstam E, Haggstrom J, Kvart C *et al.* (2000) Pulmonary artery lesions in Cavalier King Charles Spaniels. *Vet Rec* **147**:166–167.

23 McCulloch KM, Osipenko ON, Gurney AM (1999) Oxygen-sensing potassium currents in pulmonary artery. *Gen Pharmacol* **32**:403–411.

24 Tucker A, McMurtry IF, Reeves JT *et al.* (1975) Lung vascular smooth muscle as a determinant of pulmonary hypertension at altitude. *Am J Physiol* **228**:762–767.

25 Glaus TM, Grenacher B, Koch D *et al.* (2004) High altitude training of dogs results in elevated erythropoietin and endothelin-1 serum levels. *Comp Biochem Physiol A Mol Integr Physiol* **138**:355–361.

26 Gust R, Schuster DP (2001) Vascular remodeling in experimentally induced subacute canine pulmonary hypertension. *Exp Lung Res* **27**:1–12.

27 Schulman DS, Matthay RA (1992) The right ventricle in pulmonary disease. *Cardiol Clin* **10**:111–135.

28 King RR, Mauderly JL, Hahn FF *et al.* (1984) Pulmonary function studies in a dog with pulmonary thromboembolism associated with Cushing's disease. *J Am Anim Hosp Assoc* **21**:555–562.

29 Voelkel NF, Tuder RM (1995) Cellular and molecular mechanisms in the pathogenesis of pulmonary hypertension. *Eur Respir J* **8**:2129–2138.

30 Kim H, Yung GL, Marsh JJ *et al.* (2000) Endothelin medates pulmonary vascular remodeling in a canine model of chronic embolic pulmonary hypertension. *Eur Respir J* **15**:640–648.

31 Channick RN, Sitbon O, Barst RJ *et al.* (2004) Endothelin receptor antagonists in pulmonary arterial hypertension. *J Am Coll Cardiol* **43**:62S–67S.

32 Cornelissen JMM, Wolvekamp WThC, Stokhf AA *et al.* (1985) Primary occlusive vascular disease in a dog diagnosed by lung perfusion scintigram. *J Am Anim Hosp Assoc* **21**:293–299.

33 Burns MG, Kelly AB, Hornof WJ *et al.* (1981) Pulmonary artery thrombosis in three dogs with hyperadrenocorticism. *J Am Vet Med Assoc* **178**:388–393.

34 Sander M, Welling KL, Ravn JB *et al.* (2003) Endogenous NO does not regulate baseline pulmonary pressure, but reduces acute pulmonary hypertension in dogs. *Acta Physiol Scand* **178**:269–277.

35 Tanus-Santos JE, Gordo WM, Udelsmann A *et al.* (2000) Nonselective endothelin-receptor antagonism attenuates hemodynamic changes after massive pulmonary air embolism in dogs. *Chest* **118**:175–179.

36 Auger WR, Kerr KM, Kim NHS *et al.* (2004) Chronic thromboembolic pulmonary hypertension. *Cardiol Clin* **22**:453–466.

37 Fullerton DA, Mitchell MB, Jones DN *et al.* (1996) Pulmonary vasomotor dysfunction is produced with chronically high pulmonary blood flow. *J Thorac Cardiovasc Surg* **111**:190–197.

38 West JB, Mathieu-Costello O (1995) Vulnerability of pulmonary capillaries in heart disease. *Circulation* **92**:622–631.

39 Cody RJ (1992) The potential role of endothelin as a vasoconstrictor substance in congestive heart failure. *Eur Heart J* **13**:1573–1578.

40 Chen EP, Craig DM, Bittner HB *et al.* (1998) Pharmacological strategies for improving diastolic dysfunction in the setting of chronic pulmonary hypertension. *Circulation* **97**:1606–1612.

41 Glaus TM, Hassig M, Baumgartner C *et al.* (2003) Pulmonary hypertension induced in dogs by hypoxia at different high-altitude levels. *Vet Res Commun* **27**:661–670.

42 Martin-Duran R, Larman M, Trugeda A *et al.* (1986) Comparison of Doppler-determined elevated arterial pressure with pressure measured at cardiac catheterization. *Am J Cardiol* **57**:859–863.

43 Uehara Y (1993) An attempt to estimate pulmonary artery pressure in dogs by means of pulsed Doppler echocardiography. *J Vet Med Sci* **55**:307–312.

44 Glaus TM, Tomsa K, Hassig M *et al.* (2004) Echocardiographic changes induced by moderate to marked hypobaric hypoxia in dogs. *Vet Radiol Ultrasound* **45**:233–237.

45 Galie N, Seeger W, Naeije R *et al.* (2004) Comparative analysis of clinical trials and evidence-based treatment algorithm in pulmonary arterial hypertension. *J Am Coll Cardiol* **43**:81S–88S.

46 Miller MS, Tilley LP, Calvert CA (1986) Electrocardiographic correlations in pulmonary heart disease. *Semin Vet Med Surg* **1**:331–337.

47 Atkins CE, Keene BW, McGuirk SM *et al.* (1994) Acute effect of hydralazine administration on pulmonary artery hemodynamics in dogs with chronic heartworm disease. *Am J Vet Res* **55**:262–269.

48 Hirakawa A, Sakamoto H, Misumi K et al. (1996) Evaluation of pulmonary vasodilatory capacity with inhaled nitric oxide in a dog with patent ductus arteriosus. *J Vet Med Sci* **58**:673–375.

49 Hirakawa A, Sakamoto H, Misumi K et al. (1996) Effects of inhaled nitric oxide on hypoxic pulmonary vasoconstriction in dogs and a case report of venae cavae syndrome. *J Vet Med Sci* **58**:551–553.

50 Kanno S, Wu YJ, Lee PC et al. (2001) Angiotensin converting enzyme inhibitor preserves p21 and endothelial nitric oxide synthase expression in monocrotaline-induced pulmonary arterial hypertension in rats. *Circulation* **104**:945–950.

51 Ono F, Nagaya N, Okumura H et al. (2003) Effect of orally active prostacyclin analogue on survival in patients with chronic thromboembolic pulmonary hypertension without major vessel obstruction. *Chest* **123**:1583–1588.

52 Tamura M, Kurumatani H, Matsushita T (2001) Comparative effects of beraprost, a stable analogue of prostacyclin, with PGE (1), nitroglycerine and nifedipine on canine model of vasoconstrictive pulmonary hypertension. *Prostaglandins Leukot Essent Fatty Acids* **64**:197–202.

53 Hashiba E, Hirota K, Yoshioka H et al. (2000) Milrinone attenuates serotonin-induced pulmonary hypertension and bronchoconstriction in dogs. *Anesth Analg* **90**:790–794.

54 Kato R, Sato J, Nishino T (1998) Milrinone decreases both pulmonary arterial and venous resistances in the hypoxic dog. *Br J Anaesth* **81**:920–924.

55 Ghofrani HA, Pepke-Zaba J, Barbera J et al. (2004) Nitric oxide pathway and phosphodiesterase inhibitors in pulmonary arterial hypertension. *J Am Coll Cardiol* **43**:68S–72S.

56 Gutierres S (2001) Pentoxifylline. *Compend Cont Educ Pract Vet* **23**:603–605.

57 Bach J, Rozanski EA, MacGregor J et al. (2005) Sildenafil (Viagra®) as a therapy for pulmonary hypertension in dogs. Abstract. *J Vet Intern Med* **19**:403.

58 Marsella R, Nicklin CF, Munson JW et al. (2000) Pharmacokinetics of pentoxifylline in dogs after oral and intravenous administration. *Am J Vet Res* **61**:631–637.

59 Wort SJ, Woods M, Warne TD et al. (2002) Cyclooxygenase-2 acts as an endogenous brake on endothelin-1 release by human pulmonary artery smooth muscle cells: implications for pulmonary hypertension. *Mol Pharmacol* **62**:1147–1153.

24
Heartworm Disease

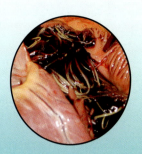

DIROFILARIA IMMITIS

OVERVIEW

Heartworm disease (HWD) is caused by the nematode *Dirofilaria immitis*. Various species of mosquitoes throughout the world serve as an obligate intermediate host and transmit the parasite. Heartworm transmission is limited by climatic conditions. For the 1st stage larvae (L1) to mature to the infective stage within a mosquito, the average daily temperature must be more than 18° C (64° F) for about a month[1]. In temperate latitudes of the Northern Hemisphere, heartworm transmission peaks in July and August; in subtropical regions, year-round transmission can occur. Microfilariae develop into infective stage larvae within two weeks at 27° C (80° F)[1]. The heartworm life cycle continues when a mosquito ingests microfilariae (L1) during a blood meal from an infected host animal. The L1 develop into the infective 3rd stage larvae (L3) within the mosquito over a 2–2.5 week period. The mosquito transmits infective larvae to the new host during a subsequent blood meal. The L3 travel subcutaneously within the new host, molting first into the 4th stage larvae (L4) in about 9–12 days, and then into the 5th stage larvae (L5). The young worms (L5) enter the vascular system about 100 days after infection; they migrate preferentially to the peripheral pulmonary arteries of the caudal lung lobes. At least 5 (usually more than 6) months pass before an infection becomes patent and gravid female worms release microfilariae. Microfilariae passed to another dog by blood transfusion or across the placenta do not develop into adult worms because the parasite life cycle requires the mosquito as intermediate host.

Dogs and other canids are the preferred host species. Although cats are also affected by HWD, they are more resistant to infection than dogs. The overall prevalence in cats is thought to be only 5–20% of that in dogs in the same geographic area; reported prevalence ranges from 0% to >16%. Infected cats generally have fewer adult worms than infected dogs because the worms mature more slowly, fewer infective larvae mature to adults, and the adults do

not live as long in cats, although live worms can persist for 2–3 years in cats. Most infected cats have <6 adult worms and often only 1 or 2; however, because of their small body size, the effects of even 1 or 2 worms can be severe (553). *D. immitis* uncommonly infects people, usually resulting in a solitary pulmonary nodule in this dead-end host[2].

PATHOPHYSIOLOGY

HWD is an important cause of PH in endemic regions. Adult worms within the pulmonary arteries incite the development of reactive vascular lesions, which precipitate PH. Pathologic changes begin within days after young adults arrive in the pulmonary arteries. Although severe disease is often associated with a large worm burden, it appears that the host–parasite interaction is more important than worm number alone in the development of clinical signs. The immune response to heartworms is thought to be modulated by intracellular endosymbiont bacteria (genus *Wolbachia*) harbored by the worms[3, 4]. Adult worms themselves are more likely to obstruct arteries in cats than in dogs

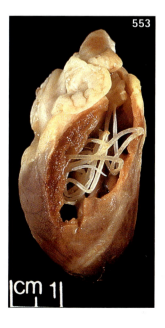

553 Opened RV outflow region, from an outdoor cat that died unexpectedly. Two heartworms were found in the heart.

because of their relative size. Little or no correlation has been found in dogs between PVR and the number of worms present. A low worm burden can lead to greater lung injury and PVR when the cardiac output is high. Exercise exacerbates the pulmonary vascular pathology because of the associated increase in pulmonary blood flow. Heartworms prefer the caudal pulmonary arteries; as the worm burden increases, some migrate toward and into the heart. The presence of worms in the caudal vena cava has been associated with heavy worm burdens. Occasionally, mechanical occlusion of the RV outflow tract, tricuspid valve, venae cavae, or pulmonary arteries occurs when there is a massive number of worms (caval syndrome). This inflow obstruction combined with consequent tricuspid insufficiency and preexisting PH causes signs of right-sided heart failure and poor left heart output (see p. 362)[5].

The characteristic lesion of infected pulmonary arteries is villous myointimal proliferation. The heartworm-induced changes begin with endothelial cell swelling, widening of intercellular junctions, increased endothelial permeability, and development of periarterial edema. Endothelial sloughing stimulates adhesion of activated white blood cells and platelets. Smooth muscle cells migrate and proliferate within the media and into the intima under the influence of various trophic factors. Villous proliferation of the intima occurs by 3–4 weeks after the arrival of adult worms. The villous projections, which consist of smooth muscle and collagen with an endothelium-like covering, narrow the lumen of the smaller pulmonary arteries and lead to further endothelial damage and proliferation. Endothelial damage promotes thrombosis as well as a perivascular tissue reaction. Periarterial edema may be severe, and partial lung consolidation develops in some animals. Dead worms incite a more intense host response, worsen the pulmonary disease, and can induce shock and coagulopathy[6–8]. Worm fragments and thrombi stimulate further reaction and lead to fibrosis. Arterial embolization and infarction, fibrosis, and hypersensitivity pneumonitis can all contribute to the development of parenchymal lung lesions. PVR is increased in the diseased, narrowed vessels. This decreases perfusion of affected lung lobes, raises pulmonary arterial pressure, and increases right heart workload. Alveolar hypoxia in consolidated lung regions exacerbates the high pulmonary resistance.

Villous proliferation (and worm distribution) is most severe in the caudal and accessory lobar arteries. Affected pulmonary arteries lose their normal tapered peripheral branching appearance and appear blunted or pruned. Aneurysmal dilation and peripheral occlusion may occur. The vessels dilate proximally and become tortuous as the increased PVR demands higher perfusion pressures.

RV dilation and hypertrophy result from the higher systolic pressure load. Chronic pulmonary hypertension can lead to secondary tricuspid valve insufficiency and RV myocardial failure, with neurohormonal activation and clinical signs of right-sided congestive failure[9, 10].

Chronic hepatic congestion secondary to heartworm disease can cause permanent liver damage and cirrhosis. Renal glomerular damage is associated with circulating immune complex deposition and, possibly, microfilarial antigens. Heartworm-induced glomerulopathy tends to worsen with the chronicity of infection, but immature worms as well as microfilariae and, possibly, adults may contribute to pathology[11]. Renal amyloidosis has also been associated with HWD in dogs, but is rare. Occasionally, aberrant worms can cause embolization of the brain, eye, or other systemic arteries[12, 13].

Cats

The immature worms, which arrive in the pulmonary arteries 4–6 months post infection, stimulate activation of pulmonary intravascular macrophages. These are specialized phagocytic cells located in the pulmonary capillary beds of cats, but not dogs. These macrophages cause acute inflammation in the pulmonary arteries and lung tissue. Interstitial lung disease occurs as in dogs; however, cats have more extensive alveolar type 2 (surfactant-producing) cell hyperplasia, which can interfere with alveolar O_2 exchange. Adventitial and perivascular inflammatory cell infiltrates consisting mainly of eosinophils and neutrophils are also seen. The parenchymal lesions probably play an important role in the development of acute respiratory distress in many cats 4–9 months after infection. This phase is fatal in some cats. In those that survive, the acute inflammation subsides. Vascular injury also causes myointimal proliferations and muscular hypertrophy in affected pulmonary arteries of cats[14]; however, these lesions tend to be focal, so clinically relevant PH is uncommon[15]. Dead and degenerating worms cause recrudescence of pulmonary inflammation and thromboembolism (TE). Disease is most severe in the caudal lung lobes. Villous proliferation, thrombi, or dead heartworms have been identified as causing caudal lobar arterial obstruction[16]. The bronchopulmonary circulation in cats is thought to prevent pulmonary infarction. Markedly dilated areas in the muscular pulmonary arteries suggests PH; however, secondary RV hypertrophy and right-sided congestive failure are uncommon in cats[17].

Sporadic vomiting occurs frequently in heartworm-infected cats. The underlying mechanism may relate to stimulation of the chemoreceptor trigger zone by inflammatory mediators, as low dose prednisone usually alleviates the vomiting[18].

CLINICAL FEATURES
Dogs

HWD disease has no specific age or breed predilection. Most affected dogs are between 4 and 8 years old, but infection in other age groups (older than 6 months) is common. Male dogs are affected 2–4 times as often as female dogs. Large breed dogs and those primarily living outdoors are at greater risk of infection than small breed or indoor dogs. The length of the haircoat does not appear to affect the risk of infection.

Many dogs are diagnosed by a positive routine screening test without showing clinical signs, but signs of HWD can include exertional dyspnea, fatigue, syncope, cough, hemoptysis, shortness of breath, weight loss, or signs of right-sided CHF. A change in or loss of a dog's bark has sometimes been reported. Aberrant worm migration occurs occasionally and causes signs related to the location (e.g. CNS, eye, femoral arteries, subcutis, peritoneal cavity, and other sites)[12, 19].

Physical examination findings can be normal in early or mild disease; however, with severe disease, poor body condition, tachypnea or dyspnea, jugular vein distension or pulsations, ascites, or other evidence of right-sided heart failure often develop. Harsh or abnormal lung sounds (wheezes and crackles), a loud and often split second heart sound (S_2), an ejection click or murmur at the left base, a murmur of tricuspid insufficiency, or cardiac arrhythmias are variably heard on auscultation. Severe pulmonary arterial disease and TE can be associated with epistaxis, DIC, thrombocytopenia, and, possibly, hemoglobinuria. Hemoglobinuria is also a sign of the caval syndrome.

Cats

Cats of any age are susceptible[18, 20]. DSH cats may be more easily affected[20]. Male cats are overrepresented in some studies but not in others[18, 20, 21]. Strictly indoor housing is not protective[22]. The infection is self-limiting in some cats. Severe clinical signs are usually associated with the arrival of L5 parasites in the pulmonary arteries (5–6 months after infection) and with TE after the death of one or more worms. Some studies have reported more cases being diagnosed in fall and winter, presumably after infection in the spring, while others have noted fewer cases in the last quarter of the year[20]. Heartworm-infected cats generally have less than 8 adult worms in the RV and pulmonary arteries, and most cats have only 1 or 2 worms, but even 1 adult worm can cause death. Unisex infections are common. Most cats have no or only a brief period of microfilaremia. Aberrant worm migration is also more common in cats than in dogs and complicates necropsy confirmation of infection[23]. Aberrant sites have included the brain, subcutaneous nodules, body cavities, and, occasionally, a systemic artery[18].

Clinical signs in cats are variable and may be transient or nonspecific. Some cats show no clinical evidence of infection. The appearance of clinical signs is usually associated with the arrival of immature heartworms in the lungs and again with death of adult heartworms. Cats may be asymptomatic at other times[18]. Well over half of symptomatic cats show respiratory signs, especially dyspnea and/or paroxysmal cough[18, 20, 22, 24]. This can mimic feline asthma, especially early in heartworm infection. Vomiting is also common and is the only sign in some cats. Vomiting is typically unrelated to eating[18]. Other complaints include lethargy, anorexia, syncope, other neurologic signs, and sudden death. Neurologic signs are common during aberrant worm migration. These signs include seizures, dementia, apparent blindness, ataxia, circling, mydriasis, and hypersalivation. Cardiopulmonary and neurologic signs rarely coexist. Sudden death is more likely in cats than in dogs and is thought to result from TE and acute respiratory distress.

Pulmonary crackles, muffled lung sounds (from pulmonary consolidation or pleural effusion), tachycardia, and, occasionally, a cardiac gallop sound or murmur may be found on auscultation. Serous pleural effusion from right-sided heart failure and syncope occur less commonly in cats than in dogs. Chylothorax, ascites, and, rarely, pneumothorax have also been associated with HWD in cats[25]. Caval syndrome develops in a few cats. Although heartworms usually cause significant pulmonary vascular disease, some infected cats have no clinical signs[20]. Peracute respiratory distress, ataxia, collapse, seizures, hemoptysis, or sudden death can occur[17, 18].

HEARTWORM TESTING
Serologic tests

Adult heartworm antigen (Ag) tests are the recommended method of heartworm screening in dogs. Heartworm Ag tests are quite accurate, and the monthly heartworm preventive drug treatment eventually eliminates microfilariae. ELISA, immunochromatographic, and hemagglutination test methods are available. Circulating Ag is detectable no earlier than about 5 months after infection, but antigenemia may not appear until after the development of microfilaremia (at about 6.5 months post infection). There is no reason to test puppies younger than 7 months for either Ag or microfilariae[1]. Likewise, it is recommended that testing of adults be done about 7 months after the end of the preceding heartworm transmission period. Depending on climate, this may require that monthly preventive drug treatment be started, or continued, prior to testing for possible infection during the preceding season. Commercially available test kits are immunoassays against Ag from the adult female heartworm reproductive tract[26]. These tests are nearly 100% specific and have good sensitivity when the manufacturer's directions are followed carefully. Most kits do not detect infections less than 5 months old, and male worms are not detected. Most serum/plasma kits can often detect infections with one live female worm, but sensitivity among available kits is variable[27, 28]. Weakly positive or ambiguous test results should be rechecked using a repeat test or a different Ag test kit, a microfilaria test, or thoracic radiographs, or a combination of these. False-positive test results usually stem from technical error; false-negative results are usually caused by a low worm burden, the presence of only immature female worms, a male unisex infection, or a cold test kit.

False-negative test results are more likely in cats because the worm burden is low and there is greater probability of male unisex infections. Therefore, heartworm Ag tests are not considered reliable for heartworm screening in cats[17]. In cats, Ag test results are negative during the first 5 months after infection and can be variably positive at 6–7 months; infections with mature female worms should be detected after 7 months.

Heartworm antibody (Ab) ELISA tests are available for cats and they use either recombinant Ag or heartworm Ag extract. These tests are used to screen for feline HWD; they have minimal to no cross-reactivity with GI parasitic infections[23, 28]. Serum Ab to both immature and adult worms is detected as early as 60 days post infection. Because heartworm larvae of either sex can provoke a host immune response, the Ab tests provide greater sensitivity than Ag tests; however, some immature heartworm larvae never develop into adults. A positive Ab test indicates exposure to migrating larvae as well as adults, not the presence of adult heartworms specifically[23]. A positive Ab test should be supported by other evidence (e.g. positive heartworm Ag, radiographs, echocardiography) before making a definitive diagnosis of HWD. The concentration of Ab does not appear to correlate well with the number of worms present, nor with the severity of clinical disease or the radiographic signs[24]. High Ab titers are often associated with death of a heartworm, and also with heavy infection. It is also unclear how long circulating Ab remains after heartworm infection is eliminated[23]. False-negative Ab tests occur in an estimated 3–14% of cases, usually in association with a single worm[20, 23, 29]. Therefore, a negative heartworm Ab test suggests either no heartworm infection, infection of less than 60 days duration, or a concentration of IgG Ab against the test Ag too low to be detected[23, 24]. If clinical findings suggest HWD despite a negative Ab test, testing can be repeated using a different Ab test and a heartworm Ag test. Chest radiographs and echocardiography are also recommended. Ab testing can also be repeated in a few months.

Detection of microfilariae

Tests for circulating microfilariae are not recommended for routine heartworm screening, but they are useful in identifying the patient as a reservoir of infection and to assess whether high numbers of microfilariae are present before administering a monthly preventive drug (see p. 367). Microfilaria testing is essential if diethylcarbamazine (DEC) is to be used as a heartworm preventive (see p. 367). The macrocyclic lactone preventive drugs, administered monthly, eventually eliminate microfilaremia by impairing female and also, possibly, male worm reproductive function. Most dogs receiving these drugs become amicrofilaremic after 6 months. An estimated 75–90% of heartworm-positive dogs that are not treated monthly with a macrolide have microfilaremia. Absence of circulating microfilariae ('occult' infection) in the remaining cases can result from immunologic destruction within the lung, unisex or sterile adult heartworms, or a prepatent infection. Occult infection is often associated with severe signs of disease. Other causes of false-negative microfilaria test results include low numbers of microfilariae and diurnal variation in the number of peripherally circulating microfilariae. Cats with HWD rarely have circulating microfilariae.

Microfilaria concentration tests use at least 1 ml of peripheral blood[28]. Nonconcentration tests, including fresh wet blood smear or spun-hematocrit-tube buffy coat examination, are more likely to miss low numbers of microfilariae, but allow microfilarial motility to be assessed[30]. *Dirofilaria* have a stationary rather than a migratory movement pattern. Concentration tests are done using either a millipore filter or by centrifugation with the modified Knott technique. Both tests lyse the RBCs and fix existing microfilariae. The modified Knott test is preferred for measuring body dimensions to differentiate *D. immitis* from nonpathogenic filarial species, such as *Acanthocheilonema* (formerly *Dipetalonema*) *reconditum* (*Table 63*)[1]. A false-positive microfilaria test can result when microfilariae are present in the absence of live adult worms.

OTHER DIAGNOSTIC FINDINGS
Dogs

Eosinophilia, basophilia, and monocytosis are inconsistent hematologic findings; <50% of dogs with HWD have eosinophilia. Mild regenerative anemia, likely from hemolysis, is present in <30% of cases. Thrombocytopenia can occur secondary to platelet consumption in the pulmonary arteries, especially after adulticide treatment. DIC also occurs with advanced disease. The immune response to the heartworms produces a polyclonal gammopathy. Mild to moderate elevation in liver enzyme activity and azotemia can occur. Proteinuria is present in

20–30% of affected dogs, especially those with advanced disease. Hypoalbuminemia can develop in severely affected animals.

Thoracic radiographs can be normal with mild disease, but changes develop rapidly in dogs with heavy worm burdens. Characteristic findings include centrally enlarged and tortuous lobar pulmonary arteries with peripheral blunting (554–557; also 55, p. 42), a pulmonary trunk bulge, and, eventually, RV enlargement[31, 32]. The caudal lobar arteries are usually affected most severely and are seen best on a DV view.

The width of these vessels is normally no larger than the 9th rib, at its intersection with the vessels. On a lateral view, the width of the cranial right lobar artery at its intersection with the 4th rib is no larger than the most narrow diameter of that rib in normal dogs. Enlargement of lobar pulmonary arteries, without concurrent venous distension, is strongly suggestive of HWD or other causes of PH. Caudal vena caval enlargement may also be seen; the reported normal maximal caval width is 0.75 +/- 0.03 times the length of the 5th thoracic vertebra[33]. Patchy pulmonary

Table 63 Morphologic differentiation of circulating microfilaria.

Smear	D. immitis	A. reconditum
Fresh smear	Undulate in one place	Move across field
Stained smear*	Straight body	Curved body
	Straight tail	Posterior extremity hook ('button hook' tail); inconsistent
	Tapered head	Blunt head
	>290 μm long	<275–280 μm long
	>6 μm wide	<6 μm wide

* Size criteria for lysate prepared using 2% formalin (modified Knott test); microfilariae tend to be smaller with lysate of filter tests. Width and morphology are the best discriminating factors.

554, 555 Lateral (554) and DV (555) views from an 8-year-old male German Shorthaired Pointer with severe heartworm-induced PA disease. Marked RV enlargement, main PA bulge (arrow, 555), and dilated lobar pulmonary arteries, especially to caudal lung lobes (arrowheads), are evident. The right caudal lobar artery is blunted. Mild peribronchial and perivascular interstitial infiltrates are also present.

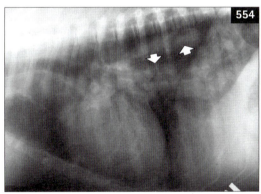

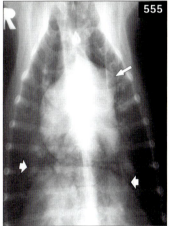

556, 557 Radiographs from an 11-year-old male mixed breed dog presented for weight loss and lethargy show mild pleural effusion, RV and main pulmonary artery enlargement, and bronchointerstitial infiltrates in the hilar and middle lung regions. The dog was positive for heartworm antibody.

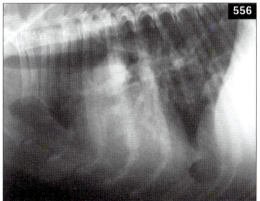

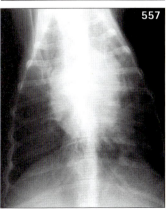

interstitial or alveolar infiltrates suggesting infarction, edema, pneumonia, or fibrosis are also common. Pulmonary opacities may be mainly perivascular. Radiographic evidence of severe pulmonary arterial disease and right heart enlargement is present when right-sided heart failure results from HWD.

The ECG is usually normal, although advanced disease may cause right axis deviation or an arrhythmia. Dogs with heartworm-induced CHF almost always have the ECG features of RV enlargement[34]. Tall P waves, suggesting RA enlargement, occur occasionally.

As with other causes of PH (see Chapter 23), echocardiographic findings in dogs with advanced HWD include RV and RA dilation, RV hypertrophy, paradoxical septal motion, a small left heart, and pulmonary artery dilation (558–560). Heartworms within the heart, proximal pulmonary artery, or vena cava appear as bright parallel linear echos, which are reflected from the parasite's body wall (559, 560)[35]. Multiple short heartworm echos are usually seen as the ultrasound beam transects various areas along the length of the worms. Suspected caval syndrome can be quickly confirmed by echocardiography (see p. 362). Any pleural, pericardial, or abdominal effusion can also be detected. Abnormal valve function and PH can be assessed using Doppler modalities (see Chapter 23, p. 344 and 561–563).

Cats

HWD is usually more difficult to diagnose in cats than in dogs. Serologic testing, thoracic radiographs, echocardiography, and, occasionally, microfilaria testing are helpful, but are not uniformly definitive. Feline heartworm Ab tests, while fairly sensitive, are not specific for adult heartworms (see above, p.354). The ELISA-based Ag tests are highly specific

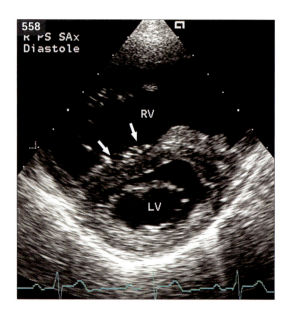

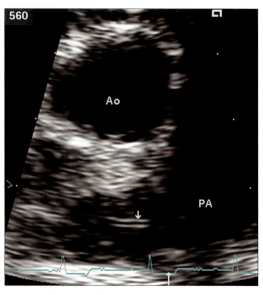

558–560 (558) 2-D echo image at end-diastole from a 6-year-old male mixed breed dog with severe HWD. RV hypertrophy and marked dilation are seen. High RV pressure caused flattening of the septum toward the LV (arrows). Echos from the open mitral and tricuspid valves are seen within their respective ventricles. (559) Echo image from the 7-year-old dam of the dog in 558. Heartworm-induced PH has dilated the RV outflow region and pulmonary arteries. Portions of heartworms are seen as bright parallel echos within the main and right pulmonary arteries (arrows). (560) A longer worm segment (arrow) is seen in the pulmonary artery from another middle-aged female dog. All images from right parasternal short-axis position. Ao = aortic root; LV = left ventricle; PA = pulmonary artery; RA = right atrium; RV = right ventricle.

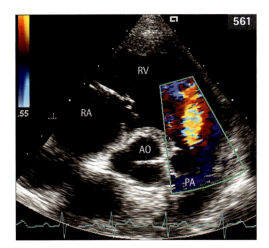

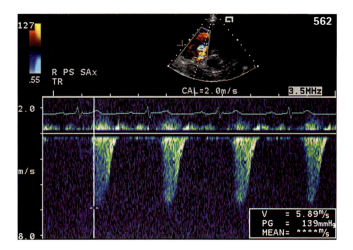

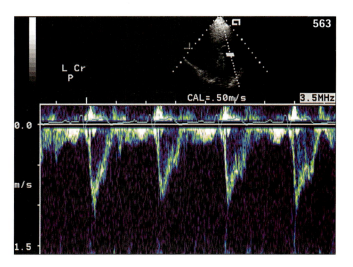

561–563 (561) Color flow Doppler image shows pulmonary insufficiency associated with heartworm-induced PH in the dog described in 558. RA and RV enlargement are also seen. Right parasternal short-axis view. (562) High velocity tricuspid valve regurgitation (TR, to almost 5.9 m/second; estimated RV-RA pressure gradient 139 mm Hg) was recorded in the same dog. (563) PW Doppler pulmonary (P) flow profile shows rapid acceleration with mild midsystolic notching consistent with the severe PH seen in this dog. 562, 563: left cranial short-axis views. Ao = aortic root; PA = pulmonary artery; RA = right atrium; RV = right ventricle.

for adult heartworm infection, but their sensitivity depends on the age, gender, and number of worms. Serologic test results may be negative early in the disease process, even when clinical signs exist. Acute death and severe clinical signs can occur in Ag-negative cats. Furthermore, postmortem diagnosis can be difficult if the worms are located in distal pulmonary arteries or aberrant sites. A positive Ag test result when no worms are found postmortem can occur with spontaneous worm death, ectopic infection, or when worms are missed during pulmonary evaluation. A low and transient microfilaremia, about 1–2 months in duration, occurs in about 50% of infected cats approximately 6.5–7 months after infection. Therefore, microfilaria concentration test results are usually negative, although a concentration test may still have value in an individual cat. A larger volume (e.g. 3–5 ml) of blood increases the probability of a positive result when microfilariae are present.

Between one and two thirds of infected cats have peripheral eosinophilia, usually between 4 and 7 months after infection[20, 24]. Often the eosinophil count is normal. Basophilia is uncommon. Mild nonregenerative anemia is found in about one third of cases[18]. Advanced pulmonary arterial disease and TE can be associated with neutrophilia (sometimes with a left shift), monocytosis, thrombocytopenia, and DIC. Hyperglobulinemia is the most common biochemical abnormality, but it occurs inconsistently. The prevalence of glomerulopathies in cats with HWD does not appear to be high[18].

Tracheal wash or bronchoalveolar lavage cytology can reveal an eosinophilic exudate consistent with allergic or parasitic disease, similar to that found with feline asthma or pulmonary parasites. Experimentally, this occurs between 4 and 8 months after infection[18]. Later in the disease, nonspecific chronic inflammation or unremarkable findings are seen on tracheal wash cytology. Pleural fluid from heartworm-induced right-sided heart failure is generally a modified transudate, although chylothorax occasionally develops.

The ECG is often normal[18], but cats that develop right-sided heart failure usually have changes suggesting RV enlargement (see *Table 11*, p. 61). Other considerations for such changes include congenital heart disease or a right bundle branch block with or without cardiomyopathy. Arrhythmias appear to be uncommon, but are more likely with advanced pulmonary arterial disease and CHF.

Radiographic findings can be similar to those in dogs with HWD, and may include pulmonary artery enlargement with or without visible tortuosity and pruning, RV or generalized cardiac enlargement, and diffuse or focal pulmonary bronchointerstitial infiltrates (**564–568**)[20, 24, 36]. The pulmonary artery and right heart changes are typically more subtle in cats.

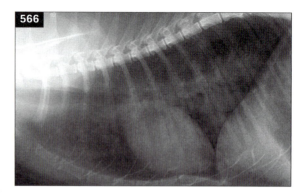

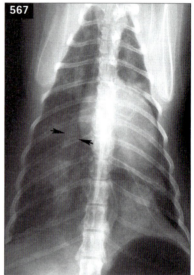

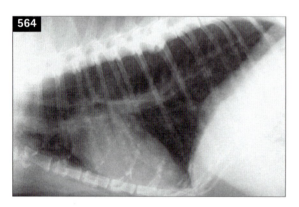

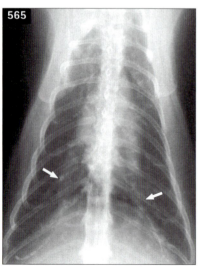

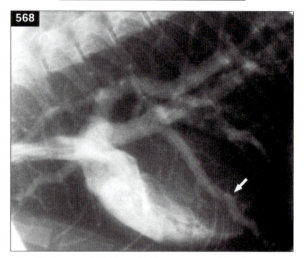

564, 565 Lateral (564) and DV (565) radiographs from a 13-year-old female cat with chronic cough and pulmonary crackles. The heart is normal size, but pulmonary artery enlargement is marked, especially in the caudal lung lobes (arrows, 565). A bronchointerstitial infiltrate is more pronounced in the caudal lobes. Heartworm serology was negative, but one adult worm was found at necropsy.

566–568 (566, 567) Radiographs from an 8-year-old male cat presented with dyspnea caused by heartworm-induced PTE. Extensive interstitial pulmonary infiltrates are seen in the caudal lobes. There is mild cardiomegaly. The right caudal pulmonary artery is markedly dilated (arrows, 567). The air-filled stomach in 567 indicates aerophagia. (568) Nonselective angiogram from a cat with HWD shows tortuous and dilated PAs. A linear filling defect is visible in the middle lobar artery (arrow).

The main pulmonary artery segment is not usually visible radiographically in cats because of its more medial location compared with dogs[36]. Experimentally, the pulmonary arteries enlarge within a few weeks to 7 months of adult worm transplantation[37]. The caudal lobar arteries appear abnormal more frequently and are best evaluated on a DV view. The right caudal lobar artery may be more prominent[36], but a left caudal pulmonary artery ≥1.6 x the width of the 9th rib at the 9th intercostal space was reported as the most discriminating radiographic finding for separating heartworm infected from noninfected cats[38]. Pulmonary artery enlargement tends to regress later in the disease process[36]. Marked right-sided heart enlargement is uncommon, but more likely when signs of right-sided heart failure (e.g. pleural effusion) are evident. Allergic pneumonitis as well as PTE cause pulmonary infiltrates; focal perivascular and interstitial changes are more common than diffuse infiltrates. Lobar consolidation, pleural effusion, or pneumothorax are uncommon findings[17]. Pulmonary hyperinflation is sometimes evident and, along with bronchointerstitial infiltrates, can mimic feline allergic bronchial lung disease[36]. Ascites occurs in some cats with HWD; it is rare in cats with heart failure from cardiomyopathy. Radiographs are normal in a small minority of heartworm-infected cats[20]. Pulmonary arteriography performed using a large-bore jugular vein catheter may confirm a suspected diagnosis of HWD in a cat with a false-negative antigen test result and normal echocardiogram. Morphologic changes in the pulmonary arteries are outlined, and worms appear as linear filling defects (568)[15, 18].

Echocardiography has allowed visualization of worms in 40–78% of positive cats, including some with negative heartworm Ab tests results[18, 20, 36, 39]. Higher numbers of worms increase the chance of echo identification, but echocardiographic findings can be normal unless worms extend into the heart, main pulmonary artery segment, or proximal right or left pulmonary arteries. Careful interrogation of the pulmonary arteries is important.

Necropsy is important for cats in which diagnosis is suspected but not confirmed and in cats with unexpected sudden death. Because single worms are easily overlooked, careful examination of the right heart, vena cavae and proximal and distal pulmonary artery segments is important. Ectopic sites, such as body cavities, systemic arteries, and CNS may harbor worms as well.

MANAGEMENT OF HEARTWORM DISEASE IN DOGS

Generally, adulticide treatment is recommended. The decision to withhold adulticide therapy in some asymptomatic dogs is controversial. Continuous monthly treatment with prophylactic doses of ivermectin kills late precardiac larvae and young adult heartworms (<7 months post infection), but this adulticide effect takes at least a year and possibly >2 years of continuous monthly treatment. Older worms are more resistant to the effects of ivermectin and may still cause clinical disease. An inactive dog with a low worm burden may not show clinical signs before the worms die naturally; however, progression of pulmonary disease or other sequelae (e.g. glomerulonephritis) may increase the risk of adulticide therapy in the future. Active dogs are probably more likely to develop clinical signs, even with a low worm burden; therefore, ivermectin is not recommended as a substitute for melarsomine unless conventional adulticide therapy is not permitted. The adulticidal effectiveness of other macrocyclic lactones appears to be less for selamectin and injectable moxidectin, and least for milbemycin oxime[40, 41]. If adulticide therapy is not provided, the dog should at least be treated continuously with ivermectin or, possibly, with selamectin or moxidectin.

The risk of postadulticide PTE is increased with preexisting signs of severe pulmonary vascular disease, especially in dogs with right-sided heart failure or a high worm burden. Pretreatment thoracic radiographs will indicate the degree of pulmonary arterial disease and parenchymal involvement. Other recommended preadulticide testing includes CBC, serum biochemistry profile, and urinalysis. A platelet count is especially important when pulmonary arterial disease is severe. A urine protein–creatinine ratio or quantification of urine protein loss can be useful if hypoalbuminemia or proteinuria is detected. A mild to moderate increase in liver enzyme activity can result from hepatic congestion related to HWD, but this does not preclude melarsomine therapy. Liver enzyme activity usually returns to normal within 1–2 months of heartworm treatment. Azotemia or severe proteinuria, or both, develop in some dogs with HWD. Prerenal azotemia should be corrected with fluid therapy before the start of adulticide treatment. Severe glomerular disease can be associated with marked hypoproteinemia, nephrotic syndrome, or renal tubular damage. Loss of antithrombin III, as well as other proteins, may increase the risk for TE in such animals. An exaggerated immune response to the dead worms may also occur.

Microfilaricide therapy is not necessary before adulticide treatment. Heartworm-positive dogs that are clinically stable may benefit from prophylactic doses of ivermectin given for 1–6 months prior to melarsomine. This reduces heartworm Ag mass by decreasing or eliminating circulating microfilariae and tissue migrating larvae, stunting immature worm growth, and damaging the adult female reproductive system. Delaying melarsomine for several months also allows late-stage larvae already present to mature more, thus increasing their susceptibility to its adulticidal effect. Microfilaria-positive dogs should be observed in the hospital after their first ivermectin dose (see p. 366). Aspirin is not recommended as a routine preadulticide treatment; convincing evidence for beneficial antithrombotic effect is lacking.

Melarsomine dihydrochloride is the preferred adulticide drug. Thiacetarsamide, its predecessor organic arsenical compound, is no longer being made. Melarsomine is effective against both immature and mature heartworms, but male worms are more susceptible. The worm kill can be controlled by adjusting the dose. Although melarsomine is a more effective adulticide than thiacetarsamide, it does not appear to cause greater risk of TE and PH[42].

The severity of disease is used to guide therapy (*Table 64*). Dogs with low risk for embolic complications (class 1 and early class 2 disease) are given the standard therapy (two doses of 2.5 mg/kg IM 24 hours apart). The drug should be given by deep IM injection into the epaxial lumbar muscles (L3 to L5 region), exactly as recommended by the manufacturer. Dogs with severe disease (class 3), or those in class 2 in which a more conservative approach is desired, are treated with the alternative dosing regimen. The alternative protocol (*Table 65*) is designed to partially reduce the worm burden with one initial injection, followed by the standard adulticide regimen 4–6 weeks later. The risk of fatal PTE from an initially heavy worm kill is reduced with this protocol. Many clinicians prefer the alternative protocol for most dogs[1, 43]. Dogs with caval syndrome (class 4) should not be given adulticide treatment until worms are surgically removed (see p. 364).

Melarsomine is rapidly absorbed from the IM injection site. Unchanged drug and a major metabolite are rapidly eliminated in the feces; a minor metabolite is excreted in the urine. The drug causes a local injection site reaction; this is clinically noticeable in about a third of treated dogs[43]. The lumbar muscle site provides good vascularity and lymphatic drainage, with minimal fascial planes. Gravity may also help prevent drug from leaking into subcutaneous tissues, where it can cause more irritation. Post-treatment coughing and (less often) dyspnea may be related to the HWD itself, although pulmonary congestion is a toxic effect of overdosing. Adverse effects in animals receiving recommended doses are generally mild. Clinical signs in dogs treated with melarsomine have usually been either behavioral (e.g. tremors, lethargy, unsteadiness and ataxia, restlessness), respiratory (panting, shallow breathing, labored respirations, crackles), or injection site related (edema, redness, tenderness, vocalization, increased AST and CK activities). Injection site reactions are generally mild to moderate and heal within 4(–12) weeks, although firm nodules can persist indefinitely at the sites. Occasional severe reaction occurs, including local neurologic complications[44]. General signs of lethargy, depression, and anorexia occur in

---

Table 64 Classification of heartworm disease severity in dogs.

1) Class 1: Asymptomatic to mild heartworm disease:

  a) Clinical signs either absent or only occasional cough, fatigue on exercise, or mild loss of condition present.

  b) No radiographic signs.

  c) No abnormal laboratory parameters.

2) Class 2: Moderate heartworm disease:

  a) Clinical signs may be absent, or occasional cough, fatigue on exercise, or mild loss of condition present.

  b) Radiographic signs present; may include RV enlargement, mild PA enlargement, circumscribed perivascular infiltrates, and/or mixed alveolar/interstitial infiltrates.

  c) Laboratory abnormalities present; may include mild anemia (PCV 0.2–0.3 l/l [20–30%]), with or without mild (2+) proteinuria.

3) Class 3: Severe heartworm disease:

  a) Clinical signs may include constant fatigue, persistent cough, dyspnea, cardiac cachexia (wasting), or other signs of right-sided heart failure (ascites, jugular distension and pulse).

  b) Radiographic signs include RV +/– RA enlargement, severe PA enlargement, circumscribed to diffuse mixed patterns of pulmonary infiltrates, +/– radiographic signs of pulmonary thromboembolism.

  c) Laboratory abnormalities include anemia (PCV <0.2 l/l [<20%]), other hematologic abnormalities, or proteinuria (>2+).

  d) Animals in class 3 should be stabilized prior to adulticide treatment and receive the alternative melarsomine protocol.

4) Class 4: Caval syndrome:

  a) See text, p. 362.

Table 65 Protocols for heartworm adulticide therapy in dogs.

1) Preparation:

    a) Confirm diagnosis.

    b) Pretreatment evaluation and management.

    c) Determine class (severity) of disease (see Table 64).

    d) Determine melarsomine dihydrochloride (Immiticide) treatment protocol.*

2) Standard treatment protocol (for class 1 and many class 2 dogs):

    a) Reconstitute melarsomine dihydrochloride as directed by manufacturer (use immediately or within 24 hours if refrigerated and protected from light).

    b) Draw 2.5 mg/kg of melarsomine into a syringe; attach a new, sterile needle: 23-gauge 2.5 cm (1 in) long for dogs <10 kg, or 22-gauge 3.75 cm (1.5 in) long for dogs >10 kg.

    c) Give by deep IM injection into lumbar (epaxial) musculature in the L3 to L5 region (record location of first injection); avoid subcutaneous leakage.

    d) Repeat steps a)–c) 24 hours after first dose; use alternative side for 2nd injection.

    e) Enforced rest for 4–6 weeks minimum; symptomatic treatment as needed.

3) Alternative treatment protocol (for class 3 and some class 2 dogs):

    a) Symptomatic treatment as needed; enforced rest.

    b) When animal's condition is stable, administer one dose of 2.5 mg/kg as described above in the standard treatment protocol.

    c) Continue enforced rest and symptomatic treatment as needed.

    d) One month (to 6 weeks) later, administer two more doses, 24 hours apart, according to the standard treatment protocol.

* See text (p. 360) for additional information.

about 15% or fewer dogs; other adverse effects, including fever, vomiting, and diarrhea, occur occasionally.

Melarsomine has a low margin of safety. Overdose can cause fatal pulmonary inflammation and edema. Collapse, severe salivation, vomiting, respiratory distress, stupor, and death occurred at triple the recommended dose in some dogs. Some clinical reversal of melarsomine toxicity can be achieved with dimercaprol (British Anti-Lewisite [BAL]) administered at 3 mg/kg IM. This will also decrease adulticide activity[45].

Strict rest should be enforced for 4–6 weeks after adulticide therapy to reduce the sequelae of adult worm death and PTE (see p. 365). The rest period for working dogs should probably be longer, because increased pulmonary blood flow in response to exercise exacerbates pulmonary capillary bed damage and subsequent fibrosis. Heartworm Ag test results should be negative by 6 months after successful treatment; testing at this time is recommended, although about 80% or more of dogs with mild to moderate HWD are heartworm Ag negative by 4 months after melarsomine. The decision to repeat treatment in a dog with persistent antigenemia is guided by the animal's overall health, performance expectations, and age. Seroconversion approaches 100% with repeated treatment; however, complete worm kill is probably not necessary and may not yield further clinical improvement.

Treatment of dogs with complicated heartworm disease

Immune-mediated pneumonitis occurs in some dogs. Manifestations of heartworm pneumonitis include a progressively worsening cough, tachypnea or dyspnea, pulmonary crackles heard on auscultation, and, sometimes, cyanosis, weight loss, and anorexia. Eosinophilia, basophilia, and hyperglobulinemia are inconsistent findings. Serologic tests for adult heartworms are usually positive. Diffuse interstitial and alveolar infiltrates are typically seen on chest radiographs, especially in the caudal lobes. These may resemble infiltrates of pulmonary edema or blastomycosis. Cardiomegaly or pulmonary lobar artery enlargement is frequently absent. Tracheal wash typically yields a sterile eosinophilic exudate with variable numbers of well-preserved neutrophils and macrophages. Glucocorticoid therapy (e.g. prednisone, 1–2 mg/kg/day initially) usually produces rapid improvement. Prednisone given in gradually tapered doses (to 0.5 mg/kg every other day) can be continued as needed and does not appear to adversely affect the adulticide efficacy of melarsomine.

Pulmonary eosinophilic granulomatosis is an uncommon syndrome that may be associated with HWD, although some affected dogs have negative heartworm tests. A hypersensitivity reaction to heartworm Ags or immune complexes, or both, is thought to contribute to its pathogenesis. Pulmonary granulomas consist of a mixed population of mononuclear and neutrophilic cells, with many eosinophils and macrophages. Bronchial smooth muscle proliferation within granulomas and abundant alveolar cells in the surrounding area are common; lymphocytic and eosinophilic perivascular infiltrates may also occur. Eosinophilic granulomas may concurrently involve lymph nodes, trachea, tonsils, spleen, GI tract, and the liver or kidneys. Clinical signs of pulmonary eosinophilic granulomatosis are similar to those of eosinophilic pneumonitis. Variable clinicopathologic findings include leukocytosis, neutrophilia, eosinophilia, basophilia, monocytosis, and hyperglobulinemia. An exudative, mainly eosinophilic, pleural effusion occasionally develops. Radiographic findings include multiple pulmonary nodules of varying size and distribution, with mixed alveolar and interstitial pulmonary infiltrates. Hilar and mediastinal lymphadenopathy may be seen. Eosinophilic granulomatosis associated with HWD is treated initially with prednisone (1–2 mg/kg q12h); however, additional cytotoxic therapy may be needed as well. Incomplete response and relapse are common, especially when therapy is reduced or discontinued. Heartworm adulticide treatment is given after pulmonary disease abates.

Severe pulmonary arterial disease is likely in dogs with a long-standing heartworm infection, with a heavy worm burden, and in active dogs. Clinical signs include severe cough, exercise intolerance, tachypnea or dyspnea, episodic weakness, syncope, weight loss, ascites, and death. Radiographic evidence of marked enlargement, tortuosity, and blunting of pulmonary arteries is common (554–557, p. 355). Pulmonary parenchymal infiltrates can lead to hypoxemia; these are treated with prednisone, as for eosinophilic pneumonitis, until resolved. Alternate day, low-dose prednisone (e.g. 0.5 mg/kg) should have beneficial antiinflammatory effects, but chronic high-dose corticosteroid therapy may reduce pulmonary blood flow, enhance the risk of TE, and inhibit vascular disease resolution. Thrombocytopenia (from platelet consumption) and hemolysis can occur in dogs with severe pulmonary arterial disease and TE; therefore, the PCV and platelet count should be monitored. DIC develops in some dogs. Conservative therapy with oxygen, prednisone, and a bronchodilator (e.g. theophylline), as for postadulticide TE (see p. 365), helps improve oxygenation and decrease pulmonary artery pressures. The alternative melarsomine protocol is used after the animal's condition is stabilized. Aspirin should be avoided, especially if hemoptysis is present. Prophylactic antibiotics are sometimes recommended because of the potential for devitalized pulmonary tissue and secondary bacterial infections to develop.

Right-sided CHF develops in some dogs with severe pulmonary arterial disease and hypertension. Typical signs include jugular venous distension or pulsation, ascites, syncope, exercise intolerance, and arrhythmias. Pleural or pericardial effusion can also develop. Other signs associated with pulmonary arterial and parenchymal disease may also be present. Treatment is as for dogs with severe pulmonary arterial disease, with the addition of furosemide (e.g. 1–2 mg/kg/day), an ACE inhibitor (e.g. enalapril, 0.5 mg/kg q12–24h), and a reduced-salt diet. The use of digoxin in this setting is controversial.

Mortality in dogs with severe HWD given melarsomine has been estimated to be 10%. This is similar to the mortality in dogs managed by strict cage confinement for 1 to more than 2 weeks before and 3–4 weeks after thiacetarsamide treatment. However, dogs treated with melarsomine can be confined at home with minimal pretreatment and post-treatment hospitalization. Historically, the survival rate in severely affected dogs treated with thiacetarsamide under similar conditions has been 53%.

Caval syndrome

The shock-like condition known as the (vena) caval syndrome occurs in heavily infected dogs when a mass of worms obstructs venous inflow to the heart and interferes with tricuspid valve function (569–571). This condition has also been called postcaval

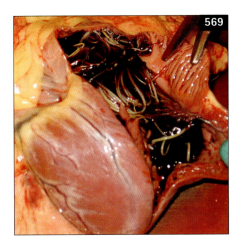

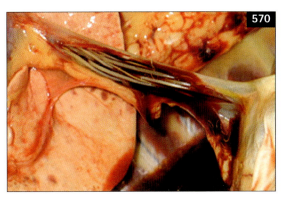

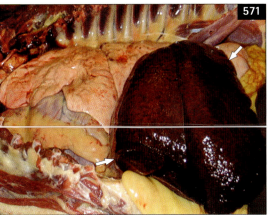

569–571 (569) Open RA (above) and RV (below) from a 9-year-old male dog with caval syndrome that was presented for a suspected abdominal mass. Numerous heartworms are seen within the intracardiac blood pool. (570) Caudal vena cava packed with heartworms from the same dog; heart is to the left, diaphragm on the right. (571) Pronounced hepatic congestion (arrows) from the caval obstruction in this dog (no other abdominal mass was found).

syndrome, acute hepatic syndrome, liver failure syndrome, dirofilarial hemoglobinuria, and vena cava embolism. Although adult heartworms prefer to be in the pulmonary arteries, as the worm burden increases, adult worms migrate upstream to the RA and caudal vena cava in rising numbers. Factors other than worm burden alone are probably also involved in the development of the caval syndrome[46, 47]. Experimentally, pulmonary artery pressures were higher in dogs that developed caval syndrome compared with dogs that did not but which had an equal worm burden[47]. This syndrome is more likely to occur in geographic areas where HWD is enzootic.

Many affected dogs have no history of heartworm-related signs. Acute collapse or weakness is common. Other signs include anorexia, tachypnea or dyspnea, pallor, hemoglobinuria, and bilirubinuria (572). A tricuspid insufficiency murmur, jugular distension and pulsations, weak pulses, a loud and possibly split S_2, and a cardiac gallop rhythm are often described. Coughing or hemoptysis and ascites sometimes occur. Partial RV inflow occlusion caused by the mass of the heartworms, in conjunction with PH and tricuspid insufficiency, lead to the development of right-sided congestive signs, severe hepatic congestion, and poor cardiac output.

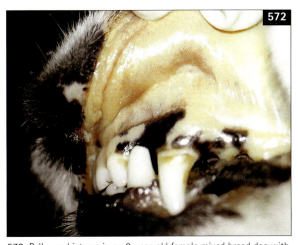

572 Pallor and icterus in an 8-year-old female mixed breed dog with hemolysis from caval syndrome.

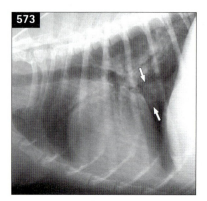

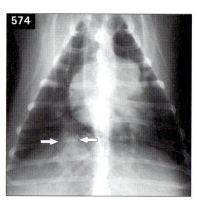

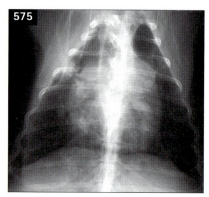

573–575 (573, 574) Radiographs from the dog in 572 on initial presentation. The caudal vena cava is markedly distended (arrows). A main pulmonary artery bulge, large and tortuous caudal right pulmonary artery, and patchy pulmonary infiltrates are also seen. (575) DV radiograph from the same dog taken within 24 hours after 10 adult heartworms were removed from the heart via jugular venotomy. Note the increase in RV filling.

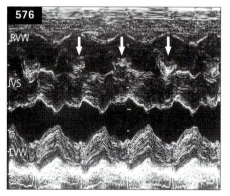

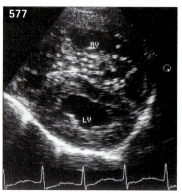

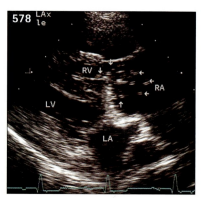

576–578 (576) M-mode echo from another, male dog with caval syndrome. The thick, irregular echos (arrows) seen in the RV in diastole are created by HWs entangled in the tricuspid valve. (577) 2-D short-axis image of RV and LV shows characteristic short, parallel echos from the mass of worms surrounding the tricuspid valve. RV hypertrophy and dilation and septal flattening are evident. (578) Long-axis view in systole from the dog in 572 shows the mass of HWs (arrows) in the RA. In diastole this mass moved into the RV. All images from right parasternal position. IVS = interventricular septum; LA = left atrium; LV = left ventricle; LVW = left ventricular wall; RA = right atrium; RV = right ventricle; RVW = right ventricular wall.

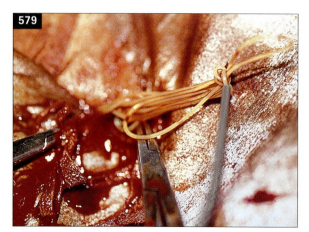

579 An endoscopic basket retrieval device was used to snare and remove heartworms from the RA via a jugular venotomy in the dog described in 573–575.

Clinicopathologic findings can include microfilaremia, Coombs-negative hemolytic anemia (from RBC trauma), azotemia, abnormal liver function with increased liver enzyme activity, and often DIC. Intravascular hemolysis causes hemoglobinemia and hemoglobinuria. Right heart and pulmonary artery enlargement are evident on thoracic radiographs (573–575). The ECG usually suggests RV enlargement. Ventricular and supraventricular premature complexes often occur[47]. Echocardiography reveals a mass of worms entangled at the tricuspid valve and in the RA, venae cavae, and, sometimes, within hepatic veins (576–578). RV dilation and hypertrophy, paradoxical septal motion, and a small LV are also features[47]. Unless treated, most dogs die within 24–72 hours from cardiogenic shock complicated by metabolic acidosis, DIC, anemia, and multiorgan failure.

The only effective therapy is physical removal of worms from the vena cava and RA as soon as possible. Usually, this is done via right jugular venotomy with the animal in left lateral recumbency (579)[19, 48]. Light sedatation, if necessary, and local anesthesia are used. Fluoroscopic guidance is preferred if available. Long alligator forceps, an endoscopic basket retrieval instrument, or horsehair brush device can be used to grasp and withdraw the heartworms through the jugular vein incision. The instrument is gently passed down the vein into the RA; some repositioning of the animal's neck or manipulation of the retrieval device may be needed to pass the instrument beyond the thoracic inlet. Resistance during withdrawal can occur if too many worms at one time, or a cardiovascular structure, has been grasped. Retrieval of as many worms as possible is the goal, with 5–6 unsuccessful attempts in sequence the end point. Survival in excess of 50–80% has been reported for dogs undergoing this procedure[49]. Right auricular cannulation performed via a thoracotomy has been described to remove worms in very small dogs[50]. Supportive care, including cautious IV fluid administration, is given during and after worm extraction. CVP monitoring helps in assessing the effectiveness of worm removal and fluid therapy. Treatment with digoxin or sodium bicarbonate is usually not necessary, but broad-spectrum antibiotic treatment is recommended. Monitoring for anemia, thrombocytopenia, DIC, and major organ dysfunction is important. Severe PTE and renal or hepatic failure are associated with poor outcome. Dogs that survive acute caval syndrome can be treated with adulticide a few weeks after being stabilized to eliminate remaining worms.

Use of flexible alligator forceps with fluoroscopic or transesophageal echo guidance has been used in heavily infected dogs without caval syndrome to reduce the worm burden in the main pulmonary artery and lobar branches before adulticide therapy. In dogs at high risk for post-treatment PTE, overall survival and recovery rate can be improved by prior physical worm removal[1]. Echocardiographic verification that worms are in accessible locations and appropriate technical facilities are needed for this procedure.

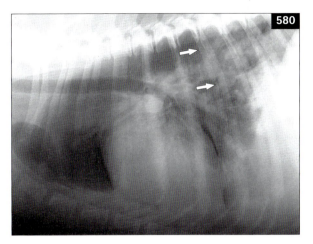

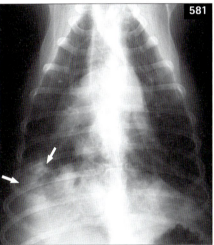

580, 581 Lateral (580) and DV (581) radiographs from a 7-year-old male Golden Retriever that had been given heartworm adulticide 1 week prior. The patchy interstitial infiltrates seen peripherally in the caudal lobes (arrows), especially on the right, are consistent with postadulticide PTE.

Postadulticide pulmonary thromboembolism

Exercise restriction during the 4–6 weeks after adulticide is critical to reducing the risk of PTE complications. Pulmonary arterial disease worsens from 5–30 days after adulticide therapy and is especially severe in dogs that had clinical signs of HWD before receiving the adulticide. Dead and dying worms cause thrombosis and pulmonary artery obstruction, with exacerbation of platelet adhesion, myointimal proliferation, villous hypertrophy, granulomatous arteritis, perivascular edema, and hemorrhage. Obstructed pulmonary flow and high vascular resistance further increase RV strain. Poor cardiac output can lead to hypotension and myocardial ischemia. Poor lung perfusion, hypoxic vasoconstriction and bronchoconstriction, pulmonary inflammation, and fluid accumulation can cause serious ventilation–perfusion mismatch. Severe pulmonary thromboembolization is most likely to occur from 7–17 days after adulticide therapy. As expected, the caudal and accessory lung lobes are most commonly and severely affected.

Clinical signs include depression, low-grade fever, tachycardia, tachypnea or dyspnea, cough, and hemoptysis, and, sometimes, right-sided heart failure signs, collapse, or death. Pulmonary crackles on auscultation result from lung inflammation and fluid accumulation. Focal lung consolidation can cause regionally muffled lung sounds. Patchy alveolar infiltrates with air bronchograms may be seen on thoracic radiographs, especially near the caudal lobar arteries (580, 581). A CBC may show thrombocytopenia or a regenerative left shift.

Symptomatic PTE is managed with strict rest (cage confinement) and glucocorticoid therapy to reduce pulmonary inflammation (prednisone, 1–2 mg/kg/day initially, then tapering). Supplemental O_2 therapy is recommended to reduce hypoxia-mediated pulmonary vasoconstriction[51]. A bronchodilator (e.g. aminophylline, 10 mg/kg PO, IM, or IV q8h; or theophylline, 9 mg/kg PO q6–8h), judicious fluid therapy, if there is evidence of cardiovascular shock, and cough suppressants may be useful. Antibiotics have been given empirically; however, their benefit is questionable unless concurrent bacterial infection is evident. Hydralazine has reduced pulmonary vascular resistance in some dogs experimentally, and some dogs seem to respond clinically to diltiazem[52], but systemic hypotension is a risk with vasodilators. Aspirin is not recommended because there is no convincing evidence that it has a beneficial antithrombotic effect or reduces pulmonary arteritis. In severe cases of PTE, heparin (see *Table 40*, p. 157) can be considered; however, excessive bleeding could be a serious adverse effect of such therapy. Low molecular weight heparin might provide a safer alternative to unfractionated heparin, but more experience is needed before definitive recommendations can be made.

In dogs that survive, endothelial changes regress within 4–6 weeks. PH and radiographic signs of arterial disease begin to resolve over the next several months.

Microfilaricide therapy

Specific microfilaricidal therapy for dogs with circulating microfilariae can be given 3–4 weeks after adulticide therapy, although the gradual micro-filaricidal effect of monthly preventive drugs has largely replaced the need for this. Ivermectin and milbemycin oxime have been used as rapid microfilaricidal drugs. Milbemycin oxime is microfilaricidal at the standard heartworm preventive dose (0.5–1.0 mg/kg). Ivermectin's microfilaricidal dose is 50 mcg/kg PO; this dose is also safe for Collies[53]. The rapid death of many microfilariae within 3–8 (and occasionally 12) hours of dosing can cause systemic effects, including lethargy, inappetence, salivation, retching, defecation, pallor, and tachycardia. Usually, such adverse effects are mild; however, dogs with high numbers of circulating microfilariae occasionally experience circulatory collapse. This usually responds to immediate IV fluid administration (e.g. 80 ml/kg over 2 hours) and shock glucocorticoid therapy (e.g. prednisolone sodium succinate, 10 mg/kg IV; or dexamethasone, 1 mg/kg IV). It is recommended that animals be observed closely for 8–12 hours after initial microfilaricide treatment with either milbemycin or ivermectin. An additional benefit of these drugs is prevention of new infection. Moxidectin and selamectin are also known to be microfilaricidal. Other drugs previously used as microfilaricides (e.g. levamisole and fenthion) are not recommended because of lower efficacy and frequent adverse effects.

MANAGEMENT OF HEARTWORM DISEASE IN CATS

Adulticide therapy is not usually recommended in light of the frequent severe complications in this species, the fact that cats are not a significant reservoir for heartworm transmission, and the potential for spontaneous cure because of a shorter heartworm life span in cats. No difference in survival was shown retrospectively between cats not given adulticide and those receiving thiacetarsamide[20]. Heartworm infected cats are managed conservatively with prednisone as needed for respiratory signs (or for radiographic evidence of pulmonary interstitial disease), a monthly heartworm preventive drug, and no adulticide treatment. Serologic heartworm testing (for both Ag and Ab) every 6–12 months is recommended to monitor infection status. Antigen-positive cats usually become negative within 4–5 months of worm death. It is unclear how long Ab tests remain positive. Serial thoracic radiographs and echocardiograms are also useful for monitoring cats with abnormal findings. Radiographically evident interstitial infiltrates usually respond to diminishing doses of prednisone (e.g. 2 mg/kg/day, reduced gradually during 2 weeks to 0.5 mg/kg every other day, then discontinued after 2 more weeks). This treatment can be repeated periodically if respiratory signs recur.

Severe respiratory distress and death may occur at any time, especially after worm death. PTE is more likely to be fatal in cats than in dogs. Clinical signs of PTE include fever, cough, dyspnea, hemoptysis, pallor, pulmonary crackles, tachycardia, and hypotension. Supportive radiographic findings include poorly defined, rounded, or wedge-shaped areas of interstitial (with or without alveolar) opacities that obscure associated pulmonary vessels. Supportive care for acutely ill cats can include IV glucocorticoids (e.g. 100–250 mg prednisone sodium succinate), fluid therapy, a bronchodilator, and supplemental O_2[17, 18]. Diuretics are not indicated. Aspirin or other nonsteroidal antiinflammatory drugs have not been shown to produce benefit, and may exacerbate pulmonary disease.

Right-sided CHF develops in some cats with severe pulmonary arterial disease. Cough, pulmonary parenchymal disease, or evidence of thromboembolic events may occur inconsistently. Dyspnea from pleural fluid accumulation and jugular venous distension or pulsation are common. RV enlargement is usually suggested by radiographic and ECG findings. Therapy for heart failure signs includes thoracocentesis as needed, cage confinement, and cautious furosemide therapy (e.g. 1 mg/kg q12–24h). An ACE inhibitor may be helpful. Digoxin therapy is not generally recommended. Other supportive care is guided by the cat's clinical progress and clinicopathologic abnormalities.

The caval syndrome occurs rarely in cats. Successful adult heartworm removal through a jugular venotomy has been reported[54, 55].

An adulticide is the therapy of last resort for cats that continue to manifest clinical signs despite prednisone treatment. Potentially fatal TE is possible even with only one worm present. About a third of adulticide-treated cats are expected to have TE complications; a higher risk is expected for heavily infected cats. Adulticide should not be given only on the basis of a positive Ag, Ab, or microfilaria test result. There is little clinical experience with using melarsomine in cats. Doses of >3.5 mg/kg appear to be toxic to cats[17]. Thiacetarsamide has been used successfully in cats, but acute respiratory failure and death can occur from dying worms or toxic effects of the arsenical drug[16, 54]. The adulticide efficacy of chronic ivermectin at prophylactic doses is unknown in cats.

Although technically challenging, several approaches have been described for removal of adult heartworms from cats. Worms in the RA and vena cava can be reached via right jugular venotomy using small alligator forceps, endoscopic grasping or basket retrieval forceps, or other devices[19, 54, 57, 58]. Worms in the pulmonary artery have been extracted using a left thoracotomy and pulmonary arteriotomy. Right thoracotomy and atriotomy have also been used successfully. Echocardiographic identification of worms in accessible locations is important prior to such a surgical procedure. Even if all the adult heartworms cannot be retrieved, surgical treatment may be a good alternative to conservative symptomatic treatment or adulticide in cats with heavy infection or persistent clinical signs. There is concern about potentially fatal anaphylactic reactions associated with worm breakage during these procedures. For this reason, pretreatment with a glucocorticoid and antihistamine has been suggested. It is unclear whether pretreatment for several days with heparin reduces thromboembolic events associated with surgical worm removal.

Microfilaricide therapy is usually not necessary since microfilaremia is brief, but ivermectin and milbemycin should be effective in this setting.

HEARTWORM PREVENTION

Dogs

Heartworm prophylaxis is indicated for all dogs in endemic areas. Because sustained warm and moist conditions are important for HWD transmission, the time of year when infection is possible is limited in many geographic areas. However, where heartworm transmission is likely during more than half the year, continuous chemoprophylaxis is generally more practical.

Several macrocyclic lactone drugs are currently available for preventing heartworm disease: the avermectins (ivermectin, selamectin) and the milbemycins (milbemycin oxime, moxidectin). Diethylcarbamazine (DEC) is also still available as a preventive agent. Preventive therapy can begin at 6–8 weeks of age. Before chemoprophylaxis is started for the first time, dogs old enough to have been previously infected should be tested for circulating heartworm Ag and, especially if DEC is to be used, for microfilariae. Retesting for circulating Ag should be done periodically; every 2–3 years is usually adequate. The avermectins and milbemycins induce neuromuscular paralysis and death in nematode (and arthropod) parasites by interacting with membrane chloride channels. They have anthelmintic activity against microfilariae, 3rd and 4th stage larvae, and, sometimes, young adult worms. They are almost 100% effective and exceptionally safe when used as directed, even in sensitive Collie dogs. Toxicosis from overdose of a macrocyclic lactone has usually been related to dose miscalculation when using a concentrated livestock preparation[1]. These agents have retroactive efficacy for at least 1 month with a single dose. The reachback effect remains high for at least an additional month.

The drugs used for monthly oral administration are ivermectin (6–12 mcg/kg), milbemycin oxime (0.5–1.0 mg/kg, which also controls hookworms), and moxidectin (3 mcg/kg). Selamectin is applied topically at the base of the neck between the shoulder blades at a monthly dose range of 6–12 mg/kg[59]. Efficacy is not affected by bathing or swimming 2 hours or longer after application[60]. All these drugs are packaged in monthly dose units according to body weight ranges. Administration should begin within 1 month of the start of the heartworm transmission season and continue to within 1 month after the transmission season ends. Year round administration may be preferable, depending on location. Sustained-release moxidectin, a subcutaneously injected suspension of drug-impregnated organic polymer microspheres, has protective effects lasting at least 6 months and possibly a year[61, 62, 63]. Safety concerns raised during postapproval experience are being investigated.

Selamectin effectively prevents HWD, kills adult fleas and prevents flea eggs from hatching, and controls ear mites in both dogs and cats. This drug also controls American dog tick infestation as well as feline hookworm and roundworm infections. A combination of milbemycin oxime with lufenuron is marketed for dogs for protection against heartworms, fleas, roundworms, hookworms, and whipworms. Ivermectin with pyrantel is available for roundworms and hookworms as well as heartworms.

DEC (3 mg/kg [6.6 mg/kg of the 50% citrate] q24h) has been used for many years for heartworm prophylaxis. In areas with cold winters the drug can be discontinued 2 months after a killing frost and reinstituted 1 month before the mosquito season in the spring. Before beginning, or restarting, DEC treatment, dogs must be negative for microfilariae (see above, p. 354). Puppies 6 months of age and older should also be tested for microfilariae. Annual microfilaria tests are strongly recommended, even in areas where the drug is given year round. DEC must be given every day to be effective. If a lapse in DEC administration of less than 6 weeks occurs, one dose of a monthly preventive drug should restore protection. With longer lapses, monthly chemoprophylaxis should be extended for a year. Dogs with microfilariae should not be given DEC because adverse reactions of variable severity can occur. These can include lethargy progressing to vomiting, diarrhea, bradycardia, hypovolemic shock, and, sometimes, death. High doses of IV dexamethasone (at least 2 mg/kg), fluids, and other supportive measures have been used to combat hypovolemia and shock; atropine is given for the control of severe bradycardia. Without clinical improvement in 3–5 hours, the condition is likely to be fatal. Adverse reactions to DEC do not occur in the absence of circulating microfilariae. Dogs on DEC prophylaxis and in which circulating microfilariae are subsequently discovered can be continued on the drug during adulticide and microfilaricide therapy.

Cats

Chemoprophylaxis is recommended for cats in endemic areas. Selamectin, ivermectin, and milbemycin oxime are marketed for heartworm prevention in cats. Selamectin is used at the same dose as for dogs (6–12 mg/kg, topically)[64]. Ivermectin is given PO at 24 mcg/kg monthly, which is four times the dose used in dogs[18]. Milbemycin oxime's minimum recommended dose is 2 mg/kg, also higher than the dose used in dogs. All are safe in kittens 6 weeks or older. Heartworm Ag testing is recommended prior to starting prophylaxis if infection could have occurred at least 8 months before. These drugs can be given to seropositive cats. The heartworm prophylactic efficacy of moxidectin and DEC in cats is unknown.

ANGIOSTRONGYLUS VASORUM

Angiostrongylus vasorum is a metastrongyloid nematode that infects dogs and a variety of wild carnivores. This parasite, sometimes known as the French heartworm, is endemic in parts of Europe, the UK, and Africa; it occurs sporadically in other parts of the world[65–69]. The adult worms live in the pulmonary arteries and right heart. Eggs are carried into the pulmonary capillaries, where they hatch. The L1 migrate through the alveolar epithelium into the airways, are coughed up, swallowed, and passed in the feces. Maturation of the L1 into the infective L3 occurs within a molluscan (slug or snail) intermediate host. Frogs can also act as intermediate or paratenic hosts[65]. When a dog, or other host, eats the intermediate host, the L3 migrate from the small intestine through abdominal lymph nodes and liver to

the heart and pulmonary arteries. Larvae can be detected in the definitive host's feces after a prepatent period of about 6 weeks[66]. Ectopic worm migration is also reported[65].

Pathologic features include pleural thickening and fibrosis, lymphadenopathy, and multifocal pulmonary hemorrhagic and granulomatous lesions, especially in peripheral lung areas. Adult worms cause intimal proliferation and thrombosis in the pulmonary arteries[66]. Signs of acute right-sided heart failure, presumably secondary to PH, are noted in occasional cases[69].

Clinical manifestations of infection can be variable and are sometimes absent. Respiratory signs, such as cough and dyspnea, related to inflammation in response to parasite eggs or migrating larvae are common. Hemorrhagic diathesis, thought to be related to intravascular coagulation and consumptive coagulopathy in response to parasite antigens, is also frequently described[70]. Lethargy, exercise intolerance, syncope, vomiting, and diarrhea can occur[65]. Neurologic signs can be associated with intracranial hemorrhage[71]. Physical findings may be nonspecific, but increased pulmonary sounds and tachypnea are common. Low-grade fever, pulmonary crackles, and cardiac murmur have been noted in some cases.

Thoracic radiographs typically show bronchial thickening and patchy alveolar and interstitial infiltrates with a peripheral or multifocal distribution[65, 72]. Pulmonary alveolar infiltrates become most severe at about 7–9 weeks, at the time the infection becomes patent[73]. Later, the interstitial pattern becomes predominant as alveolar infiltrates regress. RV enlargement and pulmonary artery blunting appear to be uncommon[69, 72, 73]. Laboratory tests may show eosinophilia or other white blood cell abnormality, thrombocytopenia, mild to moderate regenerative anemia, and/or mild to moderate hyperglobulinemia. Hypercalcemia occurs in some cases[74]. Coagulation times can be prolonged[65, 70, 71]. Airway washings can show neutrophilic or eosinophilic inflammation; larvae are more likely to be found when inflammation is present. Fecal examination using the Baermann technique is diagnostic when larvae are being shed. Larvae are about 320 μm x 18 μm in size, with a wavy tail and a cephalic button[69].

Therapy using milbemycin oxime (0.5 mg/kg weekly for 4 weeks)[67] or fenbendazole (50 mg/kg daily for 10–14 days; most effective duration unclear – a range of 5–21 days is reported)[65] has been successful. Supportive therapy, including supplemental O_2, a glucocorticoid, and a bronchodilator, may be needed. Most cases have responded well to therapy, but the infection can be fatal for dogs with severe respiratory signs[65].

REFERENCES

1 Executive Board, American Heartworm Society (2005) 2005 guidelines for the diagnosis, prevention, and management of heartworm (*Dirofilaria immitis*) infection in dogs. *American Heartworm Society*; www.heartwormsociety.org

2 Wright JC, Hendrix CM, Brown RG (1989) Dirofilariasis. *J Am Vet Med Assoc* **194**:644–648.

3 Bazzocchi C, Genchi C, Paltrinieri S *et al.* (2003) Immunological role of the endosymbionts of *Dirofilaria immitis*: the *Wolbachia* surface protein activates canine neutrophils with production of IL-8. *Vet Parasitol* **117**:73–83.

4 Morchon R, Ferreira AC, Martin-Pacho JR *et al.* (2004) Specific IgG antibody response against antigens of *Dirofilaria immitis* and its *Wolbachia* endosymbiont bacterium in cats with natural and experimental infections. *Vet Parasitol* **125**:313–321.

5 Atkins CE, Keene BW, McGuirk SM (1988) Pathophysiologic mechanism of cardiac dysfunction in experimentally induced heartworm caval syndrome in dogs: an echocardiographic study. *Am J Vet Res* **49**:403–410.

6 Kitoh K, Watoh K, Chaya K *et al.* (1994) Clinical, hematologic, and biochemical findings in dogs after induction of shock by injection of heartworm extract. *Am J Vet Res* **55**:1535–1541.

7 Kitoh K, Watoh K, Kitagawa H *et al.* (1994) Blood coagulopathy in dogs with shock induced by injection of heartworm extract. *Am J Vet Res* **55**:1542–1547.

8 Kitoh K, Katoh H, Kitagawa H *et al.* (2001) Role of histamine in heartworm extract-induced shock in dogs. *Am J Vet Res* **62**:770–774.

9 Kitagawa H, Kitoh K, Inoue H *et al.* (2000) Plasma renin activities, angiotensin II concentrations, atrial natriuretic peptide concentrations and cardiopulmonary function values in dogs with severe heartworm disease. *J Vet Med Sci* **62**:453–455.

10 Buoro IBJ, Atwell RB, Tummy T (1992) Plasma levels of renin and aldosterone in right-sided congestive heart failure due to canine dirofilariasis. *Canine Pract* **17**:21–24.

11 Paes-de-Almeida EC, Ferreira AM, Labarthe NV *et al.* (2003) Kidney ultrastructural lesions in dogs experimentally infected with *Dirofilaria immitis*. *Vet Parasitol* **113**:157–168.

12 Frank J, Nutter FB, Kyles AE *et al.* (1997) Systemic arterial dirofilariasis in five dogs. *J Vet Intern Med* **11**:189–194.

13 Carastro SM, Dugan SJ, Paul AJ (1992) Intraocular dirofilariasis in dogs. *Compend Cont Educ Pract Vet* **14**:209–217.

14 Browne LE, Carter TD, Levy JK *et al.* (2005) Pulmonary arterial disease in cats seropositive for *Dirofilaria immitis* but lacking adult heartworms in the heart and lungs. *Am J Vet Res* **66**:1544–1549.

15 Rawlings CA (1990) Pulmonary arteriography and hemodynamics during feline heartworm disease: effects of aspirin. *J Vet Intern Med* **4**:285–291.

16 Rawlings CA, Farrell RL, Mahood RM (1990) Morphologic changes in the lungs of cats experimentally infected with *Dirofilaria immitis*. *J Vet Intern Med* **4**:292–300.

17 Executive Board, American Heartworm Society (2005) 2005 guidelines for the diagnosis, prevention, and management of heartworm (*Dirofilaria immitis*) infection in cats. *American Heartworm Society*; www.heartwormsociety.org

18 Dillon R (1998) Clinical significance of feline heartworm disease. *Vet Clin North Am: Small Anim Pract* **28**:1547–1565.

19 Rawlings CA, Calvert CA, Glaus TM *et al.* (1994) Surgical removal of heartworms. *Semin Vet Med Surg* **9**:200–205.

20 Atkins C, DeFrancesco TC, Coats JR *et al.* (2000) Heartworm infection in cats: 50 cases (1985–1997). *J Am Vet Med Assoc* **217**:355–358.

21 Kramer L, Genchi C (2002) Feline heartworm infection: serological survey of asymptomatic cats living in northern Italy. *Vet Parasitol* **104**:43–50.

22 Atkins C, DeFrancesco TC, Miller MW *et al.* (1998) Prevalence of heartworm infection in cats with signs of cardiorespiratory abnormalities. *J Am Vet Med Assoc* **212**:517–520.

23 Snyder PS, Levy JK, Salute ME *et al.* (2000) Performance of serologic tests used to detect heartworm infection in cats. *J Am Vet Med Assoc* **216**:693–700.

24 Dillon AR, Brawner WR, Robertson-Plouch CK *et al.* (2000) Feline heartworm disease: correlations of clinical signs, serology, and other diagnostics – results of a multi-center study. *Vet Ther* **1**:176–182.

25 Smith JW, Scott-Moncrieff JC, Rivera BJ (1998) Pneumothorax secondary to *Dirofilaria immitis* infection in two cats. *J Am Vet Med Assoc* **213**:91–93.

26 Goodwin JK (1998) The serologic diagnosis of heartworm infection in dogs and cats. *Vet Clin North Am: Small Anim Pract* **13**:83–87.

27 Atkins CE (2003) Comparison of results of three commercial heartworm antigen test kits in dogs with low heartworm burdens. *J Am Vet Med Assoc* **222**:1221–1223.

28 Datz C (2003) Update on canine and feline heartworm tests. *Compend Cont Educ Pract Vet* **25**:30–40.

29 Robertson-Plouch CK (1998) Prevalence of heartworm infections among cats with respiratory and gastrointestinal signs: results of a multicenter study. In: *Proceedings of the American Heartworm Symposium*, Batavia. MD Soll, DH Knight (eds)., pp. 57–62.

30 Courtney CH, Zeng Qy (2001) Relationship between microfilaria count and sensitivity of the direct

smear for diagnosis of canine dirofilariasis. *Vet Parasitol* **94**:199–204.

31 Ackerman N (1987) Radiographic aspects of heartworm disease. *Semin Vet Med Surg* **2**:15–27.

32 Polizopoulou ZS, Koutinas AF, Saridomichelakis MN *et al.* (2000) Clinical and laboratory observations in 91 dogs infected with *Dirofilaria immitis* in northern Greece. *Vet Rec* **146**:466–469.

33 Litster A, Atkins C, Atwell R *et al.* (2005) Radiographic cardiac size in cats and dogs with heartworm disease compared with reference values using the vertebral heart scale method: 53 cases. *J Vet Cardiol* **7**:33–40.

34 Calvert CA, Losonsky JM, Brown J *et al.* (1986) Comparisons of radiographic and electrocardiographic abnormalities in canine heartworm disease. *Vet Radiol* **27**:2–7.

35 Badertscher RR, Losonsky JM, Paul AJ *et al.* (1988) Two-dimensional echocardiography for diagnosis of dirofilariasis in nine dogs. *J Am Vet Med Assoc* **193**:843–846.

36 Selcer BA, Newell SM, Mansour AE *et al.* (1996) Radiographic and 2-D echocardiographic findings in eighteen cats experimentally exposed to *D. immitis* via mosquito bites. *Vet Radiol Ultrasound* **37**:37–44.

37 Brawner WR, Dillon AR, Robertson-Plouch CK *et al.* (2000) Radiographic diagnosis of feline heartworm disease and correlation to other clinical criteria: results of a multicenter clinical case study. *Vet Ther* **1**:81–87.

38 Schafer M, Berry CR (1995) Cardiac and pulmonary artery mensuration in feline heartworm disease. *Vet Radiol Ultrasound* **36**:499–505.

39 DeFrancesco TC, Atkins CE, Miller MW *et al.* (2001) Use of echocardiography for the diagnosis of heartworm disease in cats: 43 cases (1985–1997). *J Am Vet Med Assoc* **218**:66–69.

40 McCall JW (2005) The safety-net story about macrocyclic lactone heartworm preventives: a review, an update, and recommendations. *Vet Parasitol* **133**:197–206.

41 Dzimianski MT, McCall JW, Steffens WL *et al.* (2001) The safety of selamectin in heartworm infected dogs and its effect on adult worms and microfilariae. In *Recent Advances in Heartworm Disease Symposium,* Batavia. RL Seward (ed). pp. 135–140.

42 Rawlings CA, Raynaud JP, Lewis RE *et al.* (1993) Pulmonary thromboembolism and hypertension after thiacetarsamide vs melarsomine dihydrochloride treatment of *Dirofilaria immitis* infection in dogs. *Am J Vet Res* **54**:920–925.

43 Atkins CE, Miller MW (2003) Is there a better way to administer heartworm adulticidal therapy? *Vet Med* **98**:310–317.

44 Hettlich BF, Ryan K, Bergman RL *et al.* (2003) Neurologic complications after melarsomine dihydrochloride treatment for *Dirofilaria immitis* in three dogs. *J Am Vet Med Assoc* **223**:1456–1461.

45 Atwell RB, Seridan AD, Buoro IBJ *et al.* (1989) Effective reversal of induced arsenic toxicity using BAL therapy. In: *Proceedings of the 1989 Heartworm Symposium*, Washington DC, pp. 155–158.

46 Hidaka Y, Hagio M, Murakami T *et al.* (2003) Three dogs under 2 years of age with heartworm caval syndrome. *J Vet Med Sci* **65**:1147–1149.

47 Atkins CE, Keene BW, McGuirk SM (1988) Investigation of caval syndrome in dogs experimentally infected with *Dirofilaria immitis*. *J Vet Intern Med* **2**:36–40.

48 Jackson RF, Seymour WG, Growney PJ *et al.* (1977) Surgical treatment of caval syndrome of canine heartworm disease. *J Am Vet Med Assoc* **171**:1065–1069.

49 Kitagawa H, Kitoh K, Ohba Y *et al.* (1998) Comparison of laboratory test results before and after surgical removal of heartworms in dogs with vena caval syndrome. *J Am Vet Med Assoc* **213**:1134–1136.

50 Kuntz CA, Smith-Carr S, Huber M *et al.* (1996) Use of a modified surgical approach to the right atrium for retrieval of heartworms in a dog. *J Am Vet Med Assoc* **208**:692–694.

51 Rawlings CA, Tackett RL (1990) Postadulticide pulmonary hypertension of canine heartworm disease: successful treatment with oxygen and failure of antihistamines. *Am J Vet Res* **51**:1565–1569.

52 Atkins CE, Keene BW, McGuirk SM *et al.* (1994) Acute effect of hydralazine administration on pulmonary artery hemodynamics in dogs with chronic heartworm disease. *Am J Vet Res* **55**:262–269.

53 Hopper K, Aldrich J, Haskins SC (2002) Ivermectin toxicity in 17 collies. *J Vet Intern Med* **16**:89–94.

54 Glaus TM, Jacobs GJ, Rawlings CA *et al.* (1995) Surgical removal of heartworms from a cat with caval syndrome. *J Am Vet Med Assoc* **206**:663–666.

55 Takehashi N, Matsui A, Sasai H *et al.* (1987) Feline caval syndrome: a case report. *J Am Anim Hosp Assoc* **24**:645–649.

56 Turner JL, Lees GE, Brown SA *et al.* (1991) Thiacetarsamide in healthy cats: clinical and pathological observations. *J Am Anim Hosp Assoc* **27**:275–280.

57 Brown WA, Thomas WP (1998) Surgical treatment of feline heartworm disease. In: *Proceedings of the 16th Annual ACVIM Scientific Forum*, San Diego, p. 88.

58 Borgarelli M, Venco L, Piga PM *et al.* Surgical removal of heartworms from the right atrium of a cat. *J Am Vet Med Assoc* **211**(1): 68–69.

59 Novotny MJ, Krautmann MJ, Ehrhart JC *et al.* (2000) Safety of selamectin in dogs. *Vet Parasitol* **91**:377–391.

60 McTier TL, Shanks DJ, Watson P *et al.* (2000) Prevention of experimentally induced heartworm (*Dirofilaria immitis*) infections in dogs and cats with a single topical

application of selamectin. *Vet Parasitol* **91**:259–268.

61 Genchi C, Rossi L, Cardini G *et al.* (2002) Full season efficacy of moxidectin microsphere sustained-release formulation for the prevention of heartworm (*Dirofilaria immitis*) infection in dogs. *Vet Parasitol* **110**:85–91.

62 Lok JB, Knight DH, Wang GT *et al.* (2001) Activity of an injectable, sustained-release formulation of moxidectin administered prophylactically to mixed breed dogs to prevent infection with *Dirofilaria immitis*. *Am J Vet Res* **62**:1721–1726.

63 Holm-Martin M, Atwell R (2004) Evaluation of a single injection of a sustained-release formulation of moxidectin for prevention of experimental heartworm infection after 12 months in dogs. *Am J Vet Res* **65**:1596–1599.

64 Krautmann MJ, Novotny MJ, De Keulenaer K *et al.* (2000) Safety of selamectin in cats. *Vet Parasitol* **91**:393–403.

65 Chapman PS, Boag AK, Guitian J *et al.* (2004) *Angiostrongylus vasorum* infection in 23 dogs (1999–2002). *J Small Anim Pract* **45**:435–440.

66 Prestwood AK, Greene CE, Mahaffey EA *et al.* (1981) Experimental canine angiostrongylosis: I. Pathologic manifestations. *J Am Anim Hosp Assoc* **17**:491–497.

67 Conboy G (2004) Natural infections of *Crenosoma vulpis* and *Angiostrongylus vasorum* in dogs in Atlantic Canada and their treatment with milbemycin oxime. *Vet Rec* **155**:16–18.

68 Bolt G, Monrad J, Koch J *et al.* (1994) Canine angiostrongylosis: a review. *Vet Rec* **135**:447–452.

69 Patteson MW, Gibbs C, Wotton PR *et al.* (1993) *Angiostrongylus vasorum* infection in seven dogs. *Vet Rec* **133**:565–570.

70 Schelling CG, Greene CE, Prestwood AK *et al.* (1986) Coagulation abnormalities associated with acute *Angiostrongylus vasorum* infection in dogs. *Am J Vet Res* **47**:2669–2673.

71 Garosi LS, Plat SR, McConnell JF *et al.* (2005) Intracranial hemorrhage associated with *Angiostrongylus vasorum* infection in three dogs. *J Small Anim Pract* **46**:93–99.

72 Boag AK, Lamb CR, Chapman PS *et al.* (2004) Radiographic findings in 16 dogs infected with *Angiostrongylus vasorum*. *Vet Rec* **154**:426–430.

73 Mahaffey MB, Losonsky JM, Prestwood AK *et al.* (1981) Experimental canine angiostrongylosis: II. Radiographic manifestations. *J Am Anim Hosp Assoc* **17**:499–502.

74 Boag AK, Murphy KF, Connolly DJ (2005) Hypercalcemia associated with *Angiostrongylus vasorum* in three dogs. *J Small Anim Pract* **46**:79–84.

25
Systemic Hypertension

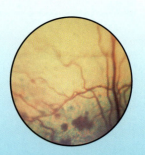

OVERVIEW

Systemic arterial hypertension in dogs and cats is associated with a number of diseases. Persistently elevated arterial pressure can have serious consequences, even though outward signs may be absent. Although the distinction between 'normal' and 'abnormally elevated' arterial pressure is not always clear, an average normal canine blood pressure (BP) across breeds is ~133/75 mm Hg (oscillometric technique)[1, 2]. Breed-related variation in BP and, sometimes, variation related to age, gender and reproductive status, or body size are reported[1–7]. The average values for systolic, diastolic, and mean BP in large and giant breed dogs are generally lower than in small breed dogs, except for sight hounds (~149/87 mm Hg)[2]. The higher pressures observed in sight hounds appear to be functional and not associated with signs of disease[1, 6, 7]. Various BP ranges have also been reported in normal cats studied noninvasively[8, 9]. An average normal BP in cats is about 124/84 mm Hg (oscillometric technique)[2]. An age-related increase in BP has been inconsistently observed, but feline BP does not appear to be influenced by breed[2, 9–11]. Variation in measured BP can be related to technique (direct and various noninvasive methods), as well as to patient anxiety[4, 12–16]. The so-called 'white coat' effect of increased BP related to anxiety at the doctor's office has been reported[17, 18]. Systolic BP can exceed 180 mm Hg in some stressed normal animals. There may be some diurnal effect on BP[19].

In general, according to the Veterinary Blood Pressure Society, repeatable (on at least 3 occasions) pressures of 150–160 mm Hg systolic and 95–100 mm Hg diastolic constitute mild hypertension; an additional 20 mm Hg is allowed for specific breed differences (e.g. for sight hounds). Moderate hypertension exists with BP between 160–180 mm Hg systolic and 100 to 120 mm Hg diastolic (plus ~30 mm Hg for specific breed differences). Arterial pressures >180/120 mm Hg (plus ~50 mm Hg for specific breeds) constitute severe hypertension[20].

Some dogs and cats clearly have clinical disease caused by hypertension, but many with 'abnormally high' BP have no evidence of related pathology, although a predisposing disease may be present. Repeated BP measurement over time is indicated before making a diagnosis of hypertension. Animals with mild hypertension and some animals with moderate hypertension may not need specific antihypertensive therapy, only treatment of the underlying disease. Severe hypertension should be treated to prevent or reduce end-organ damage. Emergency antihypertensive therapy is necessary in some animals (see p. 378).

Hypertension in dogs and cats is usually secondary to another disease, rather than a primary condition (idiopathic or essential hypertension)[20–22]. Diseases that have been associated with hypertension are listed in *Table 66*[8, 23–40]. BP should be measured when such diseases are diagnosed, and periodically thereafter, because of the increased risk for hypertension in these patients. Conversely, hypertension discovered during a routine examination may be an early marker of such underlying disease[20]. Drugs that cause vasoconstriction, including topical ocular phenylephrine, can transiently increase BP[41]. Obesity has also been associated with higher BP in dogs[1, 42]. While inherited essential hypertension has been documented in dogs and appears to occur in some cats, it is uncommon in animals[43–45]. Essential hypertension is a diagnosis of exclusion.

PATHOPHYSIOLOGY

BP is a function of cardiac output and peripheral vascular resistance (CO = P/R). There is continuous interplay between these parameters and the factors that influence them. Conditions that raise cardiac output (i.e. increased heart rate, stroke volume, and/or blood volume) or that increase vascular resistance tend to raise BP. Normally, arterial pressure is maintained within narrow limits by the actions of the autonomic nervous system (including arterial baroreceptors), hormonal systems (e.g. renin-angiotensin system, aldosternone, vasopressin/antidiuretic hormone, and

Table 66 Diseases associated with hypertension in dogs and cats.

1) Renal disease (tubular, glomerular, vascular).
2) Hyperadrenocorticism.
3) Hyperthyroidism.
4) Diabetes mellitus.
5) Liver disease.
6) Pheochromocytoma.
7) Hyperaldosteronism.
8) Intracranial lesions (↑ intracranial pressure).
9) High-salt diet (?).
10) Obesity.
11) Chronic anemia (cats).
12) Other conditions associated with hypertension in people:
    a) Acromegaly.
    b) Inappropriate antidiuretic hormone secretion.
    c) Hyperviscosity/polycythemia.
    d) Renin-secreting tumors.
    e) Hypercalcemia.
    f) Hypothyroidism with atherosclerosis.
    g) Hyperestrogenism.
    h) Coarctation (narrowing) of the aorta.
    i) Pregnancy.
    j) Central nervous system disease.

atrial natriuretic peptide), endothelial signaling mechanisms, vasodilatory prostaglandins, and blood volume regulation by the kidney[2, 21].

BP can become abnormally high with enhanced sympathetic nervous activity or responsiveness (e.g. hyperthyroidism, hyperadrenocorticism), increased catecholamine production (e.g. pheochromocytoma), or volume expansion secondary to sodium retention (e.g. renal failure, hyperaldosteronism, acromegaly, hyperadrenocorticism). Hypertension in dogs and cats with chronic renal failure may develop if decreased glomerular filtration rate (GFR) and reduced sodium excretion increase blood volume, poor renal blood flow or localized renal ischemia activates the renin-angiotensin-aldosterone cascade, or production of vasodilator substances (e.g. prostaglandins, kallikreins) decreases. Effects related to secondary hyperparathyroidism may also be involved. High BP has been associated with low serum potassium in animals with renal disease[27, 37]. Renin-angiotensin-aldosterone activation, with subsequent salt and

water retention and vasoconstriction, can also result from enhanced angiotensinogen production (e.g. hyperadrenocorticism) and diseases that increase sympathetic nervous activity or interfere with renal perfusion (e.g. hyperthyroidism, renal artery obstruction). Other conditions can also cause or facilitate hypertension.

Pathologic effects of hypertension
High perfusion pressure can damage capillary beds, but increases or decreases in arterial BP invoke vasoconstriction, or dilation, of arterioles that supply local capillary beds in most tissues. This vascular autoregulation normally protects capillaries from large pressure fluctuations and maintains constant flow when arterial BP ranges from about 60–160 mm Hg[46]; however, underlying organ disease can interfere with normal autoregulation. Also, prolonged arteriolar constriction secondary to chronic hypertension leads to vascular remodeling (e.g. medial hypertrophy), which can further increase vascular resistance. Vascular structural changes and spasm can cause local hypoxia, tissue damage, hemorrhage, and infarction[20, 47, 48]. Variable signs of organ dysfunction then result. The eye, kidney, heart, and brain are particularly vulnerable to damage from chronic hypertension and its associated vascular changes[22, 47]. These are often referred to as target organs or end-organs.

In the normal kidney, glomerular capillary pressure is maintained at 60–65 mm Hg by autoregulatory vasoconstriction or dilation of afferent arterioles. Changes in efferent arteriolar resistance also help maintain glomerular capillary pressure and promote optimal GFR[49, 50]; however, if vascular autoregulation is impaired by renal disease, glomerular pressure is likely to rise or fall directly with systemic BP. Glomerular hypertension causes hyperfiltration, which over time leads to glomerulosclerosis, atrophy, and proliferative glomerulitis. Vascular damage from chronic hypertension causes renal tubular degeneration and interstitial fibrosis. These contribute to renal function deterioration and increasing vascular resistance[8, 21, 50]; therefore, chronic hypertension tends to perpetuate itself.

In the eye, breakdown of vascular autoregulation causes dilation and leakage in precapillary arterioles, especially in the retina and choroid[47]. Focal perivascular transudate, retinal edema, arteriolarsclerosis, vascular tortuosity, focal ischemia, and retinal hemorrhages develop with hypertensive retinopathy. Similar vascular lesions and focal ischemia occur with hypertensive choroidopathy and often lead to bullous or total retinal detachment. Hypertensive optic neuropathy secondary to ischemia and edema is also described[47, 51]. Posterior segment lesions are reported in 80–100% of hypertensive cats, but most had advanced disease when diagnosed[45, 51]. Sudden blindness is common; vitreal hemorrhages, hyphema, and uveitis may also occur[26, 34, 36, 52, 53].

Cerebral blood flow autoregulation occurs in response to changes in perfusion pressure as well as $PaCO_2$ and perivascular pH changes; increased $PaCO_2$ and acidosis cause vasodilation and increased blood flow. Local disease can interfere with normal cerebral vascular autoregulation. Cerebral blood flow may increase when BP rises above 160 mm Hg, depending on several factors[54]. Conditions that increase brain intravascular pressure include systemic arterial hypertension, vascular obstruction, and abnormal cerebral autoregulation. Increased vascular pressure contributes to edema formation and increased intracranial pressure and can cause hemorrhage in and around the brain. Conversely, systemic BP can increase secondary to intracranial disease that raises intracranial pressure as a mechanism to maintain cerebral blood flow (Cushing's reflex)[54]. Therefore, hypertension can cause neurologic signs or be a secondary manifestation of elevated intracranial pressure.

High systemic arterial pressure and vascular resistance increase afterload stress on the LV, activating myocardial mechanoreceptors. This initiates a complex process leading to increased synthesis of myocardial proteins and associated tissue, which results in LV concentric hypertrophy. This can increase ventricular stiffness and may impair diastolic function. Coronary artery disease generally does not play the important role in dogs and cats with hypertension that it does in people[55], but medial hypertrophy of coronary arterioles has been noted in hypertensive cats[36]. Hypertension may decrease cardiac output but, unlike in people, hypertensive heart disease does not usually progress to CHF. This may relate to the effects of underlying disease on lifespan. Abnormal heart sounds are often heard, but they do not appear to correlate with the degree of hypertrophy[55, 56]. Aortic aneurysm and aortic dissection have only rarely been described in dogs and cats, and not always with documented hypertension[57, 58].

CLINICAL FEATURES

Clinical hypertension is more common in middle-aged to older dogs and cats, the population generally affected by associated diseases[36]. Clinical signs often relate to the underlying or associated disease process, but with severe or sustained hypertension, signs of end-organ damage can predominate.

Ocular signs are most common, especially sudden blindness, which is usually caused by acute retinal hemorrhage or detachment (582, 583). Fundic examination often reveals bullous to complete effusive retinal detachment, intraretinal edema, and hemorrhage. Vascular tortuosity, hyperreflective scars, retinal atrophy, papilledema, and perivasculitis are

other signs[26, 34, 36, 52, 53]. Vitreal or anterior chamber hemorrhage, closed-angle glaucoma, and corneal ulceration can also occur[26, 30, 34, 36, 53].

Polyuria/polydipsia is another common complaint. This is often associated with renal disease, hyperadrenocorticism (dogs), or hyperthyroidism (cats). Hypertension itself causes a so-called pressure diuresis[21].

Abnormal heart sounds are frequently heard in animals with hypertension[27, 30]. Soft systolic murmurs usually relate to abnormal LV flow dynamics or valve function. A gallop sound is heard in some cats and likely reflects increased ventricular stiffness[31]. The heart rate is usually normal, but tachycardia or arrhythmias are found in some hypertensive

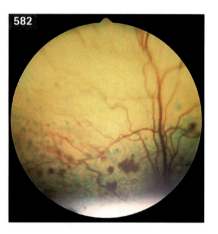

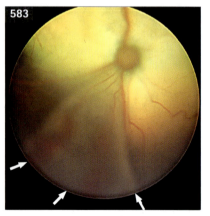

582, 583 (582) Fundic image from a dog with hypertension showing multiple retinal hemorrhages (associated with blood vessels) in the bottom (ventral) half of the image. Some vascular tortuosity is seen. Small dark spots in the 8 o'clock to 9 o'clock position were thought to be subretinal hemorrhage. Light artifact at bottom edge of image. (583) Fundus from an older, mixed breed cat with systolic BP >300 mm Hg. Partial retinal detachment is seen ventrally (arrows), with areas of hemorrhage on the detached segment. Nonuniform retinal edema is seen dorsally and around the optic disk. (Courtesy Dr D Betts.)

animals[31, 55]. Clinical heart failure is uncommon in cats and unreported in dogs[30, 36, 55, 56, 59]. Epistaxis can occur from vascular rupture in the nasal mucosa[60]. Hypertensive encephalopathy can cause behavioral changes, seizures, paresis, ataxia, collapse, vocalization, or other neurologic signs[20-22]. These may be manifestations of cerebrovascular accident (stroke) resulting from hypertensive arteriolar spasm or hemorrhage. Other nonspecific signs might include wimpering, inappetence, or behavioral changes[20].

DIAGNOSIS

BP should be measured not only when signs consistent with hypertension are found, but also when a disease associated with hypertension is diagnosed. It is important to confirm suspected arterial hypertension by measuring BP more than once and on different days. A routine hemogram, serum biochemical profile, urinalysis, and ocular examination are indicated in all hypertensive patients. Other tests may be needed to rule out certain underlying diseases or complications. These might include endocrine function tests, radiography, ultrasonography (including echocardiography), electrocardiography, and CT or magnetic resonance imaging.

The ECG sometimes shows changes suggesting LA or LV enlargement. Arrhythmias are uncommon and more likely reflect underlying disease[55].

Thoracic radiographs often indicate some degree of cardiomegaly in dogs and cats with chronic hypertension. Other findings reported in cats include a prominent aortic arch and an undulant (wavy) thoracic aorta (584–587)[36, 55, 59]. Although these findings may relate to geriatric variation, aortic

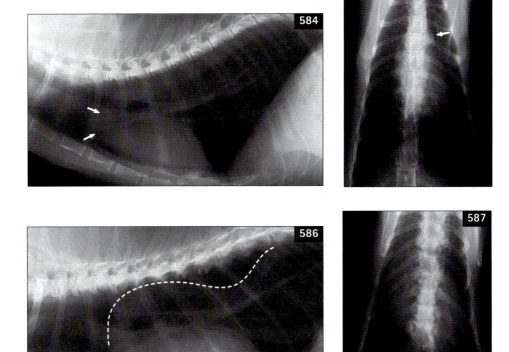

584–587 (584) Lateral radiograph from a 13-year-old male DSH cat with a systolic BP of 290 mm Hg. The aortic root and arch are enlarged (arrows); the thoracic aorta appears somewhat undulant (wavy). The heart is normal size but oriented horizontally, as is common for geriatric cats. The pulmonary parenchyma and vasculature are normal. **(585)** DV view from the same cat. The aortic arch forms a knob-like projection (arrow). **(586, 587)** Images from a 16-year-old female DSH cat (systolic BP ≥240 mm Hg) show a very horizontal heart and extremely wavy aorta (dashes outline dorsal edge) **(586)**. Cardiomegaly is evident on both views.

undulation was positively correlated with systolic BP, but not age, in one study[59]. Aortic enlargement is seen in some animals with hypertension.

Echocardiography can reveal mild to moderate LV hypertrophy (**588, 589**), but measurements within the normal reference range are common and the degree of hypertrophy is not correlated to individual BP measurements[30, 56, 59]. Normal LV wall thickness does not rule out hypertension. Mild LA enlargement, sometimes associated with MR, has been observed in cats. LV wall and septal hypertrophy can be symmetric or asymmetric[30, 56, 59]. The LV chamber diameter is typically normal, although reduced lumen size has also been reported in some hypertensive cats[30, 55, 56]. The aortic valve annulus diameter is typically normal, but the proximal aorta may be dilated (**590–592**). Correlation between ascending aortic diameter and systolic BP, but not age, is reported in cats[59]. A ratio of proximal ascending aortic diameter:aortic valve annulus diameter ≥1.25 was found in almost all hypertensive cats, but not in healthy older cats[59]. Trivial or mild aortic insufficiency may be seen with Doppler.

BLOOD PRESSURE MEASUREMENT
Several methods can be used to measure systemic arterial BP. Indirect BP measurement is easily performed given the availability of relatively accurate and inexpensive noninvasive techniques. An average of at least 3 measurements in succession is recommended to increase accuracy. When readings differ widely, the highest and lowest are discarded and an average value from 3 or more readings is used. High pressures should be confirmed by repeated measurement on separate occasions before a diagnosis of hypertension is made. Anxiety related to the clinical setting can falsely increase BP in some animals[17]. Surges in endogenous catecholamine release can rapidly raise BP. Using the least restraint

588, 589 (**588**) 2-D echo image in diastole from the cat in **586** and **587** shows mild to moderate hypertrophy of the IVS (7 mm) and LVW (6–7 mm). Right parasternal short-axis view. (**589**) M-mode image at the ventricular level from a 17-year-old cat with chronic hypertension shows mild hypertrophy of the LVW (6.5 mm) and IVS (6 mm). IVS = interventricular septum; LV = left ventricle; LVW = left ventricular wall; RV = right ventricle; RVW = right ventricular wall.

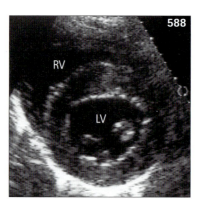
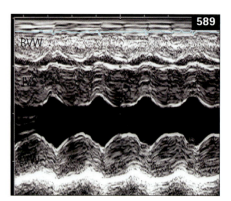

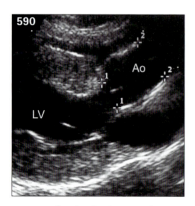
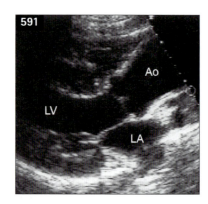
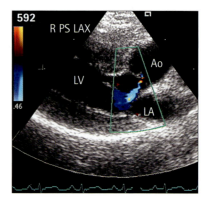

590–592 (**590**) 2-D echo image from a hypertensive cat indicates that the ascending aorta (line #2) is widened compared with the aortic valve annulus (line #1). Moderate LV hypertrophy is also seen. (Courtesy Dr OL Nelson.) (**591**) Diastolic image from the cat in **586** and **587** shows marked dilation of the ascending aorta. (**592**) Mild aortic valve regurgitation was found in the cat in **589**.

possible, a quiet and distraction-free environment, and allowing time (e.g. 5–15 minutes) for patient acclimation will minimize this. The owner's presence can have a calming effect on the patient. Consistency of technique, including choice of limb used and patient positioning, is important to minimize measurement variability.

Direct measurement

BP measurement through a needle or catheter placed directly into an artery is considered the gold standard[4, 14]; however, besides the greater technical expertise required, the physical restraint and discomfort associated with arterial puncture in awake animals can falsely increase BP. For sustained arterial pressure monitoring, an indwelling arterial catheter can be the best approach. The dorsal metatarsal artery is usually used. An electronic pressure monitor will provide continuous measurement of systolic and diastolic pressures and calculated mean pressure. The pressure transducer, for fluid-filled systems, is placed at the level of the patient's RA to avoid falsely increasing or decreasing measured pressure because of gravitational effects on the fluid within the connecting tubing. For occasional BP measurement, a small gauge needle attached directly to a pressure transducer can be used to puncture the dorsal metatarsal or femoral artery. After removal of the catheter or needle, pressure should be applied to the arterial puncture site for several minutes to prevent hematoma formation. Direct arterial pressure measurement is more accurate than indirect methods in hypotensive animals.

Indirect measurement

Noninvasive methods available for indirect BP measurement include Doppler ultrasonic flow detection, oscillometry, and photoplethysmography[18, 21, 35, 61–68]. Doppler and oscillometric methods are used most often and are the techniques recommended by the Veterinary Blood Pressure Society[14]. These methods use an inflatable cuff placed around a limb, preferably over the radial artery (most dogs) or brachial artery (small dogs and cats) or the median caudal artery of the tail, to occlude blood flow (593–595). The saphenous artery can be used, but it may be a less reliable site[14]. Controlled release of cuff pressure is monitored to detect the return of flow. Both techniques can yield measurements that correlate fairly well with direct BP measurement. Indirect methods are more reliable in normotensive and hypertensive animals. In conscious cats, greater correlation with direct BP measurement has been found using the Doppler method rather than the oscillometric method[22]. Other methods used to estimate BP (e.g. auscultation and arterial palpation) are not recommended. The auscultatory method (used to detect Korotkoff sounds in people) is not technically feasible in dogs and cats,

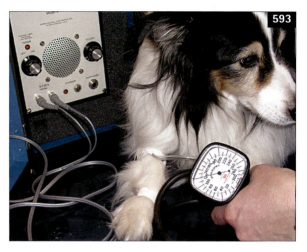

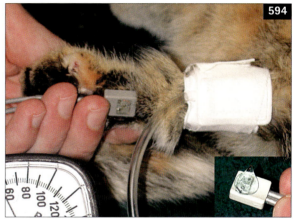

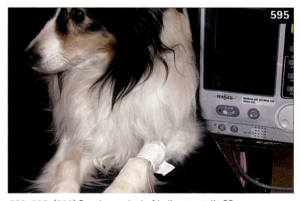

593–595 (593) Doppler method of indirect systolic BP measurement in a dog. The ultrasonic probe is positioned over the palmer common digital artery so that a clear flow signal is heard, then taped in place. The cuff (on the forearm over the radial artery) is inflated to occlude arterial flow, then slowly deflated to detect the pressure at which systolic flow recurs. (594) The Doppler flow probe can be held gently in position during BP measurement, as in this cat. It is important to shave the hair over the target artery and use sufficient ultrasonic coupling gel (inset) to achieve an air-free interface between the Doppler probe and skin. (595) Oscillometric method of indirect BP measurement using the radial artery in a dog.

mainly because of limb conformation. Direct arterial palpation is not a reliable or accurate method to estimate BP because pulse strength depends on the pulse pressure (systolic minus diastolic arterial pressure), not the absolute level of systolic or mean pressure. Pulse strength is also influenced by body conformation and other factors.

The size of cuff used is important for accurate indirect BP measurement. The width of the inflatable balloon (bladder) within the cuff should be about 30% (especially for cats) to 40% (especially for dogs) of the circumference of the extremity it encircles[69]; the length of the balloon should cover at least 60% of this circumference[14, 21]. Some of the cuff inflation pressure goes toward tissue compression. Cuffs that are too narrow are more affected by this and produce falsely increased pressure readings; cuffs that are too wide can underestimate BP. Human pediatric and infant sized cuffs can be used in dogs and cats. The cuff bladder should be centered over the target artery. The cuff should encircle the limb snugly but not be excessively tight.

Doppler method

The Doppler method uses the change in frequency between emitted ultrasound and echos reflected from moving blood cells, or vessel wall, to detect blood flow in a superficial artery. This frequency change ('Doppler shift') is converted into an audible signal. Effective locations for pressure measurement include the palmer common digital (forelimb), median caudal (tail), and dorsal metatarsal arteries. One system used commonly in animals is designed to determine systolic pressure by detecting blood cell flow (Ultrasonic Doppler Flow Detector, Model 811, Parks Medical Electronics Inc., Aloha, Oregon, US). The probe is placed distal to the occluding cuff. A small area of hair is shaved over the artery where the probe is to be placed. Ultrasonic coupling gel is applied to the flat Doppler flow probe to achieve an air-free interface with the skin. The probe is placed so that a clear flow signal is heard. The probe should be perpendicular to the target artery and not held so tightly as to occlude flow. The probe must be held still to minimize noise; it is often taped in place. A low volume setting on the Doppler unit is used to minimize patient disturbance, or a headset can be used. The flow occluding cuff is attached to a sphygmomanometer and inflated to a pressure 20–30 mm Hg above where flow stops and no audible signals are heard[62, 65]. As the cuff is slowly deflated, by a few mm Hg/second, the return of blood cell motion produces characteristic flow signals during systole. The pressure at which pulsatile blood flow first recurs, indicated by brief 'swishing' sounds, is the systolic pressure. The cuff should be completely deflated between measurements. Sometimes, a change in the flow sound from short and pulsatile to a longer, more continuous 'swishing' can be detected as cuff pressure declines. The pressure at which this occurs approximates diastolic pressure, but diastolic BP measurement is less accurate with this system because its determination is rather subjective. This change in flow sound may not be detectable, especially with small or stiff vessels. Although only systolic pressure is reliably estimated with the Doppler method, most animals are thought to have systolic rather than isolated diastolic hypertension. It may be difficult to measure BP in small or hypotensive animals. Patient movement also interferes with measurement.

Oscillometric method

The oscillometric method uses an automated system for detecting and processing cuff pressure oscillation signals (e.g. Cardell Veterinary Blood Pressure Monitor, Sharn Inc.; Memoprint, S&B Medvet and Vetline LLC). The flow occlusion cuff must be applied tightly so that oscillations are accurately detected. The cuff is inflated to a pressure above systolic pressure, then slowly deflated. The system's microprocessor measures and averages the resulting pressure oscillations characteristic of systolic, diastolic, and/or mean pressures (depending on the system). Accurate results depend on following the directions for use carefully and holding the animal still. The limb used should not be bearing any weight, because muscle contraction can produce oscillations. It is recommended that at least 5 readings are obtained, the lowest and highest being discarded, and the remaining measurements averaged. Effective use of the oscillometric method may be difficult in small dogs and cats, and underestimation of systolic BP is common[22, 68, 69].

Photoplethysmography

Photoplethysmography has been used ocasionally in small dogs (<10 kg) and cats for continuous BP estimation, but it is more commonly used in human medicine. It employs infrared light transmission to measure arterial volume, usually on a (human) finger[21, 68].

MANAGEMENT

Animals with severe hypertension, and those with clinical signs presumed to be caused by hypertension, clearly should be treated. BP is often over 200/110 mm Hg in these animals. Whether all dogs and cats with moderate hypertension (systolic pressures of 160–180 mm Hg) benefit from specific antihypertensive treatment is not clear; however, persistent hypertension after primary disease treatment with evidence or probability of end-organ damage should be treated. Hypertensive emergencies (malignant hypertension) must be treated immediately and with intensive monitoring (see below). Most hypertensive animals can be managed more conservatively, and gradual BP reduction may be safer in animals with chronic hypertension. Vascular adaptations in the cerebral autoregulatory process occur in response to sustained high BP; consequently, a sudden reduction in BP can adversely affect cerebral perfusion[21, 54]. Management of underlying or concurrent disease is indicated in all patients and is sometimes sufficient to normalize BP. In other patients, specific antihypertensive therapy is also needed. A therapeutic goal of systolic BP below (160–)170 mm Hg is usual[22, 70].

Several ancillary strategies have been used. Reduced dietary salt intake (e.g. 0.22–0.25% sodium on a dry matter basis) has been advised, but this alone is not expected to normalize BP. There is evidence that NH activation and potassium excretion are increased in cats with renal dysfunction that are fed a low-sodium diet[71]. In some cats, a high-salt diet may be involved in the development of hypertension, but dietary salt intake does not generally affect BP in normal cats[72]. Weight reduction is recommended for obese animals[70]. Drugs that can potentiate vasoconstriction (e.g. phenylpropanolamine and other alpha$_1$-adrenergic agonists) should be avoided. Glucocorticoids and progesterone derivatives should also be avoided when possible, because steroid hormones can increase BP. A diuretic (thiazide or furosemide; see Chapter 16 p. 176) may help by reducing blood volume and sodium content, but a diuretic alone is rarely effective. Diuretics should be avoided or used only with caution in azotemic animals. Serum potassium concentration should be monitored, especially in cats with chronic renal disease.

BP monitoring capability is important when antihypertensive drugs are prescribed. Serial measurements are needed to monitor therapy and avoid hypotension. In nonemergency cases, BP monitoring can be done every 1–2 weeks to assess antihypertensive treatment efficacy. Initial BP control may take several weeks to attain. Once satisfactory regulation is achieved, BP should be monitored at least every 2–3 months. Some animals become refractory to therapy that was initially effective. Increased dosage, adjunctive therapy, or a change of antihypertensive drug can be tried, as well as continued attention to the underlying disease process. Routine hemogram, serum biochemistry profile, and urinalysis are also recommended every 6 months[21, 22].

Several drugs have been used as antihypertensive agents in dogs and cats (*Table 67*, p. 380). Usually, one drug at a time is administered, starting at a low initial dose, and the animal is monitored. It may take 2 or more weeks before a significant decrease in BP is observed. The drugs most commonly used are ACE inhibitors, the calcium channel-blocker amlodipine, and beta-adrenergic blockers. In some cases, therapy with one agent is effective. Combination therapy may be needed for adequate BP control in others. The recommended initial agent for dogs is an ACE inhibitor[73]. The recommended first line treatment for cats is amlodipine, unless hyperthyroidism is the underlying cause[21, 23, 31, 45, 4]. For hyperthyroid-induced hypertension, atenolol (or another beta-blocker) is used first[31]. Adverse effects of antihypertensive therapy usually relate to hypotension, manifested by lethargy or ataxia, and reduced appetite.

The ACE inhibitors (e.g. enalapril, benazepril, captopril) diminish AT II production, thereby reducing systemic vascular resistance and volume retention (see Chapter 16, p. 178). These agents have been more effective in hypertensive dogs, although their effect would be dependent on the degree of renin-angiotensin system activation underlying the hypertension. Hypertensive cats with chronic renal failure are often not responsive to ACE inhibitors, either long term or initially[75–77]. Reduced renin activity has been identified in some cats with end-stage renal disease[75, 78], but benazepril was shown to have a small BP effect on hypertensive cats[79]. Nevertheless, ACE inhibitors may help protect against hypertensive renal damage[79]. Because AT II preferentially constricts renal efferent arterioles, ACE inhibitors tend to produce greater dilation of efferent rather than afferent arterioles; therefore, glomerular hypertension is reduced, which can especially benefit animals with renal disease, as long as adequate GFR is maintained. This benefit may be realized even without substantial reduction in systemic BP[50]. ACE inhibitors can reduce proteinuria and slow the progression of renal disease. ACE inhibitors may also inhibit growth factors associated with intrarenal AT formation that promote glomerular hypertrophy and sclerosis[50]. Veterinary experience with drugs that block AT II receptors rather than ACE (e.g. candesartan and losartan) is presently lacking. Likewise, the clinical usefulness of aldosterone antagonism (e.g. spironolactone) to help control hypertension is unclear[2, 21].

Calcium entry-blocking drugs (calcium channel-blockers) as a group decrease free calcium ion concentration in arteriolar and cardiac muscle cells, resulting in vasodilation and reduced cardiac output (see Chapter 17, p. 217). Amlodipine besylate is a long-acting dihydropyridine calcium channel-blocker that has vasodilating effects, but no appreciable cardiac effects. It is often effective as a single agent in hypertensive cats[31, 45, 74, 80, 81]. Amlodipine's effect on BP lasts at least 24 hours in cats. Amlodipine generally has minimal effect on serum creatinine concentration in cats with chronic renal failure; mild reduction in serum potassium concentration responds to oral supplementation with potassium[76]. Amlodipine is usually given q24h (*Table 67*, p. 380),

Table 67 Therapy for hypertension.*

1) ACE inhibitors (see also Chapter 16):

  a) Enalapril:

    ■ Dog: 0.5 mg/kg PO q24(–12)h.

    ■ Cat: 0.25–0.5 mg/kg PO q24h.

  b) Benazepril:

    ■ Dog: 0.25–0.5 mg/kg PO q24(–12)h.

    ■ Cat: same.

  c) Ramipril:

    ■ Dog: 0.125–0.25 mg/kg PO q24h.

  d) Captopril:

    ■ Dog: 0.5–2.0 mg/kg PO q8–12h.

    ■ Cat: 0.5–1.25 mg/kg PO q12–24h.

2) Calcium channel-blocker:

  a) Amlodipine:

    ■ Dog: 0.1–0.3 (–0.5) mg/kg PO q24(–12)h.

    ■ Cat: 0.625 mg/cat (or 0.1–0.2 mg/kg) PO q24(–12)h.

3) Beta-adrenergic blockers (see also Chapter 17):

  a) Atenolol:

    ■ Dog: 0.2–1.0 mg/kg PO q12–24h (start low).

    ■ Cat: 6.25–12.5 mg/cat PO q(12–)24h.

  b) Propranolol:

    ■ Dog: 0.1–1.0 mg/kg PO q8h (start low).

    ■ Cat: 2.5–10 mg/cat PO q8–12h.

4) Alpha$_1$-adrenergic blockers:

  a) Phenoxybenzamine:

    ■ Dog: 0.2–1.5 mg/kg PO q(8–)12h.

    ■ Cat: 0.2–0.5 mg/kg PO q12h.

  b) Prazosin:

    ■ Dog: 0.05–0.2 mg/kg PO q8–12h.

5) Diuretics (see also Chapter 16):

  a) Furosemide:

    ■ Dog: 0.5–3 mg/kg PO q8–24h.

    ■ Cat: 0.5–2 mg/kg PO q12–24h.

  b) Hydrochlorothiazide:

    ■ Dog: 1–4 mg/kg PO q12–24h.

    ■ Cat: 1–2 mg/kg PO q12–24h.

  c) Spironolactone:

    ■ Dog: 1–2 mg/kg PO q24(–12)h.

    ■ Cat: same.

6) Drugs used for hypertensive crisis:

  a) Hydralazine (see also Chapter 16):

    ■ Dog: 0.5–2.0 mg/kg PO q12h (titrate up to effect).

    ■ Cat: same.

  b) Nitroprusside (see also Chapter 16):

    ■ Dog: 0.5–1 mcg/kg/minute CRI (initial) to 5–15 mcg/kg/minute CRI.

    ■ Cat: same.

  c) Acepromazine:

    ■ Dog: 0.05–0.1 mg/kg (up to 3 mg total) IV.

    ■ Cat: same.

  d) Propranolol:

    ■ Dog: 0.02 (initial)–0.1 mg/kg slow IV.

    ■ Cat: same.

  e) Esmolol:

    ■ Dog: 200–500 mcg/kg IV over 1 minute, then 25–200 mcg/kg/minute CRI.

    ■ Cat: same.

  f) Phentolamine:

    ■ Dog: 0.02–0.1 mg/kg IV bolus, followed by CRI to effect.

    ■ Cat: same.

* See text for further information.

with or without food. It can be dosed q12h in large cats or in those that are unresponsive at the lower dose. For cats that do not respond adequately to amlodipine alone, a beta-blocker or ACE inhibitor can be added. Amlodipine has also been effective in some dogs. Amlodipine tablets are difficult to split evenly, but they can be compounded. Concerns about using calcium channel-blockers as primary antihypertensive agents in dogs are related to evidence in diabetic dogs (and people) about accelerated renal damage despite lowered BP[73, 74]. This may relate to preferential afferent arteriolar dilation with calcium channel-blockers, resulting in glomerular hypertension, but their systemic vasodilatory effect and, possibly, other nonhemodynamic effects may override this. At present, amlodipine appears safe and effective as a primary agent in cats. A calcium channel-blocker used as adjunctive therapy with an ACE inhibitor in dogs may control BP while yielding a balanced effect on glomerular pressure and GFR through equal dilation of afferent and efferent arterioles[21, 50].

A beta-blocker can be useful for adjunctive therapy. Beta-adrenergic blockers may reduce BP by decreasing heart rate, cardiac output, and renal renin release. Atenolol and propranolol have been used most often (see Chapter 17, p. 214). A beta-blocker is recommended for cats with hyperthyroid-induced hypertension, but beta-blockers are often ineffective as monotherapy in cats with renal disease[75].

Alpha$_1$-adrenergic antagonists reduce peripheral vascular resistance by opposing the vasoconstrictive effects of these adrenergic receptors; they are used primarily in treating hypertension caused by pheochromocytoma. Phenoxybenzamine is a noncompetitive alpha$_1$- and alpha$_2$-receptor blocker used for pheochromocytoma-induced hypertension (*Table 67*). A low dose is used initially, with upward titration as necessary. The alpha$_1$-blocker prazosin is better suited for use in large dogs. A beta-blocker can be used as adjunctive therapy to help control tachycardia and arrhythmias after the alpha$_1$-blocker is initiated.

Adverse effects of antihypertensive therapy usually relate to hypotension. This is usually manifested by periods of lethargy or ataxia. Reduced appetite can be another adverse effect. If antihypertensive therapy becomes unnecessary, the drug(s) should be gradually tapered then withdrawn. Rebound hypertension from sudden drug discontinuation is a concern, especially with beta- or alpha$_2$-blockers.

Because most cases of hypertension are associated with severe underlying disease, the long-term prognosis is often guarded despite apparent response to antihypertensive drugs. High BP in chronic renal failure has been associated with shorter survival time[82]. Some primary disease treatments can exacerbate hypertension, including fluid therapy, corticosteroids, and erythropoietin.

Emergency antihypertensive therapy is indicated for animals with new or progressive signs caused by high BP. These include acute retinal detachment and hemorrhage, encephalopathy or other evidence of intracranial hemorrhage, acute renal or heart failure, or aortic aneurysm. Direct vasodilating drugs such as hydralazine or sodium nitroprusside can be used for acute hypertensive crises if CRI and adequate BP monitoring (to avoid hypotension) are available (see *Table 67*, and Chapter 16, p. 173). Intravenous propranolol, esmolol, or acepromazine have also been used, especially in combination with hydralazine, if the latter has not sufficiently reduced BP within 12 hours. Once BP is stabilized below 170/110 mm Hg, long-term oral therapy can be started. Frequent BP monitoring is important.

For hypertensive crisis caused by catecholamine excess (e.g. pheochromocytoma), the alpha-blocker phentolamine is used by IV bolus (*Table 67*) followed by an infusion titrated to effect. A beta-blocker may also be indicated for pheochromocytoma-induced tachyarrhythmias, but should not be used alone or before a nonselective or selective alpha$_1$-blocker to avoid exacerbation of hypertension by unopposed alpha$_1$-receptors. Selective alpha$_2$-blockers (e.g. clonidine) are contraindicated. Antihypertensive treatment for 2–3 weeks prior to surgery for tumor excision is recommended[32]. Long-term treatment is also recommended for inoperable pheochromocytoma to avoid hypertensive emergencies.

REFERENCES

1 Bodey AR, Michell AR (1996) Epidemiological study of blood pressure in domestic dogs. *J Small Anim Pract* 37:116–125.

2 Egner B (2003) Blood pressure measurement: basic principles and practical applications. In: *Essential Facts of Blood Pressure in Dogs and Cats*. B Egner, A Carr, S Brown (eds). BE Vet Verlag, Germany, pp. 1–14.

3 Remillard RL, Ross JN, Eddy JB (1991) Variance of indirect blood pressure measurements and prevalence of hypertension in clinically normal dogs. *Am J Vet Res* 52:561–565.

4 Stepien RL, Rapoport GS (1999) Clinical comparison of three methods to measure blood pressure in non-sedated dogs. *J Am Vet Med Assoc* 215:1623–1628.

5 Meurs KM, Miller MW, Slater MR *et al.* (2000) Arterial blood pressure measurement in a population of healthy geriatric dogs. *J Am Anim Hosp Assoc* 36:497–500.

6 Bodey AR, Rampling MW (1999) Comparison of haemorrheological parameters and blood pressure in various breeds of dog. *J Small Anim Pract* 40:3–6.

7 Bright JM, Dentino M (2002) Indirect arterial blood pressure measurement in nonsedated Irish Wolfhounds: reference values for the breed. *J Am Anim Hosp Assoc* 38:521–526.

8 Bartges JW, Willis AM, Polzin DJ (1996) Hypertension and renal disease. *Vet Clin North Am: Small Anim Pract* 26:1331–1345.

9 Sparkes AH, Caney SMA, King MCA *et al.* (1999) Inter- and intraindividual variation in Doppler ultrasonic indirect blood pressure measurements in healthy cats. *J Vet Intern Med* 13:314–318.

10 Bodey AR, Sansom J (1998) Epidemiological study of blood pressure in domestic cats. *J Small Anim Pract* 39:567–573.

11 Sansom J, Rogers K, Wood JLN (2004) Blood pressure assessment in healthy cats and cats with hypertensive retinopathy. *Am J Vet Res* 65:245–252.

12 Bodey AR, Michell AR (1996) Comparison of direct and indirect (oscillometric) measurements of arterial blood pressure in conscious dogs. *Res Vet Sci* 61:17–21.

13 Chalifoux A, Dallaire A, Blais D *et al.* (1985) Evaluation of the arterial blood pressure of dogs by two noninvasive methods. *Can J Comp Med* 49:419–423.

14 Erhardt W, Henke J, Carr A (2003) Techniques of arterial blood pressure measurement. In: *Essential Facts of Blood Pressure in Dogs and Cats.* B Egner, A Carr, S Brown (eds). BE Vet Verlag, Germany, pp. 34–59.

15 Kallet AJ, Cowgill LD, Kass PH (1997) Comparison of blood pressure measurements obtained in dogs by use of indirect oscillometry in a veterinary clinic versus at home. *J Am Vet Med Assoc* 210:651–654.

16 Meurs KM, Miller MW, Slater MR (1996) Comparison of the indirect oscillometric and direct arterial methods for blood pressure measurements in anesthetized dogs. *J Am Anim Hosp Assoc* 32:471–475.

17 Belew AM, Barlett T, Brown SA (1999) Evaluation of the white coat effect in cats. *J Vet Intern Med* 13:134–142.

18 Bodey AR, Michell AR (1997) Longitudinal studies of reproducibility and variability of indirect (oscillometric) blood pressure measurements in dogs: evidence for tracking. *Res Vet Sci* 63:15–21.

19 Brown SA, Langford K, Tarver S (1997) Effects of certain vasoactive agents on the long-term pattern of blood pressure, heart rate, and motor activity in cats. *Am J Vet Res* 58:647–652.

20 Kraft W, Egner B (2003) Causes and effects of hypertension. In: *Essential Facts of Blood Pressure in Dogs and Cats.* B Egner, A Carr, S Brown (eds). BE Vet Verlag, Germany, pp. 61–86.

21 Acierno MJ, Labato MA (2004) Hypertension in dogs and cats. *Compend Cont Educ Pract Vet* 26:336–345.

22 Brown SA, Henik RA (1998) Diagnosis and treatment of systemic hypertension. *Vet Clin North Am: Small Anim Pract* 28:1481–1494.

23 Struble AL. Feldman EC, Nelson RW *et al.* (1998) Systemic hypertension and proteinuria in dogs with diabetes mellitus. *J Am Vet Med Assoc* 213:822–825.

24 Ortega TM, Feldman EC, Nelson RW *et al.* (1996) Systemic arterial blood pressure and urine protein/creatinine ratio in dogs with hyperadrenocorticism. *J Am Vet Med Assoc* 209:1724–1929.

25 Littman MP, Robertson JL, Bovee KC (1988) Spontaneous systemic hypertension in dogs: five cases (1981–1983). *J Am Vet Med Assoc* 193:486–494.

26 Lane IF, Roberts SM, Lappin MR (1993) Ocular manifestations of vascular disease: hypertension, hyperviscosity, and hyperlipidemia. *J Am Anim Hosp Assoc* 29:28–3.

27 Syme HM, Barber PJ, Markwell PJ *et al.* (2002) Prevalence of systolic hypertension in cats with chronic renal failure at initial evaluation. *J Am Vet Med Assoc* 220:1799–1804.

28 Goy-Thollot I, Pechereau D, Keroack S *et al.* (2002) Investigation of the role of aldosterone in hypertension associated with spontaneous pituitary-dependent hyperadrenocorticism in dogs. *J Small Anim Pract* 43:489–492.

29 Cowgill LD, James KM, Levy JK *et al.* (1998) Use of recombinant human erythropoietin for management of anemia in dogs and cats with renal failure. *J Am Vet Med Assoc* 212:521–528.

30 Chetboul V, Lefebvre HP, Pinhas C, *et al.* (2003) Spontaneous feline hypertension: clinical and echocardiographic abnormalities, and survival rate. *J Vet Intern Med* 17:89–95.

31 Elliot J, Barber PJ, Syme HM *et al.* (2001) Feline hypertension: clinical findings and response to antihypertensive treatment in 30 cases. *J Small Anim Pract* 42:122–129.

32 Maher ER, McNiel EA (1997) Pheochromocytoma in dogs and cats. *Vet Clin North Am: Small Anim Pract* 27:359–380.

33 Maggio F, DeFrancesco TC, Atkins CE *et al.* (2000) Ocular lesions associated with systemic hypertension in cats: 69 cases (1985–1998). *J Am Vet Med Assoc* 217:695–702.

34 Stiles J, Polzin DJ, Bistner SI (1994) The prevalence of retinopathy in cats with systemic hypertension and chronic renal failure or hyperthyroidism. *J Am Anim Hosp Assoc* 30:564–572.

35 Kobayashi DL, Peterson ME, Graves TK *et al.* (1990) Hypertension in cats with chronic renal failure or hyperthyroidism. *J Vet Intern Med* 4:58–62.

36 Littman MP (1994) Spontaneous systemic hypertension in 24 cats. *J Vet Intern Med* 8:79–86.

37 Elliot J, Barber PJ (1998) Feline chronic renal failure: clinical findings in 80 cases diagnosed between 1992 and 1995. *J Small Anim Pract* 39:78–85.

38 Flood SM, Randolph JF, Gelzer AR *et al.* (1999) Primary hyperaldosteronism in two cats. *J Am Anim Hosp Assoc* 35:411–416.

39 Turner JL, Brogdon JD, Lees GE *et al.* (1990) Idiopathic hypertension in a cat with secondary hypertensive retinopathy associated with a high-salt diet. *J Am Anim Hosp Assoc* 26:647–651.

40 Morgan RV (1986) Systemic hypertension in four cats: ocular and medical findings. *J Am Anim Hosp Assoc* 22:615–621.

41 Pascoe PJ, Ilkiw JE, Stiles J *et al.* (1994) Arterial hypertension associated with topical ocular use of phenylephrine in dogs. *J Am Vet Med Assoc* 205:1562–1564.

42 Verwaerde P, Senard JM, Galinier M *et al.* (1999) Changes in short-term variability of blood pressure and heart rate during the development of obesity-associated hypertension in high-fat fed dogs. *J Hypertens* 17:1135–1143.

43 Bovee KC, Littman MP, Saleh F *et al.* (1986) Essential hereditary hypertension in dogs: a new animal model. *J Hypertens* 4:S172–S174.

44 Bovee KC, Littman MP, Crabtree BJ *et al.* (1989) Essential hypertension in a dog. *J Am Vet Med Assoc* 195:81–86.

45 Snyder PS (1998) Amlodipine: a randomized, blinded clinical trial in 9 cats with systemic hypertension *J Vet Intern Med* **12**:157–162.

46 Berne RM, Levy MN (1997) *Cardiovascular Physiology*, 7th edn. Mosby, St. Louis, pp. 175–177.

47 Crispin SM, Mould JRB (2001) Systemic hypertensive disease and the feline fundus. *Vet Ophthalmol* **4**:131–140.

48 Finco DR (2004) Association of systemic hypertension with renal injury in dogs with induced renal failure. *J Vet Intern Med* **18**:289–294.

49 Brown S, Finco D, Navar L (1995) Impaired autoregulatory ability in dogs with reduced renal mass. *J Am Soc Nephrol* **5**:1168–1174.

50 Brown S (2003) The kidney as target organ. In: *Essential Facts of Blood Pressure in Dogs and Cats*. B Egner, A Carr, S Brown (eds). BE Vet Verlag, Germany, pp. 121–128.

51 Maggio F, Davidson MG (2003) The eye as a target organ. In: *Essential Facts of Blood Pressure in Dogs and Cats*. B Egner, A Carr, S Brown (eds). BE Vet Verlag, Germany, pp. 112–120.

52 Smith PJ (2000) Hypertensive retinopathy. In: *Kirk's Current Veterinary Therapy XIII*. JD Bonagura (ed). WB Saunders, Philadelphia, pp. 1082–1085.

53 Sansom J, Bodey A (1997) Ocular signs in four dogs with hypertension. *Vet Rec* **140**:593–598.

54 Bagley RS (2003) The brain as a target organ. In: *Essential Facts of Blood Pressure in Dogs and Cats*. B Egner, A Carr, S Brown (eds). BE Vet Verlag, Germany, pp. 129–141.

55 Stepien RL (2003) The heart as a target organ. In: *Essential Facts of Blood Pressure in Dogs and Cats*. B Egner, A Carr, S Brown (eds). BE Vet Verlag, Germany, pp. 103–111.

56 Snyder PS, Sadek D, Jones GL (2001) Effect of amlodipine on echocardiographic variables in cats with systemic hypertension. *J Vet Intern Med* **15**:52–56.

57 Waldrop JE, Stoneham AE, Tidwell AS *et al.* (2003) Aortic dissection associated with aortic aneurysms and posterior paresis in a dog. *J Vet Intern Med* **17**:223–229.

58 Wey AC, Atkins CE (2000) Aortic dissection and congestive heart failure associated with systemic hypertension in a cat. *J Vet Intern Med* **14**:208–213.

59 Nelson OL, Riedesel E, Ware WA *et al.* (2002) Echocardiographic and radiographic changes associated with systemic hypertension in cats. *J Vet Intern Med* **16**:418–425.

60 Gieger T, Northrup N (2004) Clinical approach to patients with epistaxis. *Compend Cont Educ Pract Vet* **26**:30–43.

61 Branson KR, Wagner-Mann CC, Mann FA (1997) Evaluation of an oscillometric blood pressure monitor on anesthetized cats and the effect of cuff placement and fur on accuracy. *Vet Surg* **26**:347–353.

62 Stepien RL, Rapoport GS, Henik RA *et al.* (2003) Comparative diagnostic test characteristics of oscillometric and Doppler ultrasound methods in the detection of systolic hypertension in dogs. *J Vet Intern Med* **17**:65–72.

63 Coulter DB, Keith JC (1984) Blood pressure obtained by indirect measurement in conscious dogs. *J Am Vet Med Assoc* **184**:1375–1378.

64 de Laforcade AM, Rozanski EA (2001) Central venous pressure and arterial blood pressure measurements. *Vet Clin North Am: Small Anim Pract* **31**:1163–1174.

65 Crow DT, Spreng DE (1995) Doppler assessment of blood flow and pressure in surgical and critical care patients. In: *Kirk's Current Veterinary Therapy XII*. JD Bonagura (ed). WB Saunders, Philadelphia, pp. 113–117.

66 Caulkett NA, Cantwell SL, Houston DM (1998) A comparison of indirect blood pressure monitoring techniques in the anesthetized cat. *Vet Surg* **27**:370–377.

67 Grandy JL, Dunlop CI, Hodgson DS *et al.* (1992) Evaluation of the Doppler ultrasonic method of measuring systolic arterial blood pressure in cats. *Am J Vet Res* **53**:1166–1169.

68 Binns SH, Sissons DD, Buoscio DA *et al.* (1995) Doppler ultrasonographic, oscillometric sphygmomanometric, and photoplethysmographic techniques for noninvasive blood pressure measurement in anesthetized cats. *J Vet Intern Med* **9**:405–414.

69 Pedersen KM, Butler MA, Ersboll AK *et al.* (2002) Evaluation of an oscillometric blood pressure monitor for use in anesthetized cats. *J Am Vet Med Assoc* **221**:646–650.

70 Ungemach FR (2003) Hypertension therapy. In *Essential Facts of Blood Pressure in Dogs and Cats*. B Egner, A Carr, S Brown (eds). BE Vet Verlag, Germany, pp. 143–158.

71 Buranakarl C, Mathur S, Brown SA (2004) Effects of dietary sodium chloride intake on renal function and blood pressure in cats with normal and reduced renal function. *Am J Vet Res* **65**:620–627.

72 Luckschander N, Iben C, Hosgood G *et al.* (2004) Dietary NaCl does not affect blood pressure in healthy cats. *J Vet Intern Med* **18**:463–467.

73 Brown SA, Henik RA (2000) Therapy for systemic hypertension in dogs and cats. In: *Kirk's Current Veterinary Therapy XIII*. JD Bonagura (ed). WB Saunders, Philadelphia, pp. 838–841.

74 Mathur S, Syme H, Brown CA *et al.* (2002) Effects of the calcium channel antagonist amlodipine in cats with surgically induced hypertensive renal insufficiency. *Am J Vet Res* **63**:833–839.

75 Jensen JL, Henik RA, Brownfield M *et al.* (1997) Plasma renin activity and angiotensin I and aldosterone concentrations in cats with hypertension associated with chronic renal disease. *Am J Vet Res* **58**:535–540.

76 Henik RA, Snyder PS, Volk LM (1997) Treatment of systemic hypertension in cats with amlodipine besylate. *J Am Anim Hosp Assoc* **33**:226–234.

77 Steele JL, Henik RA, Stepien RL (2002) Effects of angiotensin-converting enzyme inhibition on plasma aldosterone concentration, plasma renin activity, and blood

pressure in spontaneously hypertensive cats with chronic renal disease. *Vet Ther* **3**:157–166.

78 Taugner F, Baatz G, Nobiling R (1996) The renin-angiotensin system in cats with chronic renal failure. *J Comp Pathol* **115**:239–252.

79 Brown SA, Brown CA, Jacobs G *et al.* (2001) Effects of the angiotensin converting enzyme inhibitor benazepril in cats with induced renal insufficiency. *Am J Vet Res* **62**:375–383.

80 Arnold RM (2001) Pharm profile: amlodipine. *Compend Contin Educ Pract Vet* **23**:558–559 and 587.

81 Tissier R, Perrot S, Enriquez B (2005) Amlodipine: one of the main anti-hypertensive drugs in veterinary therapeutics. *J Vet Cardiol* **7**:53–58.

82 Jacob F, Polzin DJ, Osborne CA *et al.* (2003) Association between initial systolic blood pressure and risk of developing a uremic crisis or of dying in dogs with chronic renal failure. *J Am Vet Med Assoc* **222**:322–329.

Index